SHACKELFORD'S

SURGERY OF THE ALIMENTARY TRACT

COEDITORS

MARK B. ORRINGER
VOLUME I

ESOPHAGUS

WALLACE P. RITCHIE, JR.
VOLUME II

STOMACH AND DUODENUM
INCISIONS

JEREMIAH G. TURCOTTE
VOLUME III

PANCREAS
BILIARY TRACT
LIVER AND PORTAL HYPERTENSION
SPLEEN

ROBERT E. CONDON
VOLUME IV

COLON

LLOYD M. NYHUS
VOLUME V

MESENTERIC CIRCULATION
HERNIA
SMALL INTESTINE

SHACKELFORD'S

SURGERY OF THE ALIMENTARY TRACT

Fourth Edition

GEORGE D. ZUIDEMA, M.D.

Professor of Surgery and
Vice Provost for Medical Affairs, Emeritus
The University of Michigan
Ann Arbor, Michigan

W. B. SAUNDERS COMPANY
A Division of Harcourt Brace & Company
Philadelphia, London, Toronto, Montreal, Sydney, Tokyo

W. B. SAUNDERS COMPANY

A Division of Harcourt Brace & Company

The Curtis Center
Independence Square West
Philadelphia, Pennsylvania 19106

Library of Congress Cataloging-in-Publication Data

Shackelford's surgery of the alimentary tract. — 4th ed. / [edited by]
George D. Zuidema
    p. cm.
    Includes bibliographical references and indexes.
    Contents: v. 1. Esophagus / coeditor, Mark B. Orringer — v.
2. Stomach and duodenum ; incisions / coeditor, Wallace P. Ritchie,
Jr. — v. 3. Pancreas ; biliary tract ; liver and portal
hypertension ; spleen / coeditor, Jeremiah G. Turcotte — v.
4. Colon / coeditor, Robert E. Condon — v. 5. Mesenteric
circulation ; hernia ; small intestine / coeditor, Lloyd M. Nyhus.
    ISBN 0–7216-4982-3 (5 volume set)
    1. Alimentary canal—Surgery. I. Shackelford, Richard T.
II. Zuidema, George D. III. Title: Surgery of the alimentary
tract.
    [DNLM: 1. Digestive System - surgery. WI 900 S5241 1996]
RD540.S476 1996
617.4'3—dc20
DNLM/DLC   95-12002

ISBN Volume 1	0–7216-4983-1
Volume 2	0–7216-4984-X
Volume 3	0–7216-4985-8
Volume 4	0–7216-4986-6
Volume 5	0–7216-4987-4
5 Volume Set	0–7216-4982-3

Shackelford's SURGERY OF THE ALIMENTARY TRACT

Printed in the United States of America.

Last digit is the print number: 9   8   7   6   5   4   3   2   1

To my wife, Marcia,
who is also my best friend,
and who puts up with my attention to things like this book without complaint.

Robert E. Condon

To my wife, Joan,
who for many years has shared my interest in
and commitment to this publication,
and who has been a wonderful friend and supporter over our lifetime together.

George D. Zuidema

Contributors

VOLUME IV

HERAND ABCARIAN, M.D.
Turi Josefsen Professor and Head, Department of Surgery, University of Illinois-Chicago; Head, Department of Surgery, University of Illinois Hospital and Medical Center, Chicago, Illinois
Prolapse and Procidentia

ROBERT W. BEART, JR., M.D.
Professor of Surgery, University of Southern California School of Medicine, University Hospital, Norris Cancer Hospital, Los Angeles, California
Ileostomy and its Alternatives

SANDER R. BINDEROW, M.D.
Resident, Department of Colorectal Surgery, Cleveland Clinic Florida, Fort Lauderdale, Florida
Pilonidal Disease, Presacral Cysts and Tumors, and Pelvic and Perianal Pain

ELISA H. BIRNBAUM, M.D.
Assistant Professor of Surgery, Section of Colon and Rectal Surgery, Washington University School of Medicine; Jewish Hospital of St. Louis, Washington University Medical Center, St. Louis, Missouri
Anal Incontinence

GEORGE E. BLOCK, M.D., M.S. (Surg), F.A.C.S.[†]
Thomas D. Jones Professor of Surgery, Pritzker School of Medicine, University of Chicago, Chicago, Illinois
Abdominoperineal Resection

SCOTT J. BOLEY, M.D.
Professor of Surgery and Pediatrics, Albert Einstein College of Medicine-Montefiore Medical Center; Chief, Pediatric Surgical Services, Bronx, New York
Vascular Lesions of the Colon; Colonic Ischemia

JOHN G. BULS, M.D.
Clinical Associate Professor, Department of Surgery, University of Minnesota, Minneapolis, Minnesota
Benign Anal Strictures

STEPHEN M. COHEN, M.D.
Staff Colorectal Surgeon, Atlanta Colon and Rectal Surgery, PA, Atlanta, Georgia
Laparoscopic Appendectomy and Colectomy

ZANE COHEN, M.D., F.R.C.S.(C), F.A.C.S.
Professor of Surgery, University of Toronto; Surgeon in Chief, Mount Sinai Hospital, Toronto, Ontario, Canada
Inflammatory Bowel Disease

[†]**Deceased**

ROBERT E. CONDON, M.D., M.S., F.A.C.S.
Ausman Foundation Professor and Chairman, Department of Surgery, The Medical College of Wisconsin; Chief of Surgery, Froedtert Memorial Lutheran Hospital, Milwaukee, Wisconsin
Appendix; Resection of the Colon

THOMAS H. DAILEY, M.D.
Associate Professor of Clinical Surgery, Columbia University College of Physicians and Surgeons; Director, Division of Colon and Rectal Surgery, St. Luke's/Roosevelt Hospital Center, New York, New York
Pruritus Ani

JEROME J. DECOSSE, M.D., Ph.D.
Professor of Surgery, Cornell University Medical College; Attending Surgeon, New York Hospital, New York, New York
Polyps, Polyposis, and Benign Tumors

THEODORE E. EISENSTAT, M.D.
Clinical Professor of Surgery, UMDNJ-Robert Wood Johnson Medical School, New Brunswick, New Jersey; Senior Surgeon, Muhlenberg Regional Medical Center, Plainfield, New Jersey; John F. Kennedy Medical Center, Edison, New Jersey
Hemorrhoidal Disease

KENNETH ENG, M.D.
Professor of Surgery, New York University School of Medicine; Attending Surgeon, New York University Medical Center, New York, New York
Abdominosacral Resection

WILLIAM F. FALLON, JR., M.D.
Associate Professor of Surgery, Case Western Reserve University; Director, Trauma, Critical Care, Burns and Metro Life Flight, Metrohealth Medical Center, Cleveland, Ohio
Wounds, Foreign Bodies, and Fecal Impaction

JOHN J. FERRARA, M.D.
Professor, Department of Surgery, Chief, Section of General Surgery, Tulane University School of Medicine, New Orleans, Louisiana
Trauma to the Colon and Rectum

JAMES W. FLESHMAN, M.D.
Assistant Professor of Surgery, Section of Colon and Rectal Surgery, Washington University School of Medicine; Program Director, Jewish Hospital of St. Louis, Washington University Medical Center, St. Louis, Missouri
Anal Incontinence

PHILLIP FLESHNER, M.D.
Attending Surgeon, Division of Colorectal Surgery, Cedars-Sinai Medical Center, Los Angeles, California
Ileostomy and its Alternatives

LEWIS M. FLINT, M.D.
Regents Professor and Chairman, Tulane University School of Medicine, Department of Surgery; Chairman, Department of Surgery, Tulane Medical Center, New Orleans, Louisiana
Trauma to the Colon and Rectum

CONSTANTINE T. FRANTZIDES, M.D., Ph.D., F.A.C.S.
Associate Professor, Department of General Surgery, Medical College of Wisconsin; Staff Surgeon, Froedtert Memorial Lutheran Hospital; John L. Doyne Hospital; Columbia Hospital, Milwaukee, Wisconsin
Physiology of the Colon

ROBERT D. FRY, M.D.
Professor of Surgery, Director, Colon and Rectal Surgery, Thomas Jefferson Medical Center, Philadelphia, Pennsylvania
Anal Incontinence

STANLEY M. GOLDBERG, M.D., F.A.C.S., Hon F.R.A.C.S., Hon F.R.C.S. (Eng)

Clinical Professor of Surgery, Division of Colon and Rectal Surgery, Department of Surgery, University of Minnesota, Minneapolis, Minnesota

Low Anterior Resection

SCOTT D. GOLDSTEIN, M.D.

Assistant Professor of Surgery, Jefferson Medical Center, Philadelphia, Pennsylvania

Radiation Injury of the Rectum

PHILIP H. GORDON, M.D., F.R.C.S.(C), F.A.C.S.

Professor of Surgery and Oncology, McGill University; Director of Colon and Rectal Surgery, Vice Chairman, Department of Surgery, Sir Mortimer B. Davis Jewish General Hospital, Montreal, Quebec, Canada

Anorectal Abscesses and Fistula-In-Ano

JAY L. GROSFELD, M.D., A.B.

Professor and Chairman, Department of Surgery, Indiana University School of Medicine; Surgeon-in-Chief, J. W. Riley Hospital for Children, Director, Section of Pediatric Surgery; Indianapolis, Indiana

Anorectal Anomalies

GERALDINE M. HENEGHAN, R.N., N.S., C.E.T.N.

Rehabilitation Clinical Specialist, Hospital for Sick Children, Washington, D.C.

Ostomy Management

TERRY C. HICKS, M.D., M.S.

Clinical Instructor, Department of Surgery, Tulane Medical School; Staff Surgeon, Department of Colon and Rectal Surgery, Ochsner Clinic, New Orleans, Louisiana

Diagnosis of Anorectal Disease; Fissure-In-Ano

JAMES WM. C. HOLMES, M.D., M.S., F.A.C.S.

Associate Professor of Clinical Surgery and Colo-Rectal Surgery, Tulane University School of Medicine; Tulane University Medical Center Hospital, New Orleans, Louisiana

Antibiotics in Colon Surgery

ROGER D. HURST, M.D., F.R.C.S.(Ed)

Assistant Professor of Surgery, Pritzker School of Medicine, University of Chicago, Chicago, Illinois

Abdominoperineal Resection

RONALD N. KALEYA, M.D.

Associate Professor of Surgery, Albert Einstein College of Medicine-Montefiore Medical Center, Bronx, New York

Vascular Lesions of the Colon; Colonic Ischemia

IRA J. KODNER, M.D.

Associate Professor of Surgery, Section of Colon and Rectal Surgery, Washington University School of Medicine; Director, Section of Colon and Rectal Surgery, Jewish Hospital of St. Louis, Washington University Medical Center, St. Louis, Missouri

Anal Incontinence

LISA LINDBERG, R.D.

Senior Clinical Nutrition Specialist, Washington Hospital Center, Washington, D.C.

Ostomy Management

S. ARTHUR LOCALIO, M.D.

Johnson and Johnson Distinguished Professor Emeritus of Surgery, New York University School of Medicine, New York, New York

Abdominosacral Resection

ROBERT J. MAYER, M.D., Ph.D.

Professor of Medicine, Harvard Medical School; Clinical Director, Department of Medicine, Dana Farber Cancer Institute, Boston, Massachusetts
Adenocarcinoma of the Colon and Rectum

ROBIN S. MCLEOD, M.D., F.R.C.S.(C), F.A.C.S.

Associate Professor of Surgery, University of Toronto; Surgeon, Mount Sinai Hospital, Toronto, Ontario, Canada
Inflammatory Bowel Disease

ALAN P. MEAGHER, M.B.B.S., F.R.A.C.S.

Colorectal Surgeon, St. Vincent's Hospital, Sydney, Australia
Anatomy and Physiology of the Anus and Rectum

RONALD LEE NICHOLS, M.D., M.S., F.A.C.S.

William Henderson Professor of Surgery, Professor of Microbiology and Immunology, Tulane University School of Medicine; Attending Surgeon, Tulane University Medical Center Hospital, New Orleans, Louisiana
Antibiotics in Colon Surgery

NORMAN D. NIGRO, M.D.

Clinical Professor of Surgery, Wayne State University School of Medicine, Detroit, Michigan
Neoplasms of the Anus and Anal Canal

FRANK G. OPELKA, M.D.

Staff Surgeon, Ochsner Clinical and Medical Foundation, New Orleans, Louisiana
Diagnosis of Anorectal Disease

JOHN H. PEMBERTON, M.D.

Professor of Surgery, Mayo Medical School; Professor of Surgery, Mayo Clinic, Rochester, Minnesota
Anatomy and Physiology of the Anus and Rectum

PATRICIA L. ROBERTS, M.D., F.A.C.S.

Staff Surgeon, Department of Colorectal Surgery, Lahey Clinic, Burlington, Massachusetts
Diverticular Disease

JOSEPH L. ROMOLO, M.D.

Clinical Assistant Professor, Department of Surgery, Georgetown University School of Medicine; Attending Staff, Surgery, Washington Hospital Center, Washington, D.C.
Embryology and Anatomy of the Colon; Congenital Lesions: Intussusception and Volvulus

DAVID A. ROTHENBERGER, M.D.

Clinical Professor and Chief, Division of Colon and Rectal Surgery, Department of Surgery, University of Minnesota, Minneapolis, Minnesota
Posterior and Parasacral Approaches

EUGENE P. SALVATI, M.D.

Clinical Professor of Surgery, UMDNJ-Robert Wood Johnson Medical School, New Brunswick, New Jersey; Senior Surgeon, Muhlenberg Regional Medical Center, Plainfield, New Jersey; John F. Kennedy Medical Center, Edison, New Jersey
Hemorrhoidal Disease

THEODORE R. SCHROCK, M.D.

Professor and Interim Chairman, Department of Surgery, University of California, San Francisco, San Francisco, California
Colon and Rectum: Diagnostic Techniques

LEE E. SMITH, M.D.

Professor of Surgery, George Washington University, Washington, D.C.
Ostomy Management

GLENN D. STEELE, JR., M.D., Ph.D.

William V. McDermott Professor of Surgery, Harvard Medical School; Chairman, Department of Surgery, New England Deaconess Hospital, Boston, Massachusetts

Adenocarcinoma of the Colon and Rectum

GORDON L. TELFORD, M.D., F.A.C.S.

Professor of Surgery, Medical College of Wisconsin; Attending Surgeon, Froedtert Memorial Lutheran Hospital; Staff Physician, Milwaukee V.A. Hospital, Milwaukee, Wisconsin

Appendix

ALAN E. TIMMCKE, M.D.

Senior Staff Surgeon, Ochsner Clinic, New Orleans, Louisiana

Fissue-In-Ano

MALCOLM E. VEIDENHEIMER, M.D., C.M., F.R.C.S.C., F.A.C.S.

Vice Chairman, Department of Surgery, Chairman Division of General Surgery, Health Care International, Clydebank, Scotland

Diverticular Disease

ANTHONY M. VERNAVA, III, M.D.

Associate Professor of Surgery, Chief, Section of Colon and Rectal Surgery, Director, Colon and Rectal Surgery Residency Training Program, St. Louis University Health Sciences Center, St. Louis, Missouri

Low Anterior Resection

STEVEN D. WEXNER, M.D., F.A.C.S., F.A.S.C.R.S.

Chairman and Residency Program Director, Department of Colorectal Surgery, Cleveland Clinic Florida, Fort Lauderdale, Florida

Laparoscopic Appendectomy and Colectomy; Posterior and Parasacral Approaches; Pilonidal Disease, Presacral Cysts and Tumors, and Pelvic and Perianal Pain

Preface

It would be well to begin this book with a brief description of its history. The first edition of *Surgery of The Alimentary Tract* was edited by Dr. Richard T. Shackelford and published in 1955. It rapidly established itself as an invaluable source of information to thousands of practicing general surgeons and residents in training during the following years.

Owing to the book's success and the important contributions that it made, the W. B. Saunders Company urged Dr. Shackelford to produce a second edition. It soon became obvious that because of the rapid growth and development of surgical techniques and new approaches to the treatment of disease, the second edition would have to be expanded substantially. Dr. Shackelford completed the work on the first volume dealing with surgery of the esophagus, and I became co-editor, responsible for the completion of the succeeding four volumes.

This was accomplished with the help of several devoted faculty members at The Johns Hopkins Medical School, and the ranks of contributors were expanded to include individuals with special expertise in other, newly developing, areas. The second edition, therefore, included a total of five volumes and represented a significant step forward in the presentation of surgical science, while still including information of historical interest and related basic science. As a result, the second edition was almost totally new, but this was accomplished without departing from the approach that had been so successful in the first edition.

The third edition represented yet another important step forward. The field of Gastrointestinal Surgery had continued to advance with major and important strides, building on the many advances in surgical research that had emerged during the preceding decade. Furthermore, for this edition, I enlisted the help of a guest editor for each volume of this series. As a result, we were able to incorporate not only the fresh ideas that came from new authors but also in most cases new and contemporary illustrations.

We have now come to the fourth edition of this series. Once again this has been accomplished with the help of my colleagues who have served as guest editors for each of the five volumes. The publication of these volumes is particularly timely for there have been dramatic changes in surgical practice during the past few years. We are fortunate to be able to present these innovations, together with the contributions of many new authors.

Once again I would like to express my appreciation to the many individuals who have contributed chapters or sections to these volumes for their dedication and commitment. The contributors to the fourth edition are leaders in their fields, and I am deeply indebted to them for sharing in this commitment with great enthusiasm. I would also like to thank several individuals for their personal contributions to the enterprise.

Lisette Bralow and Hazel N. Hacker of the W. B. Saunders Company have been major sources of inspiration and help during all phases of preparation of the books.

I would also like to acknowledge the help of Barbara B. Farago and Angelina Jackson for their contributions and support here at The University of Michigan.

In addition, each of the Guest Editors has been helped immensely by his own colleagues and staff, and we would simply like to acknowledge their help as well.

It is obvious that this has been a project that all of us have enjoyed but that would not have been possible without the cheerful cooperation and goodwill of everyone involved.

GEORGE D. ZUIDEMA, M.D.

Contents

Esophageal Motor (Functional) Disorders and Esophageal Diverticula

Neoplasms and Cysts

Resectional Therapy and Complications of Esophageal Surgery

Trauma

Esophageal Varices

Miscellaneous Conditions

VOLUME II

Stomach and Duodenum

Incisions

VOLUME III

Pancreas

Liver and Portal Hypertension

VOLUME V
Mesenteric Circulation

Hernia

Small Intestine

Colon

Chapter 1

EMBRYOLOGY AND ANATOMY OF THE COLON

JOSEPH L. ROMOLO

The colon, or large intestine, is considered to begin at the ileocecal valve and extend to the peritoneal reflection at the junction of the sigmoid colon and the rectum, thus including the cecum and its vermiform appendix.

EMBRYOLOGY

Development of the Hindgut

The primitive digestive tube consists of two parts, the foregut and the hindgut. Between them is the wide opening of the yolk sac, which gradually narrows and is reduced to a small foramen leading to the vitelline duct. At first the foregut and hindgut end blindly. The anterior end of the foregut is separated from the stomodeum by the buccopharyngeal membrane; the hindgut ends in the cloaca, which is closed by the cloacal membrane. With lengthening of the primitive digestive tube, the mesoderm attaching the primitive digestive tube to the future vertebral column is thinned and drawn out to form the posterior common mesentery, which carries the blood vessels that supply the gut. The part of this mesentery that suspends the colon is termed the mesocolon.

At about the sixth week of gestation, a diverticulum of the gut appears just behind the opening of the vitelline duct and indicates the future cecum and vermiform process. That portion of the distal side of the cecal diverticulum increases in diameter and forms the future ascending and transverse portions of the large intestine. After the fifth month of gestation, the distal part of the cecal diverticulum remains rudimentary and forms the vermiform process, whereas its proximal part expands to form the cecum. At about the fifth intrauterine week of embryologic development, the small and large intestines are attached to the vertebral column by a common mesentery, with the coils of the small intestine falling to the right of the midline and those of the large intestine lying on the left side.

The development of the vascular supply of the digestive tube occurs simultaneously with the development of the gut itself. The primordium of the aorta appears in the very early embryo at about the same time as the heart. Two strands of cells arch dorsally from the endocardial mesenchyme, pass on each side of the foregut invagination, and turn caudad along the neural groove. The continuation of these strands forms the two paired dorsal aortas. After the circulation becomes functional, the circulatory system develops by (1) budding from existing trunks, (2) formation of new capillary networks, and (3) selection of parts of the network as arteries and veins.

As the bulk of an embryonic part increases, the capillaries are lengthened; this lengthening soon reaches a maximum, and the hemodynamic forces select certain channels for arterioles and arteries and others for venules and veins. The two dorsal aortas remain separate for a short time but come together when they are about 3 mm to form a single trunk caudal to the eighth or ninth aortic arch, continuing caudally from the left fourth somite. The left dorsal aorta becomes the descending aortic arch. In the early embryo, paired ventral branches of the aorta grow out on the yolk sac as the omphalomesenteric arteries. At its caudal end, the ventral branches accompany the allantois to become the umbilical arteries.

As the gut develops, a number of ventral branches grow into it. At first they are paired, but with the formation of a mesentery, the pairs fuse into single stems. These ventral branches are irregularly spaced, and by a process of shifting along a rich anastomosis, the three main trunks—the celiac, the superior mesenteric artery (SMA), and the inferior mesenteric artery (IMA)—are finally selected. The colon ultimately derives its arterial blood supply from the ileocolic, right colic, and middle colic branches of the SMA and the left colic and sigmoid branches of the IMA.

Rotation and Fixation of the Gut

The normal embryonic process of rotation and fixation of the intestinal tract takes place in three stages.[3,10] As has been mentioned previously, the primitive intestinal tract begins as a straight digestive tube suspended in a sagittal plane on a common dorsal mesentery. At some time between the fifth and eighth weeks of embryologic development, the first stage of rotation begins (Fig. 1–1). During this first stage, the primitive duct elongates on its mesentery around the SMA and bulges through the umbilical cord as a temporary physiologic herniation. At the eighth week of intrauterine life, this intraumbilical loop moves counterclockwise 90 degrees from the sagittal to the horizontal plane. Anomalies of this first stage are quite rare. They include (1) extroversion of the cloaca, (2) situs inversus, and (3) inverted duodenum.

In the second stage of gut rotation, at about the tenth week of gestation, the midgut loop returns to the peritoneal cavity from the umbilical herniation and simultaneously rotates 180 degrees counterclockwise around the mesenteric root, which serves as a pedicle. Anomalies of the second stage are relatively uncommon but are not rare. They include (1) nonrotation, (2) malrotation,

(3) reversed rotation, (4) internal hernia, and (5) omphalocele.

In nonrotation, the midgut loop returns to the peritoneal cavity without turning beyond the horizontal plane occupied at the end of the first stage. All of the small intestine is on the right side of the abdomen, and the colon is on the left side. The cecum is in the left lower quadrant of the abdomen and receives the terminal ileum from the right side. This condition may be entirely asymptomatic, but with defective fixation of the mesenteric root the entire midgut loop may twist on its pedicle at the duodenojejunal junction and the mid-transverse colon. Volvulus may involve the entire small intestine.

In malrotation, there is a failure of the cecum to migrate around the superior mesenteric vessels. The 360-degree counterclockwise rotation is not completed, and the cecum comes to rest in the right upper quadrant. The malrotated cecum is usually fixed in the right upper quadrant by lateral peritoneal reflections. These bands frequently overlie the distal portion of the duodenum and result in extrinsic compression.

In the condition of reversed rotation, the midgut rotates clockwise instead of counterclockwise, and there is a resultant retroposition of the transverse colon (Fig. 1–2). The location of all parts of the large and small bowel is normal; the only anomaly is the reverse relationship of the transverse colon and duodenum with the mesenteric artery—the colon is posterior and the duodenum is anterior.

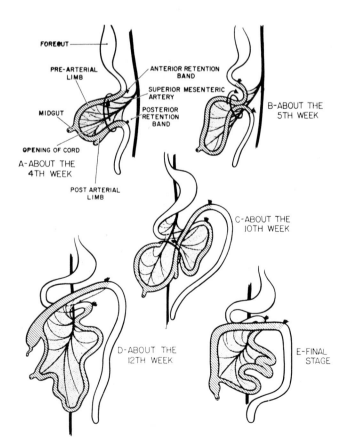

FIGURE 1–1. Normal rotation. *A,* Human embryo at fourth or fifth week. Note that the midgut, supplied by the superior mesenteric artery, has "herniated" into the cord. The foregut and hindgut derivatives do not enter this "hernia"; the retention bands are points of fixation. *B,* The prearterial segment of the midgut loop has returned into the abdomen first, as the gut has rotated counterclockwise. The duodenum thus comes to lie behind the superior mesenteric artery. Note the splenic flexure is fixed on the left. *C,* Tenth week. The postarterial segment has also reduced and comes to lie in front of the superior mesenteric artery. The cecum is in the upper abdomen and must migrate to the right lower quadrant as counterclockwise rotation continues to 270 degrees. *D,* Twelfth week. Rotation has been completed; the viscera have attained their normal relationships. *E,* Gradually, fusion of parts of the primitive mesentery occurs, fixing the duodenum and ascending and descending portions of the colon to the posterior abdominal wall. (From Haller, J.D., and Morgenstern, L.: Anomalous rotation and fixation of the left colon; embryogenesis and surgical management. Am. J. Surg., *108:*331, 1964, with permission.)

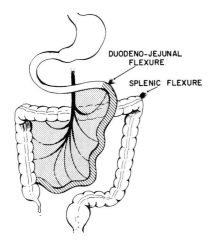

FIGURE 1-2. Reversed rotation. Note that (1) the location of all parts of the large and small bowel is normal and (2) the only anomaly is the reversed relationship of the transverse colon and duodenum with the superior mesenteric artery; the colon is posterior and the duodenum is anterior. (From Haller, J.D., and Morgenstern, L.: Anomalous rotation and fixation of the left colon; embryogenesis and surgical management. Am. J. Surg., *108*:331, 1964, with permission.)

Internal hernia is an imprisonment of the small intestine under the mesentery of the right colon during the process of fixation of the midgut loop after rotation. The wall of the sac is the mesentery of the postmesenteric arterial segment of the terminal ileum and right colon.

Omphalocele refers to the failure of rotation of the midgut beyond the first stage, with its retention in the umbilical stalk and failure of the gut to return to the peritoneal cavity.

The third stage of gut rotation and fixation continues from after return of the gut to the peritoneal cavity until birth and consists of the descent of the cecum and fusion of the mesentery. Anomalies of this stage are common and include (1) subhepatic or undescended cecum, (2) mobile cecum, (3) hyperdescent of the cecum, (4) persistent colonic mesentery, and (5) common ileocecal mesentery. During this final stage of gut rotation and fixation, the ascending and descending colons and the duodenum become fixed in their final positions. Defective fixation of the mesentery on its broad attachment to the posterior abdominal wall predisposes to volvulus of the entire mesentery.

An extremely uncommon combined error in fixation of the first stage and in rotation of the second stage of gut fixation and rotation results in the condition of anomalous rotation and fixation of the entire left colon (Figs. 1–3 and 1–4). The embryogenesis of this condition was reported by Haller and Morgenstern in 1964.[3] Their interpretation follows:

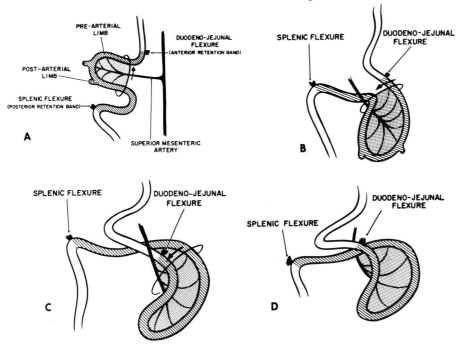

FIGURE 1-3. Mechanism for producing anomalies of rotation and fixation of the entire left colon. *A*, The splenic flexure fixes on the right side rather than on the left. This is the first and basic anomaly. *B*, Rotation begins in the normal counterclockwise direction. Since the splenic flexure is already fixed on the right, the adjacent segment of bowel, the transverse colon, reduces first and comes to lie behind the superior mesenteric artery. Thus, the first anomaly of fixation has produced the second anomaly of rotation. *C*, The next loop to reduce is the duodenum, as is normal. By projecting from this diagram, one can see that the reduction of the cecum last, as also is normal, will throw the proximal transverse colon in front of all other structures. *D*, If duodenal reduction is delayed or its rotation is incomplete, it may re-enter the abdomen later and come to lie anterior to the superior mesenteric artery. (From Haller, J.D., and Morgenstern, L.: Anomalous rotation and fixation of the left colon; embryogenesis and surgical management. Am. J. Surg., *108*:331, 1964, with permission.)

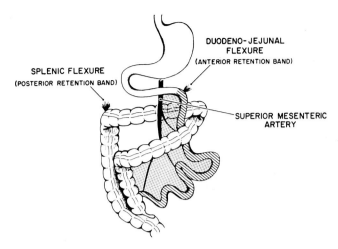

FIGURE 1-4. Anomalous rotation and fixation of the left colon. The relationships of the duodenum, superior mesenteric artery, and transverse colon: the proximal colon is most anterior, the distal colon is most posterior, and the superior mesenteric artery is behind the duodenum. The splenic flexure is ectopic on the right. An additional anomaly occurred when the cecum, the last loop to return, migrated to the right side, pulling a limb of transverse colon anterior to all other structures. This becomes apparent if the cecum and ascending colon are folded back to the left; there is then a similarity to reversed rotation. The splenic flexure, however, is on the opposite side. (From Haller, J.D., and Morgenstern, L.: Anomalous rotation and fixation of the left colon; embryogenesis and surgical management. Am. J. Surg., 108:331, 1964, with permission.)

The cause of this condition and its mechanism are primarily the fixation of the splenic flexure of the colon on the right side of the peritoneal cavity rather than on the left, which occurs during the first stage of gut rotation. After rotation begins in the normal counterclockwise direction, because the splenic flexure is already fixed on the right side, the adjacent transverse colon reduces first and comes to lie behind the superior mesenteric artery.[3]

Thus, according to these authors, the first error of fixation has produced the second anomaly of rotation. After the reduction of the transverse colon, the duodenum and cecum reduce in normal sequence. With reduction of the cecum, however, the proximal transverse colon comes to rest in front of all other structures, thus producing the condition of the entire left colon lying on the right side of the abdominal cavity.

Anomalies of Rotation

Errors occur both in the sequence of return and in the relative positions of different parts of the bowel and the SMA. Figure 1–5 demonstrates the normal topography of the abdomen of the newborn in whom rotation is successfully completed. Anything that deviates from this is termed malrotation.

A malrotation becomes clinically significant when it causes either an obstruction of the lumen of the bowel (partial or complete) or obstruction of the vascular supply of a portion of the bowel.

Anomalies of Fixation

Upon completion of the sequential rotation of the gastrointestinal tract in the latter weeks of the first tri-mester of gestation, there follows a process of fixation. The dorsal mesentery of various segments of both large and small bowel fuses with the parietal peritoneum of the posterior abdominal cavity. If the fusion of mesothelial layers is incomplete or if it occurs between structures that are abnormally rotated, two types of congenital obstruction may result: internal hernias or obstruction caused by congenital obstructive bands or adhesions.

The internal hernias resulting from abnormal fixation of the colon occur most commonly at two sites.

Right paraduodenal hernia is the result of failure of rotation of the proximal limb of the midgut beyond the initial 90 degrees, which leaves it occupying the posterior compartment of the upper right quadrant. With continuing rotation of the distal limb of the midgut, the terminal ileum, cecum, and right colon will overlie the proximal limb. Fixation of the right colon to the posterior parietal peritoneum leaves the proximal limb of the midgut trapped in a compartment bounded posteriorly by the right posterior or retroperitoneal space and anteriorly by the mesentery of the right colon. The terminal ileum will pass through an opening in this mesenteric sac to join the cecum.

Surgical treatment of the right paraduodenal hernia depends on an understanding that the abnormal location is a result of failure of rotation of the proximal part of the midgut. Release of the lateral abdominal wall attachment of the right colon allows its relocation to the left side of the abdomen. The duodenum must be completely freed of its posterior attachments so that the third portion of the duodenum and the entire jejunum lie to the right of the superior mesenteric artery. This is the essence of the Ladd procedure for congenital malrotation and offers prompt relief of the obstructive anatomic arrangement.

Left paraduodenal hernia would theoretically occur slightly later in the rotational process. With the complete 270-degree rotation of the proximal limb of the midgut, the distal duodenum and proximal jejunum lie to the left and above the SMA. If the rest of the proximal end of the midgut continues to migrate into the same area, it will occupy the compartment behind the stomach and unfixed area of the mesentery of the descending colon. The anterior wall of the hernia sac will be the stomach and the mesentery of the distal transverse and descending colon. The IMA and vein will form the medial margin of the hernia sac and will line the opening through which the terminal ileum emerges to join the cecum.

Surgical management of the more common left paraduodenal hernia can usually be accomplished by retrieving the small bowel from its retroperitoneal location, out of the hernia orifice to the left of the ligament of Treitz. If the small bowel has developed adhesions that will not allow manual reduction through the hernia's opening, the sac should be incised along its medial course, and the IMA and vein should be divided to allow a total intraperitoneal relocation of the small intestine. No other abnormality of fixation or rotation should be present.

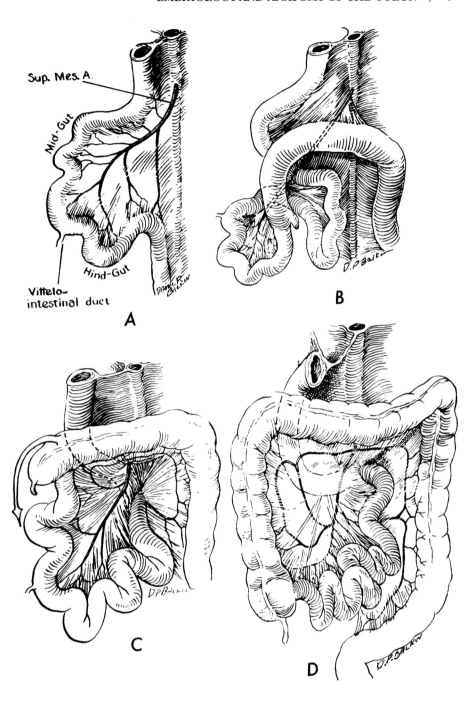

FIGURE 1-5. Normal intestinal rotation. *A*, Loop formed by midgut. *B*, Rotation of midgut and extracelomic position. *C*, Orderly return of intestinal loops into peritoneal cavity below the transverse mesocolon and further rotation of 180 degrees in counterclockwise direction. *D*, Descent of cecum and fixation of ascending colon to posterior parietal peritoneum. (From Zimmerman, L.M., and Laufman, H.: Intra-abdominal hernias due to developmental and rotational anomalies. Ann. Surg., *138*:82, 1953, with permission.)

Anomalies of Diameter and Length

Atresia of the Colon

Atresia of the colon occurs in only 5% of all forms of gastrointestinal tract atresia. It may occur at any site in the colon and varies in length. Multiple atresias are rare but do occur. Associated anomalies have been reported. Congenital colonic atresia may be confused with meconium ileus. Contrast enema studies aid in the differential diagnosis. Hirschsprung's disease has been associated with colonic atresia and has previously been reported. Colonic atresia has been classified by Louw[6] into three basic types: (1) complete occlusion of the lumen of the colon by a membranous diaphragm, (2) proximal and distal colonic segments that end blindly and are joined by a cord-like remnant of the bowel, and (3) complete separation of the proximal and distal blind colonic segments with an associated lack of a segment of mesocolon. On the basis of experimental studies in fetal dogs, Louw[6] has postulated the most accepted theory for the cause of colonic atresia. He has demonstrated that atresia of the gastrointestinal tract can be caused by a vascular accident occurring during intrauterine life.

The clinical manifestations of colonic atresia do not differ from those of other types of intestinal obstruction. A contrast enema is a necessary diagnostic procedure.

Duplication of the Colon

Duplication of the colon is a rather rare condition, and the term has been used to describe a variety of congenital abnormalities. McPherson and co-workers[7] subdivide the condition into three general groups:

The first group consists of mesenteric cysts. These anomalies lie in the mesentery of the colon or behind the rectum. They may be separable or inseparable from the bowel wall and may or may not share a common blood supply. They are similar to the duplication cysts found at other levels in the mesentery, the retroperitoneum, and the mediastinum. They are lined by intestinal epithelium, and the walls contain varying amounts of smooth muscle. The presenting symptom, resulting from the increasing size, tends to be either a palpable mass or intestinal obstruction.

The second group consists of diverticula—blind-ending pouches that are of variable lengths and arise from either the mesenteric or the antimesenteric border of the bowel and often share a common blood supply, a common wall, or both. It is significant that when a diverticulum lies in the mesocolon, the blood supply is interwoven with that of the adjoining colon. The lumen of a diverticulum is lined with intestinal mucosa, but it need not be colonic in type throughout. Gastric heterotopia is common, and pancreatic-type tissue has also been described. Because the blind-ending pouch becomes overdistended with inspissated feces, the most common presenting symptoms is an abdominal mass. In addition, if the duplication is small, it may act as a starting point of an intussusception. Because of the presence of gastric mucosa, ulceration and perfuse bleeding may occur. It has been reported that when these duplications persist into adult life, neoplastic changes may occur in the sequestered duplication of bowel.

The third group consists of long colon duplication. This is the rarest form of duplication and is unlike the two other forms in that it has no parallel in the rest of the gastrointestinal tract. The duplication almost invariably involves the whole colon and rectum; the two parts lie parallel, sharing a common wall throughout most of their length, although there is a tendency for them to separate in the pelvis. There may be two separate anal openings, but more commonly the accessory lumen, usually the inner loop, ends blindly or drains incompletely through an ectopic opening into the perineum, vagina, or posterior urethra. The mucosal lining is normal in this type of duplication, and the lesion, therefore, represents identical pairing or twinning of the colon. In approximately half the reported cases there has been an associated abnormality of the pelvic genitourinary organs as well. At birth, patients with long colon duplication may demonstrate some obvious external abnormality, such as double anus, duplication of the external genitalia, or exstrophy of the bladder. If both left and right colons can empty freely, the patient may reach adulthood with the condition remaining unnoticed; the onset of symptoms may be more insidious and result from slow distention of the blind-ending colon, with either abdominal distention or fecal leakage through an ectopic opening as the presenting symptoms.

Anomalies of Blood Supply

Congenital colonic atresia is a rare anomaly generally thought to result from occlusion of the blood supply to the atretic segment during intrauterine development. The mechanism by which the vascular occlusion occurs is thought to be accidental volvulus, malrotation, or herniation of the involved segment of bowel. Colonic atresia has been discussed briefly in the section "Anomalies of Diameter and Length," but the direct role of the vascular occlusion as the cause of the atresia as documented by Louw[6] and Abrams[1] leads to its inclusion as an anomaly of blood supply as well.

Atresia or stenosis of the colon has been reported to occur in 2 to 10% of all cases of intestinal atresia. Because the site of obstruction is distal, the diagnosis is usually delayed until significant abdominal distention and fecal vomiting occur. As a result of the delay in diagnosis, electrolyte imbalance and dehydration are usually profound, and the risk of death remains significant. Failure to diagnose colonic atresia within days after birth has uniformly resulted in the infant's death.

The clinical picture of polyhydramnois, failure to pass significant amounts of meconium, abdominal distention, and vomiting in the newborn demands a prompt and thorough evaluation of the entire gastrointestinal tract. When plain abdominal radiographs suggest a bowel obstruction, it is advisable to perform a contrast enema radiographic examination of the colon; there have been reports of several infants with combined small bowel and colon atresias in whom the distal obstruction was not recognized and a complicated postoperative period resulted. The contrast enema is the most effective means of establishing the diagnosis and localizing the site of the colonic obstruction.

ANATOMY

The colon is 120 to 200 cm long—not more than one fourth of the length of the small intestine. Its diameter diminishes gradually from 7.5 cm at its cecal extremity to 2.5 cm at the termination of the sigmoid colon. It is capable of a great increase in circumference by distention.

Three anatomic characteristics help the surgeon identify a loop of colon and distinguish it from the small intestine:

1. The taeniae coli. These are three long muscular bands that extend from the tip of the cecum to the rectosigmoid. They are approximately 6 mm in width and are situated equidistant from one another along the surface of the colon. They form the longitudinal layer of muscle fibers of the colon.

2. The haustral sacculations of the walls of the colon. These sacculations are produced by the adaptation of a greater length of bowel wall to a lesser length of the longitudinal taeniae. Internally, the haustral pouches are separated by folds that reduce the lumen of the colon to some extent.

3. The appendices epiploicae, which are small, fatty appendages of peritoneum studding the external sur-

face of the colon. They are most numerous along the taeniae and are relatively flat in the proximal colon but elongated and pedunculated in the sigmoid.

It should be added that the attachment of the greater omentum to the transverse colon is an important landmark in identifying that structure, and that generally the colon is whiter than the small intestine (Fig. 1–6).

Divisions of the Colon

The colon is anatomically divided into the cecum with its vermiform appendix, the ascending colon, the transverse colon, the descending colon, and the sigmoid colon. Descriptions of these structures follow.

Cecum

The cecum is the part of the large bowel located below a transverse line passing just above the ileocecal valve and into which open the ileum, the vermiform appendix, and the ascending colon. It is usually located in the right iliac fossa but may be found elsewhere in persons with malrotation of the intestinal tract or situs inversus. It averages 6.25 cm in length and 7.5 cm in width. Its three longitudinal taeniae converge at the tip (the point at which the appendix is attached) and serve as a guide in locating that structure. The cecum is entirely invested with peritoneum and is dependent in the

general peritoneal cavity. As a rule there is little mesocecum, and its mobility may be limited. Exceptions are common, however; the cecum may be very mobile with a long mesentery and may assume abnormal positions. A mobile cecum may twist upon its mesenteric axis to form a volvulus. It may descend into a hernial sac, or if its appendix becomes inflamed, the area of tenderness may be found on examination to be in an unusual location.

The ileocecal valve, or sphincter, is the junction of the terminal ileum with the cecum. Apparently its function is to prevent the ileal contents from entering the cecum too rapidly, thus allowing time for digestion and absorption to be completed. It is capable of preventing regurgitation of cecal contents back into the ileum, and an absolutely competent ileocecal valve in complete colonic obstruction is responsible for a closed-loop obstruction. In such instances, distention of the small bowel may be eliminated by intestinal intubation without relieving the colonic distention, and unless surgical intervention is provided, rupture of the colon may occur. The ileocecal valve is not always competent, and barium enema radiographic studies frequently reveal ileocecal incompetency in persons who have no pathologic lesions.

The vermiform appendix is attached to the posteromesial border of the cecum about 2.5 cm below the ileocecal junction, and its base always can be located by tracing the anterior longitudinal band (taenia) to the tip of the cecum. Another useful guide is the constant

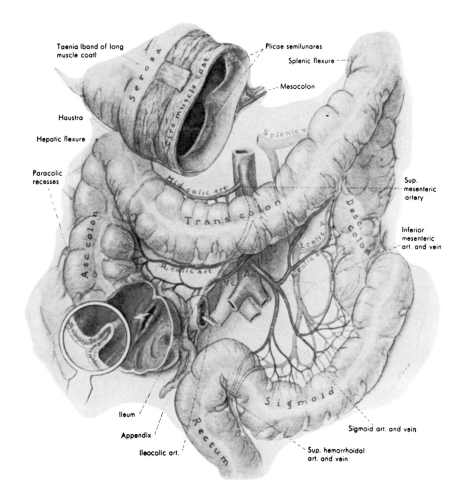

FIGURE 1–6. The large intestine. The position of the colon as shown is based on radiographic study in living humans. The anterior wall of the cecum is removed to show the ileocolic valve, characteristic folds, and opening of the appendix.

Note that the blood supply is from two sources: (1) the superior mesenteric artery through the middle, right, and ileocolic branches; and (2) the inferior mesenteric artery through the left colic, sigmoid, and superior hemorrhoidal branches. An enlarged segment of transverse colon is shown above with details of wall and plicae. A magnified portion of cecum wall is seen at lower left. (From Bockus, H.L.: Gastroenterology, Vol. II, 3rd ed. Philadelphia, W.B. Saunders, 1976, with permission.)

presence of the ileocecal fold of peritoneum and fat that connects the terminal 2.5 cm of ileum to the cecum, its inferior margin usually being attached to the base of the appendix. The appendix is a blind tube averaging about 8.75 cm in length, but varying from 2.5 to 22.5 cm. Although the relationship of the base of the appendix to the cecum is constant, the appendix may occupy a variety of positions. The five most common variations in its position are shown in Figure 1–7.

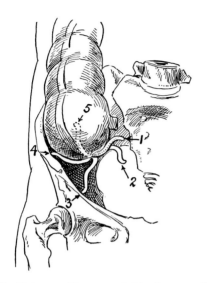

FIGURE 1-7. Various positions occupied by the appendix (Deaver).

The mesoappendix is a triangular peritoneal fold attached to the left layer of the mesentery of the terminal ileum; it contains the appendiceal vessels and their branches.

Ascending Colon

The ascending colon is that part of the colon that lies between the cecum and the right colic (hepatic) flexure. It varies from 12.5 to 20 cm in length and extends vertically upward along the right side of the abdominal wall from the cecum to the inferior surface of the right lobe of the liver (Fig. 1–8). The ascending colon is covered anteriorly and on both sides by peritoneum, which binds it to the posterior and lateral abdominal wall. Its lateral peritoneal attachment is an embryologic fusion between the visceral and parietal peritoneum. Its posterior nonperitonealized surface is bound by areolar tissue to the posterior abdominal wall. A mesentery is present in about 26% of individuals. It is separated from the right kidney, over the lower part of which it passes, by the extraperitoneal and perirenal fat and the anterior layer of perirenal fascia.

At the undersurface of the liver, just beneath the ninth and tenth costal cartilages and lateral to the gallbladder, the ascending colon turns sharply mesially and downward to form the right colic (hepatic) flexure. This flexure lies immediately over the descending duodenum. The right colic flexure is supported by the nephrocolic ligament and also, in about a third of hu-

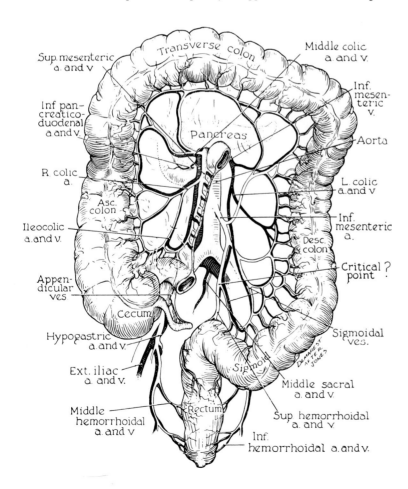

FIGURE 1–8. The colon—its anatomic divisions and its blood supply (the veins are shown, in broken black). (Modified from Jones, T., and Shepard, W.C.: A Manual of Surgical Anatomy. Philadelphia, W.B. Saunders, 1945, with permission.)

man subjects, by a cystoduodenocolic ligament. This flexure has a vertical mobility averaging 2.5 to 7.5 cm with respiration.[5]

Transverse Colon

The transverse colon is that part of the colon extending transversely across the abdomen from the hepatic flexure on the right to the splenic flexure on the left, usually with a downward curve of varying degree. It averages 40 to 50 cm in length. It is completely invested with peritoneum and has a long mesentery (transverse mesocolon) that attaches it to the posterior abdominal wall and permits it to be the most movable part of the colon. At each end, the transverse colon is supported by the relatively fixed hepatic and splenic flexures. The transverse mesocolon forms a horizontal partition across the abdominal cavity and separates the cavity of the omental bursa and supramesocolic structures from the inframesocolic compartment. It is a natural barrier to reciprocal infections between these areas.

The greater curvature of the stomach is attached to the transverse colon by the gastrocolic omentum, and the greater omentum is attached to the entire length of the transverse colon.

Just beneath the lower angle of the spleen, the transverse colon turns sharply downward to form the splenic flexure. With the exception of the rectum, the splenic flexure is the most fixed part of the large intestine. Its lateral surface is attached to the diaphragm at the level of the tenth and eleventh ribs by the phrenocolic ligament, which also supports the spleen, and to the tail of the pancreas by the left extremity of the transverse mesocolon. The splenic flexure is acute and is situated higher and deeper within the abdomen than the hepatic flexure. It is under cover of the costal margin and is partly overlain by the stomach.

Descending Colon

The descending colon is that part of the colon that extends from the splenic flexure to the brim of the pelvis, at which point the sigmoid colon begins. It averages 25 to 30 cm in length and descends vertically, inclining mesially to curve around the lower aspect of the left kidney. The anterior, lateral, and medial surfaces of the descending colon are covered by peritoneum, which fixes it to the lateral and posterior abdominal walls. Its position is fixed and immobile. Its posterior surface has no peritoneal covering but is fixed to the fascia covering the musculus quadratus lumborum. A short mesentery may be present in some persons. The descending colon is more deeply placed and much narrower than the ascending colon.

Sigmoid Colon

The sigmoid colon is that part of the colon between the descending colon and the rectum. It begins at the brim of the pelvis and ends at the rectosigmoid junction, which is at the level of the third sacral vertebra and is the point at which the peritoneal investment and mes-

entery of the sigmoid cease. The sigmoid colon is divisible into a fixed (iliac) segment and a mobile (pelvic) segment.

According to Callander,[2] the iliac segment is that part of the sigmoid flexure that lies in the iliac fossa and has no mesentery. It extends to the pelvic brim, at which point it becomes continuous with the pelvic colon. The pelvic segment is a long, omega-shaped coil that is continuous with the iliac colon above and with the rectum below. It is suspended from the posterior wall of the pelvis by a mesentery, the pelvic mesocolon. The line of mesenteric attachment resembles an inverted V. The length, location, and degree of mobility of the loop and the length of its mesentery are subject to wide variation. The intersigmoid recess is a small, funnel-shaped pouch commonly present at the junction of the two roots of the sigmoid mesocolon (Fig. 1–9). In this recess may lodge a loop of small bowel, which by a process of cleavage may insinuate itself between the mesocolon and the primitive parietal peritoneum, forming a not uncommon variety of internal or intraperitoneal hernia.

The sigmoid colon is about 40 cm in length, and its terminal 10 cm can usually be visualized during a proctoscopic examination.

The rectosigmoid junction is characterized by six anatomic features: (1) narrowing of the diameter of the bowel; (2) lack of the peritoneal investment of the gut below that point; (3) disappearance of a true mesentery below the rectosigmoid; (4) the spreading out of three longitudinal taeniae at the rectosigmoid junction to form a continuous longitudinal muscle coat for the rectum; (5) the appendices epiploicase, which are present on the sigmoid to its end but are not found below the rectosigmoid junction; and (6) internally, a gross morphologic change in the mucous membrane that can easily be seen by sigmoidoscopy (Fig. 1–10). The rectal mucosa is smooth and flat, but the mucosa of the sigmoid is seen to form prominent rugal folds. A sharp angula-

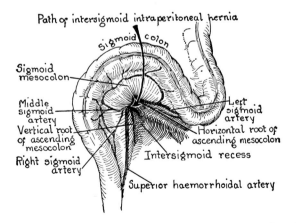

FIGURE 1–9. Sigmoid colon, its mesentery and arterial supply, and the intersigmoid recess. The sigmoid colon and mesocolon are raised forward and upward to show the vertical and horizontal attachments of its two roots. The arrow indicates the apex of the intersigmoid recess into which a loop of small bowel may insinuate and travel up behind a partially unfused descending mesocolon to form an intraperitoneal hernia. The superior hemorrhoidal artery, which is the main arterial supply to the rectum, lies between the leaves of the vertical root of the sigmoid mesocolon.

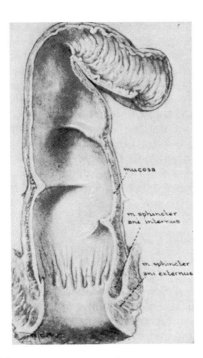

FIGURE 1-10. Longitudinal view of the anus, rectum, and lower sigmoid colon. In the lower rectum are the columns of Morgagni; the three rectal valves or valves of Houston are shown, as are the rugae of the sigmoid. (From Bacon, H.E.: Anus, Rectum, Sigmoid Colon: Diagnosis and Treatment, 3rd ed. Philadelphia, J.B. Lippincott, 1949, with permission.)

tion is invariably encountered at this level during sigmoidoscopy, and the caliber of the bowel lumen is markedly reduced.

Blood Supply

Arteries

The right half of the colon receives its arterial blood supply, in common with the small intestine, from branches of the SMA, which arises from the anterior surface of the aorta at about the level of the first lumbar vertebra and about 1.25 cm below the origin of the celiac axis (Fig. 1–8). The SMA emerges from the undersurface of the pancreas between the inferior margin of the pancreas and the upper margin of the third portion of the duodenum, and enters the mesentery of the small intestine, passing downward and to the right between the two layers of the mesentery to terminate near the ileocecal junction by anastomosing with its own ileocolic branch. Its branches supply the whole length of the small intestine, with the exception of the upper part of the duodenum, and also supply the right half of the large intestine.

The middle colic artery arises from the concave surface of the SMA a little below the origin of the inferior pancreaticoduodenal artery and before or shortly after the SMA enters the mesentery of the small intestine. The middle colic artery supplies the transverse colon and anastomoses with twigs of the right and left colic arteries. Severance of the middle colic artery usually is followed by gangrene of a considerable portion of the transverse colon.

The right colic artery arises from the concave surface of the SMA, 1 to 3 cm below the origin of the middle colic artery and either a short distance above or in common with the ileocolic artery, and supplies the ascending colon. It anastomoses with the midcolic and ileocolic arteries. Anatomic studies made by Rankin and Steward[9] showed this artery to originate from the SMA in 40% of their subjects, from the middle colic artery in 30% of their subjects, and from the ileocolic artery in 12% of their subjects. In less than 18% of the individuals they examined, no artery was found that corresponded in course or distribution to the right colic artery.

The ileocolic artery arises about halfway down the concave surface of the SMA either just below or in common with the right colic artery. It runs beneath the peritoneum toward the upper ascending colon and hepatic flexure. It supplies the cecum and gives off the appendiceal artery, which runs behind the terminal ileum to the tip of the appendix, sending off en route a series of straight branches to the appendix (see Fig. 1–8).

The appendiceal artery is a terminal vessel and does not anastomose with other arteries. The ileocolic artery anastomoses with the right colic artery and the termination of the SMA.

The left half of the colon (the dividing point between the right colon and left colon in regard to arterial blood supply is usually in the transverse colon just proximal to the splenic flexure, although this varies) receives its arterial blood supply from branches of the IMA, which arises from the anterior surface of the aorta about 2 to 4 cm above the aortic bifurcation and below the renal vessels. This artery runs subperitoneally downward and slightly to the left, enters the base of the mesosigmoid, and continues as the superior hemorrhoidal artery below the point at which it crosses the left common iliac artery. A description of the branches of the IMA follows:

1. The left colic artery arises within the first 3 cm of the IMA and passes upward and to the left (see Fig. 1–8). This divides into ascending and descending branches. The ascending branch passes between the two layers of the transverse mesocolon to anastomose at the splenic flexure and the distal transverse colon with branches from the middle colic artery. The descending branch supplies the descending colon, enters the sigmoid mesocolon, and anastomoses with branches of the sigmoid arteries.

2. The sigmoid artery may arise as a single trunk with one to four branches, or the branches may arise separately from the IMA (see Fig. 1–8). These branches fan out in the mesosigmoid and divide near the intestine into ascending and descending branches, which anastomose with similar branches of the arteries located above and below them to form arterial arches and a marginal artery in the pelvic mesocolon and to supply the sigmoid colon. The lowermost sigmoid artery does not usually anastomose with the superior hemorrhoidal artery.

3. The superior hemorrhoidal artery is the termination of the IMA and continues downward from the

level of the second or third sacral vertebra, at which point it divides into right and left branches. These branches descend along the rectum, which they supply with blood, and gradually progress anteriorly until they meet on the anterior surface of the lower rectum. They anastomose with the middle hemorrhoidal artery from the internal iliac artery and with the inferior hemorrhoidal artery from the internal pudendal artery. They may anastomose by small twigs with the last branches of the sigmoid artery.

The anastomosing of adjacent arteries forms a continuous artery that parallels the mesenteric border of the colon from the ileocecal region to the rectosigmoid, at which point it ends (see Fig. 1–8). This artery is derived from branches of the ileocolic, right colic, middle colic, left colic, and sigmoid arteries and is known as the marginal artery of the colon. The marginal artery gives off terminal vessels that run perpendicular to the wall of the colon. Short and long branches are usually formed; the former may arise from either the marginal artery or the long branches. The short branches supply the mesocolic two thirds of the circumference of the bowel. The long branches penetrate the serosal coat of the colon and encircle the bowel beneath the serosa until they reach the taeniae, beneath which they pass to supply the antimesenteric third of the circumference of the colon (Fig. 1–11). The anastomosis between these terminal branches is very slight. Those portions of the colon that are relatively fixed, such as the ascending and descending colon, have their arterial trunks in close proximity to the bowel wall, whereas those segments of the alimentary tract that have a long, freely movable mesentery, such as the transverse colon and sigmoid, have their arterial trunks located at some distance from the margin of the bowel.

Veins

Venous blood returns from the colon through veins that have names similar to those of the arteries they accompany and that drain areas supplied with arterial blood by their corresponding arteries. In general, venous blood from the right half of the colon drains into the superior mesenteric vein, which empties directly into the portal vein, and venous blood from the left half of the colon drains into the inferior mesenteric vein, which empties into the splenic or superior mesenteric veins and thence into the portal vein (see Fig. 1–8).

Specifically, the venous return from the cecum and appendix is into the ileocolic vein, which empties into the superior mesenteric vein and thence into the portal vein. This anatomic arrangement explains the occurrence of metastatic abscesses in patients who have suppurative appendicitis with pyelophlebitis and of carcinoma in the liver in those who have carcinoma of the cecoappendiceal region. The venous return from the ascending colon and hepatic flexure is by way of veins that correspond to and accompany the arteries to that region. These veins empty into the superior mesenteric vein, which drains into the portal vein. The venous return from the transverse colon is provided by the middle colic veins, which drain into the superior mesenteric vein and thence into the portal vein. The venous return from the splenic flexure is provided by the middle colic veins and also by the left colic veins, which drain into the inferior mesenteric vein and thence into the splenic vein and ultimately into the portal vein. The venous return of the descending colon is parallel with the arterial pattern and is by way of the left colic vein into the inferior mesenteric vein, thence into the splenic vein, and ultimately into the portal vein (see Fig. 1–8). The veins of the sigmoid correspond to its arteries and drain into the inferior mesenteric vein, thence into the splenic vein, and ultimately into the portal vein.

The veins draining the rectum and anus originate in two plexuses: The first is the superior hemorrhoidal (internal) plexus, which is situated in the submucosa above the anorectal line and drains into the superior hemorrhoidal vein, and thence into the inferior mesenteric vein and portal vein. Since these veins have no valves, hypertension in the portal system may be manifested by the development of internal hemorrhoids. The second plexus is the inferior hemorrhoidal plexus, which is situated outside the muscular layer and below the anorectal line (Fig. 1–12). It originates in small vessels surrounding the anal canal, which are joined by branches from the outer surface of the lower rectum and levator

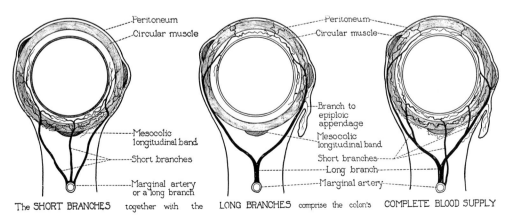

The SHORT BRANCHES together with the LONG BRANCHES comprise the colon's COMPLETE BLOOD SUPPLY

FIGURE 1-11. Terminal arteries of the large intestine. The short and long branches are shown. (From Steward, J.A., and Rankin, F.W.: Blood supply of the large intestine. Arch. Surg., 26:843, 1933, with permission.)

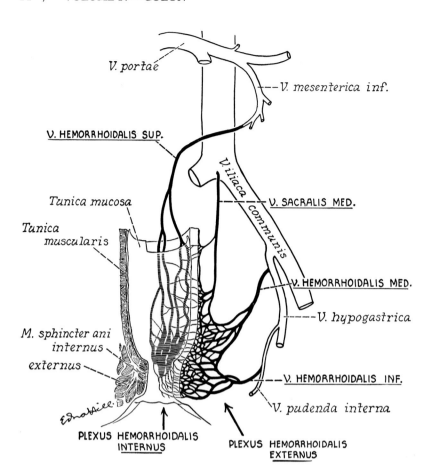

FIGURE 1-12. Venous drainage of the rectum and anus showing the internal (superior) and external (inferior) hemorrhoidal plexuses. (From Bockus, H.L.: Gastroenterology, Vol. II, 2nd ed. Philadelphia, W.B. Saunders, 1964, with permission.)

ani. The plexus is drained by two main veins: the inferior hemorrhoidal vein, which empties into the pudendal vein, and the middle hemorrhoidal vein, which empties into the hypogastric vein. Both the pudendal and hypogastric veins are part of the caval or systemic venous system (see Fig. 1–12). Venous communications between the superior and inferior hemorrhoidal plexuses are sites of the possible development of collateral circulation in persons with portal obstruction.

Lymphatic Drainage

The arrangement of the lymphatics is uniform throughout the colon. Submucous and subserous lymphatic plexuses in the wall of the colon communicate through the muscular layer and drain into the epicolic lymph nodes, which lie on the wall of the bowel beneath the serosa and in the epiploic appendices. These nodes are particularly numerous in the sigmoid colon. The epicolic nodes drain into the paracolic nodes, which lie behind the peritoneum along the mesial borders of the ascending, descending, and iliac colons, on the upper border of the transverse colon, and along the mesenteric margin of the pelvic colon. The lymph then drains into the intermediate nodes, which lie along the arteries supplying the segment of bowel involved—ileocolic, right colic, middle colic, left colic, and sigmoidal arteries (Fig. 1–13). From the intermediate nodes, the lymph from the right half of the colon proximal to the splenic flexure eventually drains into the main (principal) nodes around the origin of the superior mesenteric artery, and the lymph from the left colon distal to the splenic flexure eventually drains into the main nodes located at the origin of the inferior mesenteric artery. In both instances, ultimate lymphatic drainage is into the iliolumbar chain of lymphatics, which empties into the thoracic duct.

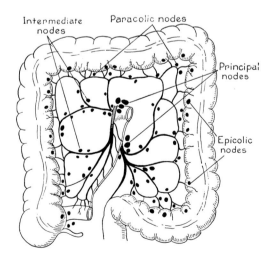

FIGURE 1-13. Diagrammatic drawing showing the epicolic, paracolic, intermediate, and principal lymph node groups accompanying the vessels of the colon. (From Grinnell, R.S.: Lymphatic metastases of carcinoid of the colon and rectum. Ann. Surg., *131*:494, 1950, with permission.)

Specifically, the appendix and cecum are well supplied with lymphatics that drain into the ileocolic group of nodes and thence to the main nodes at the root of the superior mesenteric artery. Lymphatic drainage of the ascending colon is into the intermediate nodes accompanying either the right colic or the ileocolic artery. Lymphatic drainage is more abundant from the transverse colon than from the descending colon, and the hepatic and splenic flexures are particularly well supplied with lymphatics. Lymph drainage from the transverse colon is into the nodes along the middle colic artery. Lymphatics from the transverse colon communicate with those of the omentum and may drain into the nodes in the hilum of the spleen. Jamieson and Dobson[4] found no communication in the greater omentum between the lymphatic vessels of the stomach and those of the transverse colon. The lymphatics of the descending colon are said to be not particularly well developed, but drainage from the descending colon and sigmoid passes through nodes along the left colic and inferior mesenteric arteries into the iliolumbar chain of lymph nodes and thence into the thoracic duct, which is the ultimate destination of all lymphatics of the intestinal tract.

Innervation

The intrinsic innervation and intramural nerve plexuses of the colon are believed to resemble those in the small intestine.

The colon, in common with the entire alimentary tract, is believed to be extrinsically innervated by both the parasympathetic (craniosacral) and sympathetic (thoracolumbar) divisions of the autonomic nervous system.

Parasympathetic innervation of the cecum, ascending colon, and proximal third of the transverse colon is thought by many to be derived from the vagus nerve, but others believe that the vagus has no effect beyond the ileocecal junction. The innervation of the right half of the colon is more poorly understood than that of the left half. Parasympathetic innervation of the distal colon is thought to be derived from the second, third, and fourth sacral nerves. The parasympathetics are thought to accelerate motor and secretory activity in the colon, stimulating peristalsis and opening the rectal sphincter.

The sympathetic innervation of the colon comes from the eleventh and twelfth thoracic and first and second lumbar nerves. Its fibers leave the anterior roots of those nerves and (1) pass through the ganglionated sympathetic chain to the ganglions at the origin of the superior mesenteric artery and follow that artery and its branches to the right half of the colon, or (2) pass through the sympathetic chain to the ganglions at the origin of the inferior mesenteric artery and follow the artery and its branches to supply the left half of the colon (Fig. 1–14). The sympathetic nerves are thought to have an inhibitory effect on colonic peristalsis and secretions and to cause constriction of both the ileocolic and the rectal sphincters.

The reference of intestinal pain is important to the surgeon. Nash[8] describes the results of Jones and Pierce's study of pain reference made by passing a balloon the entire length of the human intestinal tract and in-

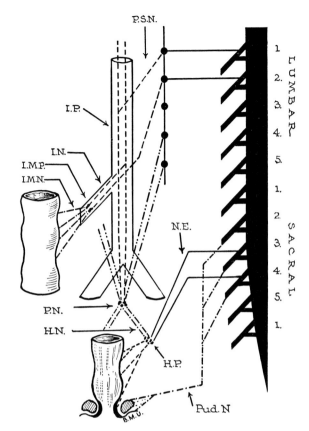

FIGURE 1-14. Nerve outflow to the distal part of the colon in humans. (H.N. = hypogastric nerve, H.P. = hypogastric plexus; I.M.N. = inferior mesenteric nerves, I.M.P. = inferior mesenteric plexus, I.N. = intermesenteric nerve, I.P. = intermesenteric plexus, N.E. = nervi erigentes, P.N. = presacral nerve, P.S.N. = pelvic splanchnic nerves, Pud. N. = pudendal nerve.) (Redrawn from Garry.) (From Quigley, J.P.: The physiology of the small and the large intestine. *In* Portis, S.A.: Diseases of the Digestive System, 3rd ed. Philadelphia, Lea & Febiger, 1953, with permission.)

flating it at different levels. This study showed that in the small intestine, pain originating at almost any level is referred to the midline immediately above or just below the umbilicus and occasionally to the back. This is in accordance with the general clinical observation. From the cecum, pain is referred to McBurney's point, with spread to the epigastrium, whereas from the hepatic flexure, it is referred to the right upper quadrant. Usually, pain from the ascending, transverse, and descending colons is referred to the lower abdomen near the midline or somewhat to the left, and pain from the rectosigmoid portion of the colon is felt in either the suprapubic or the coccygeal region. It may be stated that, in general, pain from the fixed portions of the large intestine is localized near the stimulation point, whereas pain from the more mobile portions is referred toward the midline well away from the point of stimulation.

REFERENCES

1. Abrams, J.S.: Experimental intestinal atresia. Surgery, *64*:185, 1968.
2. Callander, C.L.: Surgical Anatomy. Philadelphia. W.B. Saunders, 1935.

3. Haller, J.D., and Morgenstern, L.: Anomalous rotation and fixation of the left colon; embryogenesis and surgical management. Am. J. Surg., *108*:331, 1964.

4. Jamieson, J.K., and Dobson, J.F.: The lymphatics of the colon. Proc. R. Soc. Med., Sect. Surg. (Pt. 3) *2*:149, 1909.

5. Kantor, J.L., and Schechter, S.: Colon-studies VIII: variations in fixation of the cecocolon; their clinical significance. Am. J. Roentgenol., *31*:751, 1934.

6. Louw, J.H.: Investigations into the etiology and congenital atresia of the colon. Dis. Colon Rectum, *7*:471, 1964.

7. McPherson, A.G., Trapnell, J.E., and Airth, G.R.: Duplication of the colon. Br. J. Surg., *56*:138, 1969.

8. Nash, J.: Surgical Physiology. Springfield, IL, Charles C. Thomas, 1942.

9. Rankin, F.W., and Steward, A.J.: Quoted by Rankin, F.W., Bargen, J.A., and Buie, L.A.: The Colon, Rectum and Anus. Philadephia, W.B. Saunders, 1932, p. 30.

10. Turell, R., Pomeranz, A.A., and Denmark, S.M.: The colon and anorectum in pediatric practice. Int. Abst. Surg., *103*:209, 1956.

Chapter 2

PHYSIOLOGY OF THE COLON

CONSTANTINE T. FRANTZIDES

The colon and rectum were long regarded as merely a dynamic reservoir. Bockus[6] stated that the function of the colon may be considered physiologically to comprise two separate units, the right colon being concerned with absorption and reduction in the bulk of the excreta, and the left colon being involved with storage of feces and their expulsion. However, the colon is much more functionally sophisticated than formerly appreciated. Despite the fact that little attention was previously given to the colon, as compared with other portions of the digestive tract, the colon and rectum are now gradually being depicted physiologically.[42] The colon and rectum store, absorb, propel, and provide a socially acceptable pattern of defecation. Those functions depend on close coordination of neural, hormonal, and muscular interactions at both local and central levels.

MOTILITY

Colonic Motor Activity

Our understanding of human colonic contractile activity is based on radiologic observations of ingested barium in the colon and on manometric studies using balloons or open-tipped catheters. The classic description of normal colonic motor patterns is that of three types introduced by Templeton and Lawson[77] based on experimental work done on dogs and later applied to the human colon by Adler.[1] Type I contractions are described as simple monophasic waves of low amplitude and short duration. They are surface-dimpling contractions that create pressures of 5 to 10 cm H_2O. Their duration varies from 5 to 10 seconds and their frequency is 8 to 12/min. Type II contractions are of higher amplitude (15 to 30 cm H_2O) and of longer duration (25 to 30 seconds). When they occur in bursts, the rate is about 2/min. These two forms of contractions combine to churn or mix the feces. Type III contractions represent a change in basal pressure, usually less than 10 cm H_2O, with superimposed type I or type II waves. Larger waves lasting for 2 to 5 minutes have been described in

patients with ulcerative colitis and diarrhea as well as in individuals with normal colons, and they are referred to as type IV contractions.

Many have questioned the usefulness of this description of colonic motor activity. Several studies have demonstrated that intraluminal pressure recording devices do not provide an accurate measure of motor events in the wall of the colon.[11] Miniature strain gauges chronically implanted on the surface of the colon have recently been used in the study of colonic contractions in experimental animals. This method gives reliable and repetitive information about contractions but cannot yet be used in humans.

Colonic contractions can be divided into nonpropulsive segmental contractions and propulsive contractions.[59] Nonpropulsive segmental contractions are isolated circular muscle contractions that serve to mix and ensure good contact of contents with the colonic mucosa. They occur in a random fashion, and propulsion need not occur. They tend to delay, rather than accelerate, transit. Propulsive contractions can be divided into those progressing over short lengths of bowel and those migrating rapidly over long lengths of bowel (mass movements).[38] Propulsive activity that progresses for short distances and results in caudad or cephalad movement of bowel contents is seen chiefly in the right colon.[60] Mass movements most often begin in the transverse colon and are preceded by relaxation in the colon distal to the contractile ring.[33] This type of colonic activity is characterized by strong contractions that migrate relatively rapidly (1 cm/sec), causing propulsion of intraluminal colonic contents over long lengths of bowel. Mass movements occur three or four times/day, stimulated by food intake or physical activity.[40]

These various motility patterns are indicative of the functional differences between the right colon and the left colon. Forward and backward motion of luminal contents occurs in the right colon, permitting mixing and promoting absorption of water and electrolytes by increasing the exposure time between the liquid colonic contents and the mucosa of the right colon. At intervals, the contents of the right colon are evacuated by peristaltic movements into the transverse colon and proximal descending colon. In the left colon, mass movements result in propulsion of stool into the rectum.

A multitude of factors affect motility of the colon. Eating is one of the main physiologic stimuli, as colon activity increases after meals. The "gastrocolic reflex," as described by Hertz and Newton,[39] involves extensive propulsive activity in the colon and causes the urge to defecate after a meal, usually breakfast. The gastrocolic response is characterized by an increase of colon contractions beginning 15 to 30 minutes after ingestion of a meal. This response, however, may not depend solely on entry of food into the stomach, but may also depend on a "cephalic phase" as well as an "intestinal phase." In animal experiments, the mere sight of the anticipated food has resulted in increased colonic activity.[61] Furthermore, the colonic response is not abolished by gastrectomy[40] and can be initiated by food introduced directly into the duodenum.[17]

There is disagreement over whether this colonic response to feeding is mediated by neural mechanisms, hormonal mechanisms, or a combination of both. Gastrin, cholecystokinin, and gastric inhibitory polypeptide have been implicated as mediators of the gastrocolic response.[71] The blood levels of these hormones increase in parallel with increases in colonic motility after feeding.[68] In some studies, however, the colonic motor response was of shorter duration than the period of hormone elevation in the blood.

Neural pathways involving the vagus nerve also have been postulated as mediators of the gastrocolic response. Tansy[72,73] reported that electrical stimulation of the vagus nerve causes an increase of colon contractions through a reflex pathway involving the vagus nerve, central nervous system, and lumbar colonic nerves, whereas Collman[13] has seen the same colonic responses mediated by a vagovagal pathway. Colonic excitatory responses similar to those seen after afferent vagal stimulation are reported to occur when the stomach is distended with a balloon; this response is also believed to be mediated by a vagolumbar colonic reflex pathway. A combination of neural and hormonal mechanisms has also been suggested; the early gastrocolic response (initial 40 minutes) is blocked by cholinergic antagonists, but the later response (after 40 minutes) is not affected by these drugs.

The emotional state of the individual affects colonic motility. Hostility, anger, and resentment are associated with hypermotility, whereas anxiety and fear are associated with hypomotility. Physical activity has been shown to increase both segmental and peristaltic colonic activity, and sleep has usually been associated with depression of colonic motor activity. Distention of the colon by purely mechanical means also stimulates motility, and this effect forms the basis for the use of many laxatives. Various polysaccharides and cellulose derivatives absorb water and thus distend the colon with a soft, bulky mass of fecal material that stimulates colonic propulsive action. Any substance that will produce a sufficient osmotic effect with the resultant increase in fecal bulk will lead to enhanced colonic motility.

Colonic Myoelectric Activity

The electrical activity of gastric and small-intestinal smooth muscle is well documented. The electromechanical properties of guinea pig, rabbit, pig, cat, and dog colon have been extensively studied; those of human colonic smooth muscle remain much less well defined. Investigation of the colonic electromyogram in humans is limited; most recordings have been obtained from the most easily accessible parts of the bowel—the anal canal, rectum, and sigmoid colon. Suction electrodes or clip electrodes attached to the colonic mucosa have been the main devices used to record human colonic myoelectric activity. Few studies have been published using chronically implanted serosal electrodes in vivo.

The muscle of the colon, like that of the stomach and small intestine, generates two kinds of electrical signals: slow electrical transients, called slow waves or electrical control activity (ECA); and rapid transients, called spikes or electrical response activity. There is controversy regarding the origin, frequency, and incidence of slow waves in the colon. In some in vivo studies,[66,75] slow waves have been described as being intermittently present at two or more frequencies, whereas other investigators reported that slow waves are always present. We have shown that slow waves are present continually in humans.[27] Spike activity in the human colon has been recorded by several investigators.[7,15,24,64,66,76]

Multiple pacesetters of different frequencies are thought to exist in the colon, with dominance between these pacesetters varying over time. In general, most investigators agree that slow waves are present in two dominant frequency ranges; a lower range of 2 to 9 cycles/min and a higher frequency range of 9 to 13 cycles/min. There is an increase in slow wave frequency from more proximal to distal sites along the colon. The rectal slow wave frequency is approximately 20 cycles/min, and a gradient is observed between the colon and rectum.

Slow waves may be phase-locked or phase-unlocked. When phase-unlocked, smooth muscle cell depolarizations occur randomly. When phase-locked, individual smooth muscle cells generating slow waves do so in such a way that depolarizations in adjacent cells occur with a constant time lag and along a directional gradient that permits the related slow waves to cause coordinated contractions. The factors that control phase-locking are presumed to be neurohumoral but have not been precisely identified. Slow waves in the colon are poorly coupled compared to the small intestine. Most of the time, the right colon is phase-unlocked and motor activity is random, with twitches and dimpling occurring continuously in an uncoordinated fashion similar to brownian movement. Such nonpropulsive activity serves, however, to permit maximal absorption of fluid and electrolytes by the right colon.

Circumferential phase-locking occurs intermittently, resulting either in a standing ring contraction (haustra) or in a migrating contraction, which serves to propel stool distally. Migrating contractions are uncommon in the right colon, and when they occur usually are limited to a relatively short distance. Phase-locking is seen somewhat more frequently in the left colon, but is not the dominant state. Phase-unlocked random contractions also predominante in this bowel segment, but phase-locked coordinated contractions do occur more frequently in the left colon compared to the right colon, and more frequently are migratory. Migrating contractions usually are in the transverse colon (sometimes even in the right colon) and migrate rapidly distally to propel stool into the distal sigmoid and rectosigmoid colon.

In vivo, colonic spike potentials occur as short bursts, as in the small intestine and stomach, but they also occur as long bursts. The principal spike activity of the colon consists of independent spike bursts occurring at random. Long as well as short spike bursts, however, may occur in clusters. the long spike bursts occur in series of 2 to 3 bursts/min, whereas the short spike bursts appear in clusters of up to 12 bursts/min. Individual spike bursts or clusters of spike bursts occasionally migrate in an orad or aborad direction. Long spike bursts that migrate rapidly and exclusively in the aborad direction are accompanied by passage of flatus or defecation.[27] The relationship of slow waves to spikes is unclear; short spikes are thought to be controlled by slow waves and are superimposed on slow waves. Long spike bursts are claimed to be unrelated to slow waves.

Studies in our laboratory suggest that long spike bursts occur when the slow wave frequency is low (2 to 3 cycles/min).[16] Alternatively, shorter spike bursts occur when the slow wave frequency is higher (9 to 12 cycles/min). It is now reasonably clear that phase-locking of the ECA in a short segment of bowel usually results in segmentation, whereas phase-locking in a long segment produces a propulsive movement.

Clinical Motility Disorders

A number of clinical disorders are believed to originate from perturbations in bowel motility. Abnormalities of colonic motility appear to be important in the pathogenesis of irritable bowel syndrome, diverticular disease, idiopathic megacolon, and constipation or diarrhea. Certain differences in colonic slow wave frequency are reported to exist between normal persons and patients with the irritable bowel syndrome. A predominance of slower (3 cycles/min) activity in patients with the irritable bowel syndrome was reported by Snape[66,67] and confirmed by Taylor.[74] Manometric studies of the sigmoid colon showed that patients with the painless diarrhea variant of the irritable bowel syndrome have decreased sigmoid motility. In contrast, patients with the spastic colon–constipation variant exhibit a hypermotility pattern. The same pattern was noted in patients with constipation and diverticulosis. There is some evidence that diverticular disease occurs more frequently in patients with the irritable bowel syndrome, and therefore the underlying mechanism may be the same.[35] It has been suggested that uncoordinated smooth muscle function, followed by increased intraluminal pressure, may play some causative role in the pathogenesis of colonic diverticula.[50,51] High segmental pressures have been recorded in the sigmoid colon of patients with the

irritable bowel syndrome after the injection of morphine or neostigmine (Prostigmin). It has also been reported by Chaudhary and Truelove[10] that all classes of patients with the irritable bowel syndrome show a pronounced colonic response to intramuscular neostigmine whether or not they are having symptoms.

Postoperative ileus is characterized by temporary impairment of intestinal motility. An accumulating body of evidence implicates the colon as the primary or most persistent site of postoperative ileus.[80] It has been stated repeatedly in the past that the duration of postoperative ileus is proportional to the severity of the surgical trauma and the type of operation. The results obtained from experiments on monkeys[32] and humans,[15,79] however, showed that the duration and pattern of postoperative ileus is independent of the extent, magnitude, and duration of the operative procedure.

The mechanism responsible for postoperative ileus is unclear. One popular hypothesis is that postoperative ileus is mediated by "stress-induced" sympathetic hyperactivity, which inhibits bowel contractions. Other factors thought to be associated with ileus are peritoneal irritation caused by foreign materials, electrolyte imbalance, and the effects of analgesics and anesthetics. Peritoneal irritation and peritonitis could have a direct effect on the bowel, or the effect could be mediated through the adrenosympathetic or parasympathetic systems. The role of the sympathetic nervous system and circulating catecholamines in the etiology of postoperative ileus is still a matter of debate. Catchpole[9] and Neely and Catchpole[49] reported that total blockade of the adrenergic system with guanethidine, or a combination of alpha-receptor blockade by phentolamine and parasympathetic stimulation by neostigmine, resolved postoperative ileus. These findings were disputed by Heimbeck and Crout,[37] who found that sympathetic blockade combined with neostigmine stimulation did not resolve postoperative ileus any faster than did neostigmine alone. Circulating epinephrine and norepinephrine levels are elevated postoperatively.[21,70] Epinephrine levels return to normal after 1 to 2 days, whereas norepinephrine levels may remain elevated for up to 5 days postoperatively. The increase in epinephrine is probably due to abnormal medullary secretion, whereas norepinephrine may be produced from both sympathetic nerve activity and the adrenal medulla. Dubois[21] demonstrated an increase in the synthesis of norepinephrine within the bowel postoperatively.

Most postganglionic adrenergic sympathetic fibers innervating the intestine appear to terminate in intramural ganglions or on blood vessels. Only a few sympathetic nerves are found to terminate on smooth muscle cells and are thought to act primarily to modulate the activity of intrinsic cholinergic nerves by inhibiting release of acetylcholine. The action of norepinephrine on these cholinergic nerves is mediated through alpha$_1$-receptors. Activation of alpha$_1$-receptors causes inhibition of gastrointestinal smooth muscle contractions. Alpha$_2$-receptors are also present in postganglionic sympathetic nerve terminals and act as a negative feedback mechanism to inhibit release of norepinephrine. The smooth muscle of the gastrointestinal tract also contains adrenergic receptors of the beta$_1$ and beta$_2$ types. Stimulation of each receptor using an appropriate agonist causes relaxation of gastrointestinal smooth muscle.

Electrolyte imbalance, particularly hypokalemia, is widely accepted as a cause of prolonged ileus. Although this hypothesis is theoretically sound, surprisingly little data support it. A recent study in monkeys suggests that hypokalemia significantly reduces fasting colon contractions and could play a role in the prolongation of postoperative ileus.[65]

Cannon and Murphy, in 1906,[8] reported that diethyl ether slowed the movement of food through the gastrointestinal tract. Miller[48] showed that both ether and chloroform inhibited bowel contractions, with rapid recovery after administration of these agents was stopped. Subsequent investigations demonstrated that ethylene, cyclopropane, and halothane inhibited small bowel motility during their administration, but the effect was short-lived and normal bowel contractions returned soon after these agents were discontinued. Recent studies showed that halothane and enflurane administration profoundly decrease colon contractions: nitrous oxide is associated with increased colon contractions related to excitement in some animals. These effects were of short duration, with rapid return to normal contractile activity once the agents were withdrawn. It appears that these anesthetics play little, if any, role in postoperative ileus.[14]

Studies of the effects of analgesics on bowel motility in primates[28] and humans[15,29] clearly demonstrate that morphine affects colonic motility. The effect is variable and dose related. At low to moderate doses of morphine, there is an increase in the number of nonmigrating phasic random colonic contractions. In contrast, there is inhibition of colonic phasic myoelectric and contractile activity following higher doses. Morphine at all doses uniformly inhibits the aborad migrating contractions, which are known to be the propulsive force in the large bowel, and thus delays intestinal transit.

WATER AND ELECTROLYTE TRANSPORT

In healthy persons, the colon receives approximately 1,500 ml of chyme every 24 hours. Most of the water and electrolytes in the chyme are absorbed in the colon, leaving less than 100 ml of fluid and about 1 mEq of sodium and chloride to be lost in the feces. Under normal conditions, the colon absorbs water, sodium, and chloride while secreting potassium and bicarbonate. The maximum absorptive capacity of the colon has been calculated to be 5 to 6 l of water and 800 to 1,000 mEq of sodium and chloride daily.

It was recognized from early studies that sodium absorption in the colon occurs against an electrochemical gradient, indicating active sodium transport, whereas chloride absorption was thought to be almost entirely due to passive diffusion. Recent studies, however, have demonstrated that absorption of both sodium and chloride involves active transport mechanisms. It is now known that the mechanisms of electrolyte transport are not homogeneous throughout the large intestine[12,63]

and that differences exist among different species. In the human colon, sodium and water are absorbed primarily in the ascending and transverse colon. Active sodium absorption is a process involving electrogenic transport, neutral sodium chloride absorption, or a combination of these mechanisms. Electrogenic sodium absorption is the primary transport mechanism in the rabbit.[31] In contrast, neutral sodium chloride absorption is the primary mechanism in the rat.[5,26] It appears that both mechanisms are responsible for sodium transport in the human colon.[36,56,78] The net flux of sodium into and out of the lumen of the colon is regulated mainly by the intraluminal and intracellular sodium concentrations and by aldosterone activity.

Chloride absorption in the colon is the result of passive transport along favorable electrochemical gradients as well as active[18,52] neutral chloride-bicarbonate exchange or neutral sodium chloride absorption. The neutral chloride-bicarbonate exchange mechanism is responsible for approximately 25% of the overall chloride absorption in the human colon.[19]

It has been known for many years that the driving force for potassium secretion is the intraluminal negative potential difference (20 to 30 mv). Not until recently, however, was it realized that both active potassium secretion[26] and active potassium absorption[47] in the colon also occur. A variety of substances and factors can influence and modify water and electrolyte absorption. Aldosterone and glucocorticoids facilitate sodium and water absorption by increasing apical membrane permeability to sodium and by stimulating both active and passive potassium secretion.[25,34,43,45,62] Adrenergic and cholinergic agonists affect electrolyte transport in the large bowel. Epinephrine, for example, increases active sodium and chloride absorption and enhances active potassium secretion.[30,55] In contrast, bethanechol, a muscarinic cholinergic agonist, inhibits active sodium and chloride absorption.[82]

A number of heterogeneous agents can stimulate fluid and electrolyte secretion in the colon, including bacteria, enterotoxins, hormones, neurotransmitters, and laxatives.[4] Shigellosis and salmonellosis are two characteristic clinical entities in which diminished absorption or increased secretion of water, sodium, and chloride results in diarrhea.[57,58] During the last decade, evidence has been accumulating indicating hormonal regulation of fluid and electrolyte secretion in the small intestine and the colon. Both in vivo and in vitro studies have shown a potent effect of vasoactive intestinal polypeptide on colonic fluid and electrolyte transport.[53,81] The infusion of vasoactive intestinal polypeptide in humans results in complete blockade of colonic water absorption.[44] Similarly, the intravenous administration of antidiuretic hormone to normal subjects decreases net fluid and electrolyte absorption in the colon.[46] Prostaglandins have been implicated as important factors in the mechanism of diarrhea associated with ulcerative colitis[69] and with laxative-induced net water secretion.[2] Recent studies have shown that the increased fluid and electrolyte absorption induced by four laxatives (bisacodyl, dioctyl sodium sulfosuccinate, phenolphthalein, and ricinoleic acid) is associated with an increase of prostaglandin E in the lumen of the colon. Furthermore, pretreatment with indomethacin (a prostaglandin synthesis inhibitor) cancelled the effects of these laxatives on fluid and electrolyte movement.[3] Up to a decade ago, investigations on the effects of laxatives on the colon focused primarily on the effects of those agents on colonic motility. More recently, this focus has been redirected to the effects of laxatives on water and electrolyte transport. It is now clear that laxatives increase net water secretion and alter electrolyte movement in the colon.[20,22,23,55]

REFERENCES

1. Adler, H.F., Atkinson, A.J., and Ivy, A.C.: Supplementary and synergistic action of stimulating drugs on motility of human colon. Surg. Gynecol. Obstet., 74:809, 1942.
2. Beubler, E., and Juan, H.: Effect of ricinoleic acid and other laxatives on net water flux and prostaglandin E release by the rat colon. J. Pharm. Pharmacol., 31:681, 1979.
3. Beubler, E., and Kollar, G.: Stimulation of PGE2 synthesis and water and electrolyte secretion by senna antraquinones is inhibited by indomethacin. J. Pharm. Pharmacol., 37:248, 1985.
4. Binder, H.J.: Net fluid and electrolyte secretion: The pathophysical basis for diarrhea. In Binder, H.J. (ed.): Mechanisms of Intestinal Secretion. New York, Alan R. Liss, 1979, p. 1.
5. Binder, H.J., and Rawlins, C.L.: Electrolytic transport across isolated large intestinal mucosa. Am. J. Physiol., 225:1232, 1973.
6. Bockus, H.L.: Gastroenterology. Philadelphia, W.B. Saunders, 1956.
7. Bueno, L., Fioramonti, J., Ruckebusch, Y., et al.: Evaluation of colonic myoelectric activity in health and functional disorders. Gut, 21:480, 1980.
8. Cannon, W.B., and Murphy, F.T.: The movement of the stomach and intestine in some surgical conditions. Ann. Surg., 43:512, 1906.
9. Catchpole, B.N.: Ileus: Use of sympathetic blocking agents in its treatment. Surgery, 66:811, 1969.
10. Chaudhary, N.A., and Truelove, S.C.: Human colonic motility. A comparative study of normal subjects, patients with ulcerative colitis, and patients with the irritable colon syndrome. II. The effect of prostigmin. Gastroenterology, 40:18, 1961.
11. Christensen, J.: Motility of the colon. In Johnson, L.R. (ed.): Physiology of the Gastrointestinal Tract. New York, Raven Press, 1987.
12. Clauss, W., Schafer, H., Horch, I., et al.: Segmental differences in electrical properties and Na-transport of rabbit caecum, proximal and distal colon in vitro. Pflugers Arch., 403:278, 1985.
13. Collman, P.I., Grundy, D., Scratcherd, T., et al.: Vago-vagal reflexes to the colon of the anesthetized ferret. J. Physiol., 352:395, 1984.
14. Condon, R.E., Cowles, V., Ekbom, G., et al.: Effects of halothane, enflurane and nitrous oxide on colon motility. Surgery, 101:81, 1987.
15. Condon, R.E., Frantzides, C.T., Cowles, V., et al.: Resolution of postoperative ileus in humans. Ann. Surg., 203:574, 1986.
16. Condon, R.E., Frantzides, C.T., and Cowles, V.: Electrical activity of human colon. J. Gastr. Motility 3:177, 1991.
17. Connell, A.M., and Logan, C.J.H.: The role of gastrin in gastro-ileocolic responses. Am. J. Dig. Dis., 12:277, 1967.
18. Curran, P.F., and Schwartz, G.F.: Na, Cl and water transport by rat colon. J. Gen. Physiol., 43:555, 1960.
19. Davis, G., Morawski, S., Santa Ana, C., et al.: Evaluation of chloride/bicarbonate exchange in the human colon in vivo. J. Clin. Invest., 71:201, 1983.
20. Donowitz, M., and Binder, H.J.: Effects of dioctyl sodium sulfosuccinate on colonic fluid and electrolyte movement. Gastroenterology, 69:941, 1975.
21. Dubois, A., Weise, V.K., and Kopin, I.J.: Postoperative ileus in the rat: Physiopathology, etiology and treatment. Ann. Surg., 178:781, 1973.
22. Ewe, K.: Effects of rhein on transport of electrolyte, water and carbohydrates in the human jejunum and colon. Pharmacology, 20(Suppl.1):27, 1980.
23. Ewe, K.: Influence of diphenolic laxatives on water and electrolyte permeation in man. In Kramer, M., and Lauterbach, F. (eds): Intestinal Permeation. Excerpta Medica Amsterdam, 1977, vol. 4 p. 420.
24. Flexino, J., Beuno, L., and Fioramonti, J.: Diurnal changes in myoelectric spiking activity of the human colon. Gastroenterology, 88:1104, 1985.
25. Foster, E.S., Sandle, G.I., Hayslett, J.P., et al.: Cyclic AMP stimulates active potassium secretion in the rat colon. Gastroenterology, 84:324, 1983.
26. Foster, E.S., Zimmerman, T.W., Hayslett, J.P., et al.: Corticosteroid alteration of active electrolyte transport in rat distal colon. Am. J. Physiol., 245:G668, 1983.
27. Frantzides, C.T., Condon, R.E., and Cowles, V.: Early postoperative colon electrical response activity. Surg. Forum, 38:163, 1985.
28. Frantzides, C.T., Condon, R.E., Schulte, W.J., and Cowles, V.: Effects of morphine on colonic myoelectric activity in subhuman primates. Am. J. Physiol., 21:247, 1990.
29. Frantzides, C.T., Cowles, V., Salaymeh, B.M., et al.: Morphine effects on human colonic myoelectric activity in the postoperative period. Am. J. Surg., 163:144, 1992.
30. Frizzell, R.A., Halem, D., and Krasny, E.: Active secretion of chloride and potassium across the large intestine. In Skadhauge, E., and Heintze, K. (eds.): Intestinal Absorption and Secretion. Lancaster, MTP Press Limited, 1983, p. 313.
31. Frizzell, R.A., Koch, M.J., and Schultz, S.G.: Ion transport by rabbit colon. Active and passive components. J. Membr. Biol., 27:297, 1976.
32. Graber, J.N., Schulte, W.J., Condon, R.E., et al.: Relationship of duration of postoperative ileus to extent and size of operative dissection. Surgery, 92:87, 1982.
33. Hagihara, P.F., and Griffen, W.O., Jr.: Physiology of the colon and rectum. Surg. Clin. North Am., 52:797, 1972.
34. Halery, J., Boulpaep, E., Binder, H.J., et al.: Aldosterone stimulates maximal sodium transport capacity across basolateral membrane (Abstract). Gastroenterology, 88:1410, 1985.
35. Havia, T.: Diverticulosis of the colon. A clinical and histological study. Acta Chir. Scand., 415:1, 1971.
36. Hawker, P.C., Mashiter, K.E., and Turnberg, L.A.: Mechanisms of transport of Na, Cl, and K in the human colon. Gastroenterology, 74:1241, 1978.
37. Heimbeck, D.M., and Crout, J.R.: Treatment of paralytic ileus with adrenergic neuronal blocking drugs. Surgery, 69:582, 1971.
38. Hertz, A.F.: The passage of food along the human alimentary canal. Guy's Hosp. Rep., 61:389, 1907.
39. Hertz, A.F., and Newton, A.: The normal movements of the colon in man. J. Physiol. (Lond.), 45:57, 1913.
40. Holdstock, D.J., and Misiewicz, J.J.: Factors controlling colonic motility: Colonic pressures and transit after meals in patients with total gastrectomy, pernicious anemia and duodenal ulcer. Gut, 11:100, 1970.
41. Holdstock, D.J., Misiewicz, J.J., Smith, T., et al.: Propulsion (mass-movements) in the human colon, and its relationship to meals and somatic activity. Gut, 11:91, 1970.
42. Johnson, L.R.: Physiology of the gastrointestinal tract. New York, Raven Press, 1987.
43. Jorkasky, D., Cox, M., and Feldman, G.M.: Differential effects of corticosteroids on Na transport in the rat distal colon in vitro. Am. J. Physiol., 248:G424, 1985.
44. Krejs, G.: Effect of VIP infusion on water and electrolyte transport in the human intestine. In Said, S.I. (ed.): Vasoactive Intestinal Peptide. New York, Raven Press, 1982, 193.
45. Levitan, R., and Ingelfinger, F.J.: Effect of d-aldosterone on salt and water absorption from the intact human colon. J. Clin. Invest., 44:801, 1965.
46. Levitan, R., and Mauer, I.: Effect of intravenous antidiuretic hormone administration on salt and water absorption from the human colon. J. Lab. Clin. Med., 72:739, 1968.
47. McCabe, R., Cooke, H., and Sullivan, L.: Potassium transport by rabbit descending colon. Am. J. Physiol., 242:C81, 1982.
48. Miller, G.M.: The effects of general anethesia on the muscular activity of the gastrointestinal tract. J. Pharm. Exp. Ther., 27:41, 1926.

49. Neely, J., and Catchpole, B.: The restoration of alimentary tract motility by pharmacological means. Br. J. Surg., *58:*21, 1971.

50. Painter, N.S., and Truelove, S.C.: The intraluminal pressure patterns in diverticulosis of the colon. Gut, *5:*201, 1964.

51. Painter, N.S., Truelove, S.C., Andran, G.M., et al.: Segmentation and the localization of intraluminal pressures in the human colon, with special reference to the pathogenesis of colonic diverticula. Gastroenterology, *49:*169, 1965.

52. Parsons, D.S., and Paterson, C.R.: Fluid and solute transport across rat colon mucosa. Q.J. Exp. Physiol., *50:*220, 1965.

53. Racusen, L.C., and Binder, H.J.: Alteration of large intestinal electrolyte transport by vasoactive intestinal polypeptide in the rat. Gastroenterology, *73:*790, 1977.

54. Racusen, L.C., and Binder, H.J.: Adrenergic interaction with ion transport across colonic mucosa: Role of both a and b adrenergic agonists. *In* Binder, H.J. (ed.): Mechanisms of Intestinal Secretion. New York, Alan R. Liss, 1979, p. 201.

55. Racusen, L.C., and Binder, H.J.: Ricinoleic acid stimulation of active anion secretion in colonic mucosa of the rat. J. Clin. Invest., *63:*743, 1979.

56. Rask-Madsen, J., and Hjelt, K.: Effect of amiloride on electrical activity and electrolyte transport in human colon. Scand. J. Gastroenterol., *12:*1, 1977.

57. Rout, W.R., Formal, S.B., Giannella, R.A., et al.: Pathophysiology of *Shigella* diarrhea in the rhesus monkey: Intestinal transport, morphological and bacteriological studies. Gastroenterology, *68:*270, 1975.

58. Rout, W.R., Formal, S.B., Dammin, G.J., et al.: Pathophysiology of *Salmonella* diarrhea in the rhesus monkey: Intestinal transport, morphological and bacteriological studies. Gastroenterology, *67:*59, 1974.

59. Ritchie, J.A.: Colonic motor activity and bowel function. I. Normal movements of contents. Gut, *9:*442, 1968.

60. Ritchie, J.A., Truelove, S.C., Ardan, G.M., et al.: Propulsion and retropulsion of normal colonic contents. Am. J. Dig. Dis. *16:*697, 1971.

61. Ruckebuch, Y., Grivel, M.L., and Fargeas, M.J.: Activite electrique de l'intestin et prise de nourriture conditionelle chez le lapin. Physiol. Behav., *6:*359, 1971.

62. Sandle, G.I., Hayslett, J.P., and Binder, H.J.: Effect of chronic hyperaldosteronism on the electrophysiology of rat distal colon. Pflugers Arch., *401:*22, 1984.

63. Sandle, G.I., Wills, N.K., Alles, W., et al.: Electrophysiology of the human colon: Evidence of segmental heterogeneity. Gut, *27:*999, 1986.

64. Sarna, S.K., Latimer, P., and Campbell, D.M.: Electrical and contractile activities of the human rectosigmoid. Gut, *23:*698, 1982.

65. Schulte, W.J., Cowles, V., and Condon, R.E.: Hypokalemia and the gastrocolic response (Abstract). Dig. Dis. Sci., *29:*551, 1984.

66. Snape, W.J., Carson, G.M., and Cohen, S.: Colonic myoelectric activity in the irritable bowel syndrome. Gastroenterology, *75:*326, 1976.

67. Snape, W.J., Carlson, G.M., Matarazzo, S.A., et al.: Evidence that abnormal myoelectric activity produces colonic motor dysfunction in the irritable bowel syndrome. Gastroenterology, *72:*383, 1977.

68. Snape, W.J., Matarazzo, S.A., and Cohen, S.: Effect of eating and gastrointestinal hormones on human colonic myoelectric and motor activity. Gastroenterology, *75:*373, 1978.

69. Sharon, P., Ligumsky, M., Rachmilewitz, D., et al.: Role of prostaglandins in ulcerative colitis: Enhanced produciton during active disease and inhibition by sulfasalazine. Gastroenterology, *76:*638, 1978.

70. Smith, J., Kelly, K.A., and Weinshilbaum, R.M.: Pathophysiology of postoperative ileus. Arch. Surg., *112:*203, 1977.

71. Strom, J.A., Condon, R.E., Schulte, W.J., et al.: Glucagon, gastric inhibitory polypeptide and the gastrocolic response. Am. J. Surg., *143:*155, 1982.

72. Tansy, M.F., and Kendall, F.M.: Experimental and clinical aspects of gastrocolic reflexes. Am. J. Dig. Dis., *18:*521, 1973.

73. Tansy, M.F., and Kendall, F.M., and Mackowiak, R.C.: The reflex nature of the gastrocolic propulsive response in the dog. Surg. Gynecol. Obstet., *135:*404, 1972.

74. Taylor, I., Darby, C., and Hammond, P.: Comparison of rectosigmoid myoelectrical activity in the irritable colon syndrome during relapses and remissions. Gut, *19:*923, 1978.

75. Taylor, I., Duthie, H.L., Smallwood, R., et al.: Large bowel myoelectrical activity in man. Gut, *16:*808, 1975.

76. Taylor, I., Duthie, H.L., and Smallwood, R.: The effect of stimulation on the myoelectrical activity of the rectosigmoid in man. Gut, *15:*599, 1974.

77. Templeton, R.D., and Lawson, H.: Studies in motor activity of large intestine. Am. J. Physiol., *96:*667, 1931.

78. Wills, N.K., and Alles, W.P., Sandle, G.I., et al.: Apical membrane properties and amiloride binding kinetics of the human descending colon. Am. J. Physiol., *247:*G749, 1984.

79. Wilson, J.P.: Postoperative motility of the large intestine in man. Gut, *16:*689, 1975.

80. Woods, J.H., Erickson, L.W., Condon, R.E., et al.: Postoperative ileus: A colonic problem? Surgery, *54:*527, 1978.

81. Wu, Z.C., O'Dorisio, T.M., Cataland, S., et al.: Effects of pancreatic polypeptide and vasoactive intestinal polypeptide on rat ileal and colonic water and electrolyte transport in vivo. Dig. Dis. Sci., *24:*625, 1979.

82. Zimmerman, T.W., Dobbins, J.W., and Binder, H.J.: Mechanism of cholinergic regulation of electrolyte transport in rat colon in vitro. Am. J. Physiol., *242:*G209, 1982.

Chapter 3

COLON AND RECTUM:
Diagnostic
Techniques

THEODORE R. SCHROCK

The diagnosis of diseases of the colon and rectum is based on history, physical examination, laboratory tests, endoscopic procedures, radiographic and radionuclide imaging, intraoperative findings, and the pathologist's examination of tissues. The relative importance of various pieces of information depends on many factors, perhaps especially on the particular disease involved. This chapter discusses preoperative techniques of diagnosis. Important related conditions—for example, liver metastases—will receive only passing reference.

Much attention has focused on the early detection of neoplasms of the colon and rectum. Experts make a distinction between screening and case finding in discussions of this subject.[14,102] Screening consists of testing large asymptomatic populations. Case finding is the early diagnosis of disease in symptomatic patients or detection of lesions in asymptomatic individuals who consult a physician for routine testing. The benefits of screening are difficult to prove rigorously, but case finding is established practice. Most of the discussion in this chapter pertains to case finding.

HISTORY

Symptoms of diseases of the colon and rectum are not specific, and seldom is a clinician certain of a diagnosis from the history alone.

Symptoms

BLEEDING. Rectal bleeding may be sudden, dramatic, and life-threatening. Bleeding may be gross but slow, it may be scanty, and it may be occult. It is important to ascertain the amount of blood, its color, the presence of clots, the relationship of bleeding to defecation, and streaking on the stool or mixing in it. Sometimes, however, a bleeding pattern that seems to indicate an anal

source can be misleading. A bleeding site in the colon can coexist with anal bleeding lesions such as hemorrhoids.[62,78]

MUCUS SECRETION. Neoplasms (especially villous tumors and carcinomas) and inflammatory diseases (e.g., ulcerative colitis) can cause excessive mucus production that is visible to the patient.[79]

ALTERED BOWEL HABIT. Constipation, diarrhea, or an alternating pattern of the two is associated with many diseases. Most significant is a change from the previous pattern.

APPEARANCE OF STOOL. Consistency and caliber of the stool are helpful clues.

ABDOMINAL PAIN. Chronic abdominal pain can be caused by inflammation of colon that is in contact with parietal peritoneal surfaces. Chronic intermittent pain is typical of gradually obstructing cancers and strictures from benign causes. Tenesmus (sensation of incomplete evacuation of the rectum) is produced by rectal tumors or inflammation.

ABDOMINAL DISTENTION. Obstruction of the colon or small intestine, tumor bulk, and ascites are mechanisms of abdominal distention related to colonic diseases. Ileus and intestinal pseudo-obstruction dilate the colon and must be differentiated from mechanical obstruction.

MASS. The patient may be aware of a palpable mass. An inflammatory mass in the right lower quadrant is often sensed by patients with ileocecal Crohn's disease. Large tumors and diverticular abscesses are sometimes noted by patients.

NONMETASTATIC SYSTEMIC SYMPTOMS. Malignant colorectal disease can cause anorexia, weight loss, and fatigue. Fever suggests inflammation. Malaise results from many chronic diseases. Unusual systemic manifestations of colorectal cancer include dermatomyositis, neuropathy, ectopic adrenocorticotropic hormone production, thrombophlebitis, and Raynaud's phenomenon.

METASTATIC SYMPTOMS. Metastatic deposits in liver, lung, central nervous system, bone, or other sites may be symptomatic.

NONMETASTATIC LOCAL PROGRESSION. Acute appendicitis, colovesical fistula, pararectal abscess, ureteral obstruction, and other conditions may be present initially or may appear later during the course of colon cancer.

Other History

The assessment of risk factors for neoplastic disease is important. Age, sex, and family history of neoplasms or inflammatory bowel disease should be noted. Familial adenomatous polyposis and other polyposis syndromes should be sought. Other cancers that are associated with familial colon cancer or cancer family syndromes include cancer of the endometrium, the ovaries, and the breasts. Crohn's disease or ulcerative colitis in the family is significant.

A past history of neoplasm or inflammatory bowel disease, other gastrointestinal diseases, and previous surgical procedures are obviously important. A thorough review of systems detects the systemic manifestations previously discussed.

PHYSICAL EXAMINATIONS

The general physical examination often yields clues to colon disease, including anemia, loss of skin turgor, and weight loss. An acutely ill patient usually has systemic signs, such as fever and evidence of hypovolemia.

Abdominal examination is revealing in patients with acute abdominal pain, but chronically ill patients often have few findings. A mass is palpable in about 50% of patients with carcinoma of the cecum; about 10% of patients with cancer of the left colon have a palpable mass. The abdomen may be distended, tender, or entirely normal, depending on the circumstances. Bowel sounds may be helpful in patients with obstruction. Nodes in the groin and neck are sometimes diseased.

A digital rectal examination is essential.[79] Palpable rectal neoplasms should be assessed for depth of invasion, and retrorectal nodes are sometimes detectable. The accuracy of staging by digital rectal examination varies in different reports. In women, the anterior pelvic peritoneal reflection is located about 7 cm above the anal verge, and in men, it is located about 8 to 10 cm above this landmark. Tenderness in the cul-de-sac is common in patients with acute abdominal conditions. A mass in the cul-de-sac may be an abscess or tumor.

LABORATORY TESTS

Routine blood tests and urinalysis are helpful in the diagnosis of some diseases of the colon and rectum. Chemical markers, occult fecal blood, and several other tests deserve discussion here.

Chemical Markers

Numerous chemical markers for the presence of colorectal cancer are under investigation, but carcinoembryonic antigen (CEA) is the most common marker in clinical use today.[41,54,97] CEA is a glycoprotein found in the cell membranes of many tissues, including malignant neoplasms of the colon and rectum. Tissue CEA concentrations are lower in poorly differentiated colorectal cancers than they are in well-differentiated ones. Some of the antigen enters the circulation and is detected by radioimmunoassay of the serum. CEA is also found in urine, stool, and other body fluids.

Elevation of serum CEA levels is not specific for colorectal cancer. Malignancy in other gastrointestinal sites, cancers of other organ systems, and various benign diseases also produce abnormal CEA levels. Serum CEA levels are greater than normal in 70% of patients with colorectal cancer, but less than 50% of patients with localized disease have elevated levels. Therefore, CEA is not a useful screening procedure, nor is it an accurate diagnostic test for curable colorectal cancer.[54,97]

Preoperative CEA levels correlate well with the rate of recurrence after curative resection. If serum CEA levels do not return to normal after operation, the prognosis is poor. If CEA levels return to normal and then rise during the follow-up period, the patient should be examined for recurrence. In some patients, a second-look operation is probably justified if the work-up is unrevealing and CEA levels remain high.[8,50]

Occult Fecal Blood

Fecal occult blood tests (FOBT) are applied both to screening and to case finding. The benefits of screening large populations has been difficult to substantiate, but there are now data from a prospective controlled clinical study demonstrating a survival benefit in patients screened annually with FOBT compared with those who were not screened.[48] The lower death rate from colorectal cancer was the result of detecting cancers at an earlier stage.

The most common method of testing uses Hemoccult guaiac-impregnated slides. The peroxidase-like activity of hemoglobin catalyzes the phenolic oxidation of guaiac-impregnated filter paper to a blue dye. Positive tests are found in 2 to 6% of participants in screening programs; colorectal cancer is detected in 5 to 10% and adenomas in 10 to 43% of people with positive tests in these circumstances.[25,70] The false-positive rate in large screening studies varies from 3 to 5%.[14,25,70] Overall, the positive predictive value for invasive cancer is 11 to 24%, and for adenomas it is 36 to 41%.[25] False-positive results are generally the consequence of drugs or dietary substances.

The insensitivity of FOBT for cancer represents the major obstacle to screening efficacy.[1] In general, the false-negative rate is about 30 to 40%.[1,14,25] False-negative tests reflect inadequate sampling in some patients, but in many cases the test is negative because the neoplasm does not shed enough blood to be detected.[1] Generally, carcinomas must ulcerate before they bleed. Small polypoid adenomas (<1 cm) are unlikely to bleed, and even polyps as large as 2 cm do not bleed in every instance.[1,28] Detection of small adenomas by FOBT is almost certainly serendipity.[72] FOBT are significantly more sensitive for carcinoma of the sigmoid and descending colon (81%) than for rectal cancer (45%) or right-sided cancer (47%).[92] Rehydration of slides increases the sensitivity but lowers the specificity of FOBT.[37]

Because many chemical influences on guaiac contribute to false results, other methods have been developed. HemoQuant is a quantitative assay of fecal hemoglobin by fluorimetry of porphyrins derived from heme in the assay reaction or during intestinal transit.[22] Another method of testing for fecal occult blood is immunologic determination of fecal hemoglobin and transferrin levels.[56] It remains to be seen whether these more complex and expensive tests are sufficiently advantageous to replace Hemoccult.

The value of testing for occult blood on stool samples obtained during routine digital rectal examination is dubious, particularly in hospitalized patients. If it is important to test for fecal occult blood, it is probably worthwhile to do so under proper conditions.

Other Tests

Examination of stool for ova and parasites and the preparation of bacterial cultures, viral cultures, and stool smears for leukocytes are useful in some situations. CEA can be present in stool, but it is not routinely measured. Fecal electrolytes are quantitated in diarrheal states. A variety of breath tests are available to evaluate malabsorption of fat, bile salts, and other substances. Most disease states requiring these studies involve the pancreas or small intestine rather than the colon. The DNA content in colorectal neoplasms can be measured by flow cytometry.[40,85] Since aneuploid tumors are more aggressive in general than are diploid tumors, the results of flow cytometry may correlate with prognosis.

ENDOSCOPY

Endoscopic examination of the anus, rectum, and colon is an extension of the physical examination. Although treated separately here, anoscopy and perhaps rigid proctosigmoidoscopy are performed at the same time as digital rectal examination in the initial evaluation of patients with suspected disease of the large intestine. Flexible sigmoidoscopy and colonoscopy are done later after preparation.

Anoscopy

Anoscopy allows inspection of the anal canal and the distal few centimeters of rectum.[79] Mucosal inflammation and distal rectal tumors can be seen. Anoscopy in the diagnosis of anorectal diseases is discussed in Chapter 23.[79] Proctosigmoidoscopy, rigid or flexible, does not reliably permit examination of the entire anal canal.

Rigid Proctosigmoidoscopy

INDICATIONS. Although flexible sigmoidoscopy has advantages in certain situations, rigid proctosigmoidoscopy is preferred for other purposes (Table 3–1). Symptoms referable to the anus or rectum call for rigid proctosigmoidoscopy before flexible sigmoidoscopy, if indeed both examinations are required. Locating the position of a rectal cancer is important in planning treatment, and the rigid instrument is more accurate for this purpose. When measurements from the anal verge to various points in the rectum by rigid proctosigmoidoscopy and flexible sigmoidoscopy are compared, the measurements are identical in only 5% of patients.[16] In 80% of patients, the distance measured with the flexible scope was at least 3 cm longer than that measured with the rigid instrument. Such differences may be critical in determining the surgical approach.

If it is necessary to examine the colon in patients with idiopathic or infectious inflammatory bowel disease, the rigid instrument suffices well. Some large benign rectal polyps can be excised through a rigid scope. Flexible scopes are more expensive to clean, and rigid proctosigmoidoscopes are preferable in some patients with transmissible infections.

There are no absolute contraindications to rigid proctosigmoidoscopy.

PREPARATION. Rigid proctosigmoidoscopy is often performed without enema preparation because it is done after digital examination and anoscopy when the patient is first seen.[79] Also, enemas may wash away blood, pus, and mucus and may evoke mucosal erythema and edema. Conversely, a substantial percentage of unprepared patients have so much stool in the rectum that rigid proctosigmoidoscopy cannot be carried out. If it is essential to obtain a clear view on the first attempt, a sodium biphosphate–sodium phosphate (Fleet) enema can be used.

Premedication is required rarely. If the patient has a painful anal lesion, a topical anesthetic lubricant may make examination possible. Rigid proctosigmoidoscopy can be performed with the patient in the left lateral decubitus (Sims') position (Fig. 3–1). Elderly or debilitated patients tolerate this position well, and some examiners prefer it routinely. The prone jackknife position is also used, particularly if a special examining table is available. Draping reduces the patient's sense of vulnerability.

TECHNIQUE. The lubricated instrument in inserted,

TABLE 3–1. INDICATIONS FOR RIGID PROCTOSIGMOIDOSCOPY*

Preceding flexible sigmoidoscopy
Locate position of rectal cancer
Rectal biopsy
Monitor activity of colitis
Evaluate infectious colitis
Rectal polypectomy
Avoid contamination of flexible scope

*From Schrock, T.R.: *In* Sleisenger, M., and Fordtran, J.S. (eds.): Gastrointestinal Disease: Pathophysiology, Diagnosis, Management, 4th ed. Philadelphia, W.B. Saunders, 1989, p. 1570, with permission.

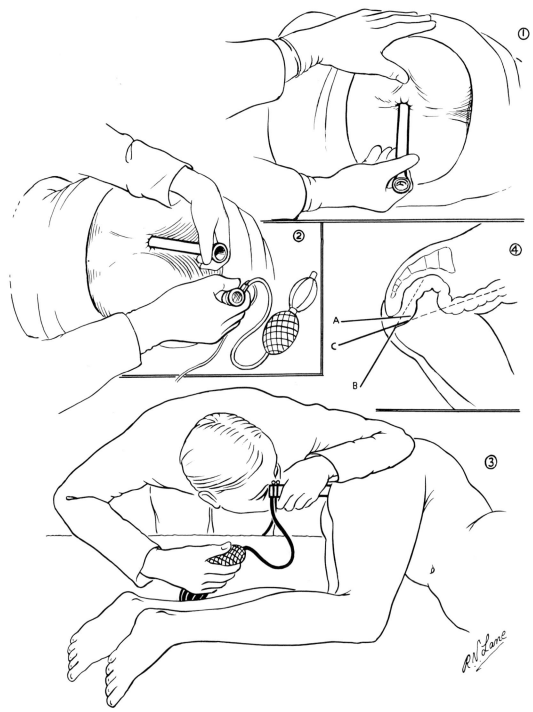

FIGURE 3-1. Technique of proctosigmoidoscopy. *1*, Introduction of proctosigmoidoscope directed toward the umbilicus until the top of the anal canal is reached. *2*, Attachment of light to instrument after withdrawal of obturator. *3*, Viewing with the proctosigmoidoscope. *4*, Alterations in the axis of the instrument during rigid proctosigmoidoscopy: *A*, axis toward umbilicus; *B*, axis toward sacral concavity when rectal ampulla is inspected; *C*, negotiation of rectosigmoid junction. (From Goligher, J.C.: Surgery of the Anus, Rectum, and Colon, 5th ed. London, Bailliere Tindall, 1984, p. 68, with permission.)

the obturator is removed, and the instrument is advanced, with the lumen in view at all times.[79] Air insufflation causes discomfort and should be used sparingly. Negotiation of the rectosigmoid junction about 16 cm above the anal verge requires that the angle be straightened (Fig. 3–1). The rectosigmoid junction often appears to be a cul-de-sac, but anterior pressure with the side of the scope, *not the tip*, may reveal the entrance into the sigmoid colon. The examination should be terminated if there is severe discomfort because of the risk of perforation. The examination is performed on withdrawal, sweeping the tip of the instrument around the lumen circumferentially. The rectal valves of Houston, two on the left and one on the right, should be smoothed out so that lesions on their cephalad surfaces are not overlooked or missed.

Biopsies are most safely obtained posteriorly. Anteriorly, the pelvic peritoneal reflection is about 7 to 8 cm above the anal verge, and a biopsy above that point has the potential to perforate into the peritoneal cavity. Small mucosal lesions can be fulgurated. Polypectomy with a snare can be carried out. The snare has a rigid outer sheath, which is different from the flexible snares used for colonscopic polypectomy.

The average depth of insertion of the rigid proctosigmoidoscope is 16 to 20 cm.[16] About one half of male patients can be examined with the rigid scope to a depth greater than 20 cm, but only one third of female patients can be examined that far because gynecologic diseases and operations increase the likelihood of pelvic fixation of the sigmoid colon, which may prevent straightening of the rectosigmoid angle.

COMPLICATIONS. Perforation complicates 0.005 to 0.01% of rigid proctosigmoidoscopy procedures.[35] Perforation by the tip of the scope occurs at angles or at sites of weakness in the bowel wall (e.g., diverticula, inflammation, ischemia, or radiation injury). Fixation of the sigmoid colon in the pelvis predisposes to perforation.

Bacteremia is demonstrable in 6.9% of rigid proctosigmoidoscopies; antibiotic prophylaxis is not required for diagnostic procedures. Therapeutic maneuvers (e.g., polypectomy) may call for antibiotics in susceptible individuals (see section "Colonoscopy").

Flexible Sigmoidoscopy

Short flexible sigmoidoscopes (30 to 35 cm) have been replaced almost entirely by longer instruments (60 to 65 cm) because they allow inspection of more mucosa and thus have a higher yield of pathologic findings.[77,79] Videoendoscopic equipment is now routine for colonoscopy, but expense limits its availability in small facilities such as physicians' offices where many of the sigmoidoscopic procedures are performed.

INDICATIONS. Flexible sigmoidoscopy is preferred for the situations listed in Table 3–2. Flexible sigmoidoscopy examines two to three times more length of bowel, and therefore it is superior to rigid proctosigmoidoscopy for screening or case finding of neoplasms.[61,77,79,83] Neoplasms are found in about 10% of flexible sigmoidoscopies performed for various indications, a yield two to six times greater than that of rigid proctosigmoidoscopy. Within the portion of colon and rectum examined, flexible sigmoidoscopy has a sensitivity for neoplasia of almost 94% and a positive predictive value of 100%. It is possible that flexible sigmoidoscopy and testing for fecal occult blood diagnose different neoplasms, so both tests are recommended. Because only the distal bowel is examined by flexible sigmoidoscopy, this procedure detects only two thirds of polyps and two thirds of all cancers of the large intestine.[80] Fifty per cent of colon cancers above the reach of the rigid proctosigmoidoscope cannot be detected by flexible sigmoidoscopy either.

Most neoplasms in the sigmoid and rectum are benign, but because carcinomas likely evolve from adenomas, the detection and removal of adenomas is believed to lower the risk of cancer.[48,80,102] Studies of screening sigmoidoscopy to detect cancer in average-risk FOBT-negative patients have reached equivocal conclusions, in part because most of the data are uncontrolled.[60,83] Carcinomas detected by screening flexible proctosigmoidoscopy typically are in an early stage, but it is unclear whether screening improves survival.[24] Two recent retrospective case-control studies concluded that the risk for death from colorectal cancer was reduced among individuals who had a single screening sigmoidoscopic examination compared with the risk for those who never had one.[61,83] The risk of death from distal cancers was markedly reduced for 10 years after a single examination, and fatal colon cancer above the reach of the sigmoidoscope did not show this difference.

Patients prefer flexible sigmoidoscopy over rigid proctosigmoidoscopy. The time required for examination is 5 to 6 minutes for rigid proctosigmoidoscopy and 8 to 15 minutes for flexible proctosigmoidoscopy. Complication rates are about the same.[35] Initial capital costs and expenses to clean and maintain the instruments are higher for flexible scopes.

PREPARATION. One or two sodium biphosphate–sodium phosphate enemas are sufficient preparation for flexible sigmoidoscopy. These outpatient examinations require no sedation or anesthesia. The patient is placed in the left lateral decubitus position.

TECHNIQUE. The technique of flexible sigmoidoscopy is well described in other tests.[77,79] The instrument is advanced with the lumen in view, taking advantage of torque, which is applied to the shaft and tip from the head of the instrument. Counterclockwise torque tends to cause a loop in the sigmoid colon, and clockwise rotation straightens it. These maneuvers and others are learned from instruction and experience. Advancement of the tip of the 60-cm instrument to the descending colon is possible in about 80% of patients.

Neoplastic lesions can be biopsied but polypectomy should not be performed. Two sodium biphosphate–sodium phosphate enemas are inadequate for safe polypectomy because there is an explosion hazard. Further, every patient with a polyp discovered in the rectum or sigmoid colon should have total colonoscopy, and polypectomy is best deferred until that time.

COMPLICATIONS. Perforation occurs in about 0.01% of flexible sigmoidoscopy procedures.[35] Other complications are rare.

TABLE 3–2. INDICATIONS FOR FLEXIBLE SIGMOIDOSCOPY*

Screening for neoplasms
Rectal bleeding: chronic gross bleeding
Radiographic lesion in sigmoid
Suspected colitis, normal rectum
Complicated sigmoid diverticular disease

*From Schrock, T.R.: *In* Sleisenger, M., and Fordtran, J.S. (eds.): Gastrointestinal Disease: Pathophysiology, Diagnosis, Management, 4th ed. Philadelphia, W.B. Saunders, 1989, p. 1570, with permission.

Colonoscopy

Colonoscopy permits examination of the entire colon from the anus to the cecum and often into the distal ileum as well. Surgeons are learning colonoscopy during residency, and this technique is increasingly becoming part of surgical practice.

INDICATIONS. Colonoscopy is diagnostic and in certain situations therapeutic. Polypectomy, control of bleeding, decompression of obstruction, removal of foreign bodies, and dilation of strictures are among the therapeutic applications. Diagnostic indications for total colonoscopy are listed in Table 3–3 and will be discussed here. Figure 3–2 shows a variety of colonoscopic findings.

Surveillance for Neoplasms. The discovery of a polyp or cancer by rectal examination, sigmoidoscopy, or barium study is an indication for total colonoscopy.[10,18,80,103] Barium enema is less accurate for detecting synchronous lesions, especially lesions 1 cm or smaller, and cannot be relied on to clear the colon preoperatively.[18,64,80] Patients who have had a polyp removed previously should undergo periodic colonscopic surveillance for metachronous tumors every 3 years.[103] New adenomas are significantly more common in patients who had carcinoma in situ or a villous component in the index polyp.[14,103] The frequency of follow-up colonoscopy after curative resection for cancer is unclear, but perhaps 1 year after the index lesion was treated and every 3 years thereafter is a sensible schedule.[36,80,87] Surveillance programs are also advised in patients with inherited colon cancer syndromes, in patients with chronic inflammatory bowel disease, and in patients with a ureterosigmoidostomy.[30,43,45,65,93,105]

TABLE 3-3. DIAGNOSTIC INDICATIONS FOR TOTAL COLONOSCOPY*

Surveillance for neoplasms
Presence of polyp or cancer
Past history of polyps or cancer
Familial colon cancer syndromes
Inflammatory bowel disease
Ureterosigmoidoscopy
Rectal bleeding
   Occult
   Acute severe hemorrhage
Radiographic lesion above sigmoid
Inflammatory bowel disease
   Initial detection
   Differential diagnosis
   Extent and severity
   Response to treatment
   Evaluation of complications (neoplasms, strictures)
   Detect recurrence
   Postoperative (anastomoses, stomas)
Diverticular disease
   Right-sided
   Exclude carcinoma
Ischemia
Obstruction, pseudo-obstruction, volvulus
Strictures
Radiation injury
Foreign bodies
Endometriosis
Pneumatosis cystoides intestinals

Rectal Bleeding. A positive fecal occult blood test can be investigated by total colonoscopy alone or by a combination of flexible sigmoidoscopy and barium enema. Colonoscopy is the best choice in most cases. It examines the entire mucosa in more than 90% of patients, it is more sensitive and more specific for neoplasm, and concurrent biopsy or polypectomy is possible.[11,21,32] Further, if barium enema is performed in a patient with occult rectal bleeding and no lesion is seen, colonoscopy is required. Conversely, if a lesion is discovered on barium enema, colonoscopy is necessary anyway to biopsy or remove the lesion and to look for synchronous tumors.

Acute severe hemorrhage from the lower gastrointestinal tract resulting from angiodysplasia, diverticula, or other causes is an indication for total colonoscopy in some patients. If bleeding stops, the colon can be prepared and the examination carried out electively. If bleeding continues, examination is undertaken without preparation.[23,78,98] Initially, endoscopists were reluctant to do colonoscopy in the presence of active bleeding because of concern about perforation and restricted visibility. Blood is a cathartic, however, and patients with massive hemorrhage can undergo colonoscopy immediately if an expert is available. A bleeding site is found, or at least the region is localized, in up to 85% of patients.[78] If the patient bleeds more slowly and can undergo mechanical bowel preparation, colonoscopy identifies the bleeding site in about 70% of patients.[31]

Radiographic Lesion Above Sigmoid. Radiographic demonstration of a lesion, even an obvious neoplasm, usually requires total colonoscopy. An exception is the patient with a left-sided obstructing lesion that does not permit passage of the colonoscopy through it.

Inflammatory Bowel Disease. Colonoscopy is an accurate means of detecting and monitoring inflammatory bowel disease.[81] Endoscopic differentiation of infectious colitis is sometimes possible. Other aspects of management that are assisted by colonoscopy are listed in Table 3–3.

Diverticular Disease. Right-sided diverticulitis is a clinical puzzle, and colonscopic evaluation may help if operation is not urgently required. Sigmoid diverticulitis requires thorough endoscopic examination before the possibility of carcinoma can be excluded.

Ischemia. Colonic ischemia often spares the rectum and cannot be seen on rigid proctosigmoidoscopy. Barium enema radiographs demonstrate edema, but the findings are nonspecific, and direct inspection of the mucosa is more accurate. The extent of involvement is mapped and its evolution over time can be monitored. Colonoscopy can perforate an ischemic colon.

Obstruction. Obstruction, volvulus (particularly sigmoid volvulus), and pseudo-obstruction can be investigated and sometimes decompressed by colonoscopy.[81]

Strictures. Strictures resulting from carcinoma, ischemia, spasm, trauma, radiation, diverticular disease, adhesions, inflammatory bowel disease, infectious conditions, or extrinsic compression are indications for colonoscopy. If the colonoscope can be passed entirely through the stricture, a diagnosis can be made, or at least carcinoma can be excluded.[69,101] If a stricture is so

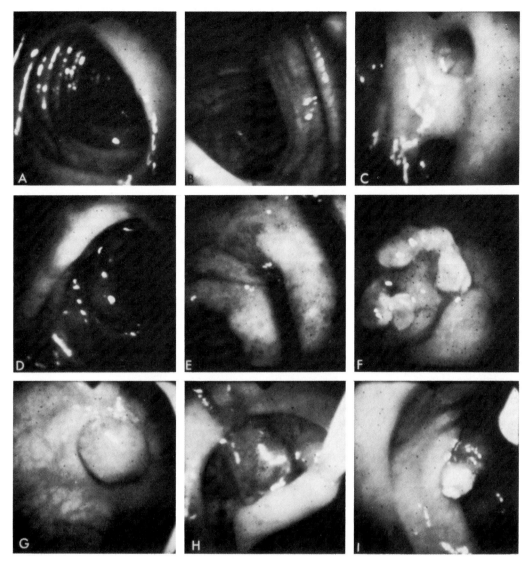

FIGURE 3-2. Colonoscopic photographs. *A*, Normal transverse colon. *B*, Normal ascending colon. *C*, Diverticula in sigmoid colon. *D*, Carcinoma of the transverse colon. *E*, Active ulcerative colitis in sigmoid colon. *F*, Pseudopolyp in chronic ulcerative colitis. *G*, Small sessile polyp. *H*, Snare secured around pedicle of polyp. *I*, Amputated polyp free in lumen. (From Schrock, T.R.: Fiberoptic colonoscopy. *In* Sleisenger, M.H., and Fordtran, J.S. [eds.]: Gastrointestinal Disease: Pathophysiology, Diagnosis, Management, 3rd ed. Philadelphia, W.B. Saunders, 1983, p. 1618, with permission.)

tight that the instrument cannot pass through it, brushings and biopsies may diagnose carcinoma. Unless a tight stricture can be dilated and a colonoscope passed through it, the diagnosis comes only after colonic resection.

OTHER INDICATIONS. Radiation injury, foreign bodies, endometriosis, pneumatosis cystoides intestinalis, and other rare colon diseases may be diagnosed by colonoscopy.

CONTRAINDICATIONS. Contraindications to colonoscopy include fulminant colitis, suspected colonic perforation, recent colonic anastomosis, an uncooperative patient, and severe associated medical conditions. Many of these contraindications are relative, and their importance depends on the necessity for colonoscopy as well as on the seriousness of the contraindication.

PREPARATION. Colonoscopy is an outpatient procedure

unless the patient is already hospitalized. Intraoperative colonoscopy is an unusual variation.[44,73]

Prophylactic antibodies are given before colonoscopic polypectomy in patients with cardiac valve prostheses, valvular heart disease, pacemakers, history of previous endocarditis, implanted orthopedic prostheses, and perhaps peritoneal shunts.[35] Since a polyp can be encountered at any time, it may be advisable to give antibiotics to most of these patients, but this issue is controversial. Prophylactic antibiotic regimens are detailed in texts.[35] Informed consent must be obtained.

Mechanical bowel preparation using polyethylene glycol sodium sulfate solution is successful and well tolerated by most patients.[80] Table 3–4 lists one effective routine. Preparation is started at 4:00 P.M. so that it will be completed before bedtime in most instances. The preparation should be modified if the patient has an intes-

TABLE 3-4. PREPARATION FOR COLONOSCOPY

Clear liquid diet all day before.
Metoclopramide, 10 mg by mouth at 4 P.M.
Polyethylene glycol and electrolyte solution, chilled, beginning 20 minutes after the dose of metoclopramide. Drink one glass every 10 minutes until 4 l are consumed.
Colonoscopy the next morning.

tinal stoma, gastrointestinal tract obstruction, any acute abdominal emergency, inflammatory bowel disease, or any other diarrheal state. An alternative method of preparation is one bottle (240 ml) of magnesium citrate at 3:00 P.M. and tap water enemas in the evening before colonoscopy the next day.

Although colonoscopy can be performed with no medication, conscious sedation with meperidine (25 to 100 mg intravenously [IV]), diazepam (2.5 to 15 mg IV), or midazolam (1 to 2.5 mg IV) is customary. The medication should be titrated so that a very light level of sedation results. Glucagon (1 mg IV) relaxes the colonic musculature and may be useful in patients with irritable colon or diverticular disease.[13,71]

TECHNIQUE. Description of the technique of colonoscopy can be found in standard texts. Fluoroscopy is not required routinely. Insufflation of carbon dioxide instead of air has advantages because carbon dioxide is absorbed more rapidly, it does not support combustion, and it may interfere less with local colonic blood flow. Air is still used by most endoscopists.

Biopsies, brushings, and washings for cytologic examination are obtained during colonoscopy if indicated. Standard pinch biopsy forceps or hot biopsy forceps can be used to excise small neoplastic lesions. Snare polypectomy is an integral part of colonoscopy, removing all of a polyp in one or more pieces for histologic examination.

Expert endoscopists require an average of about 15 minutes to perform diagnostic total colonoscopy from insertion to completion. Perhaps 30 minutes is a more realistic estimate for the average experienced colonoscopist, and beginners take much longer. Failure to examine the entire colon is the major source of error, and the rate of successful total colonoscopy improves with experience.[3,10,74,90,99,100] About 30% of colonoscopies are technically difficult, but an incomplete examination rate of 10% for experienced colonoscopists is expected with today's instruments. There are blind spots in colonoscopy in which neoplastic lesions can be missed: just proximal to flexures, in large haustra, in segments with diverticula, and below the ileocecal valve on the medial wall.

COMPLICATIONS. Major complications occur in 0.4% and deaths in 0.02% of patients who undergo diagnostic colonoscopy.[35] Difficult emergencies and therapeutic procedures increase the risks. Perforation occurs in 0.2 to 0.4% of patients as a result of diagnostic colonoscopy.[35] Mechanisms include perforation by the tip of the instrument at sites of weakness, perforation by the shaft of the endoscope if the instrument is flexed sharply, and pneumatic perforation of the colon or the ileum from distention by insufflated air. Diastatic serosal tears are also the result of colonic distention. These partial-thickness injuries usually go unrecognized unless laparotomy is performed for some other reason.

Free perforation is obvious during the procedure if the endoscopist sees abdominal viscera through the instrument. In most situations, persistent abdominal distention, pain, and a lack of dullness over the liver prompt the ordering of x-ray studies, which reveal pneumoperitoneum. The symptoms of perforation may be delayed for several days if the leak is tiny and well localized. Retroperitoneal perforation gives rise to subcutaneous emphysema and retroperitoneal and subcutaneous air.

Large lacerations require emergent operation. If no defect is seen endoscopically, and plain abdominal x-ray films show pneumoperitoneum, a water-soluble contrast enema x-ray study could be obtained to determine if the leak is still patent. If contrast does not extravasate and the patient is not ill, nonoperative treatment with antibiotics and close observation may be satisfactory for some of these presumed microperforations.

Hemorrhage, the other major complication, is essentially limited to therapeutic colonoscopy.[35] Clinically significant respiratory depression from sedation may be seen in as many as 0.5% of subjects, but arterial oxygen desaturation, occasionally severe, occurs in the majority of patients undergoing colonoscopy.[65] Other complications include transmission of infection and bacteremia. Explosion can be avoided by thorough mechanical preparation. Fluid shifts from preparation, and general and systemic complications may occur.

Other Endoscopic Procedures

Upper gastrointestinal endoscopy may be needed in some patients. Diagnostic laparoscopy is used increasingly to stage carcinoma of the colon or rectum and to evaluate other pathologic conditions, especially if the surgeon plans to proceed with laparoscopic colon resection if the findings make it appropriate. Cystoscopy is performed in patients with suspected colovesical fistula, neoplastic disease involving the bladder, and pelvic trauma.

RADIOGRAPHY

Although colonoscopy has become the initial diagnostic procedure of choice for colorectal neoplasms in the view of many clinicians, radiologic techniques—old and new—play an important role in the full evaluation of neoplasms and other pathologic conditions.

Plain Radiography of the Abdomen

Supine and erect plain films of the abdomen are routinely obtained in patients with acute abdominal diseases; oblique projections and lateral views are sometimes helpful.[53,104] The distribution of intestinal gas, edema, masses, calcifications, and the size and position of solid viscera are noted. An erect chest radiograph centered at the diaphragm is the most sensitive view for detection of pneumoperitoneum (Fig. 3–3). A lateral decubitus film substitutes in a patient who is too ill to stand.

Barium Enema

Barium enema was the mainstay of diagnosis of diseases of the colon until the advent of colonoscopy.[49,86] Barium is safe, nearly always complete, and relatively inexpensive compared to colonoscopy.[82] Preparation of the colon for barium enema must be thorough. One regimen begins with a low-residue or liquid diet for at least 24 hours.[20] A saline cathartic is given, followed by an irritant cathartic several hours later. The cleansing enema is believed to be a crucial step—1,500 ml of warm tap water is administered in three stages: 500 ml with the patient on the left side, then 500 ml with the patient prone, and 500 ml with the patient on the right side. Enemas may best be performed in the radiology department so that proper diligence is observed, but most radiologists do not follow this practice because of the logistic difficulties.[20]

In the past, there was great concern about performing barium enema soon after colonoscopic biopsy because of the risk of perforation. The interval between these studies has been shortened recently in some practices. Much depends on the depth of the biopsies; it is advisable to wait 1 week before performing a barium enema study after deep colonoscopic biopsy or polypectomy. Superficial biopsies do not require as lengthy a waiting period.

SINGLE-CONTRAST VERSUS DOUBLE-CONTRAST BARIUM ENEMA. Not all barium enemas are the same. Single-contrast barium enema (SCBE) and double-contrast barium enema (DCBE) are the two principal methods. Although DCBE often is said to be painless, many patients suffer minor pain and abdominal distention associated with air insufflation.[89,91] SCBE uses a low-density barium suspension, high kilovoltage, and vigorous fluoroscopic compression of the accessible portion of the colon. A DCBE is performed with viscous barium sulfate suspension of moderately high density. After barium reaches the splenic flexure, air is insufflated to provide a gas-filled lumen contrasting with the barium-coated mucosa. Multiple views are obtained as the patient is repositioned to allow coverage of recesses and flexures.

SCBE was the standard radiographic technique when colonoscopy was introduced.[49,86] SCBE, as it was performed 20 years ago, was not very sensitive or specific, and colonoscopy soon showed it superiority. False-positive findings were common; as many as 30% of filling defects believed to be present on SCBE were artifacts when the site was examined by colonoscopy. Specificity improved with more careful attention to colonic cleansing. False-negative results of SCBE are a problem also. Double-contrast barium enema (DCBE, air-contrast barium enema) has steadily replaced SCBE in many centers over the last three decades, but there is controversy over the relative merits of SCBE and DCBE.[27,49,67] The advantages and disadvantages of SCBE are listed in Table 3–5, and the same considerations for DCBE are found in Table 3–6.

SCBE (Fig. 3–4) is the method of choice for the very young, very old, seriously ill, or disabled patient, and it should be used also for suspected obstruction or fistula.[49] A properly performed SCBE can demonstrate the majority of neoplasms larger than 1 cm, but it is less effective for smaller lesions.[67,82] Because DCBE (Fig. 3–5) is more sensitive than SCBE in showing lesions smaller than 1.0 cm, DCBE is preferred for any patient with a positive fecal occult blood test (FOBT), a family history of polyps or cancer, a history of colorectal neoplasm, or anemia and weight loss of unknown cause.[49,82] Both SCBE and DCBE can be used as a biphasic examination even on the same day. Water-soluble contrast ma-

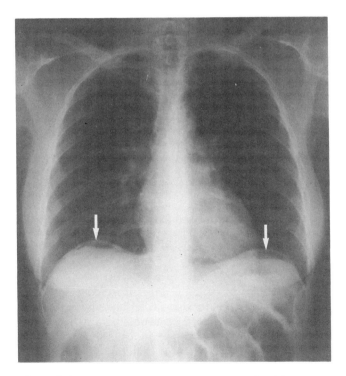

FIGURE 3–3. Erect chest film showing free air in the abdomen under the diaphragm (*arrows*). (Courtesy of Ruedi F. Thoeni, M.D.)

TABLE 3-5. SINGLE-CONTRAST BARIUM ENEMA*

ADVANTAGES
1. Easy on the patient
2. Can be performed on any patient, no matter how debilitated
3. Takes little time
4. Inexpensive
5. Little radiation exposure
6. Excellent for large neoplasms and advanced inflammatory disease

DISADVANTAGES
1. Fails to show mucosal detail and misses small lesions
2. Requires sophisticated high-resolution fluoroscopic equipment
3. Requires experienced examiner
4. Small technical margin of error in obtaining optimal overhead films
5. Does not completely evaluate the rectum

*From Margulis, A.R., and Thoeni, R.F.: The present status of the radiologic examination of the colon. Radiology, 167:1, 1988, with permission.

TABLE 3-6. DOUBLE-CONTRAST BARIUM ENEMA*

ADVANTAGES
1. Shows fine mucosal detail
2. Detects small lesions
3. Large technical margin of error for overhead films
4. Evaluates the rectum well

DISADVANTAGES
1. Difficult to perform in debilitated patients
2. Some patients do not tolerate it well
3. Takes a long time
4. Requires many radiographs
5. Expensive
6. More radiation exposure than SCBE
7. Small adherent particles are a diagnostic problem

*From Margulis, A.R., and Thoeni, R.F.: The present status of the radiologic examination of the colon. Radiology, *167*:1, 1988, with permission.

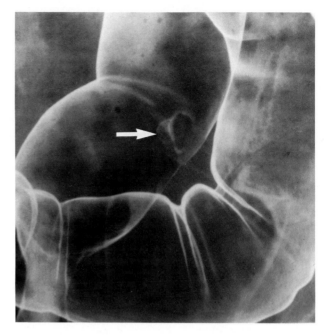

FIGURE 3-5. Double-contrast barium enema showing a colonic polyp (*arrow*). (Courtesy of Ruedi F. Thoeni, M.D.)

terial should be used in patients with suspected perforation or immediately after surgery.[49]

COMPLICATIONS. More than 3 million barium enema examinations are performed each year in the United States, and 250,000 barium enemas are done annually in England and Wales. The rate of complications or death in patients having barium enemas is very low. Three published reviews with a total of 283,500 patients indicate a perforation rate of 1 in 10,000 and a mortality rate of 1 in 50,000.[21] The morbidity and mortality rates of barium peritonitis are high. Perforation is caused by overinflation of a rectal balloon, traumatic insertion of an enema tip, weakness of the colon wall resulting from the underlying disease, or excessive hydrostatic pressure.

COLONOSCOPY OR BARIUM ENEMA? Today, barium enema (especially combined with flexible sigmoidoscopy) and colonoscopy are complementary.[15,82,86] Both tests miss lesions, but they do not miss the same lesions, and together they are more sensitive and specific than either alone. Colonoscopy is more expensive, more hazardous, and less often complete, but it finds more neoplastic lesions and it permits removal or biopsy of the lesions at the same time. In today's environment of attention to control of costs, it is not possible to perform both tests in all patients who require diagnostic evaluation of the large intestine, so which test should be performed?[12] Endoscopists argue that the most logical approach is colonoscopy first, thus avoiding the repetition of bowel preparation and the cost of barium enema in all but 10% of patients.[68] Radiologists maintain that DCBE is the most cost-effective initial approach to the early detection of cancer in most patients.[15] The answer may depend on the indication for the study (Table 3–7).[82]

Water-Soluble Contrast Enema

Contamination of the peritoneal cavity with barium can be avoided in patients with suspected colonic perforation by using water-soluble iodinated contrast media. Patients with clinical diverticulitis and those with recent colonic anastomoses are in this category. Another use of water-soluble contrast is to loosen and remove impacted feces or meconium. Some radiologists recommend water-soluble media in the presence of obstruction, a fistula, or sinus tract.[9,49]

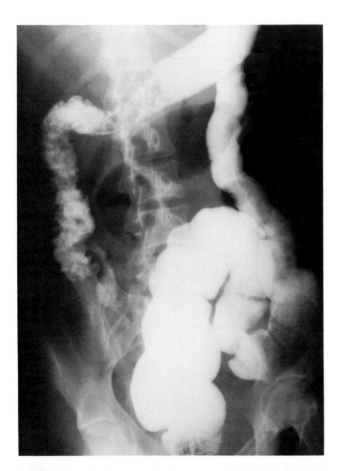

FIGURE 3-4. Single-contrast barium enema demonstrating Crohn's disease involving right colon and distal ileum. Oblique view. (Courtesy of Henry I. Goldberg, M.D.)

TABLE 3-7. INDICATIONS FOR COLONOSCOPY OR BARIUM ENEMA*

Indication	Colonoscopy	Barium Enema and Flexible Sigmoidoscopy
FOBT-positive	X	
Acute limited hematochezia	X	X
Acute severe bleeding	X	
Adenoma on sigmoidoscopy	X	
Follow-up after resection of cancer or polyps	X	Periodically
Colonic obstruction		X
Surveillance of IBD	X	Periodically
Irritable bowel syndrome		X
Chronic abdominal pain		X

*From Shrock, T.R.: Colonoscopy versus barium enema in the diagnosis of colorectal cancers and polyps. Gastrointestinal Endoscopy Clinics of North America. Vol. 3, No. 4. Philadelphia, W.B. Saunders, October, 1993, p. 604, with permission.

Defecography

Abnormal defecation associated with disorders of the pelvic floor can be evaluated by defecography.[17,34] A thick barium paste is instilled into the rectum, and lateral radiographs are obtained with the patient seated on a special commode. Internal rectal intussusception, rectal prolapse, and various other disorders can be diagnosed in this fashion.

Computed Tomography

Indications for computed tomography (CT) in the diagnosis of diseases of the colon and rectum are listed in Table 3-8. CT is used to stage rectal cancers, but unfortunately the sensitivity is too low for the clinician to rely on negative findings.[12] Abdominal CT may show the primary colonic tumor (Fig. 3-6), nodal metastases, or liver metastases.[12,51,66] Preoperative knowledge of these tumors may modify treatment (e.g., hepatic artery perfusion chemotherapy). Pelvic recurrence of rectal cancer may be seen on CT before it becomes clinically apparent, and CT-guided biopsy of tumors and CT-guided aspiration of abscesses are useful techniques.

CT yields the best results if 300 to 500 ml of contrast medium are given orally 4 to 6 hours before the examination. Sweetened water-soluble contrast or a 1% solution of barium sulfate is employed. A pelvic CT scan in women requires a vaginal tampon to identify the cervix.

TABLE 3-8. INDICATIONS FOR CT IN COLORECTAL DISEASE*

1. Stage neoplasms
2. Distinguish between locally resectable and nonresectable colorectal cancer
3. Detect recurrent cancer
4. Study the effects of extracolonic cancer or inflammatory disease of the colon
5. Diagnose abscesses and determine their extent
6. Guide percutaneous biopsy or aspiration
7. Outline sinuses and fistulas

*From Margulis, A.R., and Thoeni, R.F.: The present status of the radiologic examination of the colon. Radiology, *167*:1, 1988, with permission.

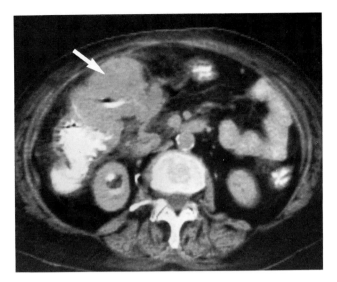

FIGURE 3-6. Abdominal CT showing carcinoma of hepatic flexure of the colon (*arrow*). (Courtesy of Ruedi F. Thoeni, M.D.)

Rectal administration of contrast material such as 200 to 300 ml of 1% diatrizoate (Gastrografin) is helpful in identifying and distending the sigmoid colon and rectum. Intravenous glucagon helps retention of air and minimizes spasm.

Magnetic Resonance Imaging

Magnetic resonance imaging (MRI) is used increasingly in the diagnosis of benign and malignant colorectal diseases.[12,49,88] MRI has proved useful in the evaluation of complex abscesses and fistulas, and it may be very helpful in complications of inflammatory bowel disease and diverticular disease.[84] The widest application of MRI at present, however, is the staging of cancer, especially rectal cancer.[12,49] A T1-weighted sequence enhances contrast between the primary tumor and adjacent perirectal fat; T2-weighted images are less useful. MRI makes it possible for the first time to assess the intactness of Denonvilliers' fascia. MRI is more accurate than CT in the diagnosis of recurrent rectal cancer because it more successfully distinguishes between fibrosis and tumor (Fig. 3-7). MRI and CT have about equal sensitivity for detecting hepatic metastases.[12]

Ultrasonography

Transabdominal ultrasound has value in the diagnosis of colonic diseases, especially diverticulitis, although other modalities are usually selected in these situations in order to avoid duplication of studies.[53] Because scattering of the sound beam by gas and loops of bowel reduces the efficiency of ultrasound, it is most useful in the pelvis. Ultrasound can detect thickening of the bowel wall, gynecologic abnormalities, hepatic metastases, and abscesses.

Transabdominal ultrasonography after intrarectal instillation of water, termed colonic sonography, is a promising new technique, but not much experience has been published to date.[96] Transrectal (endorectal) ultrasound

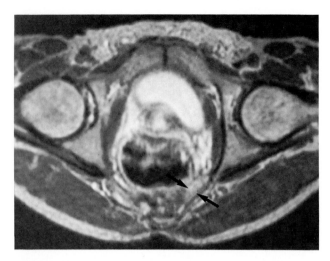

FIGURE 3-7. MRI of pelvis demonstrating recurrent carcinoma (*arrows*) after anterior resection of rectal adenocarcinoma. (Courtesy of Ruedi F. Thoeni, M.D.)

is a different type of test that is performed by positioning a transducer through the anus into the rectal lumen. It is proving to be useful for staging of rectal cancer because it is more sensitive and specific than CT or MRI in judging the depth of rectal wall invasion and spread into regional lymph nodes.[12] This test is not infallible, however.[63]

Endoscopic ultrasound involves placement of a tiny transducer through the biopsy channel of a colonoscope.[26] Experience with this procedure is growing. The obvious advantage is the ability of the colonoscope to reach areas that lie beyond the limits of transrectal ultrasonography. Staging of colonic cancer and the evaluation of mural and extramural lesions are the conditions most applicable to this procedure.[26]

The value of intraoperative ultrasound is principally in the evaluation of the liver for metastases.[39]

Angiography

Angiography is used mainly for the localization and treatment of bleeding from the colon or small intestine.[5,57] Angiography is obtained less often to diagnose colonic ischemia and to evaluate large tumors of uncertain origin and extent.

Angiography is sometimes capable of diagnosing vascular lesions in patients who are not bleeding at the time, but in general, the study is most valuable in the presence of active hemorrhage (Fig. 3–8). Angiography can detect bleeding if the rate is greater than 0.5 ml/ min, but that figure varies with how selectively the catheter is positioned. Some radiologists prefer that radionuclide scintigraphy (see further on) be obtained first because scintigraphy is more sensitive than angiography; if the scintigram is normal, there is nothing to be gained by angiography in the localization of acute bleeding. If angiography shows a bleeding site, infusion of vasopressin may stop the bleeding, at least temporarily.

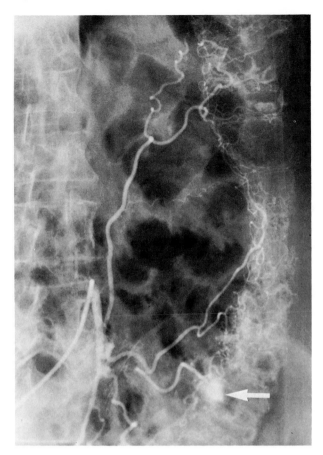

FIGURE 3-8. Selective inferior mesenteric arteriogram demonstrating bleeding site in sigmoid colon (*arrow*). (Courtesy of Ernest J. Ring, M.D.)

Fistulography

External abdominal fistulas can be traced by injection of contrast into the tracts. Interventional radiologists are skilled at manipulating catheters through fistulas to drain associated abscesses.

Urography

Excretory urography is not often needed to evaluate colorectal disease, since the position of the kidneys and the course of the uterers are seen well on CT. Retrograde ureteral studies are helpful in selected patients. Cystography is performed if a colovesical fistula is suspected.

Colonic Transit Study

The progress of ingested radiopaque markers through the gastrointestinal tract is helpful in the evaluation of patients with chronic idiopathic constipation.[55] In the single-marker bolus technique, the subject is asked to ingest a capsule containing 20 radiopaque markers on day 0 and abdominal radiographs are taken every day until all markers are passed. To make the test more practical, some clinicians just obtain a film at 5 days and avoid the interval radiographs. Most normal subjects pass all markers within 5 days. Patients with diffuse colonic inertia have markers scattered through the colon on day 5, and all of the markers typically are seen in the rectum on day 5 in patients with obstructive defecation.

Alternatively, the multiple marker bolus technique may be used.[55] The patient ingests 20 markers each day at a specified time for 3 sequential days. An abdominal radiograph is obtained on day 5 and then at 3-day intervals until all markers are passed. Calculations allow estimation of transit times through various segments of the colon.[55]

Radionuclide Scintigraphy

ACUTE LOWER GASTROINTESTINAL BLEEDING. A radionuclide "bleeding scan" is sometimes obtained in patients who appear to be bleeding actively from the lower gastrointestinal tract. Two methods are in use. ^{99m}Tc sulfur colloid is injected intravenously and cleared rapidly by the reticuloendothelial system. Sequential scintigrams are obtained for 15 to 30 minutes after injection. Bleeding rates as slow as 0.05 to 0.1 ml/min are detectable in animal studies. Localization of a bleeding site to the colon or small bowel is unreliable, although movement of extravasated material on sequential scans may help. Uptake in the liver or spleen may mask bleeding in the hepatic or splenic flexure.

The other technique involved injection of autologous red blood cells labeled in vitro with ^{99m}Tc. Sequential images of the anterior portion of the abdomen are obtained at 5-minute intervals for the first 30 minutes and every 2 to 4 hours thereafter, up to 24 hours. Focal activity indicates a bleeding site (Fig. 3–9). Only the images obtained in the first hour are relevant in patients with ongoing hemorrhage. ^{99m}Tc red blood cells are less sensitive than sulfur colloid at slow bleeding rates, but most experts favor the use of red blood cells for gastrointestinal hemorrhage. ^{99m}Tc sulfur colloid can be injected through a selectively positioned angiography catheter; this is an extremely sensitive method of detecting very slow bleeding.

Radionuclide bleeding scans are 30 to 90% accurate in various studies.[7,29,76,95] In one study, 42% of patients who underwent a surgical procedure based on localization of bleeding by radionuclide scan had the wrong operation performed.[29]

ABDOMINAL INFLAMMATION. Scintigraphy following injection of autologous leukocytes is used for detection of abscesses and other inflammatory processes (Fig. 3–10). ^{111}In was the isotope of choice for leukocyte labeling, but more recently ^{99m}Tc labeling of granulocytes has been recommended because this radiopharmaceutical is more readily available and the procedure is technically simpler.[4,42] These studies are sensitive, detecting more than 80% of abscesses, but there are many false-negative results. Leukopenia impairs the reliability of leukocyte scans. Inflammation in incisions and around surgical drains may be misleading.

Leukocyte scans are sometimes helpful in the diagnosis of inflammatory bowel disease, particularly Crohn's disease. Labeled cells accumulate in Crohn's lesions over 2 to 3 hours and can be detected by scintig-

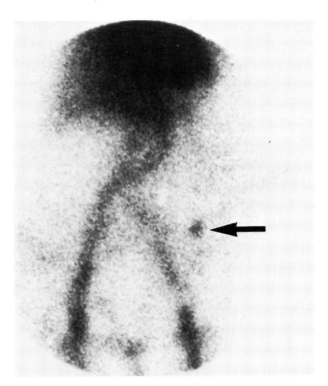

FIGURE 3–9. ^{99m}Tc red blood cell scan showing abnormal activity in area of sigmoid colon (*arrow*) 10 minutes after injection. Lesion subsequently proved to be a bleeding diverticulum. (Courtesy of Barry L. Engelstad, M.D.)

raphy. ^{111}In-labeled leukocytes are used most commonly, but other radiopharmaceuticals have been proposed for inflammatory bowel disease, including ^{67}Ga-citrate–labeled leukocytes, ^{99m}Tc sucralfate, and ^{99m}Tc-labeled porphyrins. ^{99m}Tc hexamethyl propylene amine oxine may be the best of the agents that have been studied to date.[2,4]

COLONIC TRANSIT. This is quantitated more accurately by scintigraphy than by serial radiographs to trace the progress of ingested markers.[33] ^{99m}Tc-diethylenetriaminepentaacetic acid is instilled into the right colon through a nasocecal tube, and serial scintigrams are obtained. ^{99m}Tc-labeled resin pellets mixed with standard meals is another means of studying intestinal transit.[94] Chronically constipated patients may have a pattern of slow transit through the entire colon, or only the distal colon may be affected. Scintigraphy is also used to evaluate defecation in various diseases and after rectal operations.

HEPATIC SCINTIGRAPHY. Scintigraphy following injection of ^{99m}Tc sulfur colloid generally has been abandoned in favor of other methods to detect hepatic metastases.

RADIOIMMUNOLOCALIZATION. Recurrent and metastatic carcinoma of the large intestine can be detected by immunoscintigraphy after injection of labeled monoclonal antibodies.[19] Numerous radiopharmaceuticals and many antigens have been studied, and there is no agreement at present regarding the best combination; controlled trials are underway in several institutions.[52] Single-photon emission computed tomography (SPECT) antibody images may become reliable, perhaps in combi-

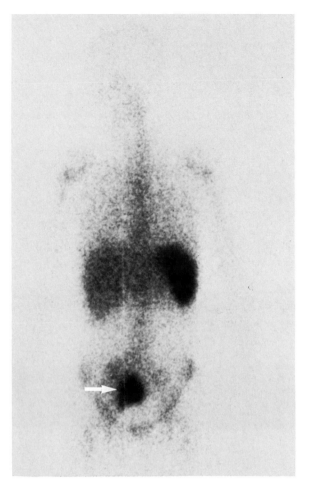

FIGURE 3-10. Anterior view 24 hours after injection of ^{111}In-labeled leukocytes showing focal activity in right lower quadrant at site of abscess related to Kock pouch. (Courtesy of Barry L. Engelstad, M.D.)

nation with standard CT.[46] Hepatic lesions are demonstrated more effectively than are extrahepatic tumors.

Intraoperative detection of tumor deposits by a hand-held probe after injection of radiolabeled antibodies is termed radioimmunoguided surgery (RIGS).[38] Its precise role has not been defined.[75]

REFERENCES

1. Ahlquist, D.: Occult blood screening. Obstacles to effectiveness. Cancer, 70:1259, 1992.
2. Allan, R.A., Sladen, G.E., Bassingham, S., et al.: Comparison of simultaneous 99mTc-HMPAO and 111 In oxine labelled white cell scans in the assessment of inflammatory bowel disease. Eur. J. Nucl. Med., 20:195, 1993.
3. Anderson, M.L., Heigh, R.I., McCoy, G.A., et al.: Accuracy of assessment of the extent of examination by experienced colonoscopists. Gastrointest. Endosc., 38:560, 1992.
4. Arndt, J.W., van der Sluys Veer, A., Blok, D., et al.: Prospective comparative study of technetium-99m-WBCs and indium-111-granulocytes for the examination of patients with inflammatory bowel disease. J. Nucl. Med., 34:1052, 1993.
5. Baba, S., and Hiramatsu, K.: Selective angiography for diagnosis and treatment for intestinal bleeding. Gastroenterol. Jpn., 3: 116, 1991.
6. Bearn, P., Persad, R., Wilson, N., et al.: 99m Technetium-labelled red blood cell scintigraphy as an alternative to angiography in the investigation of gastrointestinal bleeding: Clinical experience in a district general hospital. Ann. R. Coll. Surg. Engl., 74:192, 1992.
7. Bentley, D., and Richardson, J.: Role of tagged red blood cell imaging in the localization of gastrointestinal bleeding. Arch. Surg., 126:821, 1991.
8. Bleday, R., and Steele, G., Jr.: Second-look surgery for recurrent colorectal carcinoma: Is it worthwhile? Semin. Surg. Oncol., 7: 171, 1991.
9. Chapman, A., McNamara, M., and Porter, G.: The acute contrast enema in suspected large bowel obstruction: Value and technique. Clin. Radiol., 46:273, 1993.
10. Church, J.M.: Analysis of the colonoscopic findings in patients with rectal bleeding according to the pattern of their presenting symptoms. Dis. Colon. Rectum, 34:391, 1991.
11. Clayman, C.: Mass screening for colorectal cancer: Are we ready? (Editorial). JAMA, 261:609, 1989.
12. Collier, B.D., and Foley, W.D.: Current imaging strategies for colorectal cancer. J. Nucl. Med., 34:537, 1993.
13. Cotton, P., and Williams, C.: Practical Gastrointestinal Endoscopy. Boston, Blackwell Scientific Publications, 1990.
14. Decosse, J.: Early cancer detection: Colorectal cancer. Cancer, 62: 1787, 1988.
15. Dodd, G.D.: The role of the barium enema in the detection of colonic neoplasms. Cancer, 70(Suppl. 5):1271, 1992.
16. Dunaway, M., Webb, W., and Rodning, C.: Intraluminal measurement of distance in the colorectal region employing rigid and flexible endoscopes. Surg. Endosc., 2:81, 1988.
17. Falconio, M.A., Prasad, M.L., and Mulopulos, S.J.: Defecography as part of the evaluation of anorectal dysfunction. Gastroenterol. Nurs., 14:91, 1991.
18. Fleischer, D., Goldberg, S., Browning, T., et al.: Detection and surveillance of colorectal cancer. JAMA, 261:580, 1989.
19. Galandiuk, S.: Immunoscintigraphy in the surgical management of colorectal cancer. J. Nucl. Med., 34:541, 1993.
20. Gelfand, D., Chen, M., and Ott, D.: Preparing the colon for the barium enema examination. Radiology, 178:609, 1991.
21. Gelfand, D., and Ott, D.: The economic implications of radiologic screening for colonic cancer. Am. J. Roentgenol., 156:939, 1991.
22. Goldschmeidt, M., Ahlquist, D., Wieand, H., et al.: Measurement of degraded fecal hemoglobin-heme to estimate gastrointestinal site of occult bleeding: Appraisal of its clinical utility. Dig. Dis. Sci., 33:605, 1988.
23. Gostout, C., Wang, K., Ahlquist, D., et al.: Acute gastrointestinal bleeding. Experience of a specialized management team. J. Clin. Gastroenterol., 14:260, 1992.
24. Gupta, T.P., Jaszewski, R., and Luk, G.D.: Efficacy of screening flexible sigmoidoscopy for colorectal neoplasia in asymptomatic subjects [see comments]. Am. J. Med., 86:547, 1989.
25. Hardcastle, J., Winawer, S., Burt, R., et al.: Screening for colorectal neoplasia. In Working Party Reports. Melbourne, Blackwell Scientific Publications, 1990, p. 27.
26. Hawes, R.H.: New staging techniques. Endoscopic ultrasound. Cancer, 71:4207, 1993.
27. Heilamn, R.S.: Diagnosis of colon disease in the 1990s: Radiologists should take a stand (Editorial). Radiographics, 12:730, 1992.
28. Herzog, P., Holtermuller, K., Preiss, J., et al.: Fecal blood loss in patients with colonic polyps: A comparison of measurements with [51]chromium-labelled erythromycin and with the Haemoccult test. Gastroenterology, 83:957, 1990.
29. Hunter, J., and Pezim, M.: Limited value of technetium 99m-labeled red cell scintigraphy in localization of lower gastrointestinal bleeding. Am. J. Surg., 159:504, 1990.
30. Itoh, H., Houlston, R., and Slack, J.: Risk of cancer death in first-degree relatives of patients with hereditary non-polyposis cancer syndrome (Lynch type II): A study of 130 kindreds in the United Kingdom. Br. J. Surg., 77:1367, 1990.
31. Jensen, D., and Machicado, G.: Diagnosis and treatment of severe hematochezia: The role of urgent colonoscopy after purge. Gastroenterology, 95:1569, 1988.
32. Jensen, J., Kewenter, J., Asztely, M., et al.: Double contrast barium enema and flexible rectosigmoidoscopy: A reliable diagnostic

combination for detection of colorectal neoplasm. Br. J. Surg., 77:270, 1990.

33. Kamm, M.A.: The small intestine and colon: Scintigraphic quantitation of motility in health and disease [published erratum appears in Eur. J. Nucl. Med., 20(4):362, 1993] Eur. J. Nucl. Med., 19:902, 1992.

34. Karasick, S., Karasick, D., and Karasick, S.: Functional disorders of the anus and rectum: Findings on defecography. Am. J. Roentgenol., 160:777, 1993.

35. Keeffe, E., and Schrock, T.: Complications of gastrointestinal endoscopy. In Sleisenger, M., and Fordtran, J. (eds.): Gastrointestinal Disease. Pathophysiology/Diagnosis/Management, 5th ed. Philadelphia, W.B. Saunders, 1993, p. 301.

36. Kelly, C., and Daly, J.: Colorectal cancer: Principles of postoperative follow-up. Cancer, 70:1397, 1992.

37. Kewenter, J., Engaras, B., Haglind, E., et al.: Value of retesting subjects with a positive Hemoccult in screening for colorectal cancer. Br. J. Surg., 77:1349, 1990.

38. Kim, J.A., Triozzi, P.L., and Martin, E., Jr.: Radioimmunoguided surgery for colorectal cancer. Oncology, 7:55, 1993.

39. Knol, J.A., Marn, C.S., Francis, I.R., et al.: Comparisons of dynamic infusion and delayed computed tomography, intraoperative ultrasound, and palpation in the diagnosis of liver metastases. Am. J. Surg., 165:81, 1993.

40. Kouri, M., Laasonen, A., Mecklin, J.P., et al.: Diploid predominance in hereditary nonpolyposis colorectal carcinoma evaluated by flow cytometry. Cancer, 65:1825, 1990.

41. Kouri, M., Pyrhonen, S., and Kuusela, P.: Elevated CA 19-9 as the most significant prognostic factor in advanced colorectal carcinoma. J. Surg. Oncol., 49:78, 1992.

42. Laitinen, R., Tahtinen, J., Lantto, T., et al.: Tc-99m labeled leukocytes in imaging of patients with suspected acute abdominal inflammation. Clin. Nucl. Med., 15:597, 1990.

43. Lanspa, S.J., Lynch, H.T., Smyrk, T.C., et al.: Colorectal adenomas in the Lynch syndromes. Results of a colonoscopy screening program. Gastroenterology, 98:1117, 1990.

44. Lau, W.: Intraoperative enteroscopy—indicatings and limitations. Gastrointest. Endosc., 36:268, 1990.

45. Lennard-Jones, J.: Cancer surveillance in ulcerative colitis appears to work and can be made to work better. In Riddell, R. (ed.): Dysplasia and Cancer in Colitis. New York, Elsevier, 1991, p. 11.

46. Loats, H.: CT and SPECT image registration and fusion for spatial localization of metastatic processes using radiolabeled monoclonals. J. Nucl. Med., 34:562, 1993.

47. Longo, W.E., Dean, P.A., Virgo, K.S., et al.: Colonoscopy in patients with benign anorectal disease. Dis. Colon Rectum, 36:368, 1993.

48. Mandel, J.S., Bond, J.H., Church, T.R., et al.: Screening for fecal occult blood reduces mortality from colorectal cancer: Results from the Minnesota Colon Cancer Control Study. N. Engl. J. Med., 328:1365, 1993.

49. Margulis, A., and Thoeni, R.: The present status of the radiologic examination of the colon. Radiology, 167:1, 1988.

50. Martin, E., Jr., and Carey, L.C.: Second-look surgery for colorectal cancer. The second time around. Ann. Surg., 214:321, 1991.

51. McDaniel, K.P., Charnsangavej, C., DuBrow, R.A., et al.: Pathways of nodal metastasis in carcinomas of the cecum, ascending colon, and transverse colon: CT demonstration. AJR, 161:61, 1993.

52. McKearn, T.J.: Radioimmunodetection of solid tumors. Future horizons and applications for radioimmunotherapy. Cancer, 71:4302, 1993.

53. McKee, R.F., Deignan, R.W., and Krukowski, Z.H.: Radiologic investigation in acute diverticulitis. Br. J. Surg., 80:560, 1993.

54. Meling, G.I., Rognum, T.O., Clausen, O.P., et al.: Serum carcinoembryonic antigen in relation to survival, DNA ploidy pattern, and recurrent disease in 406 colorectal carcinoma patients. Scand. J. Gastroenterol., 27:1061, 1992.

55. Metcalf, A.: Transit time. In Smith, L. (ed.): Practical guide to anorectal testing. New York, Igaku-Shoin, 1990, p. 17.

56. Miyoshi, H., Ohshiba, S., Asada, S., et al.: Immunological determination of fecal hemoglobin and transferrin levels: A comparison with other fecal occult blood tests. Am. J. Gastroenterol., 87:67, 1992.

57. Moncure, A., Tompkins, R., Athanasoulis, C., et al.: Occult gastrointestinal bleeding; newer techniques of diagnosis and therapy. Adv. Surg., 22:141, 1989.

58. Morrissey, J.F., and Reichelderfer, M.: Gastrointestinal endoscopy (second of two parts). N. Engl. J. Med., 325:1214, 1991.

59. Neugut, A.I., Garbowski, G.C., Waye, J.D., et al.: Diagnostic yield of colorectal neoplasia with colonoscopy for abdominal pain, change in bowel habits, and rectal bleeding [see comments]. Am. J. Gastroenterol., 88:1179, 1993.

60. Neugut, A., and Pita, S.: Role of sigmoidoscopy in screening for colorectal cancer: A critical review. Gastroenterology, 95:492, 1988.

61. Newcomb, P.A., Norfleet, R.G., Storer, B.E., et al.: Screening sigmoidoscopy and colorectal cancer mortality. J. Natl. Cancer Inst., 84:1572, 1992.

62. Newstead, G.L.: Logical clinical decisions in the investigation and management of nonurgent rectal bleeding. Gastroenterol. Jpn., 3:107, 1991.

63. Nielsen, M.B., Qvitzau, S., and Pedersen, J.F.: Detection of pericolonic lymph nodes in patients with colorectal cancer: An in vitro and in vivo study of the efficacy of endosonography. AJR, 161:57, 1993.

64. Norfleet, R.G., Ryan, M.E., Wyman, J.B., et al.: Barium enema versus colonoscopy for patients with polyps found during flexible sigmoidoscopy. Gastrointest. Endosc., 37:531, 1991.

65. Nugent, F., Haggitt, R., and Gilpin, P.: Cancer surveillance in ulcerative colitis. Gastroenterology, 100:1241, 1991.

66. Ohlsson, B., Tranberg, K.G., Lundstedt, C., et al.: Detection of hepatic metastases in colorectal cancer: A prospective study of laboratory and imaging methods. Eur. J. Surg., 159:275, 1993.

67. Ott, D.J., Scharling, E.S., Chen, Y.M., et al.: Positive predictive value and posttest probability of diagnosis of colonic polyp on single- and double-contrast barium enema. Am. J. Roentgenol., 153:735, 1989.

68. Parithivel, V.S., Pandya, G.P., and Gerst, P.H.: Which one first? Barium enema or colonoscopy. Am. Surg., 55:417, 1989.

69. Petras, R.: Dysplasia and cancer in Crohn's disease. In Bayless, T. (ed.): Current Management of Inflammatory Bowel Disease. Philadelphia, B.C. Decker, 1989, p. 360.

70. Petrelli, N., Palmer, M., Michalek, A., et al.: Massive screening for colorectal cancer. A single institution's public commitment. Arch. Surg., 125:104, 1990.

71. Ponsky, J.: Atlas of Surgical Endoscopy. St. Louis, Mosby Year Book, 1992.

72. Ransohoff, D., and Lang, C.: Small adenomas detected during fecal occult blood test screening for colorectal cancer. The impact of serendipity. JAMA, 264:76, 1990.

73. Ress, A., Benacci, J., and Sarr, M.: Efficacy of intraoperative enteroscopy in diagnosis and prevention of recurrent, occult gastrointestinal bleeding. Am. J. Surg., 163:94, 1992.

74. Rex, D.K., Weddle, R.A., Lehman, G.A., et al.: Flexible sigmoidoscopy plus air contrast barium enema versus colonoscopy for suspected lower gastrointestinal bleeding. Gastroenterology, 98:855, 1990.

75. Ryan, J.W.: Immunoscintigraphy in primary colorectal cancer. Cancer, 71:4217, 1993.

76. Ryan, P., Styles, C.B., and Chmiel, R.: Identification of the site of severe colon bleeding by technetium-labeled red-cell scan. Dis. Colon Rectum, 35:219, 1992.

77. Schapiro, M., and Lehman, G.: Flexible Sigmoidoscopy. Techniques and Utilization. Baltimore, Williams & Wilkins, 1990.

78. Schrock, T.: Lower gastrointestinal bleeding. In Sivak, M.J. (ed.): Gastroenterologic Endoscopy, 2nd ed. Philadelphia, W.B. Saunders, 1992 (in press).

79. Schrock, T.: Examination of anorectum and diseases of anorectum. In Sleisenger, M., and Fordtran, J. (eds.): Gastrointestinal Disease. Pathophysiology/Diagnosis/Management, 5th ed. Philadelphia, W.B. Saunders, 1993, p. 1494.

80. Schrock, T.: Colonoscopy in the diagnosis and treatment of colorectal malignancy. In Greene, F., Ponsky, J., and Nealon, W. (eds.): Endoscopic Surgery. Philadelphia, W.B. Saunders, 256–258, 1993.

81. Schrock, T.: Conceptual developments through colonoscopy. Surg. Endosc., 2:240, 1988.

82. Schrock, T.: Colonoscopy versus barium enema in the diagnosis of colorectal cancers and polyps. Gastrointest. Clin. North Am. 3:585, 1993.

83. Selby, J.V., Friedman, G.D., Quesenberry, C.P.J., et al.: A case-control study of screening sigmoidoscopy and mortality from colorectal cancer. N. Engl. J. Med., 326:653, 1992.

84. Shoenut, J., Semelka, R., Silverman, R., et al.: Magnetic resonance imaging in inflammatory bowel disease. J. Clin. Gastroenterol., *17*:73, 1993.

85. Silvestrini, R., D'Agnano, I., Faranda, A., et al.: Flow cytometric analysis of ploidy in colorectal cancer.: A multicenter experience. Br. J. Cancer, *67*:1042, 1993.

86. Simpkins, K.: What use is barium? Clin. Radiol., *39*:469, 1988.

87. Solomon, M.J., and McLeod, R.S.: Screening strategies for colorectal cancer. Surg. Clin. North Am., *73*:31, 1993.

88. Soyer, P., Levesque, M., Caudron, C., et al.: MRI of liver metastases from colorectal cancer vs. CT during arterial portography. J. Comput. Assist. Tomogr., *17*:67, 1993.

89. Steine, S.: Will it hurt, doctor? Factors predicting patients' experience of pain during double contrast examination of the colon. BMJ, *307*:100, 1993.

90. Stevenson, G.W., Wilson, J.A., Wilkinson, J., et al.: Pain following colonoscopy: Elimination with carbon dioxide. Gastrointest. Endosc., *38*:564, 1992.

91. Taylor, P., and Beckly, D.: Use of air in double contrast barium enema—is it still acceptable? Clin. Radiol., *44*:183, 1991.

92. Thomas, W., Pye, G., Hardcastle, J., et al.: Screening for colorectal carcinoma: An analysis of the sensitivity of Haemoccult. Br. J. Surg., *9*:833, 1992.

93. Vasen, H., Griffioen, G., Offerhaus, G., et al.: The value of screening and central registration of families with familial adenomatous polyposis. A study of 82 families in The Netherlands. Dis. Colon Rectum, *33*:227, 1990.

94. Vassallo, M., Camilleri, M., Phillips, S.F., et al.: Transit through the proximal colon influences stool weight in the irritable bowel syndrome. Gastroenterology, *102*:102, 1992.

95. Voeller, G., Bunch, G., and Britt, L.: Use of technetium-labeled red blood cell scintigraphy in the detection and management of gastrointestinal hemorrhage. Surgery, *110*:799, 1991.

96. Walter, D.F., Govil, S., William, R.R., et al.: Colonic sonography: Preliminary observations. Clin. Radiol., *47*:200, 1993.

97. Ward, U., Primrose, J.N., Finan, P.J., et al.: The use of tumour markers CEA, CA-195 and CA-242 in evaluating the response to chemotherapy in patients with advanced colorectal cancer. Br. J. Cancer, *67*:1132, 1993.

98. Waye, J.: Diagnostic endoscopy in lower intestinal bleeding. *In* Sugawa, C., Schuman, B., and Lucas, C. (eds.): Gastrointestinal Bleeding. New York, Igaku-Shoin, 1992, p. 407.

99. Waye, J., and Bashkoff, E.: Total colonoscopy: Is it always possible? Gastrointest. Endosc., *37*:152, 1991.

100. Webb, W.: Colonoscoping the "difficult" colon. Am. Surg., *57*:178, 1991.

101. Williams, C., and Price, A.: Colon polyps and carcinoma. *In* Sivak, M.J. (ed.): Gastroenterologic Endoscopy. Philadelphia, W.B. Saunders, 1987, p. 921.

102. Winawer, S., and Kerner, J.: Sigmoidoscopy: Case finding versus screening (Editorial). Gastroenterology, *95*:527, 1933.

103. Winawer, S.J., Zauber, A.G., O'Brien, M.J., et al.: Randomized comparison of surveillance intervals after colonoscopic removal of newly diagnosed adenomatous polyps. N. Engl. J. Med., *328*:901, 1993.

104. Wittenberg, J.: The diagnosis of colonic obstruction on plain abdominal radiographs: Start with the cecum, leave the rectum to last. AJR, *161*:443, 1993.

105. Woolrich, A.J., DaSilva, M.D., and Korelitz, B.I.: Surveillance in the routine management of ulcerative colitis: The predictive value of low-grade dysplasia. Gastroenterology, *103*:431, 1992.

Chapter 4

TRAUMA TO THE COLON AND RECTUM

JOHN J. FERRARA / LEWIS M. FLINT

Surgeons have long recognized that traumatic perforations of the colon are more dangerous than other gastrointestinal injuries. The mortality rate approximates 4 to 10% for isolated colon injuries, with additional concomitant injuries within the abdomen acting synergistically with the colon wound to quadruple the risk of mortality or major complication.[21,34]

The high mortality and morbidity rates relate to anatomic, physiologic and microbiologic differences of the colon compared to other parts of the gut. The colon is a thin-walled viscus with its longitudinal muscle fibers gathered into taeniae running the length of the organ, while the small bowel has, in the main, a thicker circular muscle as well as a circumferentially distributed longitudinal muscle. In addition, the strong contractions occurring in the colon produce relatively high intraluminal pressures that may exude feces through perforations and place stress upon closures and anastomotic lines. Because the primary component of the colon content is bacteria, infection is a constant threat following both elective and emergency colon operations.

Injuries to the colon, except endoscopic perforations (see further on), never occur in a prepared, clean colon, and operations done for repair of injuries are frequently associated with shock and delays encountered between injury and definitive operation. Thus, the patient is subject to the immunosuppressive effects of hypovolemia and bacterial peritonitis, which increase in severity with delay. In addition, removal of other injured organs, particularly the spleen, may predispose to postinjury infection.[9]

ESTIMATING INJURY SEVERITY

Moore and colleagues[23] and others[12] have attempted to quantify the impact of the degree of intra-abdominal organ injury, the presence of associated injuries, shock, and delay on outcome. The resultant penetrating abdominal trauma index (PATI) has been developed and field tested. Using this index (Table 4–1), the surgeon can assign a risk factor for each organ injured. The risk factor integers are summed and the result multiplied by the surgeon's estimate of the severity of injury to each organ. The resultant number is statistically related to both mortality and morbidity. A synthesis of the data regarding colon and rectal injuries confirms the fact that many systemic and injury-specific factors combine to influence morbidity. These factors are listed in Table 4–2. Since most of the morbidity following colon and rectal trauma is related to bacterial infection, surgeons have been tempted to ascribe to fecal contamination the principal role in deciding outcome. No single factor, however, including the method of managing the injury, decides outcome, and precise judgments are necessary to evaluate and choose the proper mode of management for each patient.

RELATION OF INJURY SEVERITY AND MANAGEMENT TO OUTCOME

The challenge for the surgeon managing colon wounds is to choose an approach that will yield safety with a minimum of disability. During World War I, the operative treatment for colon injuries consisted of suture repair alone and there was little experience with colostomy or injury exteriorization. Mortality rates exceeded 60%.[20] It was not until Ogilvie's report[26] of experiences using colostomy and exteriorization for combat wounds incurred during World War II that these procedures became the standard approach, with mortality rates improving rapidly. Additional improvements in these results accompanied a complete understanding of the role of shock and treatment delay in adversely affecting outcome and the importance of minimizing the impact of these variables to the greatest possible extent.

While colostomy continues as the standard of care in the management of a colon injury incurred during military service, the differences between combat and civilian ("peacetime") wounds have stimulated efforts to de-

TABLE 4-1. PENETRATING ABDOMINAL TRAUMA INDEX (PATI)*

Organ risk factor × injury severity estimate = Score
Scores for each organ are summed to obtain PATI

*From Moore, E., Dunn, E., Moore, J., and Thompson, J.: Penetrating abdominal trauma index. J. Trauma, *21*:439, 1981, with permission.

TABLE 4-2. FACTORS CONTRIBUTING TO COLON INJURY MORBIDITY

Shock
Fecal spillage with gross evidence of peritonitis
Hemoperitoneum >1,000 ml
Additional organ injury
Treatment delay >4 hours
Extensive colon damage, especially with blunt injury or shotgun blast
Abdominal wall loss

velop alternatives. Civilian colon wounds (with three notable exceptions: blunt injuries, shotgun wounds and high-velocity missile wounds) are usually much less severe than combat injuries. The desire of patients to avoid colostomy and of surgeons to eliminate the additional morbidity of colostomy closure have enhanced and sustained efforts to show the feasibility of primary repair for an increasing proportion of patients with intraperitoneal colon injuries. As early as 1951, Woodhall and Ochsner[43] reported that, given a hemodynamically stable civilian with a small colon wound, minimal peritoneal soiling, and few associated injuries, primary closure of the wound could be carried out with morbidity rates no different from that associated with colostomy.

Decades later, Stones[35] randomized patients to receive colostomy or primary repair. Mandatory colostomy was reserved for patients with (1) severe shock, (2) more than two organs injured, (3) extensive fecal spillage, (4) delay of more than 8 hours, (5) a colon injury requiring resection and anastomosis, or (6) extensive abdominal wall loss. No increase in complications was seen in the patients receiving primary repair. In fact, specific complications occurring in the *favorable* patients randomized for colostomy suggested that diversion could be harmful if there were stoma complications or if wound infection occurred because of fecal discharge into an adjacent healing incision. Burch and colleagues,[4] reporting one of the largest clinical series in the literature, could identify no differences in mortality or morbidity between pa-

tients treated with colostomy versus primary suture of colon injuries. Because this study was retrospective, and inferences concerning overall morbidity and mortality were drawn by extracting data from records of selected patients whose injuries were graded in retrospect, interpretation of the data must be done with caution. Overall, however, it would appear from their study that primary repair of many civilian colon injuries can be carried out safely and with outcomes equivalent to colostomy.

Recently reported data from our own institution[37] support this central conclusion. In groups of patients equally matched according to age, injury severity score (ISS), PATI, and presence of shock, primary repair proved as safe as colostomy. We also noted that the complication rate in each group increased in direct proportion to the severity of injury. A survey of results reported by other investigators shows similar patterns and conclusions.[6,8,14,32] Moreover, in a prospective trial of 102 patients whose colon injury was almost uniformly managed by primary repair, George[15] found that nearly all injuries could be repaired primarily, despite risk factors.

From these studies it would appear that the technique of repair, be it by colostomy or primary suture, assumes critical importance less frequently than was initially considered. However, even those surgeons who most avidly espouse primary closure of colon injuries reserve a place for colostomy—generally in instances when the aforementioned risk factors converge in a single patient. Finally, with the increasing use of high-velocity military weaponry "on the streets," the surgeon must remain flexible in this decision-making process and be familiar with the history of colon injury treatment—especially regarding the role of colostomy combined with techniques that improve the outcome of patients who are in shock.

In this light, we recommend the use of one of the available scoring systems (Table 4–3) combined with an assessment of local factors, particularly the gross appearance of the peritoneal membrane. If scoring reveals a severe risk injury *with* signs of peritoneal inflammation, we would use colostomy. As such, we estimate that over 60% of patients with penetrating injuries can be managed with primary closure; the established frequencies of primary repair in several recent series are shown in Table 4–4. Clearly, as surgeons have learned to use primary repair, the frequency of its use has, not surprisingly, increased. The fact that well-trained surgeons can select patients who are good candidates for primary clo-

TABLE 4-3. COMPARISON OF COLON INJURY SEVERITY SCALES

Moore et al.[23]	Flint et al.[12]
Grade 1 = Serosa only	Grade 1 = Isolated colon injury No contamination No shock or delay
Grade 2 = Single-wall injury	Grade 2 = Through-and-through perforation
Grade 3 = <25% single-wall laceration	Grade 3 = Severe tissue loss Heavy contamination Shock or delay
Grade 4 = >25% single-wall laceration	
Grade 5 = Wall injury + impaired blood supply	

From Moore et al.: J. Trauma *21*:439, 1981 *and* Flint et al.: Ann. Surg. *193*:619, 1981, with permission.

TABLE 4-4. RESULTS OF TREATMENT OF COLON INJURIES*

AUTHOR	MORTALITY (%)	COLOSTOMY (%)
Steele and Blaisdell, 1972[34]	3.0	71
Flint et al., 1981[12]	6.0	77
Shannon and Moore, 1985[32]	2.0	36
Burch et al., 1986[4]	2.7	33
George et al., 1988[14]	2.5	42
George et al., 1988[15]	3.0	7

*Selected series reporting more than 100 patients.

sure is not mysterious, and merely suggests the relative accuracy of their judgments and the utility of risk factor assessment.

Mention must be made of so-called compromise approaches to the management of the injured colon, born out of concern for the mortality associated with breakdown of a primarily closed colon injury. The most popular of these is an exteriorized suture repair, with dropback of the repaired colon into the peritoneal cavity several days thereafter.[2,18,24] An understanding of the contribution of the intraperitoneal environment to the healing of intestinal suture lines suggests that this is an inferior approach, and clinical experience bears out this suggestion.[28,29] Breakdown of the exteriorized repair is frequent (50% in our experience) unless great care is taken to keep the portion of colon that lies on the abdominal wall moist and protected. Given the documented efficacy of primary closure of the types of colon injury for which exteriorization is recommended, we have abandoned this approach in our unit.

DIAGNOSIS OF COLON INJURY

Since the colon is an intra-abdominal organ, its injury can only be inferred by external examination. Therefore, primary emphasis is placed upon making the decision whether the patient meets criteria for exploratory laparotomy (i.e., hemodynamic instability, signs of peritoneal irritation, suspicious mechanism of injury, and positive diagnostic peritoneal lavage). Extensive efforts to diagnose a colon perforation per se are limited to hemodynamically stable patients, generally with stab wounds of the back—where a retroperitoneal colon perforation may have occurred—who, on physical examination, are otherwise good candidates for nonoperative therapy and observation (see further on).

Penetrating Colon Injury

The diagnostic process for patients suspected of suffering a penetrating injury to the torso between the nipples and the perineum is fairly well standardized, though a few points are worth highlighting. Given a responsive patient, a rapid history should be taken concerning the details of the mechanism of injury. Upon physical examination, one must assiduously survey the entire body surface for evidence of entrance and exit wound sites; notably, if the anorectum is in the potential path of the injuring agent or if there is blood found on digital rectal examination, rigid sigmoidoscopy is added to the evaluation. If possible, a chest roentgenogram is obtained to assess whether the thoracic cavity has been violated.

Virtually all *gunshot* wounds in proximity to the peritoneal cavity mandate formal exploration of the abdomen. On occasion, we do elect to perform local wound exploration on a patient who presents with a tangential, low-velocity injury to the anterior abdomen; staining of the peritoneum underlying the tract of the missile warrants laparotomy. Conversely, we uniformly subject patients with *stab* wounds to the anterior abdomen to laparotomy if clinical signs of peritoneal irritation or refractory shock or both are present, or (regardless of hemodynamic stability) if documentation of peritoneal penetration is forthcoming. Peritoneal penetration is obvious if a portion of omentum or a viscus has prolapsed through the wound. Without these signs, we employ a local anesthetic agent to explore the entrance wound under direct visualization, extending it to three times its original length if necessary. If penetration of the peritoneum is seen or strongly suspected, laparotomy is performed; all other patients are observed after appropriate local wound care.

Patients with deep stab wounds of the flank and lower chest are traditionally taken directly to the operating room because local exploration of these wounds is not dependable. However, given the increased facility of surgeons with laparoscopy and thoracoscopy, selected patients with stab or gunshot wounds to the lower chest are now being submitted to these procedures in order to assess whether diaphragmatic penetration has occurred or if intraperitoneal injury is significant.

Thoracoscopy may serve to reduce the morbidity of thoracic injury and improve diagnosis of diaphragm penetration, as a report from our unit suggests.[17] On the other hand, laparoscopy for the evaluation of acute abdominal injury remains controversial. Recent reports in the literature describe its efficacy in terms of safety, reduction of "negative" laparotomies, and cost savings.[3] Despite these promising data, it would appear that, on balance, the use of laparoscopy under these conditions should be considered investigational.

Because its thick muscle layers greatly reduce the frequency of visceral injury, many stab wounds of the back can be managed nonoperatively, given a clinical assessment that discloses no signs of visceral injury. Like anyone suspected of suffering a penetrating abdominal injury, these patients must undergo sequential clinical examinations, with diagnostic procedures and operation performed for symptoms that may subsequently develop.

Recently reported experiences with computed tomography (CT) in patients with stab wounds of the flank and back may prove of value to the clinician. Phillips,[27] reasoning that injuries to the extraperitoneal colon and urinary tract were the most important clinical consequence of stab wounds to the flank and lower back, employed rectal contrast-enhanced computed tomography to improve diagnostic accuracy and avoid nontherapeutic laparotomy. Although preliminary, these data suggest improved detection of injury by this method. Such findings await confirmation from other centers before the technique can be recommended.

Shotgun wounds represent a broad spectrum of potential injury patterns.[11] Close-range blasts to the abdomen are very destructive and uniformly mandate exploratory laparotomy. As distance from the weapon increases, the potential for serious injury decreases to the point that selected patients—those with less than three pellets within the peritoneal cavity and without clinical signs of peritoneal irritation—may be managed expectantly.

Colon Injury Due to Blunt Trauma

Although blunt abdominal trauma causes only 5% of colon injuries, these injuries present a broad spectrum of challenging problems. Diagnostic difficulty is increased because of the lack of dependability of the abdominal physical examination in patients who have multiple injuries or in whom consciousness has been altered by brain injury, alcohol, or other drugs. Large mesenteric tears and lacerations of the colon wall may result from the transfer of shear and compression forces, some of which result from the lifesaving restraint of the victim by seat belts.[36]

The diagnostic process for patients with blunt injuries proceeds simultaneously with resuscitation. In similar fashion to those with penetrating trauma, patients who are rapidly bleeding from blunt injury may require exploratory laparotomy as an integral component of initial resuscitation. In virtually all circumstances, there is time to complete a digital rectal examination; given a hemodynamically stable patient in whom blood is present in the rectal vault, sigmoidoscopy is indicated.

Radiologic studies, except for cervical spine and chest films, are best deferred until hemodynamic stability is assured. At that time, supine and upright abdominal roentgenograms (a left lateral decubitus view is taken when the patient cannot sit up) are taken to search for fractures (particularly the axial spine and pelvis) and for the presence of extraluminal gas.

Diagnostic peritoneal lavage is very useful to detect bleeding within the peritoneal cavity. The white blood cell count of the lavage fluid may be elevated in intestinal perforation, which is typically associated with minimal bleeding. In this regard, it must be noted that while some surgeons employ peritoneal lavage only in selected penetrating trauma patients, this has not been our practice.

GENERAL PREOPERATIVE MANAGEMENT PRINCIPLES

Broad-spectrum antibiotics (we typically employ a second-generation cephalosporin) are administered intravenously as soon as the decision for laparotomy is made.[10] Antibiotics are not continued beyond 24 postoperative hours unless extensive contamination and tissue loss are encountered, in which case therapy is continued for 7 days. Even under these circumstances, there is little evidence that such measures lower intra-abdominal infec-

tion risk, though infections at the site of the surgical incision are reduced.

GENERAL INTRAOPERATIVE MANAGEMENT PRINCIPLES

We have used midline incisions for blunt and penetrating trauma victims because it can be rapidly performed and provides ready access to virtually all abdominal organs and structures. In addition, this incision can be extended to a median sternotomy or anterolateral thoracotomy for extended exposure of the upper abdomen and retroperitoneum. The first priority on entering the abdomen is to control hemorrhage. Laparotomy sponges are packed into the four quadrants to tamponade bleeding and left in place until the anesthesia team can "catch up" with transfusion and fluid infusions. These packs are sequentially removed to assess each location for specific sites of bleeding, keeping in mind that, where hemorrhage is ongoing, control of vascular injuries takes priority over actively bleeding solid organ injuries. When penetrating trauma has occurred, the entire potential path of the injuring agent must be exposed; this search must be carried out with the understanding that the agent may have taken a circuitous route between entrance and destination sites. In blunt trauma patients, one must perform an exploration of the entire abdomen, including the retroperitoneal portions of the colon and duodenum as well as the pancreas.

Control of contamination from perforations of the bowel is the second priority, with expeditious (often temporary) suture closure of each site until all perforations are assessed. Once leakage is controlled, repair of vascular injuries may proceed. Definitive repair of alimentary tract injuries is completed later.

Clinical experience has shown that the surgeon's persistence in attempts to complete definitive repair of all injuries in the face of shock, hypothermia, and coagulopathy all too often leads to the death of the patient. Given prompt recognition of impending dire circumstances, the astute surgeon might alternatively tamponade bleeding with laparotomy packs, tie off any open ends of bowel with umbilical tapes, and temporarily close the abdominal incision. The patient is rapidly transported to a critical care environment in which aggressive measures can be undertaken to treat the shock-related conditions and prepare the patient for a return to the operating room for completion of definitive repairs at a later time. The choice of this strategy represents sound surgical judgment.

MANAGEMENT OF ABDOMINAL COLON INJURIES

Primary Closure

In patients with injuries amenable to primary repair (see previously), the injury will usually have been a consequence of low-velocity penetrating trauma. The site of abdominal colon injury has no bearing on our decision to use primary closure, as we have found no demonstrable difference in the risk of morbidity when closure of wounds to the right and left colon are compared. We débride only obvious devitalized tissue, and use interrupted nonabsorbable sutures to perform a single-layer closure. We avoid primary closure of lacerations on the mesenteric border of the colon if the laceration exceeds 1 inch in greatest dimension, preferring to perform a colostomy or, less commonly, resection and anastomosis.

Colostomy

This procedure is reserved for the more severe colon injuries, particularly those caused by blunt trauma and close-range shotgun wounds that tend to require extensive soft tissue débridement and removal of shell wadding fragments. Under these conditions, resection of the injured colon with end colostomy is usually required. A distal mucous fistula is preferred unless the residual colonic segment consists of extraperitoneal rectum, in which case a Hartmann procedure (extraperitoneal closure of the distal rectal stump) is necessary. Selection of the stoma site is important, giving thought to the location and fit of a stoma appliance as well as to the absolute need to prevent discharge of fecal material onto or near healing incisions or wounds. We prefer to position our stomata at lateral lower quadrant sites using oblique incisions separated by a width of skin sufficient to allow unimpeded placement of a stoma appliance. However, excessive mobilization of the colon trying to "reach" the lower abdomen is discouraged in favor of exteriorization of the colon at more convenient sites.

Our current approach to colostomy formation is to mature the stoma using interrupted absorbable dermal sutures to evert each end of the colon at the time of the initial operation. In so doing, one must perform a Brooke-type raised stoma, rather than secure the colon flush with the skin. With 1 to 1½ inches of colon protruding above the skin of the abdomen, it is simple to secure a tight seal around the colostomy with a stoma appliance, decreasing the risk of wound contamination.

As an alternative, we have managed the ends of the colon in the following manner. The mesentery from the distal 2 inches of colon is cleared, preserving the marginal artery on each limb. The ends of each limb are approximated with colostomy clamps (Stone or De-Martel) and each "chimney" is placed at the lateral or medial end of the oblique wound. The fascia is closed between the limbs with at least 1 inch of colon protruding above the skin surface. The serosa is wrapped in greased gauze to provide a vapor barrier and the incision dressed with moist dressings. The clamps are removed 3 or 4 days later; no formal eversion of the stomas to "mature" the openings is necessary.

Wound Exteriorization

When a sufficient length of colon can be mobilized, a temporarily sutured colon wound may be brought out to the surface as part of a conventional loop colostomy. We suspend the loop on soft rubber tubing or an atrau-matic plastic suspension device, and in 2 to 3 days open the temporarily sutured colon wound as a colostomy.

Resection with Anastomosis

This technique is used primarily for wounds of the right colon that are not amenable to primary closure and that can be encompassed by a standard right hemicolectomy. With severe wounds, particularly those associated with significant collateral damage, consideration of diverting ileostomy may be theoretically appealing, though the available data do not confirm the value of this strategy.[39]

Proximal "Protective" Colostomy

This approach is reserved for the few carefully selected patients with a low sigmoid colon or upper rectal injury that is amenable to resection and anastomosis. Under these circumstances, a colostomy fashioned proximal to the anastomosis effectively diverts the fecal stream until healing has occurred. Closure of the colostomy is done at a later date, generally after 4 to 6 weeks.

MANAGEMENT OF ANORECTAL INJURIES

Rectal injury is suspected in patients with penetrating wounds of the buttocks, lower back, flanks, and suprapubic area. The presence of blood in the rectum or hematuria are clinical indicators that ought to alert the surgeon to the possibility of rectal laceration. Patients who sustain compound pelvic fractures, straddle injuries of the perineum, and explosive concussion injuries (especially underwater explosions) are also at risk for rectal perforation. In such high-risk injuries, the threshold to perform diverting colostomy should be low, as the morbid consequences of a missed injury are significant.

Sigmoidoscopy will usually help in confirming the diagnosis, though some rectal lacerations are minute and may not be readily visible.[13,41] If rectal injury is documented or strongly suspected, the operative protocol illustrated in Figures 4–1 and 4–2 should be carried out. The patient is positioned in low (St. Mark's) stirrups, unless extremity fractures preclude this maneuver. A sigmoid loop colostomy is performed and the distal portion is stapled shut with a TA device to provide complete diversion of the fecal stream.[31] The anus is digitally dilated, then held open with anorectal retractors while the fecal material is irrigated from the rectum. Although the value of rectal irrigation has been repeatedly debated, the weight of evidence supports the employment of this maneuver.[19,22,40] Visible anorectal lacerations are closed, if possible, but this is not absolutely necessary. Closed suction presacral suction drains are inserted via perineal incisions placed laterally between the anus and coccyx, and are left in place for a minimum of 5 days.

Patients with mental illness or unique sexual habits are presenting with rectal perforations at an alarmingly increased frequency. These injuries, which usually lead to hematochezia and clinical signs of peritonitis, are managed according to the principles outlined above.

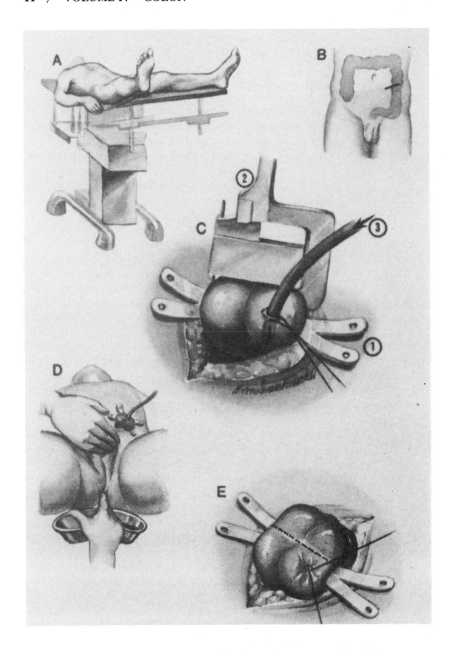

FIGURE 4-1. Principles of the intraoperative management of rectal injuries. *A*, position of patient. *B*, site of incision. *C(1)*, loop colostomy suspension device. *C(2)*, 90-mm stapler for partition of colon loop. *C(3)*, Foley catheter (20 French) inserted via pursestring suture. *D*, anus is dilated digitally followed by irrigation. *E*, pursestring closure of insertion site. From Maull, K., Sachetello, C., and Ernst, C.: The deep perineal laceration—an injury frequently associated with open pelvic fracture. J. Trauma, *17*:685, 1977, with permission.

While reported series[7,33] do contain anecdotal references to patients who present with no more than perianal fistulas resulting from contained extraperitoneal rectal injuries that occurred days previously, these "experiments of nature" do not justify the omission of a diverting colostomy when such patients are seen early after injury.

In similar fashion, it should no longer be surprising that large foreign bodies can be retained following their insertion through a widely dilated anus. Subsequent sphincter spasm entraps the object. Clinical strategy is dictated by the condition of the patient. If clinical signs of peritonitis are present, laparotomy guided by the principles outlined above is mandatory. Without signs indicating intra-abdominal injury, a combination of digital examination and roentgenography is performed to determine whether the object can be reached by sigmoidoscopy. If so, the patient is positioned in stirrups and, under general anesthesia, the anus is dilated. The foreign body may be manipulated manually or with adjunctive devices such as Foley balloon catheters that are inflated after they are passed beyond the object. Obstetric forceps may be useful as well. Such maneuvers are almost uniformly successful. However, we do not attempt to fragment solid foreign bodies, particularly glass or metal, preferring instead to perform celiotomy with colotomy to retrieve the object.

MANAGEMENT OF ENDOSCOPIC INJURIES

Colon or rectal injury may occur during sigmoidoscopy, colonoscopy, routine cleansing, and barium contrast enemas. Nelson and associates[25] reported perforation rates of 0.02, 0.24, and 0.02% for sigmoidoscopy, colonoscopy, and barium enema, respectively. Of note, they reported a 100% mortality following perforation during barium enema, due to the severity of the ensuing

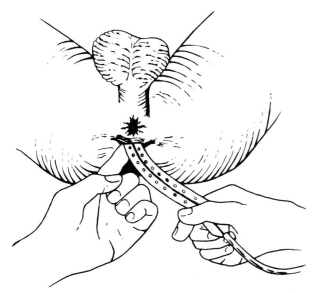

FIGURE 4-2. Suction drains are placed in the presacral space in all patients with injury to the rectum.

In all instances, if an endoscopic perforation results in clinically evident peritonitis, laparotomy is mandatory. The nonsurgeon endoscopist should have a good working relationship with a surgeon so that consultation is readily available, as delay in operation increases morbidity.[1,16,42] Since under most conditions the colon has been mechanically cleansed, perforations within or in proximity to diseased intestine can be managed by resection of that segment and anastomosis; primary closure of perforations that occur in normal intestine are preferred when conditions are favorable.

It is becoming increasingly more common that, under certain conditions, selected patients with minimal clinical signs and limited pneumoperitoneum visible on roentgenograms of the abdomen (Fig. 4–3) may be managed nonoperatively under the watchful eye of *both* the endoscopist and a surgeon. The patient is kept without food or drink, and placed on intravenous fluids and presumptive broad-spectrum antibiotic therapy (generally a second-generation cephalosporin). Resumption of diet is considered only after all symptoms and signs of peritoneal irritation have resolved (3 to 5 days).

peritonitis. Ali-Ghazi[16] categorized endoscopic perforations into two groups, according to whether the perforation occurred in diseased or in healthy intestine. The frequency of perforation in healthy intestine was directly related to the inexperience of the endoscopist. Moreover, perforations that complicated endoscopic polypectomy or cauterization of bleeding sites were generally considered avoidable.

MANAGEMENT OF THE MIDLINE WOUND

During the operation, we routinely protect the skin and subcutaneous tissues with gauze strips moistened with a 1% cephalothin solution. These are changed hourly. Upon completion of the operation, the midline fascia is closed with interrupted sutures; some prefer nonabsorbable monofilament suture, other surgeons

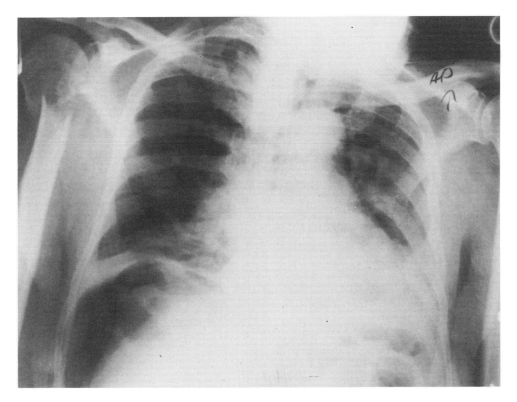

FIGURE 4-3. Pneumoperitoneum appearing 4 hours after colonoscopy in an otherwise asymptomatic patient. Progression of physical signs mandated an operation in this patient.

use absorbable monofilament or braided material. Skin and subcutaneous tissues are left open; under favorable conditions, many of these wounds can be approximated (using adhesive strips) several days later.

On rare occasions, closure of the fascia may be impossible to achieve, typically due to massive swelling of the abdominal organs and tissues. It is important to avoid attempting to close the abdomen under undue tension. Rather, we suture a generous piece of synthetic material (polypropylene or polytetrafluoroethylene) to the edges of the fascia using a running monofilament suture. When conditions are favorable and the edema has diminished, the patient is returned to the operating room (usually a few days later), the synthetic prosthesis is removed, and primary closure of the fascia is performed.

POSTOPERATIVE COMPLICATIONS

Stomal Retraction and Necrosis

Given our adherence to the practices outlined above, we have rarely encountered stomal retraction or ischemic necrosis. When this does occur, the patient is typically quite obese or is so severely injured that resuscitation-associated edema literally pulls the stoma internally or causes pressure necrosis of the stoma. As long as we can confirm that the stoma is secure at the level of the fascia, and its viability at that level can be assured, we do not routinely perform revision unless fecal soilage of the stoma wound and adjacent wounds is a threat. However, if there is any doubt as to these criteria, the best management is formal revision of the stoma.

Wound Infections

Even with the skin left open, superficial infections do occur and can be managed by simply ensuring the wound is adequately drained and débrided of necrotic tissue. Deeper fascial and subfascial infections often suggest that an intra-abdominal abscess is present. Diagnostic steps to localize and deal with these infections must be carried out, including reoperation as indicated.

Intra-abdominal Abscesses

Single, localized abdominal and pelvic abscesses may be amenable to percutaneous drainage. However, when multiple abscesses or an anastomotic leak is suspected, formal re-exploration is preferred.

COLOSTOMY CLOSURE

We plan on performing colostomy closure 4 to 6 weeks following an uncomplicated convalescence out of the hospital. Recent data suggest that selected patients may undergo colostomy closure during the same admission.[30] The data confirming the value of this approach are weak, however, because of the small number of patients reported.

Prior to operation, the mucous fistula or Hartmann pouch is endoscopically inspected for obvious areas of persistent injury. Contrast studies of the distal colon are done only if unrepaired lacerations were left at the time of the original operation. A standard preoperative mechanical and antibiotic bowel preparation is used.

While a loop colostomy usually can be closed through the colostomy incision, totally diverting stomas often require formal laparotomy. In either circumstance, we have found that our own results compare favorably with results of other reported series of patients undergoing colostomy closure, in that this procedure is associated with a very low complication rate (0% mortality and 10 to 15% morbidity).[37,38] Therefore, concern over the morbidity associated with colostomy closure should not be a major factor in the surgeon's decision regarding whether to perform primary closure or colostomy to manage a colon wound.

REFERENCES

1. Adair, H., and Hishon, S.: The management of colonoscopic and sigmoidoscopic perforation of the large bowel. Br. J. Surg., 68: 415, 1981.
2. Adkins, R., Zirkle, P., and Waterhouse, G.: Penetrating colon trauma. J. Trauma, 24:491, 1984.
3. Berci, G., Sackier, J.M., Paz-Parlow, M.: Emergency laparoscopy. Am. J. Surg., 161:332, 1991.
4. Burch, J., Gevirtzman, L., Jordan, G., et al.: The injured colon. Ann. Surg., 203:701, 1986.
5. Busch, D., and Starling, J.: Rectal foreign bodies: Case reports and a comprehensive review of the world's literature. Surgery, 100: 312, 1986.
6. Cook, A., Levine, B., Rusing, T., et al.: Traditional treatment of colon injuries. Arch. Surg., 119:591, 1984.
7. Crass, R., Tranbaugh, R., Kudsk, K., and Trunkey, D.: Colorectal foreign bodies and perforation. Am. J. Surg., 142:85, 1981.
8. Dang, C., Peter, E., Parks, S., and Ellyson, J.: Trauma of the colon. Arch. Surg., 117:652, 1982.
9. Dawes, L., Aprahamian, C., Condon, R., and Malangoni, M.: The risk of infection after colon injury. Surgery, 100:796, 1986.
10. Dellinger, E., Wert, M., Lennard, E., et al.: Efficacy of short-course antibiotic prophylaxis after penetrating intestinal injury: A prospective randomized trial. Arch. Surg., 121:23, 1986.
11. Flint, L.M., Cryer, H.M., Howard, D.A., and Richardson, J.D.: Approaches to the management of major shotgun injuries. J. Trauma, 24:415, 1984.
12. Flint, L.M., Vitale, G.C., Richardson, J.D., and Polk, H.C.: The injured colon: Relationships of management to complications. Ann. Surg., 193:619, 1981.
13. Garrison, R., Shively, E., Baker, C., et al.: Evaluation of management of the emergency right hemicolectomy. J. Trauma, 19:734, 1979.
14. George, S., Fabian, T., and Mangiante, E.: Colon trauma: Further support for primary repair. Am. J. Surg., 156:16, 1988.
15. George, S.M., Fabian, T.C., Voeller, G.R., et al.: Primary repair of colon wounds. A prospective trial in nonselected patients. Ann. Surg., 209(6):728, 1988.
16. Ghazi, A., and Grossman, M.: Complications of colonoscopy and polypectomy. Surg. Clin. N. Am. 62:889, 1982.
17. Jones, J.W., Kitahama, A., Webb, W.R., and McSwain, N.: Emergency thoracoscopy: A logical approach to chest trauma management. J. Trauma, 31:280, 1991.
18. Kirkpatrick, J.R.: The exteriorized anastomosis: Its role in surgery of the colon. Surgery, 82:362, 1977.
19. Lavenson, G., and Cohen, A.: Management of rectal injuries. Am. J. Surg., 122:225, 1971.
20. Lee, B.L.: Wounds of the colon in the medical department of the United States Army in the World War. Washington, DC, Government Printing Office, Vol. 11, 1927.

21. Malangoni, M., and Flint, L.: Abdominal injuries. *In* Richardson, J.D., Polk, H.C., and Flint, L.M. (eds.): Trauma, Clinical Care and Pathophysiology. Chicago, Year Book Medical Publishers, 1987.
22. Maull, K., Sachetello, C., and Ernst, C.: The deep perineal laceration—an injury frequently associated with open pelvic fracture. J. Trauma, *17*:685, 1977.
23. Moore, E., Dunn, E., Moore, J., and Thompson, J.: Penetrating abdominal trauma index. J. Trauma, *21*:439, 1981.
24. Nallathambi, M., Ivatury, R., Rohman, M., and Stahl, W.: Penetrating colon injuries: Exteriorized repair vs loop colostomy. J. Trauma, *27*:879, 1987.
25. Nelson, R., Abcarian, H., and Prasad, M.: Iatrogenic perforation of the colon and rectum. Dis. Colon Rectum, *25*:305, 1982.
26. Ogilvie, W.H.: Abdominal wounds in the western desert. Surg. Gynecol. Obstet., *78*:225, 1944.
27. Phillips, T., Sclafani, S., Goldstein, A., et al.: Use of the contrast-enhanced CT enema in the management of penetrating trauma. J. Trauma, *26*:593, 1986.
28. Ravitch, M.M.: Observations on healing of wounds of the intestines. Surgery, *77*:665, 1975.
29. Ravitch, M.M., Brolin, R., Kolter, J., and Yap, S.: Studies in the healing of intestinal anastomoses. World J. Surg., *5*:627, 1981.
30. Renz, B.M., Feliciano, D.V., and Sherman, R.: A new approach to rectal wounds—same admission colostomy closure. Ann. Surg., *218*:279, 1993.
31. Robertson, H., Ray, J., Ferrari, B., and Gathright, J.: Management of rectal trauma. Surg. Gynecol. Obstet., *154*:161, 1982.
32. Shannon, F.L., and Moore, E.E.: Primary repair of the colon: When is it a safe alternative? Surgery, *98*:851, 1985.
33. Shannon, R., Moore, E.E., Moore, F., and McCroskey, B.: Value of distal colon washout in civilian rectal trauma—reducing gut bacterial translocation. J. Trauma, *28*:989, 1988.
34. Steele, M., and Blaisdell, F.: Treatment of colon injuries. J. Trauma, *17*:557, 1972.
35. Stone, H.H., and Fabian, R.C.: Management of perforating colon trauma. Ann. Surg., *193*:619, 1979.
36. Strate, R., and Grieco, J.: Blunt injury to the colon and rectum. J. Trauma, *23*:384, 1983.
37. Taheri, P.A., Ferrara, J.J., Johnson, C.E., Lamberson, K.A., Flint, L.M.: A convincing case for primary repair of penetrating colon injuries. Am. J. Surg. *166*:39–44, 1993.
38. Thal, E.R., and Yeary, E.C.: Morbidity of colostomy closure following colon trauma. J. Trauma, *20*:287, 1980.
39. Thompson, J.S., Moore, E.E., and Moore, J.B.: Comparison of penetrating injuries of the right and left colon. Ann. Surg., *193*:414, 1981.
40. Trunkey, D., Hays, R., and Shires, G.: Management of rectal trauma. J. Trauma, *13*:411, 1973.
41. Tuggle, D., and Huber, P.: Management of rectal trauma. Am. J. Surg., *148*:806, 1984.
42. Vincent, M., and Smith, L.: Management of perforation due to colonoscopy. Dis. Colon Rectum, *26*:61, 1983.
43. Woodhall, J.P., and Ochsner, A.: The management of perforating injuries of the colon and rectum in civilian practice. Surgery, *29*(2):305, 1951.

Chapter 5

CONGENITAL LESIONS: Intussusception and Volvulus

JOSEPH L. ROMOLO

INTUSSUSCEPTION

Intussusception accounts for 80% of cases of intestinal obstruction in the pediatric population. In contrast, intussusception in adults is relatively rare; it is responsible for only 5% of mechanical intestinal obstructions that occur in adults. The usual site of intestinal intussusception in children is the small intestine; it is rather rare for intussusception to involve the colon. Although the cause of intussusception is idiopathic in almost all pediatric cases, it has a demonstrable cause in 80% of adult cases. Intussusception of the colon in adults is most often secondary to a malignant lesion, usually carcinoma, although unusual tumors such as plasmacytoma have been reported.[4] Among the benign lesions reported to cause intussusception of the colon are adenomatous polyps, leiomyomas, appendocele stump granulomas, and villous adenomas of the appendix. A normal appendix is seldom involved in intussusception; rather, the appendix that forms the lead point of an intussusception usually is inflamed or infested or bears a neoplasm or a deposit of endometriosis. The intussuscepted appendix has even been reported to be carried to or through the anus.[7]

Therapy of colonic intussusception is directed to the reduction of the intussusception and resection of the lead point in order to prevent recurrence. The specific operative procedure to be performed depends upon the site of the intussusception. If the lesion is located on the right side of the colon, primary resection with anastomosis is feasible. If the lesion is located on the left side of the colon, most patients are able to be treated by primary anastomosis. If the viability of the colon is questioned or if there is significant intra-abdominal sepsis or contamination, a primary anastomosis should not be performed. An exteriorization resection with colostomy should be performed; colonic continuity would be restored at a second operation.[8]

VOLVULUS

Volvulus is torsion of the bowel on its mesentery to a degree sufficient to cause symptoms. The symptoms are caused by narrowing of the bowel or strangulation of the blood vessels or both. The two areas of the colon with sufficiently long mesenteries to permit volvulus are the cecum and the sigmoid colon. Volvulus of the colon is a common surgical condition, with a mortality rate ranging from 10 to 50%. It accounts for 5% of all intestinal obstructions and 10% of all colonic obstructions.

Two major predisposing factors necessary for colonic volvulus to occur are (1) a segment of redundant mobile colon and (2) relatively fixed point or points around which the volvulus may occur (Fig. 5–1). Kerry and Ransom[10] report four main contributing factors: (1) distention of the colon by feces or gas, (2) increased muscular activity and changes in intraperitoneal relationships such as seen in pregnancy and parturition, (3) previous abdominal surgery resulting in adhesions, and (4) congenital abnormalities such as malrotation and acquired obstructing lesions in the distal colon.

There are four classic symptoms in colonic volvulus that are important to diagnosis. They are, in order of frequency, pain, distention, constipation or obstipation, and vomiting. The four most common physical findings, in order of frequency, are abdominal distention, a palpable mass, shock, and temperature elevation.

The typical diagnostic radiographic findings include the following:

1. There is abdominal and colonic distention, often to enormous proportion, occurring at the time of pain; the "bird beak" deformity at the site of torsion is pathognomonic if present. In many cases, distended loops of colon form a "bent inner tube" appearance. The curved loop usually points away from the obstruction, and the narrow pointed bowel points toward the obstruction.

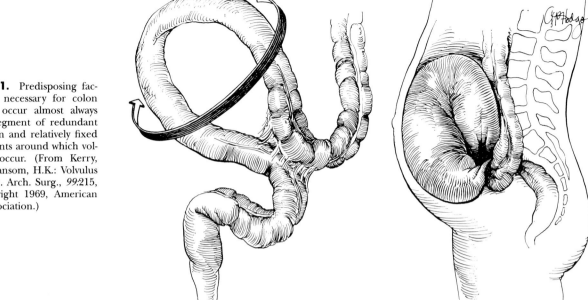

FIGURE 5–1. Predisposing factors usually necessary for colon volvulus to occur almost always consist of segment of redundant mobile colon and relatively fixed point or points around which volvulus may occur. (From Kerry, R.L., and Ransom, H.K.: Volvulus of the colon. Arch. Surg., *99*:215, 1969. Copyright 1969, American Medical Association.)

2. There is an air-fluid level, which tends to be single in cecal volvulus and double in transverse colon and sigmoid volvulus, owing to the "double closed loop obstruction." Distended small bowel with air-fluid levels suggests proximal colonic volvulus.

Treatment of volvulus of the colon consists of two basic types: (1) conservative (usually nonoperative and often emergent) and (2) definitive or operative. Conservative management usually includes reduction of the volvulus by use of a long, soft, well-lubricated rectal tube introduced through a rigid sigmoidoscope. If rigid proctosigmoidoscopy is unsuccessful in achieving decompression, flexible sigmoidoscopy or colonoscopy should be utilized.[2,3,8,9,15] There is an appreciable incidence of recurrence (59%) after this method of conservative therapy. Definitive surgical therapy includes both internal fixation and resection and anastomosis. For clarity, surgical treatment will be discussed in regard to the specific site of colonic volvulus: the right colon, the cecum and ascending colon, and the transverse and left colons, including the sigmoid colon.

Cecal Volvulus

Volvulus of the cecum is actually a somewhat misleading designation because the terminal ileum, as well as the ascending colon, is usually involved with the twisting or folding of the cecum on its mesentery. Volvulus of the cecum occurs less commonly than does volvulus of the sigmoid, but it is not rare.

A distinctive factor in development of a cecal volvulus is the incomplete peritoneal fixation of the right colon to the right abdominal wall. This results in an abnormally mobile ascending colon and the possibility of rotation around a fixed point, producing volvulus. Studies on cadavers demonstrate the presence of this anatomic variant in 10 to 22% of the population. With so great a

proportion of the population possessing a mobile cecum, it is surprising that cecal volvulus does not occur more frequently. Given a mobile cecum, one of a number of precipitating factors may initiate the pathologic process. Such precipitating factors include distention of the cecum, obstructing lesions of the left colon, a high-roughage diet, chronic constipation and frequent purgation, pregnancy, artificial ventilation, and previous abdominal surgery. It is imperative that the possibility of a lesion in the distal colon be ruled out in all patients suspected of having cecal volvulus. The twisting of the bowel upon its mesentery is more often in a clockwise direction, but a counterclockwise twist is sometimes present. The severity of the circulatory embarrassment caused by cecal volvulus depends on the tightness of the twist. The venous return is obstructed first, followed by the arterial supply, with transudation of fluid into the lumen of the bowel and edema of the wall followed by necrosis and perforation.

In most cases, the diagnosis of cecal volvulus can be made by roentgenographic examination with the use of both plain abdominal films and barium studies of the colon. Barium studies, of course, are contraindicated if peritonitis is present or perforation is suspected. Characteristically, with cecal volvulus a plain abdominal film demonstrates a large air-filled loop of colon occupying the left upper quadrant of the abdomen, with its convex surface facing the left lower quadrant (owing to clockwise rotation). In most cases, the cecal shadow is not in its normal position. A picture of small bowel obstruction is often present, and the distal colon is usually collapsed. A single air-fluid level is usually present in cases of cecal volvulus, in contradistinction to sigmoid volvulus in which multiple air-fluid levels are often present. Usually there are distended loops of small bowel in the right iliac fossa. Gas is usually lacking in the transverse colon and beyond; however, this does not apply if the volvulus has been precipitated by a distal obstruction. Following barium enema, the cecum is not visualized and a bird's beak deformity is seen at the site of torsion in the right lower quadrant. Obviously, free air in the peritoneal cavity signifies perforation and precludes barium enema evaluation. The size and configuration of the volvulus may simulate those of a distended stomach. Differentiation of the cecal volvulus from gastric distention can easily be accomplished by the passage of a nasogastric tube and aspiration of the gastric contents, followed by re-examination of the patient with plain radiographs or a barium swallow study using a small amount of barium to identify the stomach.

Cecal volvulus may be difficult to diagnose preoperatively and occurs in a region that is difficult to decompress by colonoscopy. Emergent surgical intervention is almost invariably necessary when dealing with cases of cecal volvulus.[12] Anderson and Welch have presented an analysis of 69 patients with acute volvulus of the right colon and have advocated a concise plan of surgical therapy based upon the findings at operation.[1] In their series, the overall mortality was 19%. If nonviable colon was present (20 patients, 29%), the mortality rate in this group was 40%. They have advocated that in the presence of viable bowel, a combination of simple cecopexy combined with tube cecostomy was as effective as resection in preventing long-term recurrence after an average follow-up of 9.8 years. Decompression of the dilated colonic segment together with fixation in two planes at 90 degrees to each other appeared to be responsible for this success. When perforation of the cecum is present or when there is a large area of confluent gangrene, wide resection with the formation of an ileostomy and a distal mucous fistula is advised. In patients without perforation and in whom the areas of gangrene are patchy, right colon resection and primary ileocolic anastomosis can be safely accomplished.

Volvulus of the Transverse Colon

Volvulus of the transverse colon is rather uncommon. Kerry and Ransom[10] state that in 306 cases of colonic volvulus in the literature they reviewed, the transverse colon was involved in 4%; in their own series of 81 cases, the transverse colon was involved in 11%. In a review of 52 patients with colonic volvulus, Eisenstat and co-workers[5] found an incidence of 9.6%.

Abdominal films may suggest the diagnosis of transverse colon volvulus by revealing a "double closed loop" with air-fluid levels in the twisted transverse colon and also in the ascending colon caused by obstruction at the hepatic flexure and a competent ileocecal valve. Barium enema confirms the diagnosis of transverse colon volvulus when the contrast material cannot pass beyond the splenic flexure or shows a redundant, unusually mobile, or malpositioned transverse colon. The final diagnosis in most instances is made at exploratory laparotomy. Unlike treatment for sigmoid volvulus, conservative nonoperative treatment of transverse colon volvulus is unsuccessful because the focus of torsion is simply not accessible.

Jones and Fazio report that the diagnosis of transverse colonic volvulus is usually made at laporotomy and that

resection is the preferred treatment.[9] Extended right colectomy and ileocolic anastomosis may be undertaken, unless gangrene or fecal soiling are present. If gangrene or soiling are found, then anastomosis should not be performed; instead, an end ileostomy and colonic mucous fistula are appropriate.

Sigmoid Volvulus

Sigmoid volvulus presenting as acute intestinal obstruction is rare in the western world, accounting for only 2% of all cases of obstruction. The disease is more common in eastern Europe and Asia, accounting for 18% of cases of acute intestinal obstruction. Racial and environmental differences are apparent in that American blacks, African Bantus, and Indians seem more prone to acute sigmoid volvulus. It has previously been stated that the disease more commonly affects men of middle and old age; however, there are series of cases reporting that sigmoid volvulus in younger patients is not uncommon, and indeed some series show a preponderance of females.

The essential anatomic features predisposing to sigmoid volvulus are (1) a long and freely mobile sigmoid colon, (2) a long and freely mobile mesosigmoid, and (3) a short mesenteric attachment of the proximal and distal mesocolic limbs, forming a narrow inverted V. Given these predisposing factors, the colon is thought to rotate intermittently around its narrow mesenteric attachment, either clockwise or counterclockwise between 180 and 360 degrees.[14] In addition, the bowel twists along its long axis to a variable degree. The result of such rotation is a closed loop obstruction that eventually leads to a more proximal distention of the colon. The extent of this distention depends upon the competence of the ileocecal valve. The twisted sigmoid loop is liable to ischemic change of varying severity. Repeated volvulus leads to the formation of fibrous striae, which are characteristically seen at the base of the mesosigmoid.

In a volvulus of the sigmoid, the twist usually occurs in a counterclockwise direction around the axis of the sigmoid mesentery and is accompanied by an axial torsion around the axis of the bowel. The axial torsion is always twice as great as a torsion of the mesentery. This twisting at the axis of the mesentery and the corresponding degree of torsion around the axis of the bowel cause a mechanical obstruction that may be simple or strangulated. Those cases with only a moderate torsion produce a simple obstruction in which the most important pathologic changes are caused by the bowel distention and obstruction. The colon wall remains viable, and peristalsis forces gas and fluid into the portion of the bowel involved in the volvulus, at which point they are trapped, as the twist prevents their escape; thus, rapid distention of the involved loop takes place. Occasionally, bowel contents are forced into the rectum so that diarrhea may occur in spite of other symptoms of obstruction. If the condition is unrelieved, necrotic changes occur in the bowel wall, being most marked at the site of torsion, and perforation and peritonitis ensue. In cases with torsion of greater degree, strangulation occurs. The veins are occluded first and later the arteries. Thrombosis of the mesenteric vessels occurs, and rapid infarction of the loop of bowel takes place, producing perforation with peritonitis.

Clinically, volvulus of the sigmoid colon may be manifested as an episode with acute, abrupt onset; as recurring episodes of subacute attacks that subside spontaneously; or as a chronic disorder in which the symptoms are relatively mild despite complete constipation and marked abdominal distention.

The acute type usually begins suddenly and abruptly with generalized abdominal cramps associated with a steady continuous pain and tenderness in the left lower quadrant. There is usually complete constipation for both feces and flatus; occasionally, one small stool empties the rectum after the onset, but a repeated desire to defecate is present with an inability to do so. Vomiting may occur, but when it occurs it is neither frequent nor copious. This is the least common type of volvulus of the sigmoid colon.

In the recurring subacute type there are recurrent attacks of acute abdominal colicky pain. After such milder attacks, a more severe and relatively acute attack requires medical attention. This attack may subside before the necessary studies have been completed and the diagnosis has been established. This type of volvulus of the sigmoid is common.

The chronic type of volvulus of the sigmoid is seen often in institutions for chronic psychiatric patients, homes for the aged, and similar institutions. An insidious onset of recurrent episodes of extreme abdominal distention are associated with constipation and little or no abdominal pain or discomfort. There is usually no vomiting. Abdominal distention is usually the only complaint, and otherwise the patient does not look or feel sick. Between these episodes of extreme distention, the abdominal enlargement may disappear entirely or be reduced in size. The sigmoid colon is usually thickened in the older patient, accounting for its ability to withstand massive distention and high intraluminal pressures without perforation, and despite the closed loop obstruction, it may remain viable for a few days. The younger patient does not have the protection of a thickened sigmoid, and gangrene develops more rapidly.

Differentiating between viable and gangrenous colon in sigmoid volvulus is difficult unless the gangrenous segment can be observed through the colonoscope. The history seldom aids the distinction. Physical examination is similar, with abdominal pain to palpation being either lacking or minimal regardless of viability or gangrene, and rebound tenderness is seldom elicited. With or without gangrenous bowel, the average temperature has been reported to be normal, with ranges up to 101°F. The pulse rate is moderately elevated in patients with a viable colon, but a frank tachycardia is usually present in those with gangrene. In a series reported by Sharpton and Cheek,[13] when hypotension was present on admission, there was a 50% mortality rate even though these patients had viable colons. Gangrenous bowel produces a persistently higher white blood cell count, usually greater than 20,000/cu mm with a marked shift to the left.

The diagnosis is established by radiographic examination made first without contrast material and then with barium. In the plain film of the abdomen, volvulus of the colon may be suggested by the following findings: (1) marked gaseous distention of the sigmoid, which is situated on the right side of the abdomen, giving a characteristic "bent inner tube sign" or "omega sign"; (2) air-fluid levels within the distended sigmoid loop; and (3) moderate gaseous and fluid distention of the remainder of the colon. Barium enema was useful as an emergency procedure only when the plain films and sigmoidoscopy had failed to substantiate the diagnosis. After plain films of the abdomen have been taken and after sigmoidoscopy has been performed and one is fairly certain that gangrene of the bowel mucosa does not exist, a barium enema is then administered. With this study, volvulus of the sigmoid is demonstrated by a characteristic outline of the proximal part of the rectum, which narrows down with a smooth silhouette to a beak-like projection at the site of the obstruction, giving what is called a bird's beak deformity. Occasionally, a double point of obstruction can be demonstrated. In some instances, the torsion and obstruction are released by the barium enema, in which case the radiograph will show a large, redundant sigmoid colon filled with barium. This is a common finding in patients with chronic sigmoid volvulus or with moderate torsion producing only partial obstruction.

Proctoscopic or colonoscopic examination will usually reveal spiral folds of twisted mucosa just proximal to the rectal side of the obstruction. This examination should be done with a great degree of care because of the danger of bowel perforation. If the bowel mucosa appears nonviable or gangrenous, no further attempt at nonoperative reduction of the volvulus by passage of a rectal tube should be made, and operative intervention should be planned. If the mucosa of the bowel appears viable, an attempt at nonoperative reduction should be carried out.

The treatment of acute volvulus of the sigmoid colon is both nonoperative and surgical. When treating volvulus of the sigmoid colon, it is well to keep in mind some statistics regarding patient survival and recurrence. Moseson and associates[11] reviewed their experience with 41 patients who had and were treated for 80 episodes of volvulus of the sigmoid colon. It is their belief that treating the initial episode with nonoperative reduction followed by elective resection significantly decreased both overall mortality and morbidity related to volvulus. They thought that this was true even in patients who were elderly, had serious concomitant disease, and were poor surgical candidates. In their series, death was directly related to sigmoid volvulus in 11 of their 41 patients (26%). There were 3 deaths associated with the initial episode of volvulus (7.3%), and 7 deaths in the 24 patients with recurrent volvulus (29%). A patient had the least chance of dying with the first episode of sigmoid volvulus (7.3%), a greater chance with the second episode (17%), and the greatest chance with subsequent episodes (38%). Mortality for elective surgery for sigmoid volvulus has been reported to range from 3 to 15%; in this series, one death occurred in the 14 patients in whom elective surgery was performed (7.2%).

Of the eight patients undergoing emergency operation, five died (62%). Recurrence rates after nonoperative reduction have been reported in the literature as ranging from 46 to 90%; the rate was 77% in the experience of Moseson and associates.[11] The recurrence rate following surgical procedures such as laparotomy and detorsion or detorsion plus fixation has ranged from 27 to 42%. In view of these statistics, it is the opinion of Moseson and associates that there would be a significant decrease in morbidity and mortality if all patients with sigmoid volvulus were first treated with nonoperative reduction and then underwent elective resection during the same hospitalization for the initial episode.

The procedure for nonoperative reduction is as follows: A rigid or flexible sigmoidoscope is inserted and passed under direct observation to the site of obstruction. This point is usually 15 to 25 cm from the anus and can be recognized by seeing the spiral folds caused by the torsion. If the mucosa looks ulcerated or necrotic, the procedure should be abandoned; if, however, the mucous membrane looks healthy and viable, the procedure can be continued. When the point of obstruction is reached, a large, soft 60-cm rectal tube (No. 32 French) should be gently advanced. When the procedure has been successful and the tube has passed the point of obstruction, there is an immediate, forceful evacuation of flatus and thin stool, and the patient experiences prompt relief from discomfort. The tube should be sutured to the perianal region under local anesthesia, and another upright radiograph of the abdomen should be obtained.

If the volvulus has been reduced, the tube should be used to cautiously administer repeat return-flow enemas. It is important that the rectal tube be sutured to the anal ring to maintain its position for 2 to 3 days, for if the tube is removed earlier, volvulus often recurs promptly. In addition, the patient should be observed closely over the ensuing period in order to make certain that there has been no perforation of the bowel or necrosis of previously unrecognized strangulated bowel. It cannot be stressed strongly enough that this method of treatment must not be employed if there is any possibility that serious circulatory changes exist in the bowel, either at the site of torsion or elsewhere. This method of therapy is not definitive; recurrence of sigmoid volvulus are common. However, it does relieve the acute stage of the lesion, following which the bowel can be properly prepared for safer surgical treatment later during that same hospital stay, sigmoid resection with primary anastomosis then being performed.

In those patients with acute sigmoid volvulus in whom nonoperative treatment was unsuccessful or in whom proctoscopy with passage of a rectal tube is contraindicated because strangulation is suspected, laparotomy is required.

Bloody colonic contents or dark blue or black colonic mucosa are reliable signs of ischemia or impending necrosis and mandate laparotomy.[15]

If at operation the bowel is found to be viable and noncompromised, controversy exists as to the correct surgical therapy.[6,8,9,16] Generally, resection is the best procedure. Primary anastomosis is possible with the addition of colonic lavage during operation.[6,8] An alternative would be a Hartmann's procedure and the necessity to perform a second operation in order to restore bowel continuity.[9]

If gangrenous colon is present or if there is doubt about its viability or if there is intra-abdominal infection or contamination, few surgeons recommend primary anastomosis; resection, however, is mandatory. Unfortunately, the area most likely to become gangrenous is at the site of the twist, which is just above the rectosigmoid, a point too low to exteriorize. The proximal colon is brought out as an end colostomy, the compromised sigmoid colon is removed, and the rectal stump is oversewn (Hartmann's procedure).[6,8] Surgical intervention to restore intestinal continuity at a later time will be necessary.

REFERENCES

1. Anderson, J.R., and Welch, G.H.: Acute volvulus of the right colon: An analysis of 69 patients. World J. Surg., 10:336, 1986.
2. Arigbabu, A.O., Badejo, O.A., and Akinola, D.O.: Colonoscopy in the emergency treatment of colonic volvulus in Nigeria. Dis. Colon Rectum, 28:795, 1985.
3. Brothers, T.E., and Eckhauser, F.E.: Endoscopy in colonic volvulus. Ann. Surg., 206:1, 1987.
4. Budd, D.C., Cochran, R.C., and Metildi, L.A.: Extramedullary plasmacytoma of the colon: A rare cause of intussusception. Am. Surg., 43:528, 1977.
5. Eisenstat, T.E., Raneri, A.J., and Mason, G.R.: Volvulus of the transverse colon. Am. J. Surg., 134:396, 1977.
6. Gibney, E.J.: Volvulus of the sigmoid colon. Surg. Gynecol. Obstet., 173:243, 1991.
7. Ho, L., and Rosenman, L.D.: Complete invagination of the veriform appendix with villous adenoma, intussuscepting to the splenic flexure of the colon. Surgery, 77:505, 1975.
8. Jones, D.L.: ABC of colorectal diseases: Large bowel volvulus. BMJ, 305:358, 1992.
9. Jones, I.T., and Fazio, V.W.: Colonic volvulus. Dig. Dis., 7:203, 1989.
10. Kerry, R.L., and Ransom, H.K.: Volvulus of the colon. Arch. Surg., 99:215, 1969.
11. Moseson, D.L., Lindell, T., Brant, B., et al.: Sigmoid volvulus. Am. Surg., 42:492, 1976.
12. Pahlman, L., Enblad, P., Rudberg, C., and Krog, M.: Volvulus of the colon. Acta Chir. Scand., 155:53, 1989.
13. Sharton, B., and Cheek, R.C.: Volvulus of the sigmoid colon. Am. Surg., 42:436, 1976.
14. Smith, R.B., Kettlewell, M.G., and Gough, M.H.: Intermittent sigmoid volvulus in the younger age groups. Br. J. Surg., 64:406, 1977.
15. Strodel, W.E., and Brothers, T.: Colonoscopic decompression of pseudo-obstruction and volvulus. Surg. Clin. North Am., 69:1327, 1989.
16. Welch, G.H., and Anderson, J.R.: Acute volvulus of the sigmoid colon. World J. Surg., 11:258, 1987.

Chapter 6

INFLAMMATORY BOWEL DISEASE

ZANE COHEN / ROBIN S. MCLEOD

ULCERATIVE COLITIS

Ulcerative colitis is an inflammatory disease of unknown etiology involving the mucosa of the colon and rectum. Although psychosomatic factors were once thought to be important in its etiology, data supporting this are uncontrolled and anecdotal. Ulcerative colitis is most likely caused by a combination of genetic and environmental factors. Heredity may play a role in the cause, as there is a 5 to 15% incidence of the disease occurring in families, compared with a 0.1% occurrence in the general population.[53] The disease has been observed to occur in both members of monozygotic twins. It is more prevalent in whites than in blacks and in Jews than in non-Jews.

An infectious cause of ulcerative colitis has been postulated, but as yet no bacterial or viral agents have been isolated. It is possible, however, that an infectious agent may incite the initial damage and then be eliminated by local defense mechanisms. The lesion may be perpetuated by a defective mucosal immune response. An immunologic cause for the disease was considered as early as 1945. This mechanism is supported by the fact that ulcerative colitis is associated with a variety of autoimmune disorders such as systemic lupus erythematosus, ankylosing spondylitis, and chronic active hepatitis. In addition, circulating immune complexes may be found in the serum of these patients. If it is an immune mechanism, it is likely that it is a cell-mediated, rather than a humoral, response.[17]

Pathologic Features

Ulcerative colitis is usually present in the rectum and progresses proximally to involve the remainder of the colon in a continuous manner. The disease process most commonly ends abruptly at the ileocecal junction. In some individuals, there is mucosal inflammation of the terminal ileum. This has commonly been known as "backwash ileitis." Whether this is a real entity remains controversial. The extent of the disease may vary from involvement of the rectum and sigmoid alone to total colonic involvement. In a small group of patients, segmental involvement of one or more portions of the colon without evidence of the disease in the rectosigmoid region can occur, but this is very rare.

On gross examination, the lesions of ulcerative colitis begin as pinpoint hemorrhagic spots associated with a hyperemic and edematous mucosal reaction. This friability of the mucosa produces the bleeding that is seen with the disease. Ulcerations may be superficial and smooth or ragged and undermined. Eventually the entire mucosa of the colon and rectum may be replaced by these ulcers. With chronicity, marked narrowing, thickening, and rigidity of the bowel occur as the muscular coats are replaced with scar tissue (Fig. 6–1). Polypoid masses or pseudopolyps, caused by hyperplasia of remaining small islands of mucosa and by the margins of ulcerations, may be present and may persist or recede as the inflammatory process becomes quiescent. Microscopic examination of the inflamed colon shows diffuse macroulcerations and microulcerations with adjacent edema, polymorphonuclear leukocyte infiltration, and eosinophilic cellular invasion of the mucosa. There is also destruction of villi. Microscopic crypt abscesses are common and penetrate just into the submucosa with the production of wide areas of ulceration of the overlying mucosa. There is usually a definite increase in the number of Paneth's cells in the colonic crypts, which is thought to be more likely a response to ulcerative colitis than a factor in its cause.[54] Granulomas, typically seen in Crohn's disease, are conspicuously lacking in ulcerative colitis.

Clinical Course

Ulcerative colitis is highly variable in severity, clinical course, and ultimate prognosis, although in general the severity of the disease varies with the extent and severity of the changes in the bowel wall. It has a peak incidence in persons 20 to 40 years old and is slightly more common in females. After its onset, the disease may take one

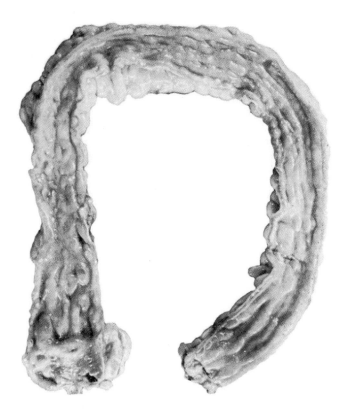

FIGURE 6-1. Nonspecific ulcerative colitis. The colonic lumen is greatly narrowed throughout, particularly in the upper left (proximal transverse colon). Even more striking is the degree of thickening of the wall and total lack of any semblance of normal mucosa. (From Roth, J.A.: Ulcerative colitis. *In* Bockus, H.L., et al. [eds.]: Gastroenterology, Vol. 2, 3rd ed. Philadelphia, W.B. Saunders, 1974, with permission.)

of several courses. It may be fulminating and reach its peak in 2 to 3 weeks or it may pass into a chronic stage with remissions and exacerbations. The chronic form of ulcerative colitis presents as three clinical types. Approximately 60 to 75% of patients have intermittent attacks of symptoms with complete symptomatic remissions between attacks. A few patients (5 to 15%) are troubled by continuous symptoms without any remission. Only a small proportion of patients (5 to 10%) have only one attack with no subsequent symptoms.

The most common symptoms are diarrhea and the passage of blood and mucus. Unlike Crohn's colitis, in which hematochezia is often lacking, bloody diarrhea is the hallmark of ulcerative colitis. The amount of blood may vary from a small amount of bright red blood, which is mistaken for hemorrhoidal bleeding, to massive bleeding.

The diarrhea may be minimal, or patients may have 10 to 20 bowel movements per day. Occasionally, patients may complain of constipation. These are usually patients with inflammation limited to the rectum and sigmoid, and the disease causes a type of functional obstruction. In addition to passing watery stools, patients may have tenesmus and pass a bloody mucous discharge.

In patients with acute colitis, abdominal pain is a frequent manifestation. It tends to be colicky. On examination of the abdomen, there may be tenderness over the colon, especially in the left lower quadrant. Large doses of steroids may mask clinical signs in acute disease.

With milder forms of distal colitis, there may be only slight impairment of general health. In severe cases, the constitutional effects can be profound and the patient may become rapidly debilitated and emaciated. Associated with these effects is pyrexia, although fever of more than 38°C is unusual except in the very rare fulminating type of colitis or in cases in which there is an intra-abdominal perforation. Loss of weight and anemia tend to occur in proportion to the severity of symptoms.

Diagnosis

The diagnosis of ulcerative colitis should be suspected in patients with a history of bloody diarrhea in whom an infectious cause has been eliminated. Barium x-ray studies, sigmoidoscopy, and colonoscopy can be used to confirm the diagnosis. Colonoscopic examination and biopsies tend to be more accurate than a barium enema in assessing the colon, particularly for detecting early changes and determining the extent of the disease. A proctosigmoidoscopy or colonoscopy reveals the typical gross features already described. There is also frequently a purulent exudate with bloody mucus, an adherent membrane, or both. Double-contrast barium enema, which is preferred over a single-contrast study, shows virtually no changes from normal in the early stages of the disease. Hence, direct visualization is preferred to make the diagnosis. With chronic disease on barium enema, one can expect to find distortion of the mucosal pattern, loss of haustral markings associated with narrowing of the lumen, and shortening of the colon (Fig. 6–2). In order to complete the gastrointestinal investigation, a small bowel study or enteroclysis should be performed to exclude the possibility of Crohn's disease of the terminal ileum. This is more accurate in assessing the terminal ileum than is reflux into the terminal ileum from a barium enema.

Natural History

Of utmost importance in treating patients with ulcerative colitis is the fact that with chronicity, ulcerative colitis carries a definite and significant risk for the development of carcinoma of the colon and rectum.[36] The observed incidence in adults with ulcerative colitis is 7 to 30 times greater than in a controlled population. The risk of cancer appears to be related to two factors: (1) the duration of the colitis and (2) the extent of colonic involvement.

It is recognized that the incidence of carcinoma increases with the duration of the disease.[31,36] However, determining the exact risk of colitis is often difficult because of many biases present in reports in the literature. One of the most important of these is lack of a well-defined inception cohort.[52] Reports tend to be retrospective, and follow-up of patients may begin at various times after the onset of their disease. Reports usually include patients who are referred by hospitals. Thus, many patients who have a benign uncomplicated course

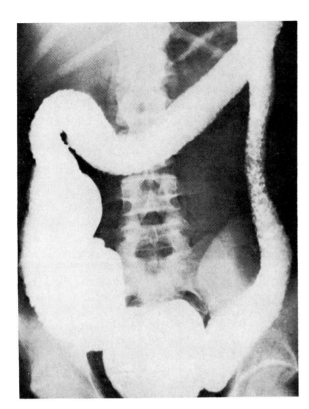

FIGURE 6-2. Barium enema film taken during the course of a recurrent chronic type of ulcerative colitis of 6 years' duration. The entire colon is involved with an extensive polypoid change, giving a honeycombed effect, which is more marked in the descending colon. (From Monaghan, J.R.: *In* Bockus, H.L., et al. [eds.]: Gastroenterology, Vol. 2. Philadelphia, W.B. Saunders, 1946, with permission.)

are not included, and follow-up is often incomplete. Kewenter and associates[31] have reported on a well-defined population of patients followed in Sweden. They calculated the accumulated incidence of carcinoma to be 3% at 10 years, 9.6% at 15 years, and 24.2% at 20 years after the onset of colitis. In contrast, much lower rates were reported by Lennard-Jones from St. Mark's Hospital.[36] He calculated a risk of only 10.8% at 20 years and 16.6% at 25 years. However, these latter results may not reflect the natural history of the disease because during this period patients underwent surveillance, and a certain number had surgery because dysplastic changes developed. If one postulates that these patients would have developed cancer, the incidence would have been much higher and more in keeping with Kewenter's series. Although there is disagreement as to the exact incidence of cancer, it is generally accepted that the risk of cancer is minimal before there has been 10 years of disease activity and that it increases after this time. The risk after 20 years may rise at a much steeper rate.

The extent of the colitis also appears important in determining the risk of carcinoma developing. Patients with only documented proctitis have a minimal risk of developing a carcinoma. Patients with pancolitis are at highest risk and patients with left-sided colitis have an intermediate risk. In a retrospective study of 267 patients,

Greenstein and co-workers[21] reported on 27 patients who developed adenocarcinoma. Twenty-one of these lesions occurred in 158 patients with total colon disease, and 5 occurred in 109 patients with left-sided disease. They also noted that the carcinoma in left-sided colitis occurred at least a decade later than that in patients with pancolitis. This study may be criticized methodologically because of biases inherent in a retrospective review.

A controversial area is the risk of colorectal cancer in patients in whom the colitis began in the prepubertal years.[11] It may be that the risk is related only to the longer duration of disease rather than to the time of onset. Similarly, it was previously believed that patients whose disease was continuously active were more at risk for carcinoma. It is our view that the activity of the disease is not important in determining the risk of carcinoma. In fact, many patients with quiescent disease often present with advanced lesions because they are asymptomatic and tend not to seek medical advice and thus come under surveillance.

In the past, prophylactic proctocolectomy was recommended for patients with longstanding disease, irrespective of their disease activity, because of the risk of cancer developing. However, with the availability of colonoscopy for surveillance of the entire colon and with increasing expertise in the evaluation of endoscopic and pathologic changes, the trend now is to recommend that patients undergo endoscopic surveillance in a search for premalignant lesions in the colonic epithelium. The objective of this course of action is to recognize premalignant changes before the onset of carcinoma. To this end, the term dysplasia has been used in reference to these precancerous epithelial abnormalities.

In 1983, a group of world experts (the Inflammatory Bowel Disease-Dysplasia Morphology Study Group) published a consensus report on the classification of dysplasia.[50] Changes were classified as positive for dysplasia, negative for dysplasia, or indeterminate. In addition, dysplasia can be classified as mild, moderate, or severe. The distinction among the grades depends largely on the degree of cytologic changes present. There is good evidence that dysplastic change precedes frank carcinoma. Unfortunately, however, carcinomas may already be present when dysplastic changes are detected. It is also recognized that the pathologist may have difficulty deciding whether microscopic changes are due to the normal regenerative changes seen in ulcerative colitis or represent dysplastic changes. This is especially true if there is disease activity at the time the biopsy is performed. An experienced pathologist is essential if patients are to be followed colonoscopically.

We perform colonoscopy on all patients with total or left-sided disease on a yearly basis starting approximately 7 years after the onset of symptoms. The patient must be properly prepared for colonoscopy so that all of the mucosa can be visualized. The colonoscopy must be complete to the cecum, and the endoscopist must search for any suspicious plaque-like or nodular lesions. Dysplasia may be present in grossly flat mucosa or may have a villous or nodular appearance. At least ten serial biopsies from around the colon and rectum are obtained for pathologic assessment. In addition, any suspicious areas are biopsied. The site of each biopsy is recorded in case early follow-up colonoscopy is indicated. With accurate endoscopic and pathologic assessment of the mucosa, a reasonable course of management can be recommended to the patient. In patients who have active disease and a diagnosis of mild dysplasia, we attempt to manage the disease medically to decrease the amount of inflammation, and we perform repeat colonoscopy and biopsy in 3 months. If there is no further dysplasia, they will undergo colonoscopy in 1 year. If mild dysplasia is again present, they will undergo repeat colonoscopy in 3 months, and if dysplasia is still present, serious consideration will be given to surgical intervention.

We have no hesitation in recommending surgical intervention in patients whose biopsy specimen shows moderate or severe dysplasia from an area of quiescent disease. We feel that there is sufficient risk in these patients to warrant resection. The objective of screening is to detect and treat the high-risk patient surgically prior to development of a cancer. Thus, the optimal result would be to find dysplastic changes in the surgical specimen but no cancer. Although this policy appears to be useful in detecting high-risk patients, it is not without its pitfalls. In our own series, we have operated on several patients in whom severe dysplasia but no invasive carcinoma was diagnosed on biopsy specimens taken at the time of colonoscopy. After colectomy, unrecognized cancers were found within the surgical specimens of these patients. Lennard-Jones has reported that in patients undergoing surgery because of mild dysplasia, 5% had unrecognized cancers found in the surgical specimen.[36] In patients with moderate dysplasia, 15% had undetected carcinomas, and if the indication was severe dysplasia, 30% of patients had undetected carcinomas. This exemplifies the difficulties in relying on colonoscopic and histologic assessment only by surveillance of these patients. As mentioned previously, the cancers can be flat and plaque-like and difficult to visualize at endoscopy.

A less aggressive policy is advocated by the group at St. Mark's Hospital in London.[36] If severe dysplasia is found on one biopsy specimen, patients undergo repeat colonoscopy in 3 months, and if the dysplasia has disappeared, they are again followed. We believe that this is inappropriate and risky in that the second biopsy may be free of dysplasia only because of a sampling error and not because of disappearance of dysplasia.

A special circumstance is the patient in whom a nodular or polypoid lesion is biopsied and is shown to have dysplastic changes histologically. These patients are at particularly high risk. Blackstone and co-workers reported that invasive carcinomas were present in 7 of 25 patients (28%) in whom mild dysplastic changes were found in so-called villous nodular lesions.[5] Thus, the presence of a polypoid mass showing any degree of dysplasia is an indication for surgery.

In summary, we feel that colonoscopic surveillance in patients with long-standing ulcerative colitis is useful. However, it has pitfalls. The exact recommendations given to patients must therefore be individualized after a full consultation outlining the potential risks.

Carcinoma in Patients With Ulcerative Colitis

The incidence of carcinoma in ulcerative colitis is the same in both sexes. Carcinoma in ulcerative colitis tends to occur early in life, with a peak incidence in the fourth decade. Tumors tend to be multicentric and evenly distributed throughout the colon, unlike those in patients without ulcerative colitis, whose lesions tend to occur more frequently within the left colon.[46] Other characteristics of these cancers are that they tend to be infiltrative, highly aggressive, and poorly differentiated. For this reason, they may escape detection colonoscopically or even at surgery. As a result, they tend to be discovered at a later stage. Another reason for their late detection is that the common symptoms of crampy abdominal pain, change in bowel habit, bleeding, and mucous discharge may be attributed to the ulcerative colitis rather than to carcinoma.

As a result of the more advanced stage of the cancer, the prognosis tends to be poor. Slaney and Brooke[56] reported an overall 5-year survival rate of 18.6% in patients who developed cancer. The Cleveland Clinic examined the long-term survival rate of 79 patients with carcinoma arising in ulcerative colitis in relation to their clinical pathologic staging and compared the survival statistics with those from a group of patients with carcinoma who did not have colitis with equivalent clinical pathologic staging. When grouped by Dukes' classification, there was no statistical difference in survival rates.[34] The overall 5-year survival rate was 41% when carcinoma and ulcerative colitis coexisted, compared with 61% when there was no colitis with the carcinoma. The overall results were worse because of the more advanced stage of the disease at diagnosis.

Acute Colitis

Although severe acute colitis is the least common form of ulcerative colitis, affecting approximately 15% of all patients with the disease, it can be life threatening. Acute colitis can occur in two forms. The first is toxic dilation of the colon with or without significant bleeding. The second is massive lower gastrointestinal hemorrhage. Toxic megacolon is defined as a severe attack of colitis with total or segmental dilation of the colon. Jalan and colleagues[27] defined toxicity as the presence of any three of the following conditions: pyrexia greater than 38.5°C, tachycardia greater than 120 beats/min, leukocytosis greater than 10,500 cells, and anemia with a hemoglobin value less than 60% of normal. In addition, one of the following conditions must be present: dehydration, mental changes, electrolyte disturbances, or hypotension. This degree of toxicity, coupled with clinical or radiologic evidence of colonic distention, completes the presentation of toxic megacolon.

Toxic megacolon can complicate long-standing disease or can occur in patients presenting with their first attack. In the latter instance, one must entertain the possibility of Crohn's disease or an infectious colitis, with the treatment varying depending on the cause. Various precipitating factors for toxic megacolon have been identified, including antidiarrheal agents, barium enema, and hypokalemia. Unfortunately, the cause is unknown but is thought to be due to a paralysis of the myenteric plexus. This, in turn, may result from a transmural type of inflammatory process that occurs in the acute colitis process.

Toxic dilation of the colon is generally considered the most serious complication of ulcerative colitis. It is a condition in which the colon loses its ability to contract and becomes widely distended, resulting in a thinned wall that is in danger of perforation. The most common sites of perforation are around the peritoneal attachments of the splenic flexure and at the cecum. The reported incidence of toxic megacolon ranges between 1 and 2.5% of patients hospitalized with ulcerative colitis.[18]

The clinical presentation of toxic dilation of the colon is dramatic. The patient may suddenly become acutely ill with rapid progression of symptoms that include fever, mental aberrations, tachypnea, tachycardia, and bloody diarrhea. Abdominal pain may be diffuse and severe, but may be lacking, particularly in those patients who are taking high-dose steroids. Sigmoidoscopy may reveal changes typical of ulcerative proctitis. The diagnosis can usually be made on a plain film of the abdomen, which shows dilation of the large bowel and, in particular, of the transverse colon with widening of the haustral folds and irregularity of the bowel wall (Fig. 6–3). More invasive studies, such as colonoscopy or barium enema, are both unnecessary and dangerous.

Patients who present with signs of localized or generalized peritonitis, radiologic evidence of perforation, or systemic instability should undergo immediate surgery. Otherwise, intensive medical management, consisting of high-dose parenteral steroids and intravenous fluids, should be initiated immediately. Patients tend to be dehydrated and may have electrolyte imbalances because of losses from vomiting and diarrhea. These imbalances must be corrected, and patients who are anemic should undergo transfusion. Restriction of oral intake is initiated along with nasogastric suction to avoid further intestinal distention. Although controversial, we believe broad-spectrum antibiotics should be administered because of the potential for bacteremia caused by the increased permeability of the colon wall and the possibility of microperforations that often exist along the peritoneal attachments.

The patient with toxic megacolon must be observed very closely with serial examinations every 2 to 4 hours. Patients who do not show any improvement in a 24-hour period, or patients who deteriorate at any time, should undergo surgical intervention. This aggressive policy is based on reports showing that although mortality increases significantly with prolonged medical treatment, the proportion of patients whose disease resolves does not.

The options of surgical therapy include subtotal colectomy and ileostomy, total proctocolectomy, and the "blowhole procedure" as advocated by Turnbull and colleagues.[60] Our own procedure of choice is subtotal colectomy and ileostomy. We feel that with this procedure, most of the disease is removed and the patient's recovery is usually rapid. Although the remaining rectal remnant discharges some small quantities of mucus and blood, it is not usually a significant problem. When performing this procedure in the presence of toxic megacolon, one must use a lengthy incision to more easily mobilize the splenic flexure without placing undue tension on it. Iatrogenic perforations of the colon most often occur when the splenic flexure is put under tension. We prefer to oversew the lower end of the sigmoid and bring it out through a separate incision in the left lower quadrant. It is buried in the subcutaneous tissue without closing the skin over it. In this way, there is no foul-smelling discharge as with a mucous fistula, but if the suture line breaks down, the rectum will not discharge into the abdomen (Fig. 6–4).

In the majority of cases of toxic megacolon, significant bleeding is not the major problem and, therefore, we have no hesitancy in leaving the remaining rectum in situ for consideration of a reconstructive procedure at a future date. If the rectal disease does become troublesome, it usually can be quite easily managed with steroid or 5-aminosalicylic acid (5-ASA) enemas. We do not advocate total proctocolectomy. Patients with toxic megacolon are often ill, septic, anemic, hypoalbuminemic, and nutritionally depleted at the time of presentation. These factors will predispose the patient to pelvic sepsis and an unhealed perineal wound if a rectal and perineal dissection is undertaken. Furthermore, total proctocolectomy is usually unnecessary to control the acute emergency, and it eliminates the possibility of a future reconstructive procedure.

The blowhole operation has not gained wide popu-

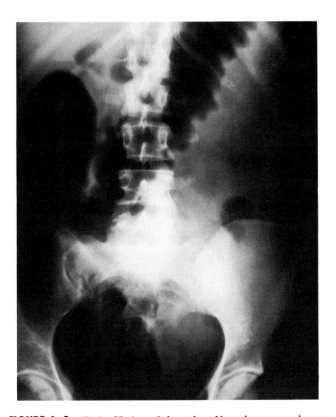

FIGURE 6–3. Toxic dilation of the colon. Note the gross enlargement, particularly of the transverse colon and cecum.

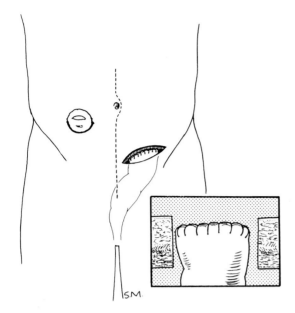

FIGURE 6-4. Anatomy following subtotal colectomy. An end ileostomy on the right side and a mucous fistula on the left. The end of the sigmoid stump has been closed and is left below the skin in the subcutaneous tissues.

larity outside of the Cleveland Clinic. The rationale for performing this operation is that there is higher mortality when a perforation occurs. Because the colon is often hugely dilated, the risk of iatrogenically perforating the colon is significant. In addition, sealed perforations may be present, and with mobilization they may be disrupted, causing fecal spillage. Turnbull and associates[60] therefore advocate the performance of a colostomy and ileostomy to decompress the colon initially, with further surgical management at a later date once the acute process has settled (Fig. 6–5). This procedure

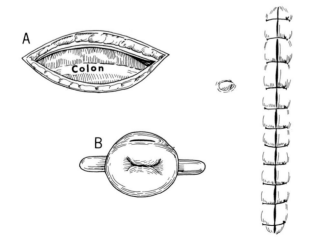

FIGURE 6-5. *A,* Short transverse epigastric incision made over the dilated proximal transverse colon allows the colon to bulge into the incision. *B,* Ileostomy completed and abdomen closed. The dilated transverse colon is identified. (From Turnbull, R., Hawk, W., and Weakley, F.: Surgical treatment of toxic megacolon, ileostomy and colostomy to prepare patients for colectomy. Am. J. Surg., *122:*325, 1971, with permission.)

should certainly be kept within the armamentarium of the surgeon. However, with careful manipulation of the colon as previously outlined, the chances of perforation are kept to a minimum, and it has been our preference to do a subtotal colectomy when possible. The blowhole procedure should be considered in acutely ill patients who have a hugely dilated and extremely friable colon. In addition, it should be considered in patients in whom a definite diagnosis of ulcerative colitis has not been made. It may also be considered in instances in which there is inadequate surgical assistance or when an operator is inexperienced in dealing with a severely diseased colon and with a high splenic flexure.

Historically, there is approximately a 25 to 30% mortality rate with medical management. This contrasts with an overall surgical mortality rate of 19%.[57] However, it is difficult to compare the medical and surgical mortality rates, as often the sicker patients come to surgery. There is an even higher mortality rate in patients with perforations. The Mayo Clinic[20] recently reported on the long-term outcome of 38 patients with toxic megacolon who were successfully treated medically. Of these patients, 47% required surgery either electively (three patients) or urgently (15 patients) at a later date. Eleven of the 38 patients (29%) subsequently suffered a second episode of fulminant acute colitis or recurrent toxic megacolon. This report supports the contention that the medical treatment of toxic megacolon should be regarded almost exclusively as preparation for imminent surgery.

Massive Hemorrhage

Although rectal bleeding is a common symptom of ulcerative colitis, massive hemorrhage necessitating rapid blood transfusion and emergency treatment is unusual, occurring in less than 5% of patients. Most frequently, it occurs in patients with acute severe colitis. Treatment of these patients usually is twofold. First, treatment of the ulcerative colitis necessitates the use of high-dose steroids and other supportive measures. Second, the bleeding must be treated expeditiously and any coagulation abnormality corrected. In most patients, hemorrhage will subside spontaneously. It is unusual that the bleeding originates from a discrete site. The indication for surgery is not arbitrary but needs to be individualized for each patient. Once the decision is made to operate, the standard procedure has been proctocolectomy. However, this procedure, as mentioned previously, can be associated with higher mortality and morbidity than subtotal colectomy and obviates the possibility of a reconstructive procedure in the future. Thus, in selected cases, one might consider a total abdominal colectomy, leaving a short rectal stump—enough to allow future reconstructive surgery. In most instances, this type of surgery will control the bleeding, although continuing massive hemorrhage can still occur in approximately 10 to 12% of patients.

Chronic Colitis

Steroids, sulfasalazine, 5-ASA compounds (Asacol, Pentasa, Rowasa, and Salofalk), and azathioprine have been the mainstays for medical treatment of ulcerative colitis. Sulfasalazine has been the most common drug used to maintain remission in ulcerative colitis. This drug is degraded into its components of sulfapyridine and 5-ASA in the colon. It is the sulfapyridine moiety to which some patients have side effects and allergic reactions. Because of this, various 5-ASA compounds have recently been developed. They have been shown to be as effective as sulfasalazine but without as many side effects. In addition to these oral medications, 5-ASA and steroid enemas have been of benefit in treating rectal disease.

The primary indication for surgical intervention in chronic colitis is the lack of response to medical management. Patients are now being considered for surgery at an earlier stage of disease mainly because of the restorative procedures that can be offered with successful results. In addition, it has been recognized that the complications and side effects of maintaining young patients on relatively high doses of steroids for a prolonged period far outweigh the complications of surgical intervention.

The absolute indications for surgery in chronic ulcerative colitis include the development of cancer or severe dysplasia in the colon, the presence of growth retardation because of the disease process or its medical treatment, and the presence of a stricture or mass lesion in the colon that precludes complete surveillance or accurate diagnosis. In addition, patients who have developed extracolonic manifestations of the disease may improve when they have undergone surgery. This applies in particular to those patients who have developed pyoderma gangrenosum and also to some patients with musculoskeletal manifestations. Some complications, such as sclerosing cholangitis, are unaffected by surgical extirpation of the colon.

At present, four procedures may be offered to the patient requiring surgery for ulcerative colitis: (1) proctocolectomy and conventional ileostomy; (2) abdominal colectomy and ileorectal anastomosis; (3) proctocolectomy and the Kock continent ileostomy; or (4) abdominal colectomy with mucosal proctectomy, ileal reservoir, and ileoanal anastomosis. Although all of these operations have certain advantages, they also have disadvantages, and it is for this reason that we believe surgeons should be familiar with and accomplished at performing all of these operations. Only in this way can they advise patients in an unbiased manner and then allow the patient to make the ultimate decision as to which procedure he or she might prefer.

With any of these procedures, the timing of the operation is important. As mentioned in the preceding section on acute colitis, a subtotal colectomy and ileostomy is our procedure of choice. Patients with more chronic forms of colitis also may be best treated initially by performing a subtotal colectomy and ileostomy. Such treatment applies especially to patients who are malnourished or are on high doses of steroids, as well as those in whom the diagnosis is in question (i.e., the possibility of Crohn's colitis is entertained). Once the general status of the patient improves or the diagnosis is confirmed, a more definitive procedure can be performed.

In patients who have carcinoma of the colon, only a subtotal colectomy and ileostomy should be considered, particularly if the disease is advanced.

Proctocolectomy and ileostomy is the standard operation against which all other operations should be compared. Its principal advantage is that it removes all of the colon and rectum so that patients are cured of the disease, no further anti-inflammatory medications are required, and there is no risk of development of carcinoma of the colon or rectum. The obvious disadvantage is that patients are left with a permanent conventional ileostomy. However, although patients are often hesitant to have a conventional ileostomy, virtually all individuals adapt quite well. Prior to undertaking surgery, it is important that the patient be seen by an enterostomal therapy nurse and a site for the ileostomy be marked, since a well-constructed stoma has been found to be the most important factor in predicting a good functional outcome.

The colectomy is performed in a standard fashion. However, the rectal dissection is performed close to the rectum to minimize the risk of pelvic nerve injury. In addition, an intersphincteric rectal excision should be performed to facilitate nerve preservation and conserve tissue for perineal closure.[15] In this way, it is hoped that the risk of perineal wound complications can be minimized. The most common early complication specifically related to this operation is perineal wound abscess, which occurs in up to 20% of patients. However, this risk is minimized by performing a strict anatomic dissection with good hemostasis. If this complication occurs, it may lead to a chronic unhealed perineal sinus. In the majority of patients with a chronic unhealed perineal sinus, minimal symptoms of mucous drainage may ensue. However, a few patients will have either recurrent perineal abscesses necessitating drainage or continuous chronic pelvic pain. In order to eradicate the problem, one must excise all of the granulation tissue and scar tissue. There is frequently a small sinus opening and a very large track extending proximally along the sacral hollow. When this track has been completely removed, the wound can be allowed to heal by secondary intention, it may be skin grafted, or a myocutaneous flap may be inserted using the gracilis or the gluteus muscle. Our preferred method is to use skin grafts in these patients.[42] It is a relatively simple technique and has a good success rate.

Another complication specific to this procedure is pelvic nerve injury. If the dissection is close to the rectum, this complication should occur in less than 1% of cases.[15] It manifests itself in difficulty with micturition, retrograde ejaculation, or impotence. Finally, ileostomy revision for prolapse or retraction is not uncommon. All of these complications should be considered when comparing the complications of newer procedures to those of proctocolectomy and ileostomy.

Total colectomy and ileorectal anastomosis is potentially an attractive surgical option in the management of patients with ulcerative colitis. It avoids the need for an ileostomy and is the simplest procedure to perform. However, it does leave the diseased rectum intact so that patients are at risk for the development of further symptoms or complications. There has been considerable controversy regarding the value of this procedure, particularly since the introduction of the ileal reservoir and ileoanal anastomosis procedure.

In selecting patients for total colectomy and ileorectal anastomosis, several factors should be considered. First, to achieve adequate functional results, the rectum should be distensible and not fibrotic. In addition, patients with evidence of dysplasia anywhere in the colon are not candidates, since dysplasia tends to be patchy, and there may be dysplastic changes in the rectum even if they are undetected on biopsy. Disease activity endoscopically does not appear to correlate with functional results after surgery. However, one would tend to perform the operation in patients in whom there is rectal sparing or minimal disease. The proportion of patients considered candidates varies depending on the proponents of the operation. Aylett[3] claimed that virtually all patients were candidates, whereas approximately 20% of patients undergoing surgery at St. Mark's Hospital were considered candidates.[44] This number has probably decreased even more since pouch procedures have become more popular.

In performing the operation, it is important to remove all of the colon and perform the anastomosis just below the sacral promontory. In doing so, functional results seem to be adequate, and continuing sigmoidoscopic surveillance of the rectum can be accomplished easily. Although some centers have recommended a temporary ileostomy, this does not seem to be necessary. With adequate patient selection, the operative mortality rate does not appear to be greater than the rates of the other procedures; the reported anastomotic leak rate has varied from 2 to 15%.

As with the other alternative procedures, patient satisfaction seems to be high. Most patients have approximately six bowel movements per day. Urgency is unusual, and most patients do not have dietary restrictions. Approximately half require occasional antidiarrheal medication to improve bowel function.

The important considerations regarding ileorectal anastomosis are (1) the rate of failure due to disease activity and (2) the risk of rectal cancer. Baker and co-workers[4] reviewed 384 patients subjected to ileorectal anastomosis by Aylett. This significant paper is the largest series of patients to have undergone an ileorectal anastomosis. Carcinoma of the rectum developed in 22 patients—a rate of 6%. The accumulated risk was determined to be 6% at 20 years, 15% at 30 years, and 18% at 35 years. Of the 22 cancers detected, 18 were poorly differentiated and 12 were Dukes' stage C lesions. At the Cleveland Clinic, 84 patients with ileorectal anastomosis were reviewed and 4.8% had cancer.[22] In this group, the accumulated risk of cancer developing in the rectal stump was 9% at 10 years, 11.1% at 15 years, 16.1% at 20 years, and 22% after 25 years. The conclusion of these papers is that the risk of cancer is markedly reduced following ileorectal anastomosis, but it points out the need for continuing surveillance. It is recommended that patients return at 6-month intervals for sigmoidoscopic examination and biopsy. If there is any suspicion of dysplasia, they should be advised to have the rectum excised. Noncompliant patients or those who are unable to return for follow-up probably should not be considered candidates for this procedure.

Although occasionally the procedure fails, it is considered beneficial in that it may postpone the need for more radical surgery. This argument, however, is not a strong one, as patients now have the alternative of a pouch procedure and do not necessarily need to have an ileostomy.

The Kock continent ileostomy is another alternative for patients who find a standard ileostomy unacceptable (Fig. 6–6). This procedure is performed mainly in patients with ulcerative colitis and familial adenomatous polyposis. One must be certain of the diagnosis and exclude the diagnosis of Crohn's disease. Thus, the patient should undergo colonoscopy preoperatively, and biopsies should be taken to prove the diagnosis of ulcerative colitis. These patients should also have a small bowel enema or enteroclysis to confirm the diagnosis and to ensure that no occult disease exists in the small bowel. In some patients, a definitive pathologic diagnosis cannot be made. In these selected patients with indeterminate colitis, a continent ileostomy may be constructed, provided the patient understands the additional risks involved.

Those patients who have had a significant small bowel resection should not be considered for a Kock pouch. If complications were to occur, necessitating removal of the reservoir, such patients might be in jeopardy of having significant malabsorption. Another consideration is the age of the patient. Generally, patients older than 50 to 60 years are not candidates because they might have to undergo later revision surgery, which would carry with it increasing morbidity. Careful patient selection is of utmost importance. Selected patients should be intelligent, well-motivated, and psychologically stable. This is particularly important if postoperative complications develop.

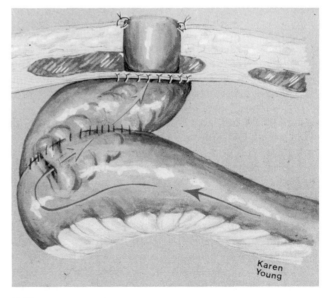

FIGURE 6–6. A completed Kock pouch constructed from approximately 45 cm of terminal ileum. Note the "nipple valve" within the pouch, which is the mechanism of continence.

The surgical technique of the continent ileostomy has undergone numerous modifications over the past 15 years. These changes are detailed in a later chapter; suffice it to say here that improvement in results has come with increasing clinical expertise, as well as with some of the modifications in the surgical technique. In our own series, the reoperation rate initially was 50%. This has been reduced over the years, and following various surgical modifications is now approximately 12 to 15%.[9]

The most frequent complication is valve slippage.[12,32] The continent ileostomy is constructed from approximately 45 cm of terminal ileum. The distal 15 cm is left undisturbed initially, and part of that is intussuscepted to act as a "nipple valve" to maintain a state of continence. This is unphysiologic, and the valve tends to slip out of position. When this does occur, the patient becomes incontinent, has difficulty intubating and emptying the pouch, and usually requires revision surgery. Another complication related to the nipple valve is valve prolapse. The nipple valve everts itself and, if complete, projects like a standard ileostomy. It requires reduction, and often reoperation to secure the valve in place. Further modifications of this procedure in an attempt to stabilize the valve have used various synthetic materials such as Marlex, Prolene, and Mersiline mesh. Initially, with the use of Marlex mesh, there was a tendency toward fistula formation from the pouch to the skin. This septic complication required a major operative revision of the nipple valve. With the use of softer weave mesh, the frequency of this complication has been greatly reduced.

Another intriguing complication of the pouch and reservoir procedures has been the development of nonspecific inflammatory change within the reservoir. This is commonly known as "pouchitis."[6] It occurs in 10 to 20% of patients. The symptoms are variable and may include abdominal pain, bloating, nausea, vomiting, fever, and malaise. The effluent usually becomes watery and the volume increases. Occasionally, patients present with anemia resulting from chronic blood loss or, rarely, they bleed acutely from the pouch. The diagnosis can usually be made by endoscopic evaluation of the pouch. The mucosa is seen to be acutely inflamed, and there may be areas of ulceration. Radiologic studies also may be of benefit. The exact cause of this condition is unknown. A single bacterial agent has not as yet been identified, but the condition is presumed to be caused by bacterial overgrowth. Antibiotics, such as metronidazole, are usually effective in alleviating the inflammation. In addition, the reservoir is placed on continuous gravity drainage to decrease stasis. In recalcitrant cases, excision of the pouch may be necessary and, if so, Crohn's disease must be excluded.

The functional results tend to be extremely good. Continence is achieved in virtually all patients in whom the continent ileostomy is functioning satisfactorily. However, some patients may require several operations to achieve this result. Satisfaction with the procedure is high among patients. In a survey of 71 patients, 96% stated that the result was as good as or better than their preoperative expectations.[43] All of these patients stated that they would again choose to undergo surgery to construct the continent ileostomy, and 97% stated that they would have revision surgery if complications should occur. Approximately 10% noted restriction in activity related to work, sports, and leisure activities. Eighty per cent felt their body image was improved, and 68% thought their sexual satisfaction was improved following conversion of their conventional ileostomy to a continent ileostomy. Thus, despite the high surgical complication rate, most patients are extremely happy with what they perceive as an improvement in their quality of life and are willing to undergo multiple procedures in order to live without an appliance. It is for this reason that the continent ileostomy should still be considered a surgical option. However, because of the relatively high complication rate, we now reserve this procedure for patients who have already undergone a total proctocolectomy and wish an appliance-free stoma. Most other patients wishing alternatives for ulcerative colitis choose the ileoanal reservoir procedure, which is known by various names including Parks' pouch, the J or S pouch, or restorative proctocolectomy (Fig. 6–7). In this operation, all the colonic and rectal mucosa to the level of the pelvic floor is excised. The remaining anal mucosa is removed via a perineal approach. In some recent reports, surgeons are now leaving up to 1 cm of anal mucosa in order to increase the sensitivity of the patient to the passage of flatus and stool.[40] A reservoir is constructed from the terminal ileum and anastomosed to the anus. As ulcerative colitis is a superficial mucosal disease, patients theoretically are cured of their disease and the sphincter mechanism is preserved allowing evacuation spontaneously via the anus.

The concept of this procedure is not new. Ravitch and Sabiston reported on its use in 1947, performing a straight ileoanal pull-through technique in two patients.[49] Both patients eventually became continent after complicated postoperative courses. However, this procedure never became popular because published series reported up to 50% incontinence and significant morbidity, including excessive stool frequency, urgency, and perianal irritation. Renewed interest in the procedure can be partially attributed to Kock, whose use of the

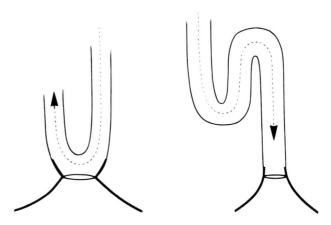

FIGURE 6-7. Schematic drawing of the J pouch described by Utsinomiya and the S pouch described by Parks. The outlet of the S pouch must be kept short to obviate need for self-catheterization.

continent reservoir stimulated others to add a reservoir to the pull-through procedure.

The indications for the ileoanal reservoir procedure are similar to those for the Kock pouch. If rectal cancer complicates ulcerative colitis, the procedure is contra-indicated if preservation of the anal musculature would compromise the chances of curing the rectal cancer. In patients in whom the cancer is situated in the colon or upper part of the rectum, an ileal reservoir and ileoanal anastomosis might be an option. However, total proc-tocolectomy and conventional ileostomy may be pref-erable, particularly if the lesion is advanced and the pa-tient's life span may be shortened. An alternative approach might be to perform a colectomy and leave the rectum in situ. At a later date, if the patient appears to be cured of the cancer, one might consider recon-structive surgery. Dysplasia without any evidence of can-cer need not necessarily alter the decision. However, the presence of severe dysplasia in the rectum might change our recommendation. As with the continent ileostomy, Crohn's disease is a definite contraindication. The risk of disease developing in the small bowel reservoir is of concern, but there is also a significant risk of perianal disease developing.

In selecting patients for the operation, excellent anal sphincter tone is essential. The stool tends to be liquid, so strong anal musculature is necessary to prevent in-continence. Because there is a gradual decline in sphincter tone with increasing years, patients older than 50 years of age should undergo careful clinical exami-nation as well as anal manometry before a final decision is made for or against this procedure. Decisions must be individualized in these patients, depending on their psy-chological and social status. In addition, patients with significant perianal disease, and patients who have had a previous fistulotomy or trauma to the sphincters, are usually not candidates for this procedure. As with the Kock pouch, ileoanal anastomosis may need to be staged in patients who are nutritionally depleted, in those on high doses of steroids or immunosuppressive drugs, or in those who require emergency surgery. In addition, careful patient selection with regard to intellectual and psychological status is as important with this operation as with the continent ileostomy.

The procedure has evolved over the years, but modi-fications have not been as frequent as with the Kock pouch. Initially, there was debate as to the length of the rectal cuff remnant, the amount, if any, of anal mucosa that should be maintained, and the type of pouch con-struction. These topics will be dealt with in a later chap-ter. The use of a temporary defunctioning ileostomy is essential. Rothenberger and colleagues have reported on six patients in whom the procedure was performed in one stage.[51] Septic complications developed in four patients, necessitating a laparotomy. At the Mayo Clinic,[45] 8 of 188 patients had the procedure performed without a defunctioning ileostomy. Although the com-plication rate was not excessive in this group, it must be noted that they were an extremely carefully selected group of patients, and the procedure was performed by very experienced surgeons.

We have recently reviewed our results of the pelvic pouch procedure performed between December 1982 and March 1992.[10] The 483 patients were divided into three groups. In group 1, there were 325 patients who had a hand-sewn ileoanal anastomosis and a defunction-ing ileostomy. In group 2, there were 87 patients with a stapled ileoanal anastomosis and a defunctioning ileos-tomy. In group 3, there were 71 patients with a stapled ileoanal anastomosis without a defunctioning ileostomy. The outcome measures in these patients included sur-gical complications, the reoperation rate, and the func-tional outcome. The factors that were analyzed for their association with an ileoanal anastomotic leak included age, sex, steroid usage, weight, intraoperative difficulty, anastomotic stapling technique, severity of disease at dis-tal margin, and whether the patient had had a previous subtotal colectomy. In the 71 patients who had no de-functioning ileostomy, there were 13 (18%) who had an ileoanal anastomotic leak. This was significantly higher than in either of the other two groups who had covering loop ileostomies. However, of interest was the fact that despite these ileoanal anastomotic leaks, only one pa-tient required a reoperation. That patient had a de-functioning loop ileostomy and subsequently has had closure of the ileostomy. The other patients were man-aged conservatively with intravenous antibiotics and rec-tal tube drainage for varying periods of time and, in all of these patients, the leak healed spontaneously. In ad-dition, the functional outcome in these 13 patients was the same as in those patients who did not have an ileo-anal anastomotic leak.

Most recently, Mattikainen[41] and associates reported only 1 failure in 25 consecutive patients done as a single-stage procedure without an ileostomy. Jarvinen[28] re-ported that there was no difference in terms of compli-cations between those patients who did or did not have a covering loop ileostomy. Launer and Sakier also re-ported no anal anastomotic leaks in a small series of eight patients in whom an intraluminal bypass tube was used in conjunction with a stapled anastomosis. In ad-dition, Sugarman and colleagues[58] reported that the functional results of a stapled ileoanal anastomosis with-out a temporary diverting ileostomy were also excellent and the morbidity low. Therefore, in our own series as well as in others, the omission of a defunctioning ile-ostomy is associated with a higher ileoanal anastomotic leak rate, but spontaneous healing occurs in almost all patients. The functional outcome is not adversely af-fected. Our results also suggest that the rate of ileoanal anastomotic leakage is greatest in men, patients who un-dergo true one-stage procedures without having had a previous subtotal colectomy, patients who are on ster-oids, and patients who are older than age 40.

If an ileostomy has been used, then prior to closure a thorough investigation by digital examination of the ileoanal anastomosis as well as contrast studies, prefer-ably through the distal limb of the loop ileostomy, are undertaken to assure that no leak exists from either the pouch or the anal anastomosis, and that the patient is continent. In doing these contrast studies, it is prefera-ble if a lateral view is taken of the pouch during filling as well as following evacuation, as most of the leaks are detected posteriorly towards the sacral hollow.

The operative mortality rate following this procedure is low. This probably relates to the fact that patients are selected carefully; if they are not in optimal condition, surgery is staged. The most significant complication that can develop is an anal anastomotic leak or dehiscence. Rates reported in the literature vary between 2 and 22%.[45] In our own series,[10] an anal anastomotic leak developed in approximately 10% of patients. Half of these patients presented with pelvic sepsis. The rest had few symptoms related to the anastomotic dehiscence, probably because the anastomosis was protected by a loop ileostomy. If a leak occurs, it is important that it be recognized early and the abscess drained if present.

In our own experience, it has been extremely helpful to use intrarectal ultrasound to localize what can be a very small abscess. Potentially, this can then be drained percutaneously with cure of the problem. Early treatment of sepsis may decrease subsequent fibrosis and result in a much better functional result.

Although treatment must be individualized in these patients, we have had only modest success with the use of an advancement flap technique.[58] In this procedure, the tissue is mobilized between the outlet and the rectal cuff. Usually, about one half to three fourths of the circumference of the outlet must be mobilized to ensure a complete tension-free suture line. Using this technique, approximately 50% of patients with a leak can have the anastomosis and pouch salvaged with an excellent functional result.

Patients who have septic complications and fistulas that have not responded well to multiple attempts at conservative approaches may require a more radical surgical approach. In a number of patients, we have done complete reconstructions of the pouch through an abdominal and a perineal approach. In one patient, we were able to mobilize the entire anastomosis through the perineum and advance the entire anastomosis and redo it. In ten patients, we have performed a complete reconstructive procedure by taking down the ileoanal anastomosis and either redoing it below the site of the fistula or excising the pouch and redoing a second pouch. The success rate in these difficult, complex patients has been very high.

Early treatment of sepsis may decrease subsequent fibrosis and result in a better functional result. Although treatment must be individualized in these patients, we now prefer to surgically repair the anastomosis using an advancement flap technique.[10] The ileal outlet is mobilized between the outlet and the rectal cuff. Usually about one half to three quarters of the circumference of the outlet must be mobilized to ensure a completely tension-free suture line. Using this technique, approximately 50% of patients with a leak can have the anastomosis and pouch salvaged, with an excellent functional result.

Other complications that occur less commonly are anal anastomotic stricture and a leak from the reservoir itself. Complications related to the loop ileostomy have been frequently reported in all series and include high ileostomy output leading to dehydration and intestinal obstruction following closure of the loop ileostomy.[16] Pouchitis also has been a relatively frequent complica-

tion with ileoanal anastomosis and is treated in the same way as described for the Kock pouch.

The assessment of functional results is difficult. The exact number of stools passed in 24 hours depends on several factors, such as daily work habits, concern over the possibility of soiling, dietary factors, and timing of eating. In addition, all reported assessments of stool frequency have been done retrospectively. Most patients cannot remember with accuracy the number of bowel movements passed, and the reported range of bowel movements tends to be arbitrary and inaccurate. Perhaps of even greater importance is the fact that many patients do not feel that the number of bowel movements is a major determinant of the success of the operation. Instead, the fact that they do not have urgency and are continent is of greater importance to them.

Most patients have erratic stool frequency for approximately 3 months after ileostomy closure. Thereafter, the pattern of bowel evacuation stabilizes and in most cases does not interfere with the daily functioning of the individual. The average 24-hour stool frequency reported 6 months after ileostomy closure is between five and six bowel movements per day. Approximately one third of patients require antidiarrheal medications.

The continent ileostomy and the ileal reservoir and ileoanal anastomosis procedures should be considered reasonable alternatives for selected patients with ulcerative colitis. Patients can expect an improved quality of life. The long-term effects of the reservoir are not completely known, but it seems unlikely that there will be long-term metabolic problems. Both procedures are still in evolution and, as such, should be confined to specialized centers in which larger experiences can be accumulated. All patients with ulcerative colitis who are being considered for surgery should be made aware of these alternative procedures. For the surgeon who does not perform these reconstructive surgical procedures, the rectum should be retained so that the patient has the option of having one of these procedures in the future. In an emergency or semiemergency situation, abdominal colectomy can be performed. Usually the disease will then settle, and decisions regarding the fate of the rectum can be made at a future date. The role of the continent ileostomy, as already mentioned, is now more limited. Given the choice, most patients prefer the pelvic pouch over a continent ileostomy. In addition, the complication rate of the continent ileostomy is higher, and it is a more technically demanding procedure to perform. Thus, at present its major role is for those patients who have had a total proctocolectomy and are not candidates for an ileoanal reservoir anastomosis but are dissatisfied with their present status.

GRANULOMATOUS COLITIS

Granulomatous colitis (Crohn's disease of the colon) is also an inflammatory disease of the large bowel of unknown etiology. Crohn and co-workers first described an entity called regional enteritis of the small intestine in 1932. In 1934, Colp described granulomatous disease of both the ileum and cecum and demonstrated that the ileocecal valve did not necessarily represent a barrier to the development of granulomatous disease of the colon. It is now well accepted that Crohn's disease of the large and small intestines is one disease but separate and distinct from ulcerative colitis. Crohn's disease is more common in Jewish patients in westernized countries, is uncommon in the black population, and appears more frequently in westernized civilizations as opposed to the African and Asian nations.

Crohn's disease primarily affects young individuals, with 80% of the cases occurring in patients less than 35 years of age. Disease in which the colon is primarily involved affects women slightly more often than men and occurs at a somewhat older age.

The colon may be involved with granulomatous disease in one of several ways. First, the colon alone may be the site of primary granulomatous disease. The large bowel may be involved in its entirety but, more commonly, there is segmental disease with sparing of the rectum and part of the sigmoid colon. In addition to granulomatous disease of the colon, there may be involvement of the small bowel. This form of ileocolitis is the most common type of Crohn's disease. The diseased area in the colon may be continuous with that in the ileum, or it may present as a skip lesion with normal intervening bowel. The colon may become involved with granulomatous disease only after surgery has been performed for regional ileitis, but this is not particularly common, as most recurrences appear at the site of or proximal to the anastomosis. Finally, the colon may be involved indirectly by fistula formation from a loop of small bowel that is the site of the primary disease. In this case, most commonly there is no primary disease in the colon but only secondary inflammation from the disease in the small intestine.

Pathologic Features

Granulomatous colitis involves all layers of the bowel wall as a transmural reaction (Fig. 6–8). This transmural reaction may be noted grossly, but is present in the earliest phases of the disease when only microscopic changes are noted.[13]

Although the gross and microscopic features of Crohn's disease are well established, there is no single pathognomonic feature. The features of ulcerative colitis and Crohn's colitis are listed in Table 6–1. In approximately 10 to 15% of patients, it may be difficult to unequivocally differentiate Crohn's disease from ulcerative colitis. The term indeterminate colitis has been used in patients in whom a definitive pathologic diagnosis cannot be made.

On macroscopic examination, the bowel wall appears to be thickened, particularly in the submucosal layer. Correspondingly, there is narrowing of the lumen. Edema, thickening, and overgrowth of the mesenteric fat encroaching on the serosal aspect of the bowel are the rule with granulomatous disease of both the large and small intestines (Fig. 6–9). The serosa tends to be hyperemic with visible vessel engorgement, and there are chronic subserosal inflammatory changes with exudate production. Mesenteric lymph nodes may be en-

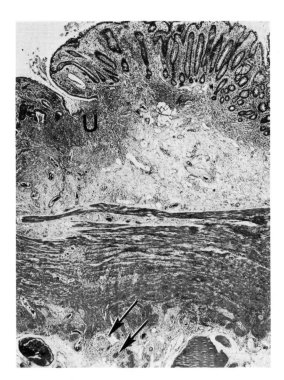

FIGURE 6-8. Crohn's disease of the colon. Transmural involvement is present with mucosal ulceration (*U*), edema of the entire bowel wall, and serosal noncaseating granulomas (*arrows*). (Hematoxylin & eosin, × 25.) (Courtesy of Stanley Hamilton, M.D., Department of Pathology, School of Medicine, Johns Hopkins University.)

larged. The gross appearance of the mucosal surface varies depending upon the extent and severity of the disease. The mucosa may appear to be normal except for hyperemia and edema, or there may be longitudinal ulcers causing the mucosal surface to have a cobblestone appearance. The ulcers vary in depth but usually extend at least to the submucosa and often to the serosa (Fig. 6–10). Because of this, frequently other loops of intestine are adherent to the involved segment, and fis-

TABLE 6-1. CHARACTERISTICS OF ULCERATIVE COLITIS AND CROHN'S COLITIS

FEATURE	CROHN'S COLITIS*	ULCERATIVE COLITIS*
Macroscopic		
Thickened bowel wall	+++	+
Narrowing of bowel lumen	+++	+
Discontinuous disease	++	o
Rectal involvement	o	+++
Deep fissures and fistulas	++	o
Confluent linear ulcers	++	o
Perianal disease	++	o
Microscopic		
Transmural inflammation	+++	+
Submucosal infiltration	+++	+
Submucosal thickening, fibrosis	+++	o
Ulceration through mucosa	+++	++
Fissures	+++	+
Granulomas	++	o

*Features are characterized as being present consistently (+++), frequently (++), infrequently (+), or rarely (o).

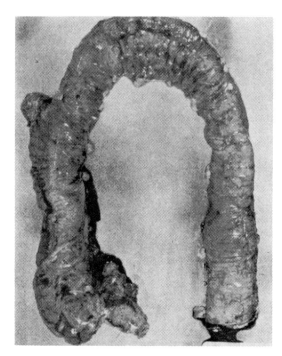

FIGURE 6-9. Serosal surface of colon resected for granulomatous colitis. (From Barnett, W.O., Mora, L.O., and Varner, J.E.: Granulomatous colitis. South. Med. J., *62*:373, 1969. Reprinted by permission from the Southern Medical Journal.)

tulization may occur. In addition, skip areas may be seen.

Microscopic changes include infiltration of inflammatory cells in all layers, and marked submucosal and subserosal thickening and intramural fissures sometimes extending through to the mesenteric fat. Criteria for the histologic diagnosis of granulomatous colitis have been classified as major and minor. The major criteria are (1) giant cell or epitheloid granulomas occurring either intramurally or within regional lymph nodes (Fig. 6–11), (2) intramural fissures or fistulas, (3) transmural mononuclear inflammation, and (4) transmural fibrosis. The minor criteria are (1) submucosal lymphangiectasia, (2) chronic serositis when there has been no prior sur-

gery, (3) muscle wall thickening (greater than twice that of normal), and (4) segmental involvement.

Clinical Features

Symptoms of granulomatous colitis include diarrhea, midabdominal and lower abdominal crampy pain, malaise, and weight loss. Other symptoms and clinical findings include fever, rectal bleeding, anemia, nausea, and vomiting. Occasionally, patients may present with symptoms suggestive of an acute abdomen. It is now recognized that toxic megacolon can complicate Crohn's colitis as well as the other forms of colitis. Extraintestinal manifestations are common, with musculoskeletal abnormalities being the most frequent.

Clinically, granulomatous colitis often has an extremely variable onset and course. Although diarrhea is a dominant feature of both ulcerative colitis and granulomatous colitis, colonic bleeding is less common with granulomatous disease. However, massive hemorrhage from acute granulomatous colitis can occur on occasion. Colonic sinuses, fistulas, and strictures are characteristic of granulomatous colitis, in distinct contrast to ulcerative colitis. However, these internal complications do not occur as frequently in colon disease as they do in terminal ileum disease.

Perianal disease is a frequent complication. It is an extremely troublesome problem and difficult to treat successfully. In the National Cooperative Crohn's Disease Study, more than 46% of patients with colon disease had associated perianal lesions, whereas the rate was 25% in those with disease localized to the small bowel.[48] The perianal lesions can precede the clinical appearance of the colitis by a variable number of years.

Buchmann and Alexander-Williams[8] have classified perianal disease into the following categories: skin lesions, anal canal lesions, fistulas, and hemorrhoids.

Skin lesions include maceration, erosion, ulceration, abscess formation, and skin tags. Because of the frequency of diarrhea in this disease, the skin around the anus may become macerated, leading to ulceration and subcutaneous abscess formation. Skin tags are frequent manifestations. They tend to be edematous and larger,

FIGURE 6-10. Crohn's disease of the colon. The mucosal surface shows serpiginous ulceration and has a cobblestone appearance. The cecum (*CE*) is less severely involved than is the remainder of the colon. (Courtesy of Stanley Hamilton, M.D., Department of Pathology, School of Medicine, Johns Hopkins University.)

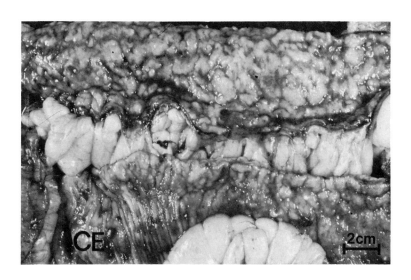

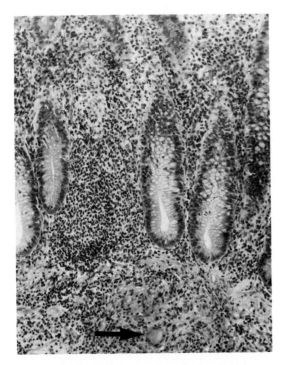

FIGURE 6-11. Crohn's disease of the colon. A noncaseating granuloma with epithelioid macrophages and a multinucleated giant cell (*arrow*) is present in the submucosa. (Hemotoxylin & eosin, × 160.) (Courtesy of Stanley Hamilton, M.D., Department of Pathology, School of Medicine, Johns Hopkins University.)

thicker, and harder than those seen in patients who do not have Crohn's disease.

Anal canal lesions include fissures, ulcers, and stenosis of the anal canal. The fissures tend to be deep and wide with undermined edges. Particularly important is the fact that they may be eccentrically placed in any position around the anal canal, in contradistinction to the uncomplicated fissure in patients who do not have Crohn's disease. The fissures in these patients usually lie in the midline. Unless there is associated sepsis, they tend to be painless.

Fistulas and abscesses are perhaps the most difficult of the perianal lesions. They may arise from an infected anal gland, as in patients who do not have Crohn's disease. However, more commonly they result from penetration by anal canal or rectal fissures or ulcers. On occasion, these fistulas are low lying and can be treated in a conventional manner. However, the more complex fistulas may have a high internal opening with multiple indirect tracks opening on the buttocks or scrotum. Some of these tracks may communicate with each other. The fistulas tend to be chronic, indurated, and cyanotic, but despite their appearance, they are often painless. If the patient does complain of pain, one should suspect an abscess.

Rectovaginal fistulas, which also complicate Crohn's disease, tend to result from direct penetration of rectal wall fissures through and into the vagina. They are a relatively frequent complication of severe perianal Crohn's disease, with rates varying from 3.5 to 20%.[61] Quite frequently these fistulas are relatively asympto-

matic, and no surgical intervention should be attempted. However, if the patient is symptomatic, surgery is indicated. Various local procedures have been described, but none is extremely successful. Some patients will require proctectomy.

Diagnosis of Granulomatous Colitis

Endoscopic evaluation of the colon and rectum is essential. Colonoscopy is particularly important to determine the extent of the disease and, in our opinion, is a more sensitive test than is radiologic examination. For gross features of the disease, endoscopy and radiology might be equivalent. However, for detecting early manifestations of the disease such as superficial aphthous ulcers, colonoscopy is superior. In addition, the discontinuous nature of the disease can be seen better with the colonoscope than on radiologic examination. It is our routine that all patients undergoing surgery for Crohn's disease, including those undergoing surgery for Crohn's disease of the small intestine, have a total colon examination prior to operation in order to fully determine the extent of their disease. The endoscopic appearance of Crohn's disease is quite different from that of ulcerative colitis. The rectum is spared in approximately 50% of patients with large bowel involvement. Depending on the extent and severity of the disease, there may be isolated aphthous ulcers with normal intervening mucosa or there may be irregular mucosal thickening, congestion, edema, and a cobblestone appearance with deep linear ulcerations and fistulas. Although biopsy specimens can be taken, microscopic features pathognomonic of Crohn's disease (i.e., granulomas) are present in only 20 to 40% of cases.[26]

Radiologic features characteristic of Crohn's colitis are similar to those seen in terminal ileal Crohn's disease.[39] The radiologic features that substantiate the diagnosis of Crohn's colitis include skip areas, longitudinal ulcerations, transverse fissures, eccentric involvement, pseudodiverticula, narrowing, strictures, pseudopolypoid changes, a cobblestone pattern, internal fistulas, sinus tracks, and the presence of longitudinal intramural fistula tracks extending parallel to the lumen of the thickened bowel (Fig. 6–12). Any portion of the colon may be involved with Crohn's colitis. The segment least frequently involved is the rectum; those segments most frequently involved are the transverse colon, cecum, and ascending colon. The skip areas must be sought carefully, since discontinuous involvement may be limited to one wall, may appear as a nodular filling defect, or may involve straightening and rigidity of a short segment of the colon. The combination of longitudinal ulcers, edematous mucosa, and transverse linear ulcers produces the cobblestone pattern previously described. Transverse linear ulcers may penetrate so deeply into the wall of the colon that they appear in contour as numerous long, thin spicules perpendicular to the long axis of the bowel or as a sinus track. They may ultimately lead to small intramural abscesses or fistulas.

A small bowel enema or enteroclysis should be included as part of the work-up in patients with Crohn's

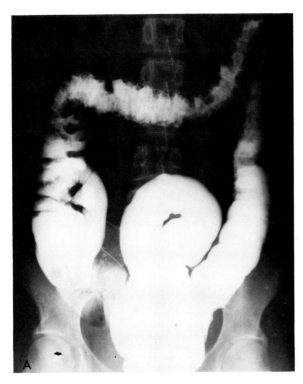
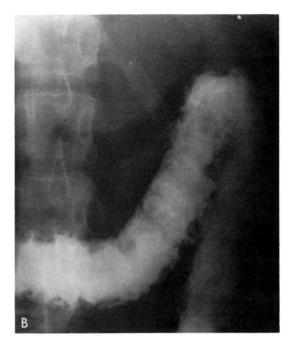

FIGURE 6-12. Granulomatous colitis. *A,* Barium enema showing segmented colonic narrowing and mucosal ulceration, especially of proximal descending colon. *B.* Barium enema showing intramural fistulous track of medial aspect of distal transverse colon.

colitis in order to document the total extent of the disease.

Granulomatous Colitis and Carcinoma

Recently, granulomatous ileocolitis has been recognized as a condition predisposing to the development of colorectal carcinoma. The exact incidence is unknown, but many case reports are documented in the literature. Carcinoma also may occur in chronic perianal fistulas. One difficulty in trying to accurately determine the incidence of carcinoma in this disease is the fact that more patients with Crohn's disease come to surgical intervention at an earlier stage of their disease than do patients with ulcerative colitis. Thus, a relatively small cohort of patients with unresected disease is followed for long periods.

A dilemma arises concerning the association of granulomatous colitis and carcinoma when one considers patient follow-up. Although some authors estimate the incidence of carcinoma in granulomatous colitis to be 20 times higher than in the general population,[62] it is still unclear how frequently these patients should be followed with either colonoscopy or a combination of endoscopy and radiologic examination of the colon. In view of the fact that there does seem to be a definite association between these two entities, our recommendation for patients with Crohn's colitis is similar to that for patients with chronic ulcerative colitis (see earlier discussion).

Therapy

The medical management of granulomatous colitis does not differ significantly from that of granulomatous small bowel disease and includes the use of anti-inflammatory agents, such as sulfasalazine and steroids, and immunosuppressive agents, such as azathioprine and 6-mercaptopurine. Additionally, in recent years, numerous 5-ASA products have been formulated; the role of these agents in the treatment of Crohn's colitis is as yet unknown. Steroid and 5-ASA enemas may be of benefit with limited distal disease. There also are some anecdotal reports about cyclosporine and antituberculous drugs being of benefit.

The evidence suggests that medical management, although often successful on a temporary basis, is certainly not curative. The majority of patients will require surgery for colon or perianal disease. Indications for surgery in Crohn's colitis include failure to respond to medical management, intestinal obstruction, fistula formation, abscess formation, and rectal stricture. The indications for surgery tend to differ somewhat from those for small bowel disease. In a review of patients who underwent surgery at the Cleveland Clinic, bowel obstruction and internal fistula or abscess formation tended to be the most common reasons for surgery in patients with small bowel disease. The indications for surgery in the 127 patients with colon disease were poor response to medical care (25%), internal fistula and abscess (23%), toxic megacolon (20%), perianal disease (19%), and intestinal obstruction (12%).[14]

Like all operations for Crohn's disease, recurrence is

the major consideration. In assessing recurrence rates, it is important to use actuarial figures, since recurrence increases over time. Rates of 5 to 16% per year,[24,29,37] depending on the criteria used to diagnose recurrent disease, have been reported. In a review of patients operated on at the Cleveland Clinic, the overall recurrence rate necessitating surgery was approximately 50% per year.[38] Patients with colon disease alone had a lower recurrence rate than did patients with either ileocolonic disease or ileitis.

The type of operation performed varies depending upon the location of the disease. Because the rectum and distal colon are often spared in Crohn's disease, colectomy with preservation of the rectum is often possible. Ileorectal or ileosigmoid anastomosis has the obvious advantage that an ileostomy is not necessary. However, to perform an ileorectal anastomosis, the rectum should be spared of disease or should be only minimally involved, there should be distensibility of the rectum on air insufflation, sphincter tone should be adequate, there should be a lack of perianal sepsis or fistula, there should be no extensive ileal disease, and patients should not have had a prior significant small bowel resection, as the functional result might be poor. None of these criteria is absolute. In fact, Alexander-Williams and Buchmann reported that the presence of perianal disease made no difference in the functional result.[1] However, they did provide the caveat that patients with perianal disease should be asymptomatic before surgery is advised. These authors found that patients who had disease in the rectum, as assessed sigmoidoscopically, fared poorly compared with those in whom the rectum was spared (55% versus 81% functioning, respectively), but they also reported that patients in whom the ileum was affected with Crohn's disease fared no worse than did those in whom the ileum was free of disease.

One option for the patient may be colectomy, ileostomy, and preservation of the rectum in a fashion similar to that described for ulcerative colitis. This procedure also allows the option for a future anastomosis if local conditions are favorable. An additional advantage of preserving the rectum is that patients may feel that they have the option to have the ileostomy closed at a later date. During this interval, the patient may be better able to become prepared psychologically for a permanent ileostomy in case removal of the rectum in the future becomes necessary or if reanastomosis appears to be unwise. If the rectum is left indefinitely, one should be aware of the possibility of the future development of carcinoma. Addressing this problem, the Cleveland Clinic reported on five patients with inflammatory bowel disease in whom cancer developed in the retained rectum. Two of these patients had Crohn's disease. Symptoms from the cancer developed 22 to 25 years after the onset of the disease.[35]

Segmental resection for Crohn's disease is controversial. It is a rare patient in whom a segmental resection is indicated, since disease usually is widespread and occurs both proximally and distally in a patchy distribution. Although experience is limited, recurrence following segmental resection appears to be increased. Nevertheless, segmental resection may be indicated in

patients who have had multiple bowel resections in the past. In addition, in that rare situation in which the remainder of the colon appears normal, one might consider a segmental resection realizing that there is an increased risk of recurrence.

Loop ileostomy may be useful in situations in which the patient may be in some danger with an unprotected anastomosis—for example, following an ileocolic or sigmoid resection for Crohn's disease associated with an abscess. We do not hesitate to do a temporary loop ileostomy if local factors warrant this approach.

Of interest are recent reports documenting the use of stricturoplasty in Crohn's disease.[2,30,55,59] Crohn's disease, particularly in the small intestine, may present with stricture formation and obstruction, which can be alleviated by a stricturoplasty if the stricture is relatively short. The results from several institutions, including our own, have been encouraging in this respect. Stricturoplasty has been used, for the most part, in Crohn's disease of the small bowel, and its role in the colon appears to be more limited. It has been used in some patients with short colonic strictures and relatively normal intervening bowel, especially when a significant amount of the intestinal tract has already been removed. However, it is unusual for a fibrotic stricture to be the principal indication for surgical intervention in Crohn's disease of the colon. In addition, if a stricture is present, one must be cautious in offering a stricturoplasty as opposed to a resection because of the possibility of carcinoma occurring at the site of the stricture. Stricturoplasty also may be performed at the site of a previous ileocolic anastomosis. To perform a stricturoplasty, the intestine is incised longitudinally and closed horizontally in one layer (Fig. 6–13).

Perianal disease often poses difficult management decisions. In view of the wide spectrum of perianal lesions, treatment will vary. In making management decisions, one must consider the nutritional status of the patient, the extent and severity of disease in the remainder of the gastrointestinal tract, and the symptomatology. Many patients will have relatively few symptoms from perianal disease, even though it may appear to be quite severe.

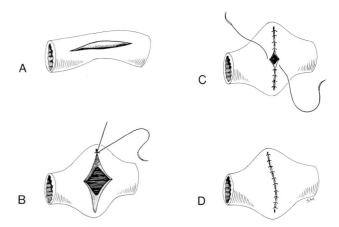

FIGURE 6-13. A short stricture can be managed by stricturoplasty without bowel resection. In this example, the bowel is opened longitudinally (A) and closed transversely (B through D) to overcome the obstruction.

One must understand the limitations of attempting to eradicate the disease. The aim of treatment of perianal disease, as in other forms of Crohn's disease, should be to provide symptomatic relief. Simple measures may be used initially to achieve palliation.

Although treatment may vary according to the specific lesion and the individual patient, certain general measures may be of benefit to most patients. They include hospitalization to improve the nutritional status, assessment of the extent and severity of any proximal disease, and treatment of the proximal disease. Local skin care includes sitz baths, anesthetic ointments, and frequent dressing changes.

Skin tags are rarely symptomatic and one should avoid excising them. If they produce symptoms, it is usually because of irritation caused by diarrhea, which results in edema of the tags and generally responds to local care and control of the diarrhea.

Only rarely is anal dilation indicated for anal stenosis. Dilation should be performed cautiously and should be limited to one or two fingers. In order to maintain a patent anal canal or lower rectum, the patient may also use a dilator on a daily basis. Long strictures, also rare occurrences, are a complication of severe rectal disease and, if symptomatic, may require proctectomy.

The typical broad-based fissure seen in Crohn's disease is often asymptomatic, and no treatment is indicated. If a fissure is painful, one should suspect associated sepsis, and an examination under anesthesia may be necessary to rule out sepsis or to drain an associated abscess. Sphincterotomy should be avoided, as the fissure or ulcer is often a sign of severe rectal or anal involvement. Wounds from Crohn's disease may heal poorly, and the disease itself often has damaged the ability of the sphincters to act reliably. Treatment with antibiotics, such as metronidazole, or with steroid suppositories may be beneficial in treating the commonly associated rectal disease.

Abscesses and fistulas tend to be the most difficult lesions to treat. We do not hesitate to examine the patient under anesthesia to assess more fully the extent of the involvement of perianal and rectal disease. Abscesses require incision and drainage similar to abscesses in patients who do not have Crohn's disease. They should be suspected in patients who complain of severe pain in previously asymptomatic fissures or fistulas. Induration is frequently present, but often only small quantities of pus are found. An examination under anesthesia is essential in these patients to assess the extent of disease. Treatment should consist of incision, unroofing, and drainage of the abscess when necessary (Fig. 6–14). Usually, primary fistulotomy should not be undertaken unless the fistula is of the low-lying variety. In some patients who have associated cellulitis, broad-spectrum antibiotics, such as metronidazole and an aminoglycoside, should be prescribed.

There are several approaches in the treatment of perianal fistulas depending on various local and general factors. The symptomatology, the complexity of the fistula, and the presence or lack of rectal disease are all important. A low fistula may be managed by fistulotomy with good wound healing. For complex fistulas with rectal

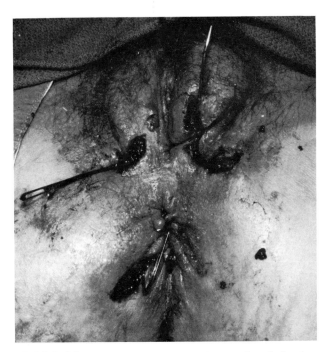

FIGURE 6–14. Conservative unroofing of external tracks has been accomplished. The vertical probe demonstrates the internal opening in the anterior midline.

involvement, treatment should first concentrate on medical management of the rectal disease. Antidiarrheal agents may be used judiciously, and nutritional improvement is important. Simple drainage of the abscesses with unroofing of the fistulas, as well as long-term drains or setons, may be used to effect drainage and keep the patient in an asymptomatic state. Metronidazole, azathioprine, and 6-mercaptopurine have been used with some success.[7,33]

Some patients in whom these treatments fail may require diversion of the intestinal tract as a loop or split ileostomy, and eventually a proctectomy may be needed. Following construction of a loop or split ileostomy to divert the fecal stream, initial improvement in the local perianal disease usually occurs. However, the ileostomy does not usually change the natural history of the disease. Relapse is common, and it is not usually possible to restore intestinal continuity. In our own limited series of 12 patients treated with a diverting loop ileostomy for proctitis or anorectal sepsis, all had temporary remission of the disease.[19] However, five patients required proctocolectomy or proctectomy because of exacerbation of the disease while defunctioning was taking place. None had successful closure of the ileostomy. Similar experiences have been reported by others. In a series of 22 patients who underwent loop ileostomy for anorectal disease, six individuals remained well for 3 to 5 years.[63] Harper and colleagues[23] reported that 21 of 29 patients with anorectal Crohn's disease treated by a split ileostomy had early improvement. However, only six patients had intestinal continuity restored. Eight patients underwent a proctocolectomy and 15 patients retained their defunctioning ileostomies. Despite these poor long-term results, there may be some merit in constructing a diverting ileostomy. First, the general and nutritional status of the patient often improves, and the perianal sepsis resolves to some extent. Therefore, at least in theory, a subsequent proctectomy or other definitive procedure can be performed with less morbidity. Second, some patients may be loathe to have definitive surgery in the form of a proctectomy as an initial procedure. A loop or split ileostomy allows them to adjust psychologically to a stoma without committing themselves to a permanent ileostomy.

If perianal disease continues and is symptomatic, proctectomy may be necessary, although it is not usually required to treat perianal disease alone. Almost always, patients have associated severe rectal involvement. Farmer and co-workers[14] reported that perianal disease was a significant indication for surgery in patients with colonic or ileocolic Crohn's disease. Prior to performing a proctectomy, it is important that the patient be in optimal condition, as this operation is associated with relatively high morbidity. In particular, perineal wound problems are common. Thus, preoperative measures to decrease local sepsis and improve healing should be undertaken. To decrease local sepsis, a staged procedure may be planned. As discussed previously, by performing a subtotal colectomy and ileostomy or ileostomy alone, temporary improvement in local perianal sepsis can be expected. The general status of the patient is improved, and steroids may be tapered prior to performing rectal excision. At the time of surgery, measures to decrease the potential for sepsis should be employed, including an adequate mechanical bowel preparation and administration of prophylactic antibiotics. An intersphincteric dissection of the anorectum along anatomic planes, when possible, and meticulous hemostasis also are important in preventing the perineal wound problems that are frequent complications following proctectomy in patients with Crohn's disease.

There are some reports suggesting that surgical treatment of proximal gastrointestinal disease may result in improvement of perianal disease. Heuman and associates[25] reviewed 20 patients who had perianal disease and underwent proximal bowel resection. Complete healing of the perianal disease occurred within 3 months of the resection in 12 patients. Healing occurred in 80% of patients in whom there was no recurrence of disease, but none of the patients in whom a recurrence subsequently developed healed. In reviewing the Mayo Clinic experience in children, Orkan and Teelander[47] noted that only 5 of 19 patients with intestinal and perianal disease experienced improvement of their perianal disease following intestinal resection and primary anastomosis. These series are retrospective, uncontrolled, and include small numbers of patients. We believe, despite these reports, that an intestinal resection should not be performed unless warranted because of primary intestinal symptoms.

REFERENCES

1. Alexander-Williams, J., and Buchmann, P.: Criteria of assessment for suitability and results of ileorectal anastomosis. Clin. Gastroenterol., 9:409, 1980.
2. Alexander-Williams, J., and Haynes, I.G.: Conservative operations for Crohn's disease of the small bowel. World J. Surg., 9:945, 1985.
3. Aylett, S.O.: Three hundred cases of diffuse ulcerative colitis treated by total colectomy and ileorectal anastomosis. BJM, 1: 1001, 1966.
4. Baker, W.N.W., Glass, R.E., Ritchie, J.K., and Aylett, S.O.: Cancer of the rectum following colectomy and ileorectal anastomosis for ulcerative colitis. Br. J. Surg., 65:862, 1978.
5. Blackstone, M.O., Riddell, R.H., Rogers, D.H.G., and Levin, V.: Dysplasia—association lesion or mass (DALM) detected by colonoscopy in longstanding ulcerative colitis: An indication for colectomy. Gastroenterology, 80:366, 1981.
6. Bonelo, J.C., Thow, G.D., and Manson, R.R.: Mucosal enteritis: A complication of the continent ileostomy. Dis. Colon Rectum, 24: 37, 1981.
7. Brandt, L.J., Bernstein, L.S., Bolui, S.J., and Frank, M.S.: Metronidazole therapy for perineal Crohn's disease: A follow-up study. Gastroenterology, 83:383, 1982.
8. Buchmann, P., and Alexander-Williams, J.: Classification of perianal Crohn's disease. Clin. Gastroenterol., 9:323, 1980.
9. Cohen, Z.: Symposium on the treatment of inflammatory bowel disease in children and adolescents. Part 4. Evolution of the Kock continent reservoir ileostomy. Can. J. Surg., 25:509, 1982.
10. Cohen, Z., McLeod, R.S., Stephen, W., et al.: Continuing evolution of the pelvic pouch procedure. Ann. Surg., 216:506, 1992.
11. Devroede, G.J., Taylor, W.F., Sawer, W.G., et al.: Cancer risks and life expectancy of children with ulcerative colitis. N. Engl. J. Med., 285:17, 1971.
12. Dozois, R.R., Kelly, K.A., Beart, R.W., and Beahrs, O.H.: Improved results with continent ileostomy. Ann. Surg., 192:319, 1980.
13. Farmer, R.G., Hawk, W.A., and Turnbull, R.B.: Regional enteritis of the colon: A clinical and pathological comparison with ulcerative colitis. Am. J. Dig. Dis., 13:501, 1968.
14. Farmer, R.G., Hawk, W.A., and Turnbull, R.B.: Indications for surgery in Crohn's disease: Analysis of 500 cases. Gastroenterology, 71:245, 1976.
15. Fazio, V.W., Fletcher, J., and Montague, D.: Prospective study of the effect of resection of the rectum on male sexual function. World J. Surg., 4:149, 1980.
16. Feinberg, S.M., McLeod, R.S., and Cohen, Z.: Complications of loop ileostomy. Am. J. Surg., 153:102, 1987.
17. Fiocchi, C.: Etiology of mucosal ulcerative colitis. In Jagelman, D. (ed.): Mucosal Ulcerative Colitis. Mount Kisco, NY, Futura Publishing Company, 1986, p. 1.
18. Gilat, T., Lilos, P., Zemishlamy, Z., et al.: Ulcerative colitis in the Jewish population of Tel Aviv–Yafo, III, clinical course. Gastroenterology, 70:14, 1976.
19. Grant, D.R., Cohen, Z., and McLeod, R.S.: Loop ileostomy for anorectal Crohn's disease. Can. J. Surg., 29:32, 1986.
20. Grant, C.S., and Dozois, R.R.: Toxic megacolon: Ultimate fate of patients after successful medical management. Am. J. Surg., 147: 106, 1984.
21. Greenstein, A.J., Sachar, D.B., and Smith, H.: Cancer in universal and left-sided ulcerative colitis—factors determining risks. Gastroenterology, 77:290, 1979.
22. Grundfest, S.F., Fazio, V.W., Weiss, R.A., et al.: The risk of cancer following colectomy and ileorectal anastomosis for extensive mucosal ulcerative colitis. Ann. Surg., 193:9, 1981.
23. Harper, P.H., Keptlewell, M.G., and Lee, E.C.: The effect of split ileostomy on perianal Crohn's disease. Br. J. Surg., 609:608, 1982.
24. Hellers, J.: Crohn's disease in Stockholm county 1955–1974: A study of epidemiology. Acta Chir. Scand., 490:31, 1979.
25. Heuman, R., Bolin, T., Sjodahl, R., et al.: The incidence and course of perianal complications and arthralgia after intestinal resection with restoration of continuity for Crohn's disease. Br. J. Surg., 68:529, 1981.
26. Hill, R.B., Kent, T.H., and Hansen, R.N.: Clinical usefulness of rectal biopsy in Crohn's disease. Gastroenterology, 77:938, 1979.
27. Jalan, K.M., Sircus, W., Card, W.I., et al.: An experience of ulcerative colitis. 1. Toxic dilatation in 55 cases. Gastroenterology, 57: 68, 1969.
28. Jarvinen, H.J., and Luukkonen, P.: Comparison of restorative proctocolectomy with and without covering ileostomy in ulcerative colitis. Br. J. Surg., 78:199, 1991.
29. Karesen, R., Search-Hanssen, A., Thoresen, B.O., and Hertzberg,

J.: Crohn's disease: Longterm results, surgical treatment. Scand. J. Gastroenterol., 16:67, 1981.

30. Kendall, G.P.N., Hawley, P.R., Nicholls, R.J., and Lennard-Jones, J.E.: Strictureplasty. A good operation for small bowel Crohn's disease? Dis. Colon Rectum, 29:312, 1986.

31. Kewenter, J., Ahlman, H., and Hulten, L.: Cancer risk in extensive ulcerative colitis. Surgery, 188:824, 1978.

32. Kock, N.G., Myrvold, H.E., and Nilsson, L.O.: Progress report on the continent ileostomy. World J. Surg., 4:143, 1980.

33. Korelitz, B.I., and Present, D.H.: Favourable effects of 6-mercaptopurine on fistulae in Crohn's disease. Dig. Dis. Sci., 30:58, 1985.

34. Lavery, I.C., Chiulli, R.A., Jagelman, D.G., et al.: Survival with carcinoma arising in mucosal ulcerative colitis. Ann. Surg., 195:508, 1982.

35. Lavery, I., and Jagelman, D.: Cancer in the excluded rectum following surgery for inflammatory bowel disease. Dis. Colon Rectum, 25:522, 1982.

36. Lennard-Jones, J.E., Morson, B.C., Ritchie, J.K., and Williams, C.B.: Cancer surveillance in ulcerative colitis: Experience over 15 years. Lancet, 2:149, 1983.

37. Lennard-Jones, J.E., and Stalder, G.A.: Prognosis after resection of chronic regional ileitis. Gut, 8:332, 1967.

38. Lock, M.R., Farmer, R.G., Fazio, V.W., et al.: Recurrence and reoperation for Crohn's disease. N. Engl. J. Med., 304:1586, 1981.

39. Marshak, R.H.: Granulomatous disease of the intestinal tract (Crohn's disease). Radiology, 114:3, 1975.

40. Martin, L.W., Fischer, J.E., Sayers, H.J., et al.: Anal continence following Soave procedure: Analysis of results in 100 patients. Ann. Surg., 203:525, 1986.

41. Mattikainen, M., Santa Virta, J., and Hiltunen, K.M.: Ileo-anal anastomosis without covering ileostomy. Dis. Colon Rectum, 33:384, 1990.

42. McLeod, R.S., Cohen, Z., and Palmer, J.A.: Management of chronic perineal sinuses by wide excision and split thickness skin grafting. Can. J. Surg., 28:315, 1985.

43. McLeod, R.S., and Fazio, V.W.: Quality of life with a continent ileostomy. World J. Surg., 8:90, 1984.

44. Medical Controversies. Ileostomy or ileorectal anastomosis for ulcerative colitis? BMJ, 1:1459, 1978.

45. Metcalf, A.N., Dozois, R.R., Kelly, K.A., et al.: "J"-pouch anal anastomosis. Ann. Surg., 202:735, 1985.

46. Ohman, U.: Colorectal carcinoma in patients with ulcerative colitis. Am. J. Surg., 144:344, 1982.

47. Orkan, B.A., and Teelander, R.L.: The effect of intra-abdominal resection of fecal diversion on perianal disease in paediatric Crohn's disease. J. Pediatr. Surg., 20:333, 1985.

48. Rankin, G.B., Watts, H.D., Melnyk, C.S., and Kelley, M.L.: National Cooperative Crohn's Disease Study: Extra-intestinal manifestations and perianal complications. Gastroenterology, 77:914, 1979.

49. Ravitch, M.M., and Sabiston, D.C.: Anal ileostomy with preservation of the sphincter. Surg. Gynecol. Obstet., 84:1095, 1947.

50. Riddell, R.H., Goldman, H., Ransohoff, D.L., et al.: Dysplasia in inflammatory bowel disease: Standardized classification with provisional clinical applications. Hum. Pathol., 14:931, 1983.

51. Rothenberger, D.A., Vermeulen, F.D., Christenson, C.E., et al.: Restorative proctocolectomy with ileoreservoir and ileoanal anastomosis. Am. J. Surg., 145:82, 1983.

52. Sackett, D.L., and Whelan, G.: Cancer risks in ulcerative colitis: Scientific requirements for the study of prognosis. Gastroenterology, 78:1632, 1980.

53. Sanford, G.E.: Genetic implications in ulcerative colitis. Am. Surg., 37:512, 1971.

54. Scott, H.W., Wimberly, J.E., Shull, H.J., et al.: Single stage proctocolectomy for severe ulcerative colitis. Am. J. Surg., 119:87, 1970.

55. Serra, J., McLeod, R.S., and Cohen, Z.: Natural history of stricturoplasty in Crohn's disease—eight year experience. (In press.)

56. Slaney, G., and Brooke, B.N.: Cancer in ulcerative colitis. Lancet, 2:694, 1959.

57. Strauss, R.J., Flint, G.W., Platt, N., et al.: The surgical management of toxic dilatation of the colon: A report of 28 cases and review of the literature. Ann. Surg., 184:682, 1976.

58. Sugarman, H.J., Newsome, H.H., DeCosta, G., and Zfass, M.: Stapled ileo-anal anastomosis for ulcerative colitis and familial polyposis without a temporary diverting ileostomy. Ann. Surg., 213:606, 1991.

59. Tjandra, J.J., Fazio, V.W., and Lavery, I.C.: Results of multiple stricturoplasties in diffuse Crohn's disease of the small bowel. Aust. N. Z. J. Surg., 63:95, 1993.

60. Turnbull, R.B., Jr., Hawk, W.A., and Weakley, F.L.: Surgical treatment of toxic megacolon: Ileostomy and colostomy to prepare patients for colectomy. Am. J. Surg., 122:325, 1971.

61. Tuxen, P.A., and Castro, A.F.: Rectovaginal fistula in Crohn's disease. Dis. Colon Rectum, 22:58, 1979.

62. Weedon, D.D., Shorter, R., Ilstrup, D., et al.: Crohn's disease and cancer. N. Engl. J. Med., 289(21):1099, 1973.

63. Zelas, B., and Jagelman, D.G.: Loop ileostomy in the management of Crohn's colitis in the debilitated patient. Ann. Surg., 191:164, 1981.

Chapter 7

VASCULAR LESIONS OF THE COLON

RONALD N. KALEYA / SCOTT J. BOLEY

During the past three decades, vascular lesions of the colon have been recognized as a major cause of rectal bleeding, especially in the geriatric patient population. However, despite the plethora of articles published on these vascular abnormalities, confusion and controversy remain concerning the pathogenesis, natural history, appropriate therapy, and proper naming of these lesions. Although many reports have grouped them together, several distinct entities (Table 7–1), each having as its common presentation the passage of blood via the rectum, can now be identified.

VASCULAR ECTASIA

Vascular ectasias of the colon are by far the most common vascular lesions found in the intestines and probably are the most frequent cause of recurrent lower intestinal bleeding in patients older than 60 years of age.[9,10] They are distinct pathologic and clinical entities,[8,30] and in our concept of their pathogenesis,[9,10] they arise from the age-related degeneration of previously normal colonic blood vessels. Vascular ectasias almost always occur in the cecum or the proximal ascending colon, are usually multiple rather than single, and are less than 5 mm in diameter. They can only rarely be identified by gross inspection or routine pathologic examination, are diagnosed by colonoscopy or angiography, and, unlike many congenital or neoplastic vascular abnormalities, they are not associated with synchronous angiomatous lesions in the skin, mucous membranes, or other viscera.

Incidence

There does not appear to be any sex predilection for vascular ectasia. Most patients are older than 50 years of age; only one patient in our series was younger than 55 years, and two thirds were older than 70 years. Several investigators[9,10,17] have shown that mucosal vascular ectasias of the the right colon can be found in more than

25% of completely asymptomatic patients older than 60 years of age. Accurate comparison of data from different investigators is difficult, however, because of the use of varying terms for the same abnormalities and the same terms to describe different lesions. For example, the terms angiodysplasia and angioectasia have been used to describe lesions that are histologically and angiographically identical to what we call vascular ectasia,[3,17,46] and also to describe vascular abnormalities of the intestinal tract in general.[18,37] There have been several reports of angiodysplasia in the small bowel,[2] in the left colon,[43] in association with Meckel's diverticulum,[20] and in adolescents, but none of these reports has contained corroborating histologic evidence. We have personally reviewed tissue sections from reported vascular ectasia or angiodysplasia in sites other than the right colon and have found morphologic changes totally different from those seen with true ectasia. Clearly, if investigators are to establish the specific occurrence of vascular ectasia in the young, in the small bowel, or in the left colon, histologic proof of the nature of these lesions is necessary. Only when inconsistencies in the terms used to describe vascular lesions are finally eliminated can the experience of many clinicians be combined and compared, further enhancing our understanding of these entities.

Etiology and Pathogenesis

Any hypothesis concerning the formation of colonic vascular ectasia must account for their prevalence in elderly persons, their small size and multiplicity, and their preponderance in the cecum and right colon. Although the cause of these lesions has not been definitively established, injection and clearing studies lead us to postulate that vascular ectasia is a degenerative lesion associated with aging and represents a unique entity distinct from previously described intestinal vascular abnormalities.[9,10] We believe that over the course of many years, normal processes of contraction and distention cause repeated, partial and intermittent, low-grade obstruction of submucosal veins, especially in areas in

72

TABLE 7-1. VASCULAR LESIONS OF THE COLON

Vascular ectasia
Hemangioma
Congenital arteriovenous malformation
Colonic varices
Telangiectasia
Syndrome—related lesions (e.g., Klippel-Trenaunay-Weber
   syndrome, Maffucci's syndrome
Others
   Vascular spiders and venous stars of liver disease
   Degenerative phlebectasia of the elderly
   Vasculitic lesions
   Focal hypervascularity of ulcerative, Crohn's, and ischemic colitis
   Neovascularity of radiation colitis
   Angiosarcoma (e.g., Kaposi's sarcoma)

which they pierce the muscle layers of the colon. These repeated episodes of transiently elevated pressure result in dilation and tortuosity, initially of the submucosal veins and then, in a retrograde manner, of the venules and the arteriolar-capillary-venular units draining into them. Ultimately, the capillary rings surrounding the crypts dilate, and the competency of the precapillary sphincters is lost, thus producing a small arteriovenous communication (Fig. 7-1). The latter is responsible for the early filling vein, which was the original angiographic hallmark of this lesion.

The presence of these abnormal submucosal veins without a mucosal lesion, or the presence of these veins underlying only a minute mucosal ectasia supplied by a normal artery, originally pointed to dilation of the submucosal vein as the primary change rather than as a secondary result of arterialization from an arteriovenous communication. Indeed, support for the theory that intramural veins can be partially obstructed by functional colonic activity can be found in previous studies. Evidence that venous flow in the bowel is diminished by colonic motility, increased tension in the wall, and increased intraluminal pressure comes from investigations by Semba and Fujii,[35] Chou and Dabney,[12] and Noer and Derr.[31] Rhythmic alterations in venous blood flow and venous pressure related to colonic contractions have also been demonstrated.[31] The prevalence of these degenerative lesions in the right colon is explained by the greater tension found in the cecal wall, as compared with other parts of the colon, according to LaPlace's law.

Approximately 25% of patients with bleeding ectasias have a history or clinical diagnosis of aortic stenosis, and some investigators ascribe a causative role in ectasia to aortic valvular disease. We do not believe that there is a causative relationship between aortic stenosis and the development of colonic ectasia. Rather, there may be some feature of aortic stenosis, perhaps the low pulse pressure or decreased systemic perfusion characteristic of this disorder, that increases the chance of bleeding in individuals who have vascular ectasia. For instance, a low flow state may well cause ischemic necrosis of the single layer of endothelium that often separates ectatic vessels from the colonic lumen. Alternately, a roughened or stenotic aortic valve could produce a mild consumptive coagulopathy or a subtle alteration in platelet function, and these defects—combined with a thin-walled, dilated, mucosal vascular lesion—may cause an ectasia to bleed.[26]

In view of these factors and contradictory evidence concerning the beneficial effect of aortic valve replacement in the treatment of bleeding ectasia, it seems prudent to consider cardiac disease and colonic lesions as separate and only potentially related entities. A rational approach would appear to be that initial therapy be directed to the colonic lesion if the patient's cardiac status does not require surgical correction. If valvular replacement is indicated, however, it should be done first and treatment of the colonic ectasia deferred until there is continuing or recurrent postoperative bleeding.

Pathologic Features

Histologic identification of vascular ectasia is difficult without special techniques, as demonstrated by our own early experience.[9,10] Of seven patients with angiographically demonstrated colonic ectasias who were studied only by routine gross examination and microscopic study of random or selected colonic sections, a mucosal ectasia could be identified in only two patients.

Our present technique for the localization and identification of vascular ectasia consists of the injection of a silicone rubber compound (Microfil) through catheters placed in one or more of the arteries supplying the colon. Specimens are then dehydrated in increasing concentrations of ethyl alcohol and are cleared with methyl salicylate. This produces a transparent specimen with a filled vascular bed that is studied by dissection microscopy, using direct light as well as transillumination.

We have used this method in 25 colons.[9,10,30] One or more mucosal ectasias, measuring 1 mm to 1 cm in diameter, were identified in all of the specimens (Fig. 7-2). Seven colons contained two lesions, and 11 colons contained three or more lesions. The ectasias were all located within the cecum and the proximal part of the ascending colon; the most distal one was 23 cm from the ileocecal valve. All of the cleared specimens had prominent dilated and tortuous submucosal veins both beneath the ectasias and in areas in which the mucosal vessels appeared normal (Fig. 7-3). The colon from the oldest patient, an 88-year-old man, contained approximately 50 mucosal ectasias of varying sizes.

Microscopically, vascular ectasias consist of dilated, distorted, thin-walled vessels, mostly lined only by endothelium and, less frequently, by a small amount of smooth muscle. Structurally, they appear to be ectatic veins, venules, and capillaries. The degree of distortion of the normal vascular architecture varies in different lesions, but the most consistent, and apparently the earliest, abnormality noted in all of the lesions we have studied is the presence of dilated, often huge, submucosal veins (Fig. 7-4A). Progressively more extensive lesions show increasing numbers of dilated and deformed vessels traversing the muscularis mucosa and involving the mucosa until, in the most severe lesions, it is replaced by a maze of distorted, dilated vascular channels (see Fig. 7-4B).

Although the typical histologic findings showed only abnormal thin-walled veins, venules, and capillaries lo-

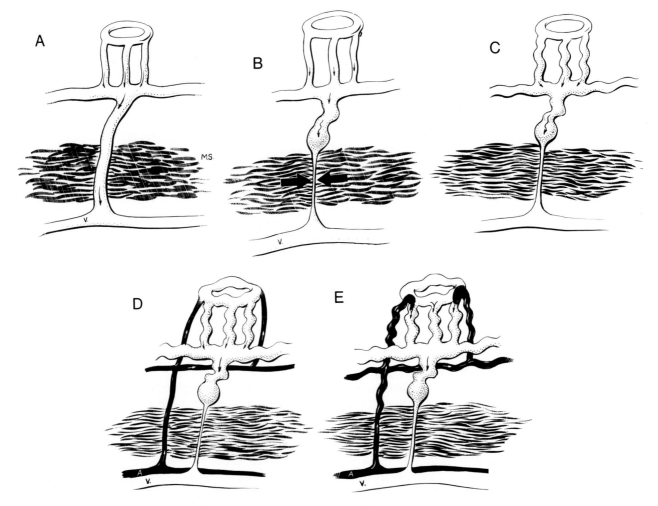

FIGURE 7–1. Diagrammatic illustration of proposed concept of the development of cecal vascular ectasia. *A*, Normal state of vein perforating muscular layers. *B*, With muscular contraction or increased intraluminal pressure, the vein is partially obstructed. *C*, After repeated episodes over many years, the submucosal vein becomes dilated and tortuous. *D*, Later, the veins and venules draining into the abnormal submucosal vein become similarly involved. *E*, Ultimately, the capillary ring becomes dilated, the precapillary sphincter becomes incompetent, and a small arteriovenous communication is present through the ectasia. (From Boley, S.J., Sammartano, R.J., Adams, A., et al.: On the nature and etiology of vascular ectasias of the colon: Degenerative lesions of aging. Gastroenterology, *72*:650, 1977, with permission.)

calized to the submucosa and mucosa, enlarged arteries and thick-walled veins were seen in a few instances. This is not a surprising finding in advanced lesions in which the dilated arteriolar-capillary-venular unit has become a small arteriovenous fistula. As classically described by Holman,[21] the artery supplying an arteriovenous fistula becomes enlarged, sclerotic, and thin walled, and the vein draining it becomes arterialized and shows both intimal and smooth muscle hypertrophy. Once the ectasia becomes an arteriovenous communication, therefore, the pathophysiologic, histopathologic, and angiographic findings change. The presence of large, thick-walled arteries is much more typical of other vascular lesions and makes the diagnosis of vascular ectasia suspect.

Clinical Aspects

Except for gastrointestinal bleeding, vascular ectasia of the colon is an asymptomatic pathologic and clinical entity. Bleeding from ectasias is most often recurrent and low grade, although approximately 15% of patients, some of whom are in shock, present with acute massive hemorrhage. The nature and degree of bleeding frequently vary in the same patient during different episodes, and patients may have bright red blood, maroon-colored stools, and melena on separate occasions. In 20 to 25% of episodes, only tarry stools are passed; in 10 to 15% of patients, bleeding is evidenced by iron-deficiency anemia and stools that intermittently contain occult blood. This spectrum reflects the variable rate of bleeding from the ectatic capillaries, venules and, in advanced lesions, arteriovenous communications. In more than 90% of patients, the bleeding stops spontaneously.

In the early series, as many as 30% of patients with colonic vascular ectasias had undergone prior surgery for other suspected sources of intestinal bleeding, including partial gastrectomy, vagotomy with antrectomy

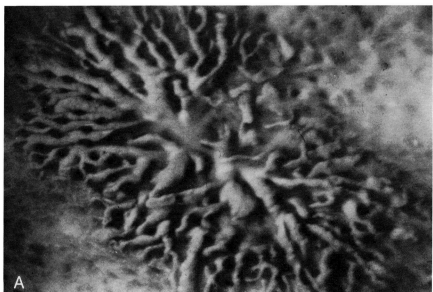

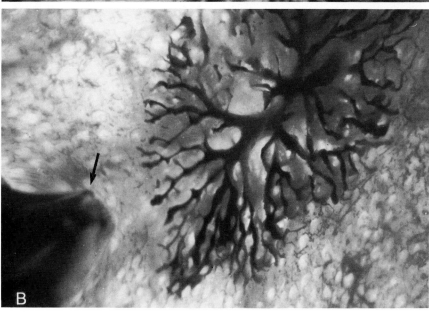

FIGURE 7-2. *A*, The "coral reef" appearance of an ectasia in an injected but not cleared colon. Normal crypts are seen surrounding the ectasia. *B*, Transilluminated, cleared colon showing ectasia involving the mucosal capillaries and venules. Pinhead shown for size comparison (*arrow*). (*A*, From Mitsudo S., Boley, S.J., Brandt, L.J., et al.: Vascular ectasias of the colon. Hum. Pathol. *10*:585, 1979, with permission. *B*, From Sprayregen, S., and Boley, S.J.: Vascular ectasias of the colon, JAMA, *239*:962, 1978. Copyright 1978, American Medical Association.)

or pyloroplasty, and left colon resection for purported diverticular bleeding.

None of the patients in our series who underwent a left colectomy had angiographic or histologic documentation of a bleeding site at the time of the prior operation. More recently, the percentage of patients having had previous operations has decreased, as the diagnosis is established earlier and physicians have been more willing to refer patients for endoscopic ablation or operation before repeated episodes of bleeding occur. The problem of differentiating blood loss from vascular ectasias or diverticulosis when bleeding is not demonstrated endoscopically or angiographically is compounded by the frequent occurrence of these lesions without bleeding in people over 60 years of age. Diverticulosis has been estimated to occur in up to 50% of the population older than 60 years of age, and we previously have shown that mucosal vascular ectasias of the right colon can be found in more than one quarter of

people the same age with no evidence of bleeding. Therefore, without a demonstrated site of hemorrhage, the only basis for determining if the bleeding is caused by identified ectasias or by diverticulosis is the indirect evidence provided by the course of the patient after resection of the suspected lesion. Furthermore, in some patients with angiographically confirmed vascular ectasias, an additional unrelated and undetected nondiverticular lesion may actually be responsible for the blood loss.[33,42] The prevalence of a second, different type of bleeding lesion in patients with vascular ectasias is not known, and the use of conflicting and inconsistent terminology again makes comparison among different studies difficult. However, several investigators have reported recurrent lower intestinal bleeding in approximately 20% of patients who have undergone right hemicolectomy for angiographically proven vascular ectasias,[8,34] suggesting that a second source may be found in as many as one fifth of affected patients.

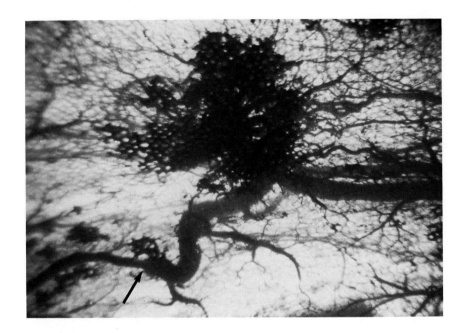

FIGURE 7–3. Transilluminated, cleared colon showing a mucosal ectasia surrounded by normal crypts with ectatic venules leading to a large, distended, tortuous, underlying submucosal vein. A sharp constriction (*arrow*) can be seen where the vein traverses the muscle layers. (From Boley, S.J., Brandt, L.J., and Mitsudo, S.: Vascular lesions of the colon. *In* Stollerman, G.H. [ed.]: Advances in Internal Medicine, Vol. 29. Copyright © 1984 by Year Book Medical Publishers.)

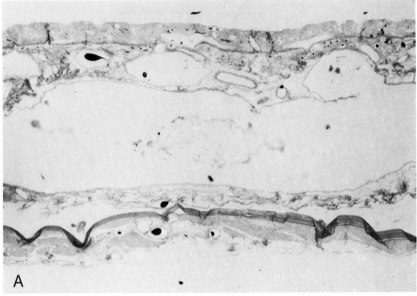

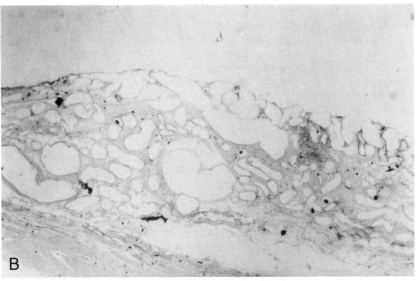

FIGURE 7–4. *A,* A large distended vein completely filling the submucosa with a few dilated venules in the overlying mucosa. This is the hallmark of early ectasia. (Hematoxylin & eosin, ×50.) *B,* Advanced lesion showing total disruption of the mucosa with replacement by ectatic vessels. Only one layer of endothelium separates the lumen of the cecum from the lumina of the dilated vessels. (Hematoxylin & eosin, ×50.) *A,* From Boley, S.J., Sammartano, R.J., Adams, A., et al.: On the nature and etiology of vascular ectasias of the colon: Degenerative lesions of aging. Gastroenterology, *72:* 650, 1977, with permission. *B,* From Boley, S.J., Brandt, L.J., and Mitsudo, S.: Vascular lesions of the colon. *In* Stollerman, G.H. [ed.]: Advances in Internal Medicine, Vol. 29. Copyright © 1984 by Year Book Medical Publishers.)

Diagnosis

The evaluation of a patient in whom bleeding from a vascular ectasia is suspected essentially is the same as that for lower gastrointestinal bleeding. The diagnostic approach that we use in these patients varies with their age, the presence or lack of active bleeding, and the severity of hemodynamic compromise caused by the blood loss.

All patients with lower gastrointestinal bleeding should have coagulation studies (including platelet count, prothrombin time, and partial thromboplastin time) performed to identify any clotting abnormalities, as well as a careful digital rectal examination to help exclude any anorectal disease. To facilitate further evaluation, patients with lower gastrointestinal bleeding are separated into those with major bleeding and those without major bleeding.

The approach to the diagnosis and treatment of patients with severe lower intestinal bleeding is outlined in Figure 7–5. Emphasis is placed upon converting an emergency situation to an elective one by stopping the bleeding, at least temporarily. The role of endoscopy has evolved from a secondary diagnostic tool to the primary diagnostic and treatment modality. The conversion of an emergent situation to an elective one can reduce the need for surgery and decrease the mortality and morbidity associated with the bleeding episode.

Major Bleeding

Major bleeding is identified either by (1) acute blood loss capable of causing the hemodynamic signs of hypovolemia to develop or by (2) the sudden passage of large amounts of bloody, maroon, burgundy, or melenic stools even when there is no hemodynamic compromise.

In these patients, nasogastric lavage is the first study to follow assessment of the clotting status and digital rectal examination, and is necessary because 10 to 15% of major lower gastrointestinal bleeding begins in the upper gastrointestinal tract.[11] The lack of blood and the presence of bile in the aspirate virtually exclude a source of bleeding proximal to the ligament of Treitz. A clear, nonbilious aspirate eliminates the possibility of an actively bleeding lesion in the esophagus or stomach, but it does not exclude the possibility of one in the duodenum, since the pylorus may be closed. Therefore, a nonbloody, nonbilious aspirate is an indication for upper gastrointestinal endoscopy in actively bleeding patients. A blood urea nitrogen (BUN) level greater than 30 mg/dl occurs in approximately two thirds of patients with major bleeding proximal to the colon and may help guide the clinician toward a putative site of bleeding. Standard proctosigmoidoscopic examination is performed to exclude the presence of an anorectal and distal sigmoid pathologic condition.

Rigid sigmoidoscopy is followed by abdominal scintigraphy in patients who are actively bleeding or in those in whom it is uncertain as to whether bleeding has ceased, and by colonoscopy in patients in whom bleeding has stopped. Abdominal scintigraphy is performed first in patients thought to be actively bleeding because it may both localize the anatomic site of blood loss and detect whether bleeding has stopped, better enabling the clinician to decide whether further evaluation should proceed using endoscopy or angiography. Scintigraphy is noninvasive, safer than angiography and colonoscopy, more sensitive in detecting active bleeding than is angiography, and capable of identifying bleeding over a 24-hour period, not just during the brief period of a colonoscopic examination or an angiographic contrast injection.[1,47] When a radioactive agent is injected into a patient who is actively bleeding, a fraction of the injected material will extravasate at the bleeding site, and each time the blood recirculates, another fraction of the radionuclide extravasates. Ideally, the radiolabeled agent should be actively cleared by a specific target organ out of the scanning field, allowing a contrast to be seen between radionuclide accumulation at the site of bleeding and the surrounding background.

Two radionuclides commonly used to detect intestinal bleeding are ^{99m}Tc-labeled sulfur colloid and ^{99m}Tc-labeled red blood cells. Previously, ^{99m}Tc-labeled sulfur colloid scanning was considered the more sensitive of the two techniques and, because it is rapidly cleared from the circulation (plasma half-life of only 2 to 3 minutes), the better agent for detecting active bleeding. Conversely, ^{99m}Tc-labeled red blood cell scanning, although it was thought be less sensitive than sulfur colloid scanning, was considered very useful for detecting intermittent bleeding, primarily because of the 24-hour half-life of technetium-labeled red blood cells. Thus, it was recommended that both agents be administered concurrently.[6] However, it now appears that only ^{99m}Tc red blood cell labeling is necessary, as both clinical and experimental studies[40] have found it and sulfur colloid equally sensitive, reliably detecting active bleeding even at rates less than 0.1 ml/min. Unlike sulfur colloid scanning, frequent serial studies can be obtained with red blood cell scintigraphy for up to 36 hours following a single injection of the radionuclide,[47] allowing lesions that bleed intermittently to be detected. Furthermore, ^{99m}Tc-labeled red blood cells are not cleared by the liver and spleen as is sulfur colloid, so bleeding in the area of these organs, often obscured with sulfur colloid, can be visualized.

Active Major Bleeding

If scintigraphy demonstrates a bleeding site in the colon and the patient is hemodynamically stable, colonoscopy is performed. In this circumstance, clotted blood within the colon often obscures visibility and increases the risks of the procedure. Because of these increased dangers, if the bleeding site is shown by the scan to be proximal to the midtransverse colon, colonoscopy should be halted promptly if technical difficulties are encountered. If a site of hemorrhage is identified distal to the midtransverse colon, extra efforts to cleanse the bowel and proceed cautiously are usually rewarding. Modern colonoscopes have a large suction capacity and allow greater amounts of blood to be aspirated. Further, newly developed variable-speed pumps substantially im-

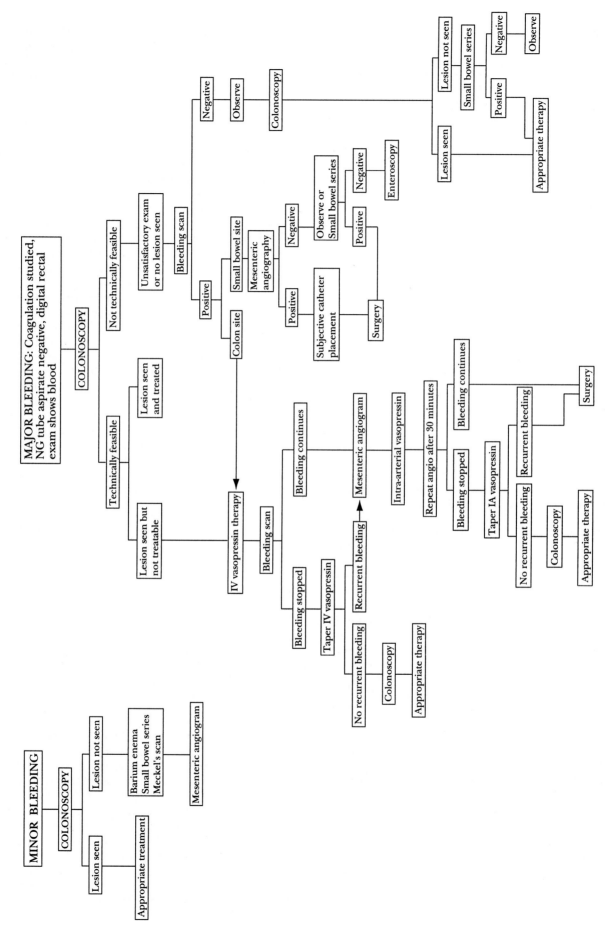

FIGURE 7-5. Diagnostic algorithm for lower intestinal bleeding.

prove the endoscopist's ability to cleanse the colon by fragmentation and dispersion of blood and debris.

Although colonoscopy is playing an increasing role in the diagnosis of colonic vascular lesions, the endoscopist's ability to diagnose the specific nature of a given lesion is limited by the similar appearance of many vascular, inflammatory, neoplastic, and iatrogenic abnormalities. Indeed, vascular ectasias can be mimicked by any of the lesions listed in Table 7–1. Thus, all vascular lesions must be evaluated as soon as they are observed, preferably on entering the colon rather than on withdrawal, in order to avoid traumatic and suction artifacts that may further limit the endoscopist's ability to identify and differentiate these lesions.[14]

If neither scintigraphy nor colonoscopy is revealing, if colonoscopy is not technically feasible, or if scintigraphy demonstrates bleeding within the small bowel and the patient continues to bleed actively, angiography is performed. Flush aortograms have not proved helpful, and therefore the initial study is a selective superior mesenteric artery angiogram. This type of arteriography is performed first because both the 6 m of small bowel between the duodenojejunal junction and the ileocecal valve and the right colon, in which the majority (50 to 80%) of diverticular bleeding and all bleeding from angiographically and histologically proven vascular ectasias occur, are served by the superior mesenteric artery. If this study produces normal results, inferior mesenteric artery and celiac axis studies are performed, in that order.

Mesenteric arteriography may be productive both in patients with active lower intestinal tract bleeding and in patients in whom the bleeding has stopped. Extravasation of contrast material represents the angiographic equivalent of active hemorrhage and can be seen with bleeding rates as low as 0.5 ml/min,[32] whereas angiographic signs of tumor neovascularization or vascular lesions may identify the presumed cause and location of the bleeding. Angiography can be diagnostic and can also provide access for treatment. In 80% of cases, active bleeding can be stopped, at least temporarily, by the transcatheter infusion of vasopressin. Transcatheter embolization of ectasia has been reported but should be employed only in desperate situations because of the danger of infarction.

Angiography is successful in identifying the source of major lower intestinal bleeding in approximately two thirds of patients. Pooling of extravasated contrast material in a diverticulum is the angiographic sign of diverticular bleeding and was present in 75% of patients with diverticular bleeding in the series by Welch and colleagues.[46] In contrast, extravasation has been shown in only 10 to 20% of patients bleeding from vascular ectasias of the colon, since the bleeding is usually episodic. However, the presence of other angiographic signs enables the diagnosis of colonic ectasia or other vascular lesions of the small and large bowel to be made even when there is no active bleeding. There are three major angiographic signs of ectasia (Fig. 7–6). The earliest sign to develop in the evolution of an ectasia, and hence the one most frequently seen, is a densely opacified, dilated, tortuous, slowly emptying intramural vein

that reflects ectatic changes in the submucosal veins. This sign is present in more than 90% of patients with ectasias. A vascular tuft, present in 70 to 80% of patients, represents a more advanced lesion and corresponds to extension of the degenerative process to mucosal venules. An early filling vein is a sign of even more advanced changes and reflects an arteriovenous communication through a dilated arteriolar-capillary-venular unit. It is a late sign, present in only 60 to 70% of patients. All three angiographic signs are present in more than one half of patients with bleeding ectasias. Intraluminal extravasation of contrast material alone is inadequate to diagnose an ectasia, but when seen in conjunction with at least one of the three signs of ectasia, it is indicative of a ruptured mucosal lesion.

On rare occasions, vigorous resuscitation with intravenous fluids and compatible blood products may fail to stabilize the patient in whom there is major bleeding. Colonoscopy is best avoided in hemodynamically unstable patients; emergent angiography is the procedure of choice. Transcatheter or intravenous vasopressin will usually control bleeding and convert an emergency procedure into an elective one, thus saving the patient unnecessary and potentially debilitating surgery.

Major Bleeding that Has Ceased

In patients in whom there is lower gastrointestinal bleeding and proctosigmoidoscopy and nasogastric aspiration produce normal results and bleeding has ceased, scintigraphy is not performed, and colonoscopy is the initial diagnostic procedure. Again, the presence of blood clots may severely limit visualization, obscure the lesion, and make passage of the colonoscope technically difficult and hazardous. In these instances, cleansing enemas and lavage carefully delivered through the colonoscope can be used in an attempt to clean the lumen and bowel wall. If these efforts fail, it is wise to postpone the examination, prepare the patient with a polyethylene glycol–based agent (Golytely, Colyte), and repeat the procedure. As discussed previously, vascular lesions must be evaluated as soon as they are observed, preferably on entering the colon.

If complete and satisfactory colonoscopic examination reveals no explanation for the bleeding other than diverticulosis, double-contrast barium studies of the colon, the upper gastrointestinal tract, and the small bowel are indicated. Selective mesenteric angiography has been the most informative study in our experience, if both colonoscopy and barium opacification studies are normal or show only the presence of diverticula. Other techniques such as sequential long-tube aspiration of the intestine and small bowel enteroscopy also may be of value.[25] During angiography, the superior and inferior mesenteric arteries and the celiac axis are injected, in that order. Arteriography, when performed in patients whose bleeding has stopped, is used primarily to diagnose tumor neovascularity or vascular lesions, many of which have characteristic angiographic findings, permitting them to be identified when extravasation is not present.

Occasionally, an initially normal ^{99m}Tc-labeled red

blood cell study, performed because it was not apparent clinically whether bleeding had stopped, may reveal extravasation during serial scanning and localize a lesion that bleeds intermittently.

Patients with recurrent or persistent major bleeding for which no site of hemorrhage is found may require exploratory laparotomy with attempts at intraoperative localization (e.g., intraoperative enterocolonoscopy) in order to avoid blind resection of part or all of the colon.

Minor Bleeding

Minor bleeding is identified either by (1) a chemical test for blood in the stool (occult lower gastrointestinal bleeding) or by (2) the passage of hemodynamically insignificant amounts of either gross blood via the rectum or melena. Although bleeding of this type has been identified in one quarter to one third of patients with ectasias, it is probably less common. Until recently, evaluation of patients with minor bleeding consisted of rigid proctosigmoidoscopy followed by a single-contrast bar-

ium enema study. However, this approach is suboptimal or inadequate in most patients, since (1) flexible fiberoptic sigmoidoscopy (sigmoidoscopy using a 60-cm flexible fiberscope) cannot visualize the right colon and will therefore miss 40% of mass lesions[11] and all vascular ectasias and (2) double- or air-contrast barium enema (the highest resolution contrast study) will be equivocal in 20% of cases[28] and will regularly miss 40% of polyps, 33% of cancers, 60% of discrete ulcerations and colitis,[16,44,45] and all mucosal or submucosal vascular lesions. Conversely, colonoscopy can reliably visualize the entire mucosal surface of the colon and should be the initial diagnostic study in patients with minor bleeding. Adequate colon preparation without fear of significant weight loss, fluid depletion, or electrolyte abnormalities is now possible within 6 hours in 90% of patients (using a polyethylene glycol solution). Retroflexion of the colonoscope in the rectal vault, combined with careful and meticulous examination of the anus during egress of the instrument, will provide sufficient examination of the anorectum, thereby replacing proctosigmoidoscopy.

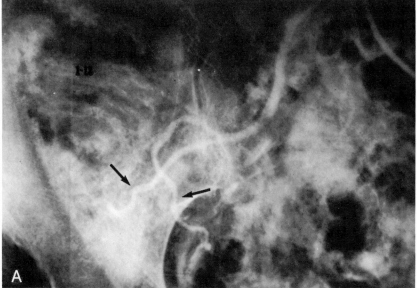

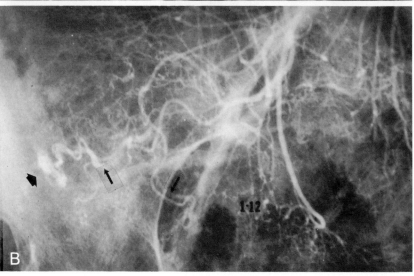

FIGURE 7-6. *A*, SMA arteriogram from a patient with vascular ectasias showing only two densely opacified, slowly emptying, dilated, tortuous cecal veins (*arrows*) at 14 seconds. Note the late visualization of the ileocolic vein after other veins have cleared. *B*, Arterial phase from the same arteriogram showing vascular tuft (*large arrow*) and two early filling veins (*small arrows*) at 6 seconds. (From Boley, S.J., Sprayregen, S., Sammartano, R.J., et al.: The pathophysiologic basis for the angiographic signs of vascular ectasias of the colon. Radiology, *125*:615, 1977, with permission.)

Barium enema is necessary only when the entire colon cannot be visualized endoscopically.

If the colonoscopic examination is normal, esophagogastroduodenoscopy is performed, preferably on the same day, in order to examine the upper gastrointestinal tract. If the results of this examination are normal, double-contrast radiography of the upper gastrointestinal tract and small bowel follows. On rare occasions, repeat endoscopic studies or a barium enema may be helpful. If these studies are repeatedly normal, but occult or slow bleeding continues, small bowel enteroscopy,[25] [111]I-platelet scintigraphy,[38] or mesenteric angiography may at times be helpful. Less commonly, exploratory laparotomy with attempts at intraoperative localization may be the only alternative and has been very effective in some studies.[4,24]

Treatment

Once a colonic vascular ectasia has been identified, management consists of controlling the acute hemorrhage and definitive treatment of the lesion itself. Major changes in management have occurred since the original descriptions of vascular ectasia and include the increasing roles of radionuclide scanning and colonoscopy in identifying the cause and site of bleeding, as well as transcolonoscopic ablation of focal lesions.

Control of Acute Hemorrhage

In most patients, the acute hemorrhage can be controlled by nonoperative means, and an emergency operation, with its increased morbidity and mortality, can be avoided. In patients in whom colonoscopy has been successful, and in whom an actively bleeding ectasia or fresh mucosal thrombus (i.e., a sentinel clot) has been identified, an effective mode of therapy is transendoscopic ablation of the lesion. In those active bleeders in whom angiography was performed because colonoscopy was unsuccessful or was not technically feasible, vasopressin infusion, either intravenously or intra-arterially through the angiographic catheter, is successful in arresting hemorrhage in more than 80% of patients in whom extravasation is demonstrated. The intravenous route appears as effective as the intra-arterial route when the bleeding is in the left colon, but intra-arterial administration has been more successful when the bleeding is in the right colon or small bowel.

Definitive Treatment

During the first 15 years after vascular ectasia was described, definitive treatment consisted of some type of colon resection. Endoscopic electrocoagulation was a therapeutic option that was reserved mainly for elderly patients with complicated medical illnesses; that is, the high-risk patient. Today, in institutions in which physicians experienced in endoscopic surgery are available, a greater number of patients are being managed endoscopically, and resection is often reserved for patients whose bleeding cannot be stopped or in whom endoscopic treatment is unsuccessful.

Numerous publications have documented the use of the argon laser, the neodymium:yttrium-aluminum-garnet (Nd:YAG) laser, endoscopic sclerosis, monopolar electrocoagulation, bipolar electrocoagulation, and the heater probe for miscellaneous vascular lesions throughout the gastrointestinal tract. However, differences in technique and study design, combined with the lack of long-term randomized studies controlled for the location and specific nature of individual lesions, preclude comparisons among them.

The presence of asymptomatic vascular ectasias, noted incidentally during colonoscopy in many elderly patients, raises concern as to their proper management. At present, most endoscopists do not recommend treating asymptomatic cecal vascular lesions, but if increasing experience with some of the newer modes of therapy (e.g., bipolar electrocoagulation and heater probes) proves them to be safe, a more aggressive approach to these lesions may be warranted.

Right hemicolectomy remains the treatment of choice in patients who have bled and in whom an ectasia of the right colon has been identified either by colonoscopy or angiography if (1) the bleeding cannot be stopped, (2) an endoscopist experienced in transcolonoscopic ablation is not available, and (3) endoscopic ablation has been unsuccessful or is not feasible for technical reasons (e.g., in large or multiple lesions). In the latter two situations, the right hemicolectomy is done as an elective procedure once active bleeding is controlled.

The extent of colon resection is not altered by the presence or lack of diverticulosis in the left colon; only the right half of the colon is removed. It is important that the entire right half of the colon be removed to ensure that no ectasias are left behind. Since up to 80% of bleeding diverticula are located in the right side of the colon, the risks of leaving the left colon are far outweighed by the increased morbidity and mortality of subtotal colectomy. Recurrent bleeding can be expected in up to 20% of patients so treated and was observed in 4 of our 27 patients with angiographically proven ectasias. Subtotal colectomy should be performed only as a last resort; that is, in a patient in whom active colonic bleeding persists, the angiogram is completely normal, and colonoscopic results either are normal or are not helpful.

OTHER VASCULAR LESIONS

As shown in Table 7–1, many vascular lesions other than ectasias can affect the lower gastrointestinal tract, some as part of a syndrome or systemic disease and others as single or multiple lesions unrelated to disease elsewhere in the body.

Hemangiomas

The second most common vascular lesion of the colon is the hemangioma. Although these lesions are considered by some to be true neoplasms, they are generally thought to be hamartomas because of their presence at birth in most cases. Colonic hemangiomas may occur as solitary lesions, as multiple growths limited to the colon, or as part of diffuse gastrointestinal or multisystem angiomatosis. Individual hemangiomas may be broadly classified as cavernous, capillary, or mixed. Most hemangiomas are small, ranging from a few millimeters to 2 cm. Larger lesions do occur, however, especially in the rectum.

Clinically, bleeding from colonic hemangiomas is usually slow, producing occult blood loss with anemia or melena. Hematochezia is less common, except in the case of large cavernous hemangiomas of the rectum, which can cause massive hemorrhage. The diagnosis is best established by colonoscopy; roentgenologic studies, including angiography, may produce normal findings. In the presence of gastrointestinal bleeding, hemangiomas of the skin or mucous membranes should suggest the possibility of associated bowel lesions.

Pathologically, hemangiomas are well circumscribed but are not encapsulated. Grossly cavernous hemangiomas appear as polypoid or mound-like reddish purple lesions of the mucosa. Sectioning of the lesion reveals numerous dilated, irregular blood-filled spaces within the mucosa and submucosa, sometimes extending through the muscular wall to the serosal surface. The vascular channels are lined by flat endothelial cells with flat or plump nuclei. Their walls do not contain smooth muscle fibers but are composed of fibrous tissue of varying thickness (Fig. 7–7). Capillary hemangiomas are plaque-like or mound-like reddish purple lesions composed of a proliferation of fine, closely packed, newly formed capillaries separated by very little edematous stroma. The endothelial lining cells are large and usually hypertrophic, and in some areas they may form solid cords or nodules with ill-defined capillary spaces. There is little or no pleomorphism or hyperchromasia. Small hemangiomas that are either solitary or few in number can be treated by colonoscopic laser coagulation. Large or multiple lesions usually require resection of either the hemangioma alone or the involved segment of colon. The hemangioma can either be palpated directly or revealed by transilluminating the bowel wall with an operative endoscope. The affected area can be resected and often this can be accomplished without opening the bowel.

Cavernous Hemangiomas of the Rectum

A distinct form of colonic hemangioma is the cavernous hemangioma of the rectum. These lesions usually are not associated with other gastrointestinal hemangiomas and are extensive, involving the entire rectum, portions of the rectosigmoid, and the perirectal tissues. They cause massive, sometimes uncontrollable, hemorrhage that often begins in infancy. The diagnosis usually can be suggested on plain films of the abdomen by the presence of phleboliths and by displacement or distortion of the rectal air column.[19] A barium enema study showing narrowing and rigidity of the rectal lumen, scalloping of the rectal wall, and an increase in the size of the presacral space further supports the diagnosis. Endoscopically, elevated nodules or vascular congestion causing a plum red coloration are seen. Ulcers and signs of proctitis may be evident. Angiography can be used to demonstrate these lesions but is rarely necessary to establish the diagnosis.

The massive bleeding resulting from these rectal hemangiomas often necessitates excision of the rectum by either abdominoperineal or low anterior resection, but because lesions occasionally involve the perirectal tissues, attempts at maintaining continence via pull-through procedures may fail. Ligation and embolization of major feeding vessels have been employed with varying degrees of success, and though local measures (e.g., electrocoagulation, sclerotherapy) usually are only temporarily effective, they have been of value in some instances.

Colonic and Extracolonic Involvement

The presence of skin or subcutaneous hemangiomas in the colon has been mentioned, and it is also not uncommon for hemangiomas of the liver to be present. Several disorders embodying multiple gastrointestinal hemangiomas have been described.

DIFFUSE INTESTINAL HEMANGIOMATOSIS. This connotes numerous (as many as 50 to 100) lesions involving the stomach, small bowel, and colon.[29] Bleeding or anemia usually leads to the diagnosis in childhood. Hemangiomas of the skin or soft tissues of the head and neck are frequently present. Continuous, slow but pernicious bleeding requiring transfusions, or an intussusception led by one of the lesions, may necessitate surgical intervention. The diagnosis may be made by endoscopy and barium studies; angiography results can be normal in spite of numerous lesions. The hemangiomas are similar in appearance to solitary lesions and are usually cavernous, although some have the histologic appearance of hemangioendotheliomas (benign lesions in children). At operation, all identifiable lesions should be excised either through enterotomies or by limited bowel resections. Transillumination and compression of the bowel wall are helpful in finding small lesions. Repeated operations may be necessary to control blood loss.

Universal (miliary) hemangiomatosis is usually fatal in infancy. It is, fortunately, a rare condition in which there are hundreds of hemangiomas involving the skin, brain, lung, and abdominal viscera. Death results from congestive heart failure caused by large arteriovenous shunts, or it may be a result of the local effects of the lesions. Colonic lesions rarely are of significance.

BLUE-RUBBER-BLEB NEVUS SYNDROME (CUTANEOUS AND INTESTINAL CAVERNOUS HEMANGIOMAS). In 1980, Gascoyen reported an association of cutaneous vascular nevi, intestinal lesions, and gastrointestinal bleeding. Bean[5] later coined the name blue-rubber-bleb syndrome and distinguished it from other cutaneous vascular lesions. A familial history is infrequent, although a few cases of transmission in an autosomal dominant pattern have been reported.

The lesions in this syndrome are distinctive. They vary in size from 0.1 to 5 cm and are blue, raised, and have a wrinkled surface. Characteristically, the contained blood can be emptied by direct pressure, leaving a wrinkled sac. The hemangiomas may be single or innumer-

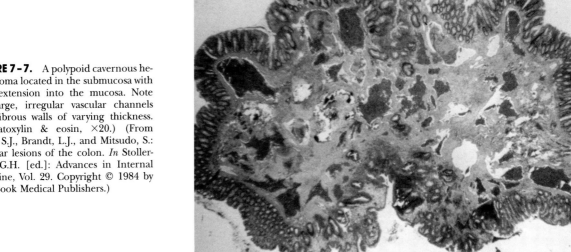

FIGURE 7-7. A polypoid cavernous hemangioma located in the submucosa with focal extension into the mucosa. Note the large, irregular vascular channels with fibrous walls of varying thickness. (Hematoxylin & eosin, ×20.) (From Boley, S.J., Brandt, L.J., and Mitsudo, S.: Vascular lesions of the colon. *In* Stollerman, G.H. [ed.]: Advances in Internal Medicine, Vol. 29. Copyright © 1984 by Year Book Medical Publishers.)

able; they are usually found on the trunk, extremities, and face but not on mucous membranes; they increase in size and number with advancing age and do not undergo malignant transformation.[48] They may be present in any portion of the gastrointestinal tract but are most common in the small bowel. In the colon, they occur more commonly on the left side and in the rectum. They are infrequently seen by barium or angiographic studies and are detected best by endoscopy if they are proximal to the ligament of Treitz or are in the colon. Microscopically, they are cavernous hemangiomas composed of clusters of dilated capillary spaces lined by cuboidal or flattened endothelium with connective tissue stroma. In the bowel, they are located in the submucosa. Resection of the involved segment of bowel is recommended for recurrent hemorrhage, although endoscopic laser coagulation is an attractive therapeutic option.

Less Common Vascular Lesions

Congenital Arteriovenous Malformations

Congenital arteriovenous malformations are embryonic growth defects and are considered to be developmental anomalies. Although they are found mainly in the extremities, they can occur anywhere in the vascular tree. In the colon, they may be small, similar to ectasias, or they may involve a long segment of bowel. The more extensive lesions are most often seen in the rectum and sigmoid.

Histologically, arteriovenous malformations are persistent communications between arteries and veins located primarily in the submucosa. Characteristically, there is arterialization of the veins (i.e., tortuosity, dilation, and thick walls with smooth muscle hypertrophy) and intimal thickening and sclerosis (Fig. 7–8). In long-standing arteriovenous malformations, the arteries are dilated with atrophic and sclerotic degeneration.

Angiography is the primary means of diagnosis. Early

filling veins in small lesions and extensive dilation of arteries and veins in large lesions (Fig. 7–9) are pathognomonic of arteriovenous malformations. Patients with significant bleeding should undergo resection of the involved segment of colon.

Colonic Varices

Varices of the colon are very rare but may be a cause of hematochezia or melena. In most cases, the varices are located in the rectosigmoid and are found progressively less often in the more proximal colon. The most common cause of colonic varices is portal hypertension; congenital anomalies, mesenteric venous obstruction, congestive heart failure, and pancreatitis account for the others.[22] Why varices form so rarely in the colon, and why they bleed, is unclear. Varices are easily diagnosed by proctosigmoidoscopy, colonoscopy, or angiography, and may be seen on conventional barium studies of the colon. Therapy consists of segmental colon resection, portocaval shunting, or local ligation or sclerosis.

Telangiectasia

Telangiectasias are small vascular lesions found on cutaneous, mucocutaneous, and mucosal surfaces throughout the body. Grossly, and at endoscopy, they are the size of millet seeds and appear as cherry red spots, vascular spiders, smooth hillocks, or lesions resembling ectasia. They may be hereditary or acquired and have been described in association with many disorders (e.g., chronic renal failure, progressive systemic sclerosis, von Willebrand's disease, CRST syndrome (calcinosis, Raynaud's phenomenon, sclerodactyly, telangiectasia),[13,27,49] but they are best known as part of Osler-Weber-Rendu disease or hereditary hemorrhagic telangiectasia.

Hereditary hemorrhagic telangiectasia is a familial disorder characterized by telangiectasias of the skin and mucous membranes and recurrent gastrointestinal

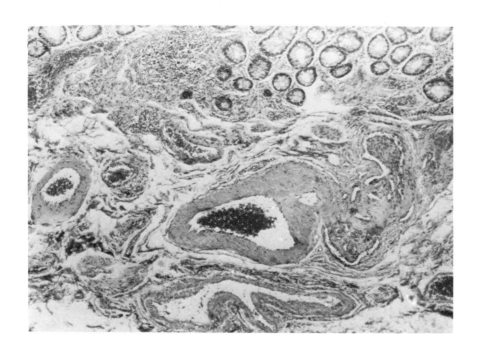

FIGURE 7–8. Arteriovenous malformation with tortuous veins, having sclerotic intima, hypertrophied muscle, and thick-walled sclerotic arteries. (Hematoxylin & eosin, ×100.) (From Boley, S.J., Brandt, L.J., and Mitsudo, S.: Vascular lesions of the colon. *In* Stollerman, G.H. [ed.]: Advances in Internal Medicine, Vol. 29. Copyright © 1984 by Year Book Medical Publishers.)

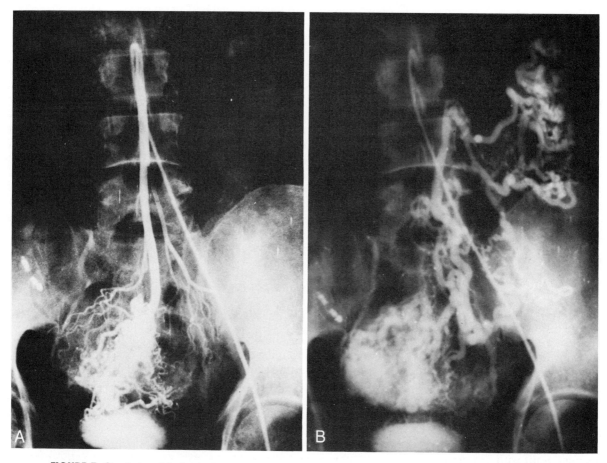

FIGURE 7–9. *A,* Arterial phase of inferior mesenteric arteriogram from a patient with a congenital arteriovenous malformation showing multiple dilated arteries going to a large segment of the rectosigmoid. *B,* Venous phase of the same arteriogram showing dilated tortuous vessels to the same segment, as well as to other more proximal areas. (From Boley, S.J., Brandt, L.J., and Mitsudo, S.: Vascular lesions of the colon. *In* Stollerman, G.H. [ed.]: Advances in Internal Medicine, Vol. 29. Copyright © 1984 by Year Book Medical Publishers.)

bleeding. Lesions are noticed frequently in the first few years of life, and recurrent epistaxis in childhood is characteristic of the disease. By the age of 10 years, about one half of patients will have had some bleeding, but severe hemorrhage is unusual before the fourth decade of life and occurs with a peak incidence in the sixth decade. In almost all patients, bleeding presents as melena, whereas epistaxis and hematemesis are less frequent. Bleeding may be quite severe and patients not uncommonly receive more than 50 transfusions in a lifetime. A family history of disease has been reported in 80% of patients with the disorder but less commonly in those with bleeding, especially when the bleeding occurs later in life.

Telangiectasias are almost always present on the lips, oral and nasopharyngeal membranes, tongue, or hand. Lack of involvement of these sites casts suspicion on the diagnosis. Lesions on the lips are more common in patients with gastrointestinal bleeding than in those without. Telangiectasia occurs in the colon but is far more common in the stomach and small bowel. Upper gastrointestinal lesions are more apt to cause significant bleeding.

Telangiectasia is not demonstrable on barium enema examination but is easily seen on endoscopy. Occasionally, in the presence of severe anemia and blood loss, the lesions transiently become less visible, but with blood replacement they again increase in prominence. Angiography results are usually normal but may demonstrate arteriovenous communications or small clusters of abnormal vessels.

Pathologically, the major changes involve the capillaries and venules, but arterioles may also be affected. The lesions consist of irregular, ectatic, tortuous, blood-filled spaces lined by a delicate single layer of endothelial cells and supported by a fine layer of fibrous connective tissue. No elastic lamina or muscular tissue is present in these vessels. The arterioles show some intimal proliferation and often contain thrombi, suggesting vascular stasis, but the most conspicuous findings are in the venules. In contrast to those in vascular ectasia, these venules are abnormally thick and have very prominent, well-developed longitudinal muscles. Apparently these abnormal venules play a major role in regulating blood flow to the telangiectasia.

Many treatments have been recommended, including oral and parenteral estrogen therapy and multiple resections of involved bowel. At present, endoscopic electrosurgery or laser coagulation appears most promising and may be performed during active bleeding or before any bleeding episodes. Although endoscopic therapy has diminished the need for bowel resection in some cases, long-term follow-up studies are needed to evaluate the ultimate course of patients so treated.

Klippel-Trenaunay-Weber Syndrome

Originally described by Klippel and Trenaunay in 1900, the Klippel-Trenaunay-Weber syndrome is characterized by unilateral congenital lesions of the lower extremities, including (1) cutaneous hemangiomas, usually of the flat, diffuse capillary type; (2) varicose veins dating from childhood; and (3) soft tissue hypertrophy and bone elongation. Involvement of the colon is uncommon and poorly defined, usually involving the rectum or rectosigmoid when it occurs.[15]

The cause of the syndrome has been variably ascribed to congenital arteriovenous fistulas or to aplasia, hypoplasia, dysplasia, atresia, or obstruction of the deep venous system. Rectal lesions usually cause bleeding during childhood and have been described by some authors as being cavernous hemangiomas (with reported biopsy documentation) or as varicosities of the rectal veins (based upon venography).[36] Recently, computed tomography (CT) and ultrasonography were found helpful in determining the extent of colon and other visceral disease.[23]

Major rectal or bladder bleeding has occurred in a few children, with one reported death. Ligation of bleeding hemorrhoids or sclerosis of rectal veins is often temporarily effective, but proctectomy may be necessary in some patients.

REFERENCES

1. Alavi, A.: Scintigraphic demonstration of acute gastrointestinal bleeding. Gastrointest. Radiol., 5:205, 1980.
2. Allison, D.J., Hemingway, A.P., and Cunningham, D.A.: Angiography in gastrointestinal bleeding. Lancet, 3:30, 1982.
3. Athanasoulis, C.A., Galdabini, J.J., Waltman, A.C., et al.: Angiodysplasia of the colon; a cause of rectal bleeding. Cardiovasc. Radiol., 1:3, 1978.
4. Athanasoulis, C.A., Moncure, A.C., Greenfield, A.J., et al.: Intraoperative localization of small bowel bleeding sites with combined use of angiographic methods and methylene blue. Surgery, 87:77, 1984.
5. Bean, W.B.: Vascular Spiders and Related Lesions of the Skin. Springfield, IL, Charles C. Thomas, 1958, p. 178.
6. Boley, S.J., and Brandt, L.J.: Vascular ectasias of the colon—1986. Dig. Dis. Sci., 31:265, 1986.
7. Boley, S.J., Brandt, L.J., and Mitsudo, S.: Vascular lesions of the colon. In Stollerman, G.H. (ed.): Advances in Internal Medicine. Chicago, Year Book Medical Publishers, 1984.
8. Boley, S.J., Dibiase, A., Brandt, L.J., et al.: Lower intestinal bleeding in the elderly. Am. J. Surg., 137:57, 1979.
9. Boley, S.J., Sammartano, R.J., Adams, A., et al.: On the nature and etiology of vascular ectasias of the colon: Degenerative lesions of aging. Gastroenterology, 72:650, 1977.
10. Boley, S.J., Sprayregen, S., Sammartano, R.J., et al.: The pathophysiologic basis for the angiographic signs of vascular ectasias of the colon. Radiology, 125:615, 1977.
11. Cello, J.P.: Diagnosis and management of lower gastrointestinal tract hemorrhage—Medical Staff Conference. West. J. Med., 143:80, 1985.
12. Chou, C.C., and Dabney, J.M.: Interrelation of ileal wall compliance and vascular resistance. Am. J. Dig. Dis., 12:1198, 1967.
13. Durray, P.H., Marcal, J.M., LiVolsi, V.A., et al: Gastrointestinal angiodysplasia: A possible component of von Willebrand's disease. Hum. Pathol., 15:539, 1984.
14. Frank, M.S., Brandt, L.J., Boley, S.J., et al.: Iatric submucosal hemorrhage. Am. J. Gastroenterol., 75:209, 1981.
15. Ghahremani, C.G., Kangarloo, H., Volberg, F., et al.: Diffuse cavernous hemangioma of the colon in the Klippel-Trenaunay syndrome. Radiology, 118:673, 1976.
16. Gilberstein, V.: Colon cancer screening: The Minnesota experience. Gastrointest. Endosc., 26:315, 1980.
17. Hamoniere, G., Grenner, A., Lalloue, C., et al.: Recherchessur l'angiectasie du colon droit. Ext Lyon Chir., 78:125, 1982.
18. Harford, W.V.: Gastrointestinal angiodysplasia: Clinical features. Endoscopy, 20:144, 1988.
19. Hellstrom, J., Hultborn, K.A., and Engstedt, L.: Diffuse cavernous hemangioma of the rectum. Acta Chir. Scand., 109:277, 1955.

20. Hemingway, A.P., and Allison, D.J.: Angiodysplasia and Meckel's diverticulum: A congenital association? Br. J. Surg., 69:493, 1982.
21. Holman, E.: Abnormal Arteriovenous Communications, 2nd ed. Springfield, IL, Charles C. Thomas, 1968.
22. Izsak, E.M., and Finlay, J.M.: Colonic varices: Three case reports and review of the literature. Am. J. Gastroenterol., 73:131, 1980.
23. Jafri, S.Z.H., Bree, R.L. and Glazer, G.M.: Computed tomography and ultrasound findings in Klippel-Trenaunay syndrome. J. Comput. Assist. Tomogr., 7:457, 1983.
24. Lau, W.Y., Fan, S.T., Wong, S.H., et al.: Preoperative and intraoperative localization of gastrointestinal bleeding of obscure origin. Gut, 28:869, 1977.
25. Lewis, B., and Waye, J.: Gastrointestinal bleeding of obscure origin: The role of small bowel enteroscopy. Gastroenterology, 94:1117, 1988.
26. Love, J.W.: The syndrome of calcific aortic stenosis and gastrointestinal bleeding. Resolution following aortic valve replacement. J. Thorac. Cardiovasc. Surg., 83:779, 1982.
27. Marshall, J.B., and Settles, R.H.: Colonic telangiectasias in scleroderma. Arch. Intern. Med., 140:1121, 1980.
28. Maxfield, R.G., and Maxfield, C.M.: Colonoscopy as a primary diagnostic procedure in chronic gastrointestinal tract bleeding. Arch. Surg., 121:401, 1986.
29. Mellish, R.W.P.: Multiple hemangiomas of the gastrointestinal tract in children. Am. J. Surg., 121:412, 1971.
30. Mitsudo, S., Boley, S.J., Brandt, L.J., et al: Vascular ectasias of the right colon in the elderly: A distinct pathologic entity. Hum. Pathol., 10:585, 1979.
31. Noer, R.J., and Derr, J.W.: Effect of distention on intestinal revascularization. Arch. Surg., 59:542, 1949.
32. Nusbaum, M., and Baum, S.: Radiographic demonstration of unknown sites of gastrointestinal bleeding. Surg. Forum, 14:374, 1963.
33. Riley, J.M., Wilson, P.C., and Grant, A.K.: Double pathology as a cause of occult gastrointestinal blood loss. BMJ, 282:686, 1981.
34. Salem, R.R., Thompson, J.N., Rees, H.C., et al.: Outcome of surgery in colonic angiodysplasia. Gut, 26:A1155, 1985.
35. Semba, T., and Fujii, Y.: Relationship between venous flow and colonic peristalsis. Jpn. J. Physiol., 20:408, 1976.
36. Servelle, M., Bastin, R., Loygue, J., et al.: Hematuria and rectal bleeding in the child with Klippel and Trenaunay syndrome. Ann. Surg., 183:418, 1976.
37. Shah, I.A.: Angiodysplasia: Morphologic diagnosis. Endoscopy, 20: 149, 1988.
38. Schmidt, K.S., Rasmussen, J.W., Grove, D., et al.: The use of indium-111-labelled platelets for scintigraphic localization of gastrointestinal bleeding with special reference to occult bleeding. Scand. J. Gastroenterol., 21:407, 1986.
39. Sidky, M., and Bean, J.W.: Influence of rhythmic and tonic contraction of intestinal muscle on blood flow and blood reservoir capacity in dog intestine. Am. J. Physiol., 193:386, 1958.
40. Smith, R., Copely, D.J., and Bolen, F.H.: 99mTc RBC scintigraphy: Correlation of gastrointestinal bleeding rates with scintigraphic findings. Am. J. Roentgenol., 148:869, 1987.
41. Sprayregen, S., and Boley, S.J.: Vascular ectasias of the colon. JAMA, 239:962, 1978.
42. Steger, A.C., Galland, R.B., and Hemingway, A.: Gastrointestinal haemorrhage from a second source in patients with colonic angiodysplasia. Br. J. Surg., 74:726, 1987.
43. Stewart, W.B., Gathright, J.B., and Ray, J.E.: Vascular ectasias of the colon. Surg. Gynecol. Obstet., 148:670, 1979.
44. Tedesco, F.J., Gottfried, E.B., Corless, J.K., et al.: Prospective evaluation of hospital bed patients with nonactive lower intestinal bleeding—timing and role of barium enema and colonoscopy. Gastrointest. Endosc., 30:281, 1984.
45. Tedesco, F.J., Waye, J.D., Raskin, J.B., et al.: Colonoscopic evaluation of rectal bleeding—a study of 304 patients. Ann. Intern. Med., 89:907, 1978.
46. Welch, C.E., Athanasoulis, C.A., and Galdabini, J.J.: Hemorrhage from the large bowel with special reference to angiodysplasia and diverticular disease. World J. Surg., 2:73, 1978.
47. Winzelberg, G.G., Froelich, J.W., McKusick, K.A., et al.: Scintigraphic detection of gastrointestinal bleeding: A review of current methods. Am. J. Gastroenterol., 78:324, 1983.
48. Wong, S.H., and Lau, W.Y.: Blue rubber bleb nevus syndrome. Dis. Colon Rectum, 25:371, 1982.
49. Zuckerman, G.R., Cornette, G.L., Clouse, R.E., et al.: Upper gastrointestinal bleeding in patients with chronic renal failure. Ann. Intern. Med., 102:588, 1985.

Chapter 8

COLONIC ISCHEMIA

RONALD N. KALEYA / SCOTT J. BOLEY

Colonic ischemia (CI) has come to be recognized as one of the most common colonic disorders of the elderly population. Although it was described more than a century ago, CI continues to be a difficult clinical problem because of the diverse outcomes associated with ischemic injury to the colon. Inadequate blood flow to all or part of the colon can produce a heterogeneous spectrum of clinical syndromes and pathologic findings ranging from completely reversible intramural and submucosal hemorrhage to transmural colonic gangrene. Although some patients develop the severe complications of gangrene, perforation, ischemic stricture, and persistent colitis, most episodes of CI are noncatastrophic with transient symptoms and pathologic changes. Colonic ischemia isolated to the right colon is often a manifestation of acute mesenteric ischemia (AMI), which has a more fulminant course, and therefore will be discussed separately.

Intestinal ischemia can be classified into four broadly defined types: (1) AMI, which is acute ischemia of major portions of the small intestine with or without involvement of the colon; (2) focal mesenteric ischemia, which is ischemia of localized segments of small bowel; (3) CI, which is ischemia involving only the colon; and (4) chronic mesenteric ischemia, which is ischemia of the small bowel without loss of tissue viability. Of these, CI is the most common in our experience.

Before 1950, colonic ischemia was considered synonymous with colonic infarction. During the 1950s, there were many reports of different forms of iatrogenic ischemic injury of the colon resulting from high ligation of the inferior mesenteric artery (IMA) in the course of aneurysmectomy or colectomy for colon carcinoma.[12,13] In 1963, Bernstein and Bernstein[1] termed the persistent colitis following iatrogenic ischemic injuries "ischemic ulcerative colitis."

Also in 1963, based on retrospective and experimental studies, Boley and associates[4,11] described the clinical, roentgenologic, and pathologic features of the previously unrecognized noniatrogenic, noncatastrophic reversible forms of ischemic colonic injury. Their later animal research,[3] reported in 1965, confirmed that spontaneous colonic ischemia could also result in irreversible pathologic colonic injury; specifically, stricture, gangrene, and chronic colitis. Subsequently, in 1966,

Marston and associates[10] applied the term ischemic colitis to a group of 16 patients, one of whom had colonic gangrene, 12 ischemic strictures, and three reversible colitis.

In comparison with AMI, CI usually produces milder symptoms and fewer physical findings and systemic derangements. Although patients with AMI usually present during the ischemic episode because of the profound hemodynamic and metabolic changes accompanying this disorder, CI is most often diagnosed only after the ischemic episode is over and the circulation has returned to normal. Thus, AMI and CI are generally very different problems; AMI is a catastrophic emergency with high mortality, whereas CI is usually not catastrophic and does not require prompt surgical intervention. In CI, however, the intestinal damage resulting from the ischemic insult persists and produces a gamut of morphologic and clinical presentations.

Many names have been applied to the various clinical forms of CI. Most characterize only one aspect of the condition, and often an overlap of the pathologic changes signified by different terms has created confusion. Moreover, as understanding of the nature of CI has increased, it has become apparent that some of the names used are inaccurate. For example, our original term of "reversible vascular occlusion of the colon" describing the transient manifestations of CI is not completely correct, since it is the effect of an occlusion rather than the occlusion itself that is reversible and, in fact, there may not be a demonstrable occlusion responsible for the ischemia. Similarly, the terms ischemic colitis and colonic infarction are suitable only for parts of the spectrum of CI, because the milder reversible ischemic episodes are not inflammatory but hemorrhagic, and true infarction (i.e., coagulation necrosis) is often lacking.

Today the term colonic ischemia is used to describe a general pathophysiologic process that causes a variety of clinical conditions. These conditions are classified as reversible and nonreversible and then further categorized as (1) reversible ischemic colopathy (submucosal or intramural hemorrhage), (2) reversible or transient ischemic colitis, (3) chronic ulcerative ischemic colitis, (4) ischemic colonic stricture, (5) colonic gangrene, or (6) fulminant universal colitis (Fig. 8–1). The adoption

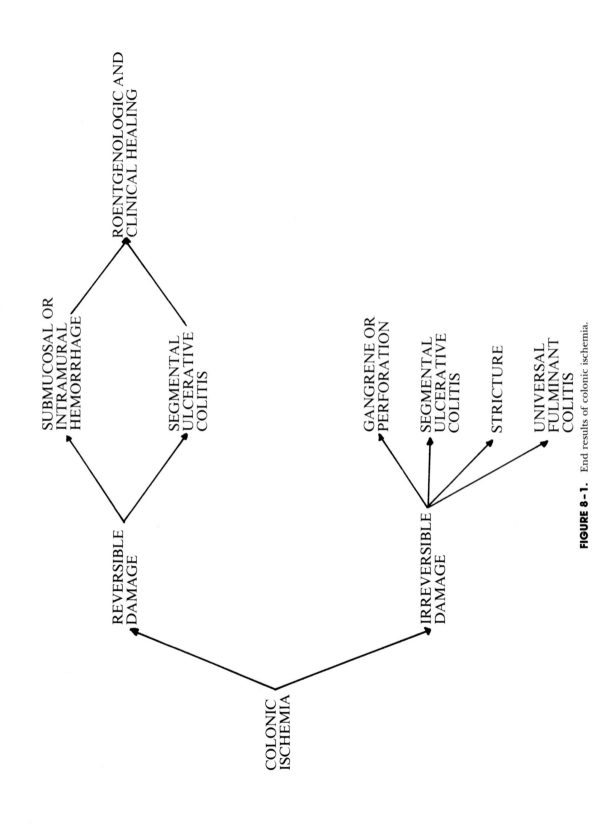

FIGURE 8–1. End results of colonic ischemia.

of this terminology and the elimination of nonspecific names would allow the experience of many clinicians to be combined and uniformly compared, broadening our understanding of these entities.

INCIDENCE

Although the clinical features of most forms of CI have been known since 1963, when the spontaneous and reversible nature of some ischemic episodes and the radiologic criteria for their early diagnosis were described, the condition is still frequently misdiagnosed, and to date no study has provided an accurate determination of the incidence of CI. Also, barium enema and colonoscopy are not always performed early in the course of the disease, and many cases of transient or reversible ischemia are probably missed.

In addition, several retrospective reviews of older clinical material have revealed many cases of CI that were either undiagnosed or misdiagnosed because the various clinical manifestations of this disorder were not recognized. Using the modern clinical, roentgenologic, and pathologic criteria for the diagnosis of colonic ischemia, two retrospective reviews of 154 patients in whom colitis was identified after the age of 50 revealed that 72 to 74% of the patients, in fact, had colonic ischemia.[5,14] Half of these patients had been previously diagnosed as having inflammatory bowel disease.

In our experience with more than 250 cases of CI, there appears to be no significant sex predilection. Although our patients have ranged in age from 1 to 87 years, more than 90% of those whose lesions were not iatrogenic were in the seventh decade of life or older. This prevalence in the older age group has been confirmed by numerous other reports and is to be expected in view of the general deterioration of the vascular tree that accompanies aging.

Ischemia may involve any portion of the colon, but most commonly it involves the splenic flexure, descending colon, and sigmoid colon (Fig. 8–2). Although the distribution and pattern of involvement do not bear any relationship to the severity of the ischemia, specific causes of ischemia do appear to more commonly affect certain areas. Iatrogenic ischemia resulting from ligation of the IMA usually involves the sigmoid colon, whereas low flow states show a predilection for the splenic flexure. Similarly, the length of bowel affected varies with the cause. For example, atheromatous emboli often result in short segment changes, and low flow states usually involve much longer ones. Irrespective of cause, however, CI recurs only rarely and has been documented in only 3 of the more than 250 patients in our experience.

Although British authors initially considered rectal involvement to be rare or nonexistent,[8] in our experience and in that of others, it occurs in more than 10% of patients. Farman[14] found that rectal ischemic disease was always accompanied by involvement of the sigmoid colon, but we have seen several instances of isolated rectal changes, including one patient in whom a short rectal stricture developed with normal bowel proximally. This wide variation in the site and degree of ischemic change is understandable in view of the plethora of causes of colonic vascular insufficiency.

ETIOLOGY

Although many associated conditions have been reported with CI, most patients have no identifiable cause for their ischemic episodes. Features of the clinical history that might suggest CI include previous episodes of either small bowel ischemia or CI or a precipitating cardiovascular event leading to a transient low flow state. Up to 20% of patients have an associated lesion, such

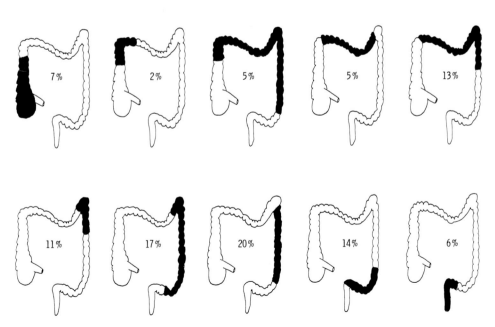

FIGURE 8-2. Distribution and length of involvement in 250 cases of colonic ischemia. More frequent involvement of the left half of the colon is apparent.

as a potentially obstructing colonic stricture, carcinoma, or diverticulitis, which may not only make the diagnosis more obscure but may also complicate treatment. Approximately 90% of patients with CI are older than 60 years of age and have other evidence of systemic atherosclerotic disease; however, oral contraceptive and cocaine use are responsible for an increasing number of cases in the younger population. Other reported causes are listed in Table 8–1.

One possible factor predisposing the colon to ischemia is that it has an inherently lower blood flow than that of the small intestine. Of even greater importance is experimental evidence suggesting that functional motor activity of the colon is accompanied by a decrease in blood flow. This is contrary to the increase in small intestinal blood flow during periods of digestion and increased peristalsis. Geber[7] has postulated that "the combination of normally low blood flow during functional activity would seem to make the colon (1) rather unique among all areas of the body where increased functional activity is usually accompanied by an increased blood flow and (2) more susceptible to pathology." Furthermore, the more pronounced effect of straining on systemic arterial and venous pressure in constipated, as compared with normal, patients provides indirect evidence that constipation may accentuate the circulatory effects of defecation. What finally triggers an ischemic episode is still conjectural in most instances—whether increased demand by the colonic tissues is superimposed on an already borderline flow, or whether flow itself is acutely diminished, has yet to be determined.

PATHOPHYSIOLOGY

Regardless of its cause, bowel ischemia produces one spectrum of pathologic, clinical, and radiologic manifestations. The pathologic changes evoked by ischemia range from simple submucosal hemorrhage and edema to colonic gangrene with perforation and peritonitis. Between these extremes, gradations of tissue damage from the basis of the diverse clinical course that individual episodes of CI may take, varying with the severity of

TABLE 8-1. CAUSES OF COLONIC ISCHEMIA

Inferior mesenteric artery thrombosis	Polycythemia vera
Arterial embolus	Parasitic infestation
Cholesterol emboli	Allergy
Cardiac failure or arrhythmias	Trauma—blunt and penetrating
Shock	Ruptured ectopic pregnancy
Digitalis toxicity	Iatrogenic causes
Volvulus	Aneurysmectomy
Periarteritis nodosa	Aortoiliac reconstruction
Systemic lupus erythematosus	Gynecologic operations
Rheumatoid arthritis	Exchange transfusions
Necrotizing arteritis	Colon bypass
Thromboangiitis obliterans	Lumbar aortography
Strangulated hernia	Colectomy with inferior mesenteric artery ligation
Drug-induced (e.g., oral contraceptives, cocaine)	

the episode. Mild ischemia produces morphologic changes that regress and ultimately disappear or heal, a sequence of events reflected clinically and radiologically by transient or reversible colonic findings. More severe ischemia may result in irreparable damage, with gangrene, perforation, or persistent colitis; if healing occurs, it does so with scarring, fibrosis, and resultant stricture.

The ultimate outcome of an episode of CI depends on many factors, including (1) the cause (i.e., occlusion or low flow), (2) the level of the occlusion, (3) the duration and degree of the ischemia, (4) the rapidity of onset of the ischemic process, (5) the adequacy of the collateral circulation, (6) the state of the general circulation, (7) the metabolic requirements of the affected bowel, (8) the presence and virulence of bacteria within the intestinal lumen, and (9) the presence of associated conditions such as colonic distention. Although the end results of the interaction of all these factors are obviously complex and may take weeks or months to develop, the initial response to ischemia may be the same regardless of its severity. It is therefore impossible to predict the progression of the ischemic process based upon the initial physical, roentgenologic, or endoscopic evaluation.

SYMPTOMS

Colonic ischemia usually presents with the sudden onset of mild abdominal pain, usually localized to the left lower quadrant and crampy in character. Less commonly, the pain is severe, or conversely, in other patients, the description of pain can only be elicited retrospectively, if at all. An urgent desire to defecate frequently accompanies the pain and is followed, within 24 hours, by the passage of either bright red or maroon blood in the stool. The bleeding is usually not vigorous and blood loss requiring transfusion is so rare that it should suggest an alternative diagnosis. Physical examination may reveal mild to severe abdominal tenderness elicited over the site of the involved segment of bowel.

Physical examination in the acute phase of illness may be remarkable only for mild abdominal tenderness over the involved colonic segment, and although transient peritonitis has been documented in patients with ultimately reversible lesions, peritoneal signs persisting longer than 2 to 3 hours are most suggestive of irreparable damage. Fever and leukocytosis are usually present and are important parameters to follow when assessing the clinical course.

CLINICAL COURSE

Most commonly, symptoms subside in 24 to 48 hours, and clinical, roentgenographic, and endoscopic evidence of healing is seen within 2 weeks. More severe, but still reversible, ischemic damage may take 1 to 6 months to resolve. Frequently, however, ischemic damage is too severe to heal, and in this situation some form of irreversible disease ultimately develops. This group of patients composes about 50% of those with CI, and their clinical course varies considerably. In approximately two thirds of these patients, CI follows a more protracted course, developing over time into either chronic ischemic colitis or an ischemic stricture. In the remaining one third of patients, signs and symptoms of a catastrophic event such as gangrene or perforation develop, often becoming obvious within hours of the patient's initial presentation.

Since the outcome of an episode of CI cannot be predicted at its onset unless the initial physical findings indicate an unequivocal intra-abdominal catastrophe, patients must be examined serially for evidence of clinical improvement or for less favorable prognostic factors such as peritonitis, rising temperature, elevation of the white blood cell count, or worsening symptoms.

Patients with diarrhea or bleeding that persists beyond the first 10 to 14 days usually experience perforation or, less commonly, a protein-wasting enteropathy. Strictures may develop over weeks to months and may be asymptomatic or produce progressive bowel obstruction. Some asymptomatic strictures resolve spontaneously over many months.

DIAGNOSIS

Appropriate management of CI requires early diagnosis, continuous monitoring of the patient, and serial radiographic or colonoscopic evaluation of the colon, or both. The more severe cases of CI may be difficult to distinguish from AMI, whereas the less severe cases may mimic acute or chronic idiopathic ulcerative colitis, Crohn's colitis, infectious colitis, or diverticulitis. A combination of radiographic, colonoscopic, and clinical findings may be necessary to establish the diagnosis of CI.

In the patient with suspected CI, if scout films of the abdomen are normal, sigmoidoscopy is unrevealing, and the patient does not have an acute abdomen, gentle barium enema or colonoscopy should be performed in unprepared bowel within 48 hours of the onset of symptoms. The most characteristic findings, representing submucosal hemorrhage and edema, appear as "thumbprinting" or pseudotumors on barium enema and hemorrhagic nodules or bullae during colonoscopy. Segmental distribution of these findings, with or without ulceration, is very suggestive of CI, but the diagnosis cannot be made conclusively from a single study (Fig. 8–3).

Repeat radiographic or endoscopic examinations of the colon, together with observation of the clinical course, are necessary to confirm the diagnosis. Segmental colitis associated with a tumor or other potentially or partially obstructing lesion also is characteristic of ischemic disease. Findings of universal colonic involvement, loss of haustrations, or pseudopolyposis are more typical of chronic idiopathic ulcerative colitis, whereas the presence of skip lesions, linear ulcerations, or fistulas suggests Crohn's colitis.

It is imperative to obtain the initial endoscopic or roentgenologic study early in the course of the disease because the thumbprinting will disappear within days, as the submucosal hemorrhages are either resorbed or evacuated into the colon when the overlying mucosa ulcerates and sloughs. Barium enema or colonoscopy performed 1 week after the initial study should reflect the evolution of the disease, either by a return to normal-appearing bowel or by replacement of the thumbprints

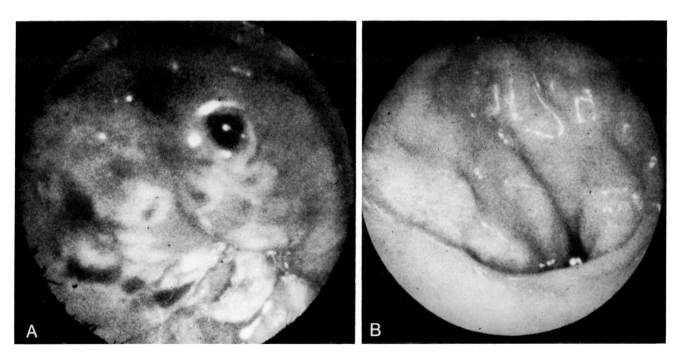

FIGURE 8–3. *A*, Endoscopic appearance of the colon during the initial evaluation of a patient with colonic ischemia. The dark nodular mass is a submucosal hemorrhage below which are ulcerations in which other areas of hemorrhage have broken down. *B*, Follow-up study 3 weeks later demonstrates complete healing of the colonic mucosa. (From Littman, L., Boley, S.J., and Schwartz, S.: Sigmoidoscopic diagnosis of reversible vascular occlusion of the colon. Dis. Colon Rectum, *6*:142, 1963, with permission.)

with a segmental ulcerative colitis pattern. Persistence of the thumbprints suggests a diagnosis other than CI; for example, lymphoma or amyloid (Fig. 8–4).

Caution is indicated if colonoscopy is chosen as the initial study. Distention of the bowel with air pressures greater than 30 mm Hg diminishes intestinal blood flow, shunts blood from the mucosa to the serosa, and causes a progressive decrease in the arteriovenous oxygen difference.[4] Kozarek and colleagues[9] have shown that pressures greater than 30 mm Hg are generated during routine colonoscopic procedures. Thus, there is a potential for induced or exacerbated CI during colonoscopy. This problem can be minimized by insufflating with carbon dioxide, which increases colonic blood flow at similar pressures.[13]

Biopsy specimens of nodules or bullae identified endoscopically early in the course of CI reveal submucosal hemorrhage, whereas biopsy specimens of the surrounding mucosa generally show nonspecific inflammatory changes. Histologic evidence of mucosal infarction, though uncommon, is pathognomonic of ischemia. Angiography rarely shows significant occlusions of other abnormalities and is not indicated in patients suspected of having CI.

The diagnosis of colonic infarction progressing to gangrene and perforation is made on the basis of abdominal tenderness, guarding, rebound tenderness, a rising fever, leukocytosis, and evidence of paralytic ileus. These signs may evolve over time or may become obvious within hours of presentation. However, they are not specific for infarction and dictate the need for emergent laparotomy. Diarrhea, bleeding, or both that persist for more than 2 weeks are also consistent with irreversible ischemic damage.

When the clinical presentation does not allow a clear distinction between CI and AMI and plain films of the abdomen do not show the characteristic thumbprinting pattern of CI, an "air enema" is performed by gently insufflating air into the colon under fluoroscopic control. The submucosa hemorrhage and edema that produce the thumbprinting pattern of CI can be identified in this manner. Once the provisional diagnosis of CI is made, a gentle barium enema is performed to determine the site and distribution of the disease and to identify any associated lesion that may have predisposed to the episode of ischemia; for example, carcinoma, stricture, or diverticulitis. If, however, thumbprinting is not observed and the "air enema" does not suggest the diagnosis of CI, a selective mesenteric angiogram is immediately performed to exclude AMI. AMI progresses rapidly to an irreversible outcome, and optimal diagnosis and treatment require emergent angiography.[5] The diagnosis of AMI must always be established or excluded prior to performing a barium study because residual barium from a contrast study of the colon may preclude adequate angiographic study.

TREATMENT

Acute Onset of Symptoms

Appropriate management of ischemic lesions of the colon requires early diagnosis, serial radiographic eval-uation, and continued monitoring of the patient. Once the diagnosis of CI has been established, and the physical examination does not suggest intestinal gangrene or perforation, the patient is treated expectantly.

A broad-spectrum antibiotic including coverage for gram-negative rods, enterococcis, and anaerobic organisms is prescribed, because antibiotic therapy reduces the length of bowel damaged by ischemia, although it will not prevent colonic infarction. Cardiac output is maximized and urine output is monitored to ensure adequate systemic perfusion. Medications that cause mesenteric vasoconstriction (e.g., digitalis and vasopressors) should be withdrawn if possible. If the colon appears distended, it is decompressed with a rectal tube and gentle saline irrigations because increased intraluminal pressure may further compromise the intestinal blood supply. Systemic corticosteroids are of no value and may be harmful, as they increase the possibility of perforation and secondary infection.

The patient should have white blood cell, hemoglobin, and hematocrit evaluations frequently during the acute episode. Blood products should be administered according to the patient's requirements, and the fluid and electrolyte status must be carefully monitored, with special attention to potassium and magnesium levels, as they are adversely affected by diarrhea and tissue necrosis. Levels of lactate dehydrogenase, creatine phosphokinase, and serum glutamic-oxaloacetic transaminase in the venous blood may reflect the degree of bowel necrosis, but they are nonspecific. Patients with significant diarrhea should receive parenteral nutrition early in the course of treatment. Narcotics should be withheld until it is clear that an intra-abdominal catastrophe is not present and that the patient is improving clinically. Cathartics are contraindicated, and no attempt should be made to prepare the bowel for surgery in the acute phase of illness because this may precipitate perforation.

As already mentioned, increasing abdominal tenderness, guarding, rebound tenderness, rising temperature, and paralytic ileus during the period of observation are consistent with CI and are indications for surgery. The appearance of an infarcted colon ranges from wet tissue paper to a mottled, thickened, and aperistaltic bowel. The resected specimen should be opened and examined immediately to determine the extent of mucosal injury. If the margins are involved, more colon should be removed until only normal bowel remains.

Reversible Lesions

In the mildest cases of CI, symptoms and signs of illness disappear within 24 to 48 hours. Submucosal and intramural hemorrhages are resorbed, there is complete clinical and radiographic resolution within 1 to 2 weeks, and no further therapy is needed. More severe ischemic insults result in necrosis of the overlying mucosa with varying degrees of ulceration and inflammation and the development of a segmental ulcerative colitis. Areas of mucosa may slough, ultimately healing over 1 to 6 months. Patients with such protracted healing may be clinically asymptomatic even in the presence of persistent radiographic or endoscopic evidence of disease.

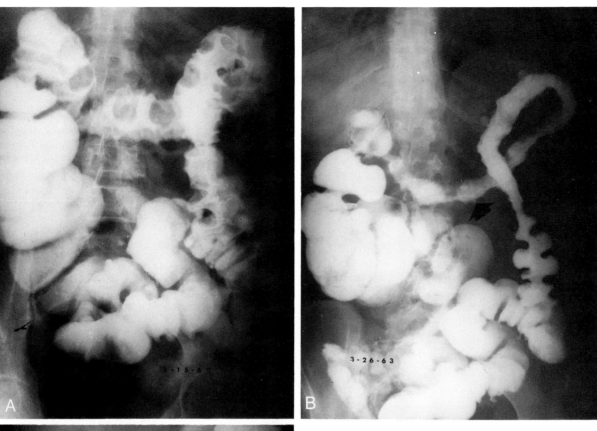

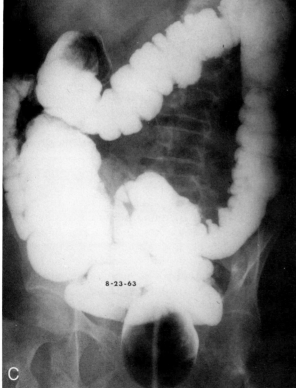

FIGURE 8-4. Ischemic changes in the transverse colon and splenic flexure. *A,* Initial study shows dramatic thumbprints throughout the area of involvement. *B,* Eleven days later, the thumbprints are gone and the involved colon has the typical appearance of segmental colitis, including ulcerations (*arrow*). *C,* Five months after the onset, there is complete return to normal. The patient was asymptomatic 3 weeks after her illness. (From Boley, S.J., and Schwartz, S.S.: Colonic ischemia: Reversible ischemic lesions. *In* Boley, S.J., Schwartz, S.S., and Williams, L.F. [eds.]: Vascular Disorders of the Intestine. New York, Appleton-Century-Crofts, 1971, with permission.)

These asymptomatic patients are managed with a high-residue diet and follow-up evaluation to identify complete healing or the development of a stricture or persistent colitis. Recurrent sepsis in asymptomatic patients with unhealed segmental colitis usually comes from the diseased segment and is an indication for resection.

Irreversible Lesions

Patients with persistent diarrhea, rectal bleeding, protein-wasting enteropathy, or recurrent sepsis lasting longer than 10 to 14 days usually experience perforation, and resection is indicated in these cases. Despite a normal-appearing serosa, there may be extensive mucosal injury, and the extent of the resection should be guided by the distribution of the disease as seen on preoperative studies rather than by the appearance of the bowel at the time of operation. As in all resections for CI, the specimen must be opened at the time of operation to ensure that the margins are free of disease.

Although patients are generally taking little or nothing by mouth when surgery is contemplated, the bowel still should be prepared prior to surgery using a polyethylene glycol–based agent along with oral and intravenous antibiotics. At no time should enemas be given to prepare the bowel.

If, at the time of surgery, the segmental ulcerative colitis involves the rectum, a mucous fistula or Hartmann's procedure with end colostomy should be performed. The mucous fistula can be fashioned through diseased bowel, and in some cases this segment will heal sufficiently to allow restoration of bowel continuity at a later date; simultaneous proctocolectomy is rarely indicated. Local steroid enemas may help healing, but parenteral steroids are contraindicated.

In patients who have had a concurrent or recent myocardial infarction, or in those in whom there are major medical contraindications to surgery, a trial of prolonged parenteral nutrition, with or without concomitant intravenous antibiotic therapy, may be considered as a temporizing measure.

Late Onset of Symptoms

CI may not manifest clinical symptoms during the acute insult but may still produce a chronic segmental ulcerative colitis. Patients with this form of CI are frequently misdiagnosed if not seen during the acute episode. Barium enema studies may show a segmental colitis pattern, a stricture simulating a carcinoma, or even an area of pseudopolyposis (Fig. 8–5). The clinical course at this stage of disease is often indistinguishable from that in other causes of colitis or stenosis. If the patient has been followed from the acute episode, the ischemic nature of the lesion should be apparent; if not, the de novo occurrence of a segmental area of colitis or stricture in an elderly patient should be considered ischemic and treated accordingly. Crypt abscesses and pseudopolyposis, usually considered histologically diagnostic of chronic idiopathic ulcerative colitis, can also be found with ischemic colitis.

The natural history of segmental colitis in elderly patients is that of CI; the involvement remains localized, resection is not followed by recurrence, and the response to steroid therapy is usually poor. Initially, patients with chronic ischemic colitis are managed symptomatically. Local steroid enemas may be helpful, but parenteral steroids should be avoided. Segmental resection of the diseased bowel should be performed in patients whose symptoms cannot be controlled by medication.

Stricture

Stenosis or a stricture of the colon may develop in patients with asymptomatic segmental ulcerative colitis. Strictures that produce no symptoms should be observed, and some will return to normal over 12 to 24 months with no further treatment required (Fig. 8–6). However, if symptoms of obstruction develop, segmental resection is indicated.

SPECIFIC LESIONS

Colonic Ischemia Complicating Abdominal Aortic Surgery

Mesenteric vascular reconstruction is not indicated in most cases of colonic ischemia, but it may be required to prevent CI during and after aortic reconstruction. A small percentage of patients develop clinically symptomatic CI, but a higher incidence, up to 10%, is noted when routine colonoscopy is performed after abdominal aortic surgery.[7] After aortic replacement, the 1 to 3% of patients who develop clinical signs of CI account for approximately 10% of the postoperative deaths.[6,9] Up to 31% of those patients who develop CI following infrarenal aneurysm repair will die.[8] Factors that contribute to the development of postoperative colonic ischemia include rupture of the aneurysm, hypotension, operative trauma to the colon, hypoxemia, arrhythmias, prolonged aortic cross-clamp time, and improper management of the IMA during aneurysmectomy.

The most important aspect of management of colonic ischemia following aortic surgery is its prevention. Collateral blood flow to the left colon after occlusion of the IMA comes from the superior mesenteric artery (SMA) via the arch of Riolan ("the meandering artery") or the marginal artery of Drummond, and from the internal iliac arteries via the middle and inferior hemorrhoidal arteries (Fig. 8–7). If these collateral pathways are intact, postoperative colonic ischemia rarely occurs. Therefore, aortography to determine the patency of the celiac axis, SMA, IMA, and internal iliac artery is advised prior to aneurysmectomy. The presence of a meandering artery does not, in and of itself, allow safe ligation of the IMA, because the blood flow in the meandering artery frequently originates from the IMA and reconstitutes an obstructed SMA. Ligation of the IMA in the latter circumstance can be catastrophic, leading to infarction of the small and large bowel. Ligation of the IMA is safe only when angiography confirms that the blood flows in the meandering artery from the SMA to the IMA. Therefore, reimplantation of the IMA and re-

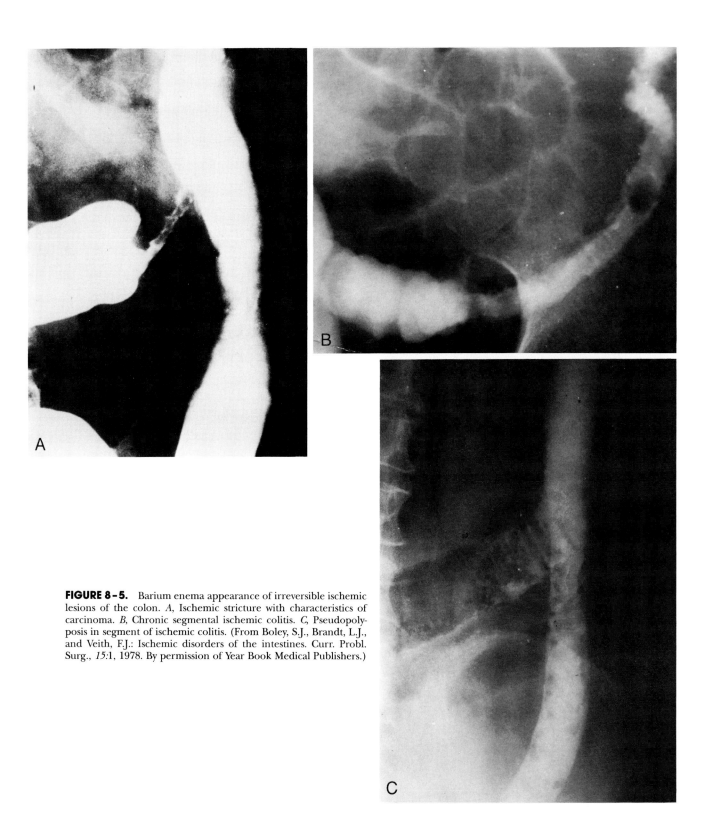

FIGURE 8–5. Barium enema appearance of irreversible ischemic lesions of the colon. *A*, Ischemic stricture with characteristics of carcinoma. *B*, Chronic segmental ischemic colitis. *C*, Pseudopolyposis in segment of ischemic colitis. (From Boley, S.J., Brandt, L.J., and Veith, F.J.: Ischemic disorders of the intestines. Curr. Probl. Surg., *15*:1, 1978. By permission of Year Book Medical Publishers.)

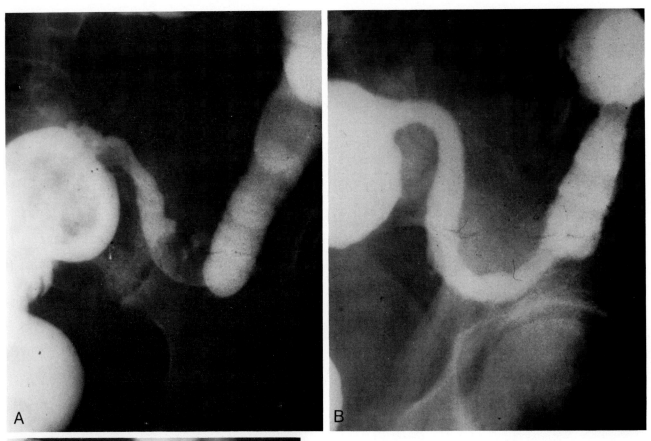

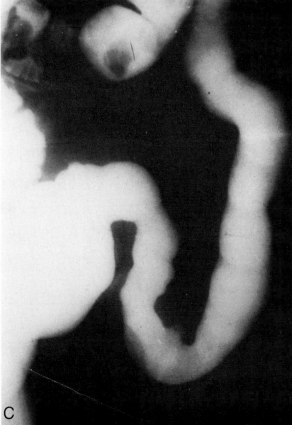

FIGURE 8-6. *A,* Ischemic stricure of the sigmoid colon. *B,* Eighteen months later, stricture is still obvious. *C,* Two years after the initial study, the colon has almost returned to normal. (From Boley, S.J., Brandt, L.J., and Veith, F.J.: Ischemic disorders of the intestines. Curr. Probl. Surg., *15*:1, 1978. By permission of Year Book Medical Publishers.)

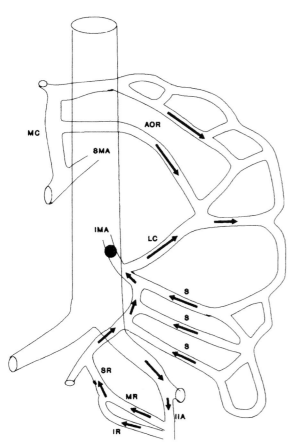

FIGURE 8-7. Collateral blood flow to the colon from the marginal artery, arch of Riolan, and internal iliac artery via the inferior and middle rectal arteries to an occluded IMA. (SMA = superior mesenteric artery, IMA = inferior mesenteric artery, MC = middle colic artery, AOR = arch of Riolan, LC = left colic artery, S = sigmoid arteries, R = superior rectal artery, MR = middle rectal artery, IR = inferior rectal artery, IIA = internal iliac artery.)

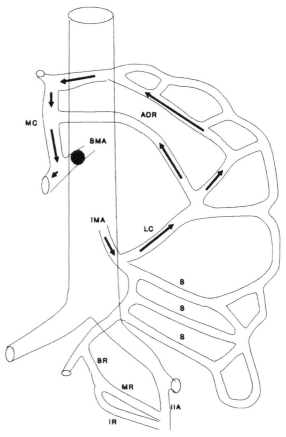

FIGURE 8-8. Collateral blood flow from the IMA via the marginal artery and arch of Riolan to an occluded SMA. (SMA = superior mesenteric artery, IMA = inferior mesenteric artery, MC = middle colic artery, AOR = arch of Riolan, LC = left colic artery, S = sigmoid arteries, R = superior rectal artery, MR = middle rectal artery, IR = inferior rectal artery, IIA = internal iliac artery.)

vascularization of the SMA is required when the SMA is occluded or tightly stenosed and the IMA provides inflow to the meandering artery (Fig. 8–8).

Occlusion of both hypogastric arteries on the preoperative arteriogram indicates that the rectal blood flow is dependent upon collateral flow from the IMA or from the SMA via the meandering artery (Fig. 8–9). In this circumstance, reconstitution of flow to one or both hypogastric arteries as well as the IMA as desirable at the time of aneurysmectomy.

At operation, cross-clamp time should be minimized, and hypotension must be avoided. If a meandering artery is identified, it is carefully preserved. Because the serosal appearance of the colon is not a reliable indicator of collateral blood flow, several methods have been suggested to determine the need for IMA reimplantation. Stump pressure greater than 40 mm Hg in the transected IMA, or an IMA/systemic mean blood pressure ratio greater than 0:40, reliably indicates adequate collateral circulation and has been used to avoid IMA reimplantation. Doppler ultrasound flow signals recorded at the base of the mesentery and at the serosal surface of the colon with temporary IMA inflow occlusion may also suggest that the IMA can be ligated safely without the need for reimplantation.

Another technique used to determine the adequacy of colonic blood flow during aneurysmectomy is tonometric determination of the intramural pH of the sigmoid colon.[2] A tonometric balloon passed prior to cross clamping the aorta enables one to evaluate the effects of cross clamping and restoration of aortic flow on the colonic intramural pH. The latter, when low, is a marker of tissue acidosis and will reflect clinically significant ischemia. Thus, the need for revascularization can be identified while the abdomen is open. When IMA reimplantation is deemed necessary, the IMA should be excised with a patch of aortic wall (Carrell's patch), and the patch should be sutured into the side of the aortic prosthesis. Revascularization of the SMA with a jump graft from the aortic prosthetic graft to the side of the SMA should be performed whenever the SMA is occluded.

The difficulty in accurately assessing the development of CI postoperatively and the significant mortality associated with its occurrence have led to a recommendation that postoperative colonoscopy be performed in high-risk patients. Patients at high risk for the development of postoperative CI following aortic reconstruction are those with (1) ruptured abdominal aortic aneurysm, (2) prolonged cross-clamp time, (3) a patent

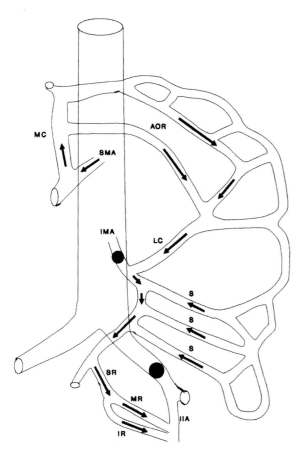

FIGURE 8-9. The entire rectal blood flow is dependent on collateral flow after occlusion of both internal iliac arteries. In this figure, the IMA is also occluded, leaving rectal blood flow dependent on collateral flow from the SMA via the arch of Riolan and the marginal artery and then via the superior rectal vessel to the middle and inferior rectal arteries. (SMA = superior mesenteric artery, IMA = inferior mesenteric artery, MC = middle colic artery, AOR = arch of Riolan, LC = left colic artery, S = sigmoid arteries, R = superior rectal artery, MR = middle rectal artery, IR = inferior rectal artery, IIA = internal iliac artery.)

IMA on preoperative aortography, (4) nonpulsatile flow in the hypogastric arteries at operation, and (5) postoperative diarrhea. Colonoscopy is performed within 2 to 3 days of the operation; if CI is identified, therapy is begun before major complications develop.

Fulminating Universal Colitis

Recently, a rare fulminating form of CI involving all or most of the colon and rectum was identified in a few patients who presented with sudden onset of a toxic universal colitis. Bleeding, fever, severe diarrhea, abdominal pain, and tenderness, often with signs of peritonitis, have been present. The clinical course is rapidly progressive and has required emergency colectomy. The appearance of the colon has been that of a combination of ischemic changes and severe colitis. The management of these patients is similar to that in other forms of fulminating colitis. They require total abdominal colectomy with an ileostomy. A second-stage proctectomy has been required in some patients within 1 month of the original operation.

Lesions Mimicking Colon Carcinoma

Ischemic colitis can present with lesions that appear, on barium enema and colonoscopy, to be similar to colon carcinoma.[1] Colonoscopy and biopsy may, in some cases, be able to distinguish malignant lesions from those resulting from ischemic cicatrization. Therefore, in patients with a history compatible with ischemic colitis, colonoscopy is advised when an annular lesion is identified on barium enema. Treatment consists of local resection and restoration of bowel continuity.

Colitis Associated with Colon Carcinoma

Colitis developing acutely in patients with carcinoma of the colon has been recognized for many years. The colitis is usually, but not always, proximal to the tumor and occurs with or without clinical obstruction. This form of colitis is of ischemic origin and has the radiologic and endoscopic appearance of ischemic colitis. Clinically, patients may present with symptoms of CI or with symptoms related to the primary cancer; that is, crampy pain of a chronic nature, bleeding, or acute colonic obstruction. In most cases, however, the predominant complaints are related to an ischemic episode—sudden onset of mild to moderate abdominal pain, fever, bloody diarrhea, and abdominal tenderness.

It is imperative for both the radiologist and surgeon to be aware of the frequent association of CI and colon cancer. The radiologist must be careful to exclude cancer in every case of CI. For the surgeon, it is vital to examine any colon resected for cancer to exclude the presence of an ischemic process in the area of the anastomosis because such involvement may lead to stricture or a leak.

Colonic ischemia localized to the right side of the colon may be the initial manifestation of interference with the SMA circulation. If a thumbprinting pattern is seen on a barium enema, or colonoscopy reveals colonic ischemia isolated to the right colon, we consider this an indication for selective mesenteric angiography before discharge from the hospital to exclude the diagnosis of some form of AMI. AMI is a spectrum of disorders affecting the SMA blood flow including superior mesenteric arterial embolus (SMAE), nonocclusive mesenteric ischemia (NOMI), superior mesenteric artery thrombosis (SMAT), and mesenteric venous thrombosis (MVT). We have seen three patients who presented with right-sided colonic ischemia and developed small bowel ischemia within 1 month. All had advanced atherosclerotic disease involving the SMA.

REFERENCES

1. Bernstein, W.C., and Bernstein, E.F.: Ischemic ulcerative colitis following inferior mesenteric artery ligation. Dis. Colon Rectum, 6:54, 1963.
2. Boley, S.J., Brandt, L.J., and Veith, F.J.: Ischemic disorders of the intestine. Curr. Probl. Surg., 15:1, 1978.
3. Boley, S.J., Krieger, H., Schultz, L., et al.: Experimental aspects of peripheral vascular occlusion of the intestine. Surg. Gynecol. Obstet., 121:789, 1965.

4. Boley, S.J., Schwartz, S., Lash, J., and Sternhill, V.: Reversible vascular occlusion of the colon. Surg. Gynecol. Obstet., *116*:53, 1963.
5. Brandt, L.J., Boley, S.J., Goldberg, L., et al.: Colitis in the elderly. Am. J. Gastroenterol., *76*:239, 1981.
6. Dahan, P., Roseau, G., Duchatele, J.P., et al.: Intestinal ischemia after surgery of the inrfarenal aorta. Apropos of 13 cases. Ann. Chir., *45*:402, 1991.
7. Ernst, C.B., Hagihara, P.F., Daugherty, M.E., et al.: Ischemic colitis incidence following abdominal aortic reconstruction: A preospective study. Surgery, *80*:417, 1976.
8. Farkas, J.C., Calvo-Verjat, N., Laurian C, et al.: Acute colorectal ischemia after aortic surgery: pathophysiology and prognostic criteria. Ann. Vasc. Surg., *6*:111, 1992.
9. Kim, M.W., Hundahl, S.A., Dang, C.R., et al: Ischemic colitis following aortic aneurysmectomy. Am. J. Surg., *145*:392, 1983.
10. Marston, A., Phiels, M.T., Thomas, M.L., and Morson, B.C.: Ischemic colitis. Gut, 7:1, 1966.
11. Schwartz, S., Boley, S.J., and Lash, J.: Roentgenological aspects of reversible vascular occlusions of the colon and its relationship to ulcerative 122:533, 1963.
12. Shaw, R.S., and Green, T.H.: Massive mesenteric infarction following inferior mesenteric artery ligation in resection of the colon for carcinoma. N. Engl. J. Med., *248*:890, 1953.
13. Smith, R.F., and Szilagyi, D.E.: Ischemia of the colon as a complication in the surgery of the abdominal aorta. Arch. Surg., *80*:806, 1960.
14. Wright, H.G.: Ulcerating colitis in the elderly. Epidemiological and clinical study of an in-patient hospital population. Submitted as thesis for M.D. degree. Yale University, 1970.

Chapter 9

DIVERTICULAR DISEASE

PATRICIA L. ROBERTS / MALCOLM C. VEIDENHEIMER

Diverticular disease is largely a disease of the twentieth century. Although diverticula were briefly described by Littre[43] in the late 1700s and by Cruveilhier[20] in 1849, it was Graser[26] in 1899 who actually described the condition of diverticulitis and Beer[6] in 1904 who correlated the histologic and clinical features of colonic diverticulitis. In 1907, William J. Mayo,[49] in a presentation to the American Surgical Association, found only 19 reported cases of diverticulitis to which he added five of his own cases.[63]

Diverticular disease occurs with relatively equal frequency in men and women, although recently an increasing incidence in females (3:2) has been suggested.[56] Rodkey and Welch[67] found that diverticular disease predominated in men 50 years of age and less, but its predominance in women occurred after the age of 70 years. Diverticulosis is distinctly uncommon before the age of 20 years; thereafter, it increases linearly with age. It is more commonly found in western countries and is said to occur in North America in one third of the population over the age of 45 years and in two thirds of the population over the age of 85 years.[84] The reported incidence of inflammatory changes with the presence of diverticula varies from 10 to 25%.[9,12,33,50,58,74,83]

The sigmoid colon is the most frequent site of involvement in up to 95% of patients. Cecal involvement occurs in about 5% of patients. In the United States, patients with left-sided diverticulitis have an incidence of diverticula in the right colon that has varied from 7 to 30%.[11] In the Far East, diverticulitis affects the right colon more commonly than the left side.[45]

ETIOLOGY

Recent advances have resulted in an improved understanding of both the cause and the physiologic changes that occur in the bowel as a result of diverticular disease. Factors contributing to the development of diverticula include a relative weakness in the bowel wall and a pressure gradient from the lumen to the serosa.

Painter and co-workers[55] studied intracolonic pressures with perfusion manometry and cineradiography and demonstrated a process called segmentation, describing the tendency of the colon to function not as a tube but as small compartments generating high pressures. Pulsion diverticula result from herniations of the mucosa through the weakest part of the bowel wall (Fig. 9–1). Through extensive anatomic dissections, Slack[72] demonstrated that these weak sites are in four different areas between the mesenteric and antimesenteric taeniae at points where intramural blood vessels penetrate. Furthermore, diverticula occur most commonly in the sigmoid colon because of its narrow caliber. Based on Laplace's law, which states that the tension in the wall of a cylinder is directly proportional to the pressure within the cylinder multiplied by the diameter and inversely proportional to the wall thickness, the intraluminal pressure is highest in the sigmoid colon where the wall is thickest and the lumen is narrowest.

Myoelectric studies[1] have shown that patients with symptomatic diverticular disease have an abnormal slow wave pattern of 12 to 18 cycles/min. This contrasts with the slow wave pattern of patients with irritable bowel syndrome; namely, 3 cycles/min.[75] Patients with symptomatic diverticula who eat bran have a motility pattern that returns to normal. No change occurs when patients with irritable bowel syndrome ingest the same diet. Furthermore, patients with asymptomatic diverticula have no change in motility pattern after eating bran.[1]

EPIDEMIOLOGY AND ROLE OF DIET

The frequency of diverticular disease correlates closely with advancing age and western civilization. In 1920, diverticula were found in 5% of autopsies performed in the United States, the United Kingdom, and Australia[54]; this number has now risen to 50%.[66] It is believed that this is the result of striking dietary changes in the twentieth century.

A steep rise in the incidence of diverticular disease

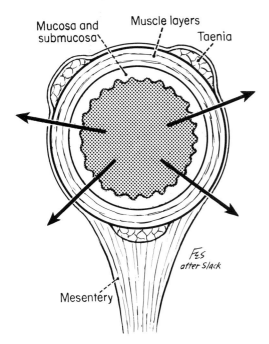

Mucosa and submucosa

Muscle layers

Taenia

Mesentery

FIGURE 9-1. Common sites of diverticula formation. (From Hackford, A.W., and Veidenheimer, M.C.: Diverticular disease of the colon: Current concepts and management. Surg. Clin. North Am. *65*:351, 1985, with permission.)

occurred in England in the early 1900s. This may have resulted in part from roller milling of wheat flour, which resulted in a decreased intake of crude cereal grain and an increased consumption of white flour and refined sugar. The death rate from diverticular disease rose steadily from 1923 to 1963, except in the years from 1939 to 1945.[1] Wartime restrictions modified the British diet during this period, and a higher intake of whole grains, fruits, and vegetables occurred.

The decrease in intake of nondigestible fiber in the western diet is believed to have played a key role in the increase in diverticular disease. It has been estimated that consumption of fiber has fallen to almost one third

of previous consumption because of modern processing techniques.[1] Resultant low-volume tenacious stools require high propulsive efforts for expulsion. This contrasts with the high bulk found in African diets, permitting passage of large volumes of stool. Thus, in countries where high-fiber diets are common, diverticular disease has been considered relatively rare. However, recent evidence has suggested that diverticular disease may be an emerging disease entity in many African countries. Ihekwaba[35] reported on 15 patients in Nigeria with diverticular disease and noted that most (73%) were young and overweight. Although these patients had not abandoned the traditional Nigerian diet, they had also had substantial intake of highly processed foods.

PATHOLOGY

Diverticula are saccular outpouchings of the colon. False diverticula or pseudodiverticula are herniations of the mucosa and submucosa and occur commonly in the sigmoid colon. True diverticula are herniations of the entire bowel wall. Both true and false diverticula occur in the proximal colon. Diverticula are usually 0.5 to 1.0 cm in size and occur along the margins of the taeniae, which represent the weakest points of the bowel wall. The muscle is weakened further by the penetration of segmental blood vessels. In the uninflamed state, diverticula are elastic and compressible and empty freely of fecal contents unless inflammation supersedes. Patients with diverticular disease may have striking changes in the muscle layer of the bowel (Fig. 9–2). Although these changes were once believed to be caused by muscular hypertrophy, careful examination has revealed no evidence of hypertrophy or hyperplasia. Rather, a significant increase is noted in the coarse and smooth elastin fibers of the taenia termed a tenia-specific elastosis by Whiteway and Morson.[85] The taeniae thus become thick and may have a cartilaginous appearance. The circular muscle may be corrugated, and its appearance has been likened to the bellows of a concertina.[37]

FIGURE 9-2. Appearance of diverticular disease with segmentation and foreshortening of sigmoid colon. (From Hackford, A.W., and Veidenheimer, M.C.: Diverticular disease of the colon: Current concepts and management. Surg. Clin. North. Am., *65*:349, 1985, with permission.)

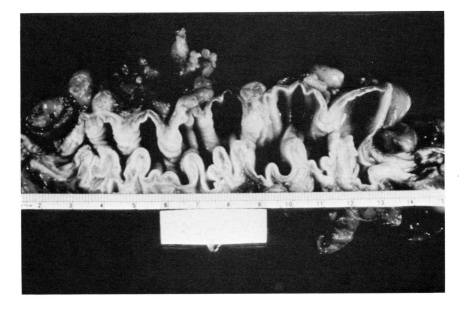

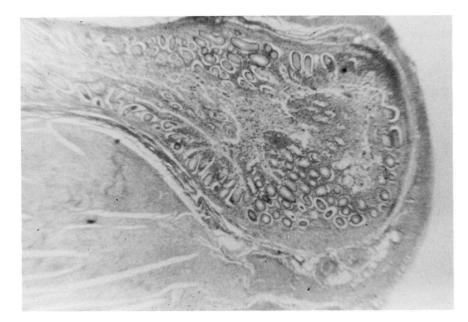

FIGURE 9-3. Microscopic view shows penetration of bowel wall by diverticulum. (From Veidenheimer, M.C.: Surgical management of diverticulitis and its complications. *In* Kodner, I.F., Fry, R.D., and Roe, J.P. [eds.]: Colon, Rectal, and Anal Surgery: Current Techniques and Controversies. St. Louis, C.V. Mosby, 1985, p. 118, with permission.)

Histologic examination of inflamed diverticula reveals a thin wall of flattened or atrophic mucosa, compressed submucosa, and an attenuated or absent mucularis (Fig. 9-3). Repeated episodes of inflammation may result in severe inflammatory changes about the colon wall and luminal narrowing. Extension of infection may lead to abscess or fistula formation or, more rarely, free perforation. Abscesses may perforate into adjacent organs or back into the colon itself, forming intramural fistulas.

DIAGNOSIS AND EVALUATION

Patients with acute diverticulitis usually have left lower quadrant abdominal pain on presentation, which is associated with fever and leukocytosis. An appreciable rate of error may occur, however, by relying on the latter two symptoms for diagnosis. Of 130 patients operated on at the Lahey Clinic for acute complications of diverticular disease, 64% had normal leukocyte counts.[29] Patients may also have tenderness and guarding with or without peritoneal signs. Pelvic or rectal examination or both may reveal a mass. Urinary tract symptoms should alert the clinician to a possible colovesical fistula. The differential diagnosis should include carcinoma, Crohn's disease, ulcerative colitis, ischemic colitis, pelvic inflammatory disease, pyelonephritis, and appendicitis.

The diagnosis of diverticulitis may be made by endoscopy, contrast enema examination, ultrasonography, or computed tomography (CT). Until recently, the barium enema study had been considered the prime diagnostic modality for evaluation of patients with diverticular disease. This study is usually performed after the acute process has subsided with conservative therapy. When a localized perforation is suspected, a water-soluble enema study should be performed. Although diverticula are easy to identify, specific findings consistent with inflammation or diverticulitis are more difficult to discern. Radiologic signs, such as an abscess cavity or intramural or

extramural fistulization, may be accepted as indicators of diverticulitis (Fig. 9-4).

Endoscopy is relatively contraindicated in the acute phase of diverticulitis because insufflation of air may convert a contained perforation into a free perforation. In the setting of acute diverticulitis, limited rigid sigmoidoscopy may be performed to exclude another diagnosis, such as inflammatory bowel disease. Sigmoidoscopy often reveals spasm and inability to advance beyond the rectosigmoid, which is indirect evidence of a diagnosis of diverticulitis. Other changes that may be seen include edema of the mucosa, an extraluminal mass, and fixation of the bowel wall. When performing

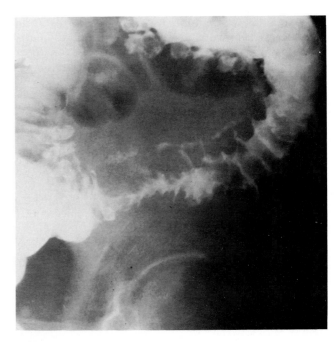

FIGURE 9-4. Contrast enema reveals intramural fistula consistent with diagnosis of diverticular disease.

sigmoidoscopy, caution should be exercised to inflate the least amount of air possible because inflamed bowel is more likely to perforate. In the elective setting, endoscopic examination of the sigmoid colon may be helpful to distinguish diverticular disease from carcinoma, particularly in the patient who is found to have a stricture. Although a long stricture with normal-appearing mucosa is more consistent with diverticulitis, and a short segment with overhanging edges and ulceration of the mucosa more consistent with carcinoma, at times, a distinction cannot be made. In these patients, flexible sigmoidoscopy or colonoscopy may aid in diagnosis. When doubt exists, resection is indicated.

Recently, initial examination with CT or ultrasonography has been advocated for the diagnosis of diverticulitis (Fig. 9–5). Ultrasonography may reveal a thickened colonic wall or cystic masses with echogenic densities consistent with abscess.[57] Bowel wall thickening, however, is not specific and may occur in Crohn's disease, carcinoma, and metastatic disease. A prospective study[70] of 130 consecutive patients with abdominal complaints evaluated by ultrasonography found sonographic signs of diverticulitis in 96% of patients. Ultrasound examinations are operator dependent, however.

Because diverticulitis is largely an extramural disease, CT, which permits evaluation of the bowel wall and mesentery, has intrinsic appeal. Computed tomography may assist in making the diagnosis of acute diverticulitis and may also have a therapeutic role in the patient who has an abscess that may be drained percutaneously. In addition, CT may enable the severity of disease to be staged and may be useful in assessing the degree of resolution of diverticulitis after a course of therapy. Clinical examination, however, may be just as effective and less expensive in assessing response to therapy in diverticulitis.

Computed tomography has been compared with contrast enema examination in a number of series. The superiority of one examination over the other has been debated. In a series of 43 CT examinations performed on patients with diverticular disease, the most common findings were inflammation of the pericolic fat (98%), diverticula (84%), thickening of the bowel wall (70%), pericolic abscess (35%), peritonitis (16%), fistula (14%), colonic obstruction (12%), and intramural sinus tracts (9%). Other findings included distant abscesses (12%) and ureteral obstruction (7%).[34] Hulnick and associates[34] found CT more accurate than contrast enema in 41% of patients and advocated CT as the initial study for the evaluation of patients with diverticular disease. A somewhat different view was espoused by Johnson and associates,[36] who compared the use of contrast enema and CT in 102 patients with diverticulitis and reported a diagnostic accuracy of 77% and 41%, respectively. They[36] concluded that CT should be reserved for patients who are unable to have adequate contrast enemas, whose condition is unresponsive to medical therapy, who are candidates for percutaneous drainage, or who are suspected of having distant or diffuse abscesses. Both series[34,36] were retrospective. In a subsequent series[15] of patients with a strong clinical suspicion of sigmoid diverticulitis in whom CT was compared with barium enema studies, results of CT were positive in 93% compared with 80% in barium enema studies, which were positive. However, the radiologist did not know the results of each study.

In the assessment of acute diverticulitis, CT and contrast enema examination should probably be viewed as complementary examinations. In particular, contrast enema examination may be useful in the patient with equivocal or misleading results on CT. Results of CT may be misleading, particularly in patients with substantial colonic wall thickening in whom a diagnosis of carcinoma must be excluded and in patients with small intramural abscesses.[5] The contrast enema examination may be more useful in such patients.

UNUSUAL PRESENTATIONS

Although patients with diverticulitis usually present with left lower quadrant abdominal pain, unusual extraperitoneal clinical presentations may appreciably delay diagnosis and the institution of proper therapy. Perforated diverticula may penetrate extraperitoneally, resulting in inflammation of the abdominal wall, flank, perineum, scrotum, buttock, vagina, hip joints, thigh, lower extremities, mediastinum, and neck. Ravo and associates[64] noted that these unusual presentations were more common in elderly women; the most common extraperitoneal location is the hip.

SPECIAL ISSUES

Recurrent Diverticulitis After Resection

Patients who undergo colonic resection for diverticular disease rarely require a second operation. Yet, a small percentage of patients may have recurrence of disease with signs and symptoms of acute diverticulitis after what had appeared to be adequate resection. This has been estimated to occur in approximately 7% of patients who have undergone resection; 20% of these patients may require another operation.[42,87]

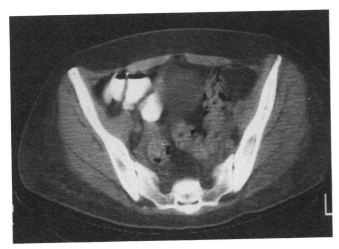

FIGURE 9–5. Computed tomographic scan reveals streaky fat in the left lower quadrant consistent with a diagnosis of sigmoid diverticulitis.

Controversy exists as to how much bowel should be resected on initial operation for diverticulitis. Diverticulitis usually involves a short segment of sigmoid colon. At the Lahey Clinic,[81] the average length of bowel resected is 17.2 cm. Resection should be sufficient to remove the inflammatory lesion and to perform an anastomosis in soft pliable bowel. All distal diverticula should be resected; however, proximal diverticula may be left in place.

Benn and associates[7] advocated total sigmoidectomy to prevent recurrent diverticulitis. In this series, recurrent diverticulitis developed after resection more commonly in patients in whom the sigmoid colon had been used for the distal margin of anastomosis as opposed to patients in whom the rectum had been used; the difference was statistically significant. Excision of all distal diverticula and anastomosis to the rectum is performed to prevent or lessen the incidence of recurrent diverticulitis after resection. An additional study[23] of 93 patients with colocutaneous fistulas further supports resecting all distal diverticula; that is, performing complete sigmoid resection. Anastomosis to the distal sigmoid was a risk factor for the development of a colocutaneous fistula, presumably because the narrow distal sigmoid acted like distal obstruction to an anastomosis.[23]

Any patient who has signs and symptoms of recurrent diverticulitis after resection should be examined for possible inflammatory bowel disease, particularly Crohn's disease and ischemic bowel disease (see section, "Crohn's Disease and Diverticulitis"). Another suggested cause of recurrent diverticulitis is the possibility that the patient did not have diverticulitis in the first place. In such patients, review of the original pathologic findings may be useful.

Diverticulitis and Immunocompromised Patients

Immunocompromised patients with diverticulitis are a special challenge for the surgeon because of a potential delay in diagnosis, with resultant increased morbidity and mortality. Such patients include those receiving steroids, patients receiving organ transplants, patients with cancer who are undergoing chemotherapy or radiotherapy, patients with diabetes, and patients who are chronic alcoholics. Rodkey and Welch[67] found that the number of immunocompromised patients with diverticulitis in their series increased from 3% in 1964 to 1973 to 11.1% in 1974 to 1983. Perkins and associates[59] compared 76 nonimmunocompromised patients with 10 immunocompromised patients who had acute diverticulitis; the immunocompromised patients were more likely to have minimal or few symptoms of diverticulitis at presentation. In all of the immunocompromised patients, medical therapy failed, necessitating surgical intervention. The authors[59] emphasized the lack of symptoms, the necessity for a high index of suspicion, and the need for aggressive surgical management in these patients. Another study[80] that compared 40 immunocompromised patients with diverticulitis with 169 nonimmunocompromised patients with diverticulitis had similar findings. Immunocompromised patients had a much higher incidence of free perforation compared with nonimmunocompromised patients (43% versus 14%) and a greater risk of requiring surgery (58% versus 33%).[80]

Patients with chronic renal failure are also a challenge for the surgeon. This includes both patients who have undergone renal transplantation and who are maintained on immunosuppression and patients undergoing dialysis. It has also been suggested[69] that patients with adult polycystic kidney disease have a higher incidence of diverticulitis. Starnes and co-workers[77] reported on 25 patients with treated chronic renal failure who underwent operation for acute diverticulitis. This group[77] represented 1.1% of the patients with chronic renal failure treated at their institution during a 22-year period. Although it is not known whether patients with chronic renal failure have an increased incidence of acute diverticulitis compared with the population at large, in this study,[77] patients with chronic renal failure tended to be much younger than nonuremic patients with acute diverticulitis; 30% of patients were 40 years of age or younger and almost half were less than 50 years of age. Another striking feature in the group of patients was that 50% had free perforation of diverticula into the peritoneal cavity with minimal surrounding inflammation. As expected, mortality and morbidity rates were high in this group. Factors correlating with the increased mortality and morbidity were increasing age of patients and longer duration of symptoms. Once again, this underscores the need for a high index of suspicion and for aggressive treatment in the immunocompromised patient.

Diverticular Disease in Young Patients

Diverticular disease of the colon is relatively rare in patients less than 40 years of age and constitutes only 2 to 5% of the total number of patients evaluated in multiple large series.[16,22,24,53,67,71] Nevertheless, diverticular disease in young patients is often more virulent than in older patients, and young patients are more likely to have complications of diverticulitis.

In young patients, diverticular disease is not often considered in the initial differential diagnosis. In a series[16] of 35 patients with diverticulitis who were less than 40 years of age, in only one third of patients was a correct diagnosis made on initial presentation. Other series[22,23] have corroborated this finding. The most common incorrect diagnosis was acute appendicitis.

As is true in the general population, young patients with acute diverticulitis most commonly have sigmoid involvement. However, diverticular disease has been found to be predominant in male patients in all series of patients with diverticular disease less than 40 years of age in contrast to the relative predominance of diverticular disease in female patients. Patients with Marfan's syndrome have a higher incidence of diverticular disease. Parks[56] has suggested that the deficiency of collagen tissue in patients with Marfan's syndrome predisposes them to mucosal herniation. Obesity in young patients has also been postulated[68] as an etiologic factor in the development of diverticular disease.

Although Parks[56] has stated that about one third of patients require operation for diverticular disease on presentation, a much higher percentage of young patients require urgent or emergent resection on initial presentation. In a series of 181 patients, Eusebio and Eisenberg[22] found that 66% required resection. Similarly, Chodak and associates[16] found that 76.5% of their patients required operation during the initial attack of diverticular disease.

Although a large number of young patients with acute diverticulitis require urgent or emergent laparotomy on initial presentation, the natural history of diverticular disease after one episode of relatively mild diverticulitis in the young patient is less clearly defined. Such patients may recover fully and never have another bout of diverticulitis; however, because a young person will have a life expectancy of an additional 30 to 40 years, long-term longitudinal follow-up studies are necessary, and no such study has been performed. In general, however, elective resection should strongly be considered in young patients after one well-documented episode of diverticulitis because elective sigmoid resection is associated with less risk than urgent or emergent resection.

Diverticular Disease and Carcinoma

Although initially it was believed that diverticular disease predisposed patients to carcinoma of the colon as a result of chronic irritation,[47,86] it is now recognized that the two conditions may commonly exist in the same patient.[39]

Rauch[62] studied 118 patients with concomitant diverticulitis and carcinoma of the colon and noted that these patients had a much poorer prognosis, which may have been the result of a delay in diagnosis. Colonic diverticula obscure the sigmoid colon, making detection of mucosal lesions difficult. Therefore, all patients with known diverticular disease and guaiac-positive stools should be investigated aggressively to rule out coincidental carcinoma. Flexible sigmoidoscopy or colonoscopy in this group of patients is superior to the barium enema study.

Crohn's Disease and Diverticulitis

Patients who undergo sigmoid resection for diverticular disease rarely undergo a second operation for recurrent disease. A subset of patients who require a second operation for recurrent pain, fever, and leukocytosis may, in fact, have Crohn's disease. Berman and associates[8] reviewed records of 25 patients who underwent initial sigmoid resection for presumed diverticular disease; all 25 patients had evidence of Crohn's disease in resected specimens. Features consistent with a diagnosis of late-onset Crohn's colitis include anorectal disease, rectal bleeding, fistula, complicated course after initial resection, multiple operations, and extraintestinal manifestations. The patients reported on by Berman and associates[8] also tended to be older than most patients with diverticular disease. Crohn's disease should be considered in the differential diagnosis of recurrent diverticular disease after resection and in the patient who appears to have a complicated course after resection.

COMPLICATIONS OF DIVERTICULAR DISEASE

Phlegmon or Abscess

Localized perforation or abscess is the most common complication of diverticulitis, occurring in 10 to 57% of patients treated surgically.[8,56,67,73] The slowly developing pericolitis associated with diverticulitis causes envelopment of the affected segment of bowel by epiploic appendices, omentum, small bowel, bladder, and uterus. Localized abscesses occur more commonly than free perforation (Fig. 9-6).

Although abscesses begin in the mesocolon, they may penetrate to the pelvis or retroperitoneum. Unusual locations have also been reported, such as in the hip and thigh.

A patient with a discrete abscess will present with continued spiking temperatures, abdominal tenderness, leukocytosis and, often, unresolved ileus. Although small pericolic abscesses often resolve with antibiotic therapy,[2] larger abscesses or distant abscesses, such as retroperitoneal or pelvic abscesses, often require surgical intervention or percutaneous drainage under ultrasound or CT guidance. When a discrete abscess is found on CT or ultrasonography, percutaneous drainage may permit stabilization of the patient and resolution of the septic process, subsequently enabling performance of single-stage sigmoid resection instead of a two-stage procedure. Stabile and associates[76] examined 19 patients with large abscesses (mean size, 8.9 cm) from diverticulitis who had undergone percutaneous drainage. In 12 patients, the condition was able to be stabilized, and they subsequently underwent single-stage resection.

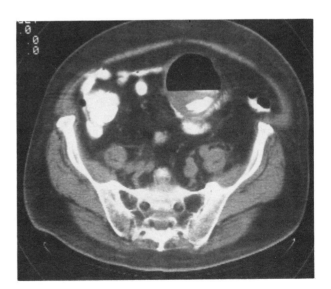

FIGURE 9-6. Large pericolic abscess in a patient with diverticulitis who underwent percutaneous drainage followed by single-stage sigmoid resection. (From Veidenheimer, M.C., and Roberts, P.L.: Colonic Diverticular Disease. Boston, Blackwell Scientific Publications, 1991, p. 72, with permission.)

Obstruction

The incidence of colonic obstruction associated with diverticular disease varies from 8 to 65%, most series[10,56,67,73] reporting an incidence of about 10%. In a series of patients with complicated diverticular disease reported on by Veidenheimer,[81] 6% had some bowel obstruction.

Repeated episodes of acute diverticulitis heal with residual fibrosis and scarring. Sufficient fibrosis may narrow the lumen, resulting in obstructive symptoms. Obstruction may also be caused by a pericolic abscess, by phlegmon, or by extrinsic compression from adherent loops of small bowel. Patients with obstruction associated with diverticular disease may have an acute onset of symptoms, but the usual course is increasing constipation, mucous discharge, abdominal distention, and narrowed caliber of stools. Obstruction associated with diverticular disease is usually incomplete and resolves with bowel rest, nasogastric suction, and intravenous feedings. On initial presentation, the main goal of treatment is fluid resuscitation of the patient. After the patient's condition has been stabilized, the cause of the obstruction is investigated further through endoscopic or barium contrast studies. Contrast studies may demonstrate complete obstruction to the retrograde flow of barium in the absence of antegrade obstruction in a patient who is improving and passing gas. Patients who have obstruction on presentation are a diagnostic challenge for the clinician to differentiate between diverticular disease or carcinoma or both.

Conservative measures and primary resection of the involved segment (usually sigmoid) will resolve the obstruction in most patients. Anastomosis may be considered when adequate bowel preparation is possible. For patients whose obstruction does not resolve, primary resection with end colostomy and either a Hartmann turn-in of the distal segment or creation of a mucous fistula may be performed. Restoration of bowel continuity should be performed several months later. An alternative treatment for selected patients whose obstruction is not resolved is on-table colonic lavage followed by sigmoid resection and primary anastomosis. Murray and colleagues[52] reported on 25 patients who underwent emergent or urgent colonic resection with on-table lavage. No patient required colostomy, and primary anastomosis was performed in all patients.

Fistula

Fistulas associated with diverticulitis result from perforation of localized pericolic abscesses and may involve the bladder, uterus, vagina, fallopian tubes, ureter, small intestine, or abdominal wall (Figs. 9–7 and 9–8). Fistulas have been reported[29,67] in 10 to 24% of patients undergoing resection for complicated diverticular disease. The diagnosis of Crohn's disease must be considered and carefully excluded.

Colovesical fistulas are most common and comprise about 50% of all fistulas associated with diverticular disease.[17,67] They are more common in men than in women

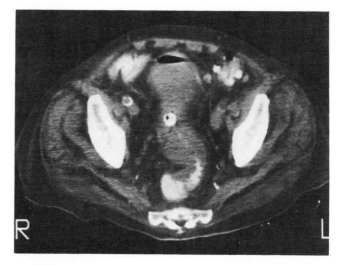

FIGURE 9–7. More than 50% of fistulas associated with diverticular disease are colovesical fistulas. They are more common in men. Computed tomography is the most sensitive test for detecting colovesical fistulas. Air is seen in the bladder. (From Veidenheimer, M.D., and Roberts, P.L.: Colonic Diverticular Disease. Boston, Blackwell Scientific Publications, 1991, p. 70, with permission.)

because of the protective effect of the intervening uterus in women. Most patients have urinary tract signs and symptoms on presentation; pneumaturia and recurrent urinary tract infections are common manifestations. Bowel complaints are usually mild because the area has been decompressed from the higher pressure colonic side into the bladder. Colovesical fistulas are rarely demonstrated on barium enema examination, intravenous pyelography, or cystography. Cystoscopy may reveal an area of bullous edema or erythema at the site of the fistula. Computed tomography is probably the best imaging study to document a colovesical fistula.[40] In the patient who has not had prior instrumentation, the finding of an air-fluid level or air bubble in the bladder is diagnostic of a fistula. The diagnosis may also be made presumptively on clinical grounds. Treatment consists of resection of the involved segment of colon (virtually always the sigmoid colon) and simple closure of the fistulous connection with the bladder. An indwelling Foley catheter is left in place for 7 to 10 days.

Colovaginal fistulas are rare and occur almost exclusively in women who have undergone hysterectomy. Patients with colovaginal fistulas often present with vaginal discharge. Treatment consists of resection of the involved segment of colon and closure of the fistulous connection. If available, the omentum may be interposed between the vagina and the trectosigmoid.

Colocutaneous fistulas occur primarily in patients who have undergone previous operations for diverticulitis and represent operative complications. They are more likely to occur in a patient who has had resection and primary anastomosis in the setting of acute inflammation. Spontaneous colocutaneous fistulas are extremely rare. Only one instance was reported[48] in a series of 27 colocutaneous fistulas. In the largest reported series[23] of 93 patients, 88 patients had fistulas after operation, and fistulas developed spontaneously in five patients.

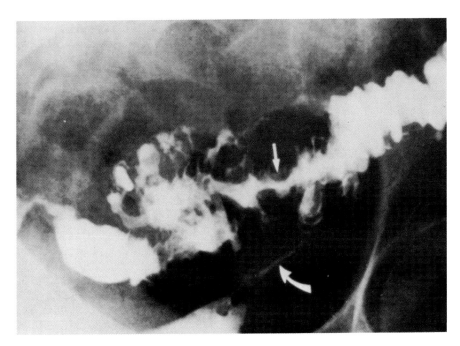

FIGURE 9-8. Colouterine fistulas are extremely rare. Endometrial carcinoma must be ruled out.

Free Perforation

Free perforation is the most morbid complication of acute diverticulitis and occurs in 4 to 15% of patients undergoing operation for complicated diverticular disease.[29,56,67] Free perforation is relatively uncommon because the slow progression of diverticulitis usually permits sealing of the inflammatory process from the peritoneal cavity. This may be the most common presenting complication in patients who are immunocompromised and particularly in patients receiving steroid therapy.

Patients with this complication on presentation are extremely ill, and after a brief period of intensive resuscitation consisting of the administration of intravenous fluids and broad-spectrum antibiotics, immediate operation is indicated. The goal of operation is removal of the septic process from the abdominal cavity. Sigmoid resection with proximal end colostomy and Hartmann closure of the rectum is the procedure of choice. Bowel continuity is restored 3 months later. A reasonable alternative may be the creation of a primary anastomosis and proximal stoma. In a series[29] of 140 patients operated on for complicated diverticular disease at the Lahey Clinic, 16% of patients who underwent this alternative procedure had generalized peritonitis (Fig. 9-9). No deaths occurred, and the morbidity rate (22%) was comparable to that of patients undergoing a Hartmann procedure (23%).[29] As another alternative, some surgeons[38] have advocated prograde colonic lavage of the proximal colon to prepare the bowel for anastomosis in an emergency setting. Three-stage procedures—consisting of initial transverse colostomy followed by sigmoid resection and, finally, colostomy closure—are mentioned only to be condemned, as they do not permit removal of the septic focus at initial operation.

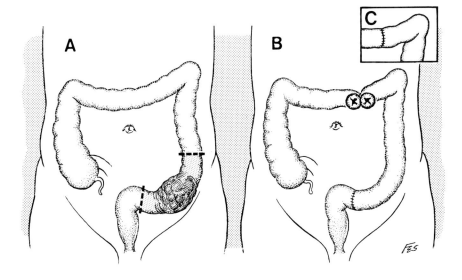

FIGURE 9-9. Operation for complicated diverticular disease. *A,* Sigmoid colon is resected at initial procedure. *B,* Primary anastomosis is performed and protected by left transverse loop colostomy. The left side is preferred because the colostomy is tethered by the splenic flexure and is less likely to prolapse. In addition, stool is more solid on the left side, facilitating care of the colostomy. *Inset,* Stoma is closed in 6 to 8 weeks. (From Veidenheimer, M.C.: Clinical presentation and surgical treatment of complicated diverticular disease. *In* Allan, R.N., Keighley, M.R.B., Alexander-Williams, J., et al. [eds.]: Inflammatory Bowel Diseases. Edinburgh, Churchill Livingstone, 1983, p. 526, with permission.)

Hemorrhage

Parks[56] estimated that 30% of patients with diverticulosis have lower gastrointestinal tract bleeding at some time, ranging in severity from an occasional guaiac-positive stool to massive lower gastrointestinal tract bleeding. This number is probably an overestimation because the greater frequency of endoscopic examinations and guaiac-positive stools attributed to diverticular disease have often been found to be caused by polyps or carcinoma. Any patient with known diverticular disease, guaiac-positive stools, and no obvious anorectal source of bleeding should be evaluated aggressively to exclude an underlying malignancy. It is believed that colonoscopy is superior to the barium enema study in this group of patients.

The evaluation of the patient who has massive bleeding must proceed rapidly and logically and is identical regardless of the cause of bleeding. Resuscitation of the patient with a balanced salt solution and blood products as indicated administered intravenously through a large-bore catheter is carried out first. A nasogastric tube should be inserted to exclude an upper gastrointestinal tract source of bleeding, and sigmoidoscopy should be performed to exclude an anorectal source of bleeding.

At the Lahey Clinic, patients with massive bleeding are treated according to the algorithm shown in Figure 9–10. A radionuclide scan for bleeding is then performed with labeled red blood cells. Radionuclide scans may detect bleeding rates as slow as 0.1 to 0.5 ml/min as opposed to angiography, which detects bleeding rates from 0.5 to 1.0 ml/min. Radionuclide scans are safe, noninvasive, and simple to perform. When results of the radionuclide scan are positive, angiography is performed. Angiography may be diagnostic as well as therapeutic. If a bleeding site is identified, as demonstrated by extravasation of contrast material (consistent with a diagnosis of bleeding diverticulosis), vasopressin is administered in a dose of 0.2 units/min and increased up to 0.4 units/min. When the bleeding stops, administration of vasopressin is stopped slowly, and the patient is observed. When bleeding continues, laparotomy is performed. Although embolization may be performed, it may be associated with infarction of the intestinal wall and, therefore, should be employed with caution.

When the site of bleeding has been localized by angiography and by radionuclide scan, segmental resection may be performed. This operation is associated with a mortality and rebleeding rate of less than 5%.[14]

Some patients may present with massive bleeding, which stops rapidly. These patients may be prepared and may undergo colonoscopy.

The patient who continues to bleed and whose bleeding site cannot be demonstrated before operation poses a particular challenge for the surgeon. Resecting only the area with the predominance of diverticula (usually the left side) is doomed to failure because the incidence of bleeding diverticula on the left side of the colon equals the incidence on the right side. Blind segmental resection in this instance has been associated with a mortality rate of 30 to 40% and a rebleeding rate of 33%.[51] When the bleeding site cannot be located, the procedure of choice is subtotal colectomy. In some instances, intraoperative colonoscopy may aid in identification of the bleeding site.

Miscellaneous

Although colonic diverticula are usually less than 1 to 2 cm in size, sigmoid diverticula may occasionally enlarge to such a degree that they are termed giant diverticula (Fig. 9–11). This is a rare manifestation of diverticular disease. The treatment of choice includes resection of the involved colon and end-to-end anastomosis.

MEDICAL MANAGEMENT

Patients with mild abdominal tenderness in the absence of systemic signs and symptoms may be treated on an outpatient basis. A low-residue diet is recommended. A broad-spectrum antibiotic (doxycycline, tetracycline, ampicillin, or metronidazole) is prescribed for 7 to 10 days, and patients are advised to take their temperatures daily. If the patient continues to improve, elective diagnostic evaluation is performed. If the patient's condition worsens, inpatient hospitalization is required.

For patients with more severe signs and symptoms, including localized pain or localized peritonitis in the absence of any evidence of free perforation or peritoneal soilage, inpatient hospitalization is indicated. Initial therapy consists of bowel rest, intravenous fluids, and antibiotics. Antibiotic coverage is aimed at covering bowel flora. Nasogastric tubes are not routinely used unless the patient has some degree of obstruction or vomiting.

Careful monitoring and frequent repeated abdominal examinations are necessary. Improvement, as manifested by decreased tenderness, leukocytosis, and fever, often occurs within 48 hours. Persistent fever and leukocytosis may represent an unresolving phlegmon or abscess. Computed tomography helps to identify patients with a discrete abscess that may be amenable to percutaneous drainage. In the patient who improves, the diet is advanced gradually from clear liquids to low-residue foods. Intravenous antibiotics are usually continued for 1 week, although patients who have rapid resolution of symptoms may be instructed to follow an oral antibiotic regimen.

In a relatively young patient (<55 years of age) who is in good health, elective sigmoid resection is considered. Patients who have complications, such as abscess or fistula, should undergo resection after one attack of diverticulitis. After one attack of diverticulitis, the chance of a second attack is approximately 30%. After a second attack of diverticulitis, about 90% of patients will continue to have symptoms.[1] In patients with a mild initial attack of diverticulitis (i.e., patients treated as outpatients or >55 years of age), disease may be managed with fiber and osmotic bulking agents. After the acute attack has subsided, the increase in fecal bulk leads to expansion of the diameter of the sigmoid and a reduction in the intraluminal pressure according to Laplace's law

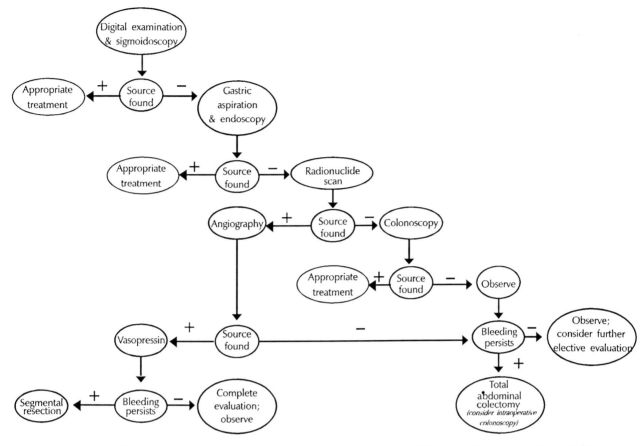

FIGURE 9-10. Proposed algorithm for treatment of massive gastrointestinal bleeding of presumed colonic origin. (From Roberts, P.L., and Veidenheimer, M.C.: Diverticulosis and hemorrhage. *In* Fazio, V.W. (ed.): Current Therapy in Colon and Rectal Surgery. Philadelphia, B.C. Decker, 1990, p. 236, with permission.)

and, therefore, offers some protection against fecal inspissation.

SURGICAL MANAGEMENT

Elective Procedures

Sigmoid Resection

Surgical intervention is mandatory for patients with complications of diverticulitis (including perforation, abscess, obstruction, fistula and, often, hemorrhage) and is associated with high morbidity and mortality. Ideally, patients should be operated on electively before complications ensue. Operations performed electively on patients with uncomplicated diverticular disease are much safer than operations performed on patients in whom complications have developed. Elective resection is advocated for patients who fulfill the following criteria:

1. Two or more attacks of proven diverticulitis associated with abdominal pain, fever, mass, or leukocytosis.
2. An attack of diverticulitis associated with leakage of contrast material at the time of barium or water-soluble enema, obstructive symptoms, urinary symptoms, or inability to differentiate between diverticulitis and carcinoma.

3. A single attack of diverticulitis in a young person (<50 years old).

Elective resection should be carried out 6 to 8 weeks after the initial attack. This enables the acute symptoms to subside and the inflammatory process to resolve. Waiting any longer increases the possibility of another attack of diverticulitis.

Myotomy

In the 1960s, myotomy for the treatment of patients with diverticular disease generated much interest. Longitudinal myotomy was described by Reilly[65] for use in patients with long-standing diverticular disease that was not responsive to medical management. Transverse myotomy was described by Hodgson[32] in 1973, and although measured intraluminal pressures decreased after this procedure was performed, enthusiasm appears to have waned.[18,32,46] Veidenheimer and Lawrence[82] were not impressed with the results of limited myotomy employed at the site of anastomosis in a small series of patients undergoing sigmoid resection.

Surgery for Acute Diverticulitis

In the patient who fails to respond to medical therapy and is not a candidate for percutaneous drainage,

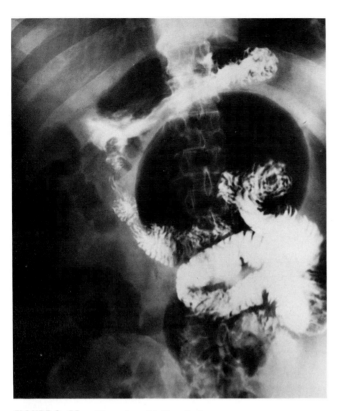

FIGURE 9-11. Giant sigmoid diverticulum.

prompt surgical intervention is indicated. The surgical management of patients with acute diverticulitis is similar to that for complications of diverticulitis. Operative approaches that have been employed for the treatment of patients with complicated diverticular disease include the following:

1. Three-stage procedures, such as transverse colostomy and drainage.

2. Two-stage procedures, such as resection with primary anastomosis and proximal colostomy, Hartmann resection, resection with proximal end colostomy and distal mucous fistula, and Mikulicz operation.

3. One-stage procedures, such as resection with primary anastomosis.

Transverse Colostomy and Drainage

Lockhart-Mummery[44] and Smithwick[74] advocated staged operation for the treatment of patients with complicated diverticular disease. An initial proximal colostomy was followed by resection of the diseased segment and later closure of the colostomy. Smithwick[74] reported a mortality rate of 5% and a morbidity rate of 12% in a series of patients treated by staged operation. Subsequent reports, however, had a much higher mortality and morbidity. Greif and associates[28] reviewed records of more than 1,300 patients operated on for perforated sigmoid diverticulitis. The combined mortality rate for patients undergoing initial colostomy and drainage was 29% compared with 12% in patients who underwent primary resection. An additional review[39] of emergency operations for perforated diverticulitis found a mortality

rate of 25% in patients treated without resection versus 11% in patients treated with resection.

Three-stage operation had several other drawbacks. Patients had to have a stoma in place for several months with the septic source left in place, providing a source for further peritoneal contamination. Drainage achieved by placing drains in the area of the sigmoid colon was often inadequate. Patients had to undergo two other operative procedures, each with attendant morbidity and mortality, while still recovering from their initial operation. The correct time to perform the second stage of the resection was difficult to determine; some patients did not undergo a second-stage or third-stage procedure.

Three-stage procedures result in a long period of hospitalization and disability, which does not fit in with the current climate of medical economics and cost containment. Ponka[60] described the 20-40-60 rule, in which 20 days of hospitalization can be anticipated for a one-stage procedure, 40 days of hospitalization for a two-stage procedure, and 60 days of hospitalization for a three-stage procedure. Three-stage procedures are currently the least commonly employed operations for the management of complicated diverticular disease.

Two-Stage Procedures

If primary resection and anastomosis is considered unsafe because of significant sepsis, resection with a proximal stoma or resection with anastomosis and a proximal stoma may be performed.

HARTMANN PROCEDURE. The Hartmann operation, originally described by Hartmann[30] in 1921 for the treatment of carcinoma of the rectum, is the most commonly performed two-stage procedure for treatment of diverticulitis. This procedure enables resection of the diseased segment and creation of a proximal stoma.

The Hartmann procedure includes mobilization and resection of the sigmoid colon and either a stapled or sutured closure of the rectum. Although the sigmoid colon is acutely inflamed and edematous, mobilization is almost always possible using blunt finger dissection. Dissection from the proximal colon, proceeding in a caudad direction, facilitates the procedure. When the diagnosis is diverticulitis, a segment of uninvolved rectosigmoid is nearly always encountered and may serve as the site for closure of the rectum. An alternative method is to use this distal end as a mucous fistula. However, when total sigmoidectomy is performed, a sufficient length of colon is rarely present to permit construction of a tension-free mucous fistula. Leaving enough inflamed distal sigmoid colon to achieve the creation of a mucous fistula also creates a potential source of infection.

The Hartmann procedure has been advocated by many surgeons and is the procedure of choice for the management of complicated diverticular disease.[21,79]

RESECTION WITH PRIMARY ANASTOMOSIS AND PROXIMAL STOMA. An alternative to the Hartmann resection involves primary resection and anastomosis with formation of a proximal diverting loop colostomy (Fig. 9-9). This operation obviates difficulty in identifying the rectal stump at the time of closure of the colostomy. Subsequent closure of the colostomy may be performed with a peristomal incision without laparotomy, thus avoiding the need for a potentially difficult pelvic dissection.

Single-Stage Procedures

When is it appropriate to perform primary resection and anastomosis when operating on a patient with acute diverticulitis? As pointed out succinctly by Byrne and Garick,[13] it is difficult to compare various series reported in the literature because it is impossible to classify the severity of disease. Toward this end, an attempt at classification was made by Hinchey and colleagues[31] and modified by Auguste and Wise[4] (Table 9–1). With use of their classification, the treatment of choice for patients with stage I or stage II diverticular disease is primary resection and anastomosis. Surgical decision making must be tailored to specific intraoperative findings. When the degree of inflammation, size of the abscess, or degree of contamination is a concern, the most prudent course is to protect the anastomosis with a stoma.

Cecal Diverticulitis

Cecal diverticulitis was first reported by Potier[61] in 1912. It is relatively rare in western countries. In a review of 338 patients with surgically treated diverticulitis, Rodkey and Welch[67] noted that the primary pathologic focus was in the sigmoid colon in 95% of patients and in the ascending colon in less than 5%. In contrast, right-sided diverticular disease is relatively common in Japan.[78]

Cecal diverticula consist of two types. The congenital variety, a true diverticulum, is usually solitary and contains all layers of the bowel wall. Acquired diverticula are usually multiple and are associated with diverticula elsewhere in the colon. Like sigmoid diverticula, they contain only mucosa and submucosa and, thus, are false diverticula.

The entity of cecal diverticulitis is relatively rare. To date, about 400 occurrences have been reported[25] in patients with a solitary diverticulum. At presentation, patients with cecal diverticulitis have a clinical picture identical to that of patients with acute appendicitis. Pain in the right lower quadrant associated with nausea, vomiting, fever, and leukocytosis is the usual presentation. Patients with cecal diverticulitis tend to be older than patients with appendicitis (average age, 40 years) and younger than patients with sigmoid diverticulitis. Radiographic signs include paracolic mass, calcified fecalith, and localized ileus. Recently, improved diagnostic accuracy using CT has been reported.[19]

At laparotomy, cecal diverticulitis may be indistinguishable from acute appendicitis or may mimic a perforated cecal carcinoma. In some reviews,[3,27,41] it has been reported that the intraoperative diagnosis has been incorrect in 60 to 70% of patients. Treatment should be dictated by intraoperative findings. In many patients with cecal diverticulitis involving a solitary diverticulum (true diverticulum), a single well-circumscribed area projecting from the cecal wall may be noted. In these patients, simple excision of the involved diverticulum and closure is adequate. More commonly, however, an inflammatory mass involving the cecum and right colon is encountered. Differentiation between perforated cecal carcinoma and cecal diverticulitis is impossible, and, in these patients, right colectomy and ileocolic anastomosis are indicated.

REFERENCES

1. Almy, T.P., and Howell, D.A.: Medical progress. Diverticular disease of the colon. N. Engl. J. Med., 302:324, 1980.
2. Ambrosetti, P., Robert, J., Witzig, J.A., et al.: Incidence, outcome, and proposed management of isolated abscesses complicating acute left-sided colonic diverticulitis: A prospective study of 140 patients. Dis. Colon Rectum, 35:1072, 1992.
3. Asch, M.J., and Markowitz, A.M.: Cecal diverticulitis: Report of 16 cases and a review of the literature. Surgery, 65:906, 1969.
4. Auguste, L.J., and Wise, L.: Surgical management of perforated diverticulitis. Am. J. Surg., 141:122, 1981.
5. Balthazar, E.J., Megibow, A., Schinella, R.A., et al.: Limitations in the CT diagnosis of acute diverticulitis: Comparison of CT, contrast enema, and pathologic findings in 16 patients. Am. J. Roentgenol., 154:281, 1990.
6. Beer, E.: Some pathological and clinical aspects of acquired (false) diverticula of the intestine. Am. J. Med. Sci., 128:135, 1904.
7. Benn, P.L., Wolff, B.G., and Ilstrup, D.M.: Level of anastomosis and recurrent colonic diverticulitis. Am. J. Surg., 151:269, 1986.
8. Berman, I.R., Corman, M.L., Coller, J.A., et al.: Late onset Crohn's disease in patients with colonic diverticulosis. Dis. Colon Rectum, 22:524, 1979.
9. Boles, R.S., Jr., and Jordan, S.M.: The clinical significance of diverticulosis. Gastroenterology, 35:579, 1958.
10. Botsford, T.W., and Zollinger, R.M., Jr.: Diverticulitis of the colon. Surg. Gynecol. Obstet., 128:1209, 1969.
11. Bova, J.G., Hopens, T.A., and Goldstein, H.M.: Diverticulitis of the right colon. Dig. Dis. Sci., 29:150, 1984.
12. Brown, P.W., and Marcley, D.M.: Prognosis of diverticulitis and diverticulosis of the colon. JAMA, 109:1328, 1937.
13. Byrne, J.J., and Garick, E.I.: Surgical treatment of diverticulitis. Am. J. Surg., 121:379, 1971.
14. Casarella, W.J., Galloway, S.J., Taxin, R.N., et al.: "Lower" gastrointestinal tract hemorrhage: New concepts based on arteriography. Am. J. Roentgenol., 121:357, 1974.
15. Cho, K.C., Morehouse, H.T., Alterman, D.D., et al.: Sigmoid diverticulitis: Diagnostic role of CT—comparison with barium enema studies. Radiology, 176:111, 1990.
16. Chodak, G.W., Rangel, D.M., and Passaro, E., Jr.: Colonic diverticulitis in patients under age 40: Need for earliest diagnosis. Am. J. Surg., 141:699, 1981.
17. Colcock, B.P., and Stahmann, F.D.: Fistulas complicating diverticular disease of the sigmoid colon. Ann. Surg., 175:838, 1972.
18. Correnti, F.S., Pappalardo, G., Mobarhan, S., et al.: Follow-up results of a new colomyotomy in the treatment of diverticulosis. Surg. Gynecol. Obstet., 156:181, 1983.
19. Crist, D.W., Fishman, E.K., Scatarige, J.C., et al.: Acute diverticulitis

TABLE 9–1. PATHOLOGIC CLASSIFICATION OF ACUTE DIVERTICULAR DISEASE*

Stage I	Pericolic abscess or phlegmon formation
Stage II	Pelvic, intra-abdominal, or retroperitoneal abscess resulting from perforation of confined pericolic abscess
Stage III	Generalized purulent peritonitis caused by rupture of stage I or stage II abscess
Stage IV	Generalized fecal peritonitis

*From Auguste, L.J., and Wise, L.: Surgical management of perforated diverticulitis. Am. J. Surg., 141:122, 1981, with permission.

of the cecum and ascending colon diagnosed by computed to-mography. Surg. Gynecol. Obstet., 166:99, 1988.

20. Cruveilhier, J.: Traité d'Anatomie Pathologique Genéralé, Vol. 1. Paris, Baillière, 1849, p. 592.

21. Eng, K., Ranson, J.H.C., and Localio, S.A.: Resection of the per-forated segment: A significant advance in treatment of divertic-ulitis with free perforation or abscess. Am. J. Surg., 133:67, 1977.

22. Eusebio, E.B., and Eisenberg, M.M.: Natural history of diverticular disease of the colon in young patients. Am. J. Surg., 125:308, 1973.

23. Fazio, V.W., Church, J.M., Jagelman, D.G., et al.: Colocutaneous fistulas complicating diverticulitis. Dis. Colon Rectum, 30:89, 1987.

24. Freischlag, J., Bennion, R.S., and Thompson, J.E., Jr.: Complica-tions of diverticular disease of the colon in young people. Dis. Colon Rectum, 29:639, 1986.

25. Graham, S.M., and Ballantyne, G.H.: Cecal diverticulitis: A review of the American experience. Dis. Colon Rectum, 30:821, 1987.

26. Graser, E.: Das falsche Darmdivertikel. Arch. Klin. Chir., 59:638, 1899.

27. Greaney, E.M., and Synder, W.H.: Acute diverticulitis of the cecum encountered at emergency surgery. Am. J. Surg., 94:270, 1957.

28. Greif, J.M., Fried, G., and McSherry, C.K.: Surgical treatment of perforated diverticulitis of the sigmoid colon. Dis. Colon Rec-tum, 23:483, 1980.

29. Hackford, A.W., Schoetz, D.J., Jr., Coller, J.A., et al.: Surgical man-agement of complicated diverticulitis: The Lahey Clinic experi-ence, 1967 to 1982. Dis. Colon Rectum, 28:317, 1985.

30. Hartmann, H.: Nouveau procédé d'ablation des cancers de la par-tie terminale du colon pelvien. Congr. Fr. Chir., 28:411, 1921.

31. Hinchey, E.J., Schaal, P.G.H., and Richards, G.K.: Treatment of perforated disease of the colon. Adv. Surg., 12:85, 1978.

32. Hodgson, J.: Transverse taeniamyotomy for diverticular disease. Dis. Colon Rectum, 16:283, 1973.

33. Horner, J.L.: A study of diverticulitis of the colon in office practice. Gastroenterology, 21:223, 1952.

34. Hulnick, D.H., Megibow, A.J., Balthazar, E.J., et al.: Computed to-mography in the evaluation of diverticulitis. Radiology, 152:491, 1984.

35. Ihekwaba, F.N.: Diverticular disease of the colon in black Africa. J. R. Coll. Surg. Edinb., 37:107, 1992.

36. Johnson, C.D., Baker, M.E., Rice, R.P., et al.: Diagnosis of acute colonic diverticulitis: Comparison of barium enema and CT. Am. J. Roentgenol., 148:541, 1987.

37. Keith, A.: A demonstration of diverticula of the alimentary tract of congenital or of obscure origin. BMJ, 1:376, 1910.

38. Koruth, N.M., Krukowski, Z.H., Youngson, G.G., et al.: Intra-operative colonic irrigation in the management of left-sided bowel emergencies. Br. J. Surg., 72:708, 1985.

39. Krukowski, Z.H., Koruth, N.M., and Matheson, N.A.: Evolving practice in acute diverticulitis. Br. J. Surg., 72:684, 1985.

40. Labs, J.D., Sarr, M.G., Fishman, E.K., et al.: Complications of acute diverticulitis of the colon: Improved early diagnosis with com-puterized tomography. Am. J. Surg., 155:331, 1988.

41. Lauridsen, J., and Ross, F.P.: Acute diverticulitis of the cecum: A report of four cases and review of one hundred fifty-three sur-gical cases. Arch. Surg., 64:320, 1952.

42. Leigh, J.E., Judd, E.S., and Waugh, J.M.: Diverticulitis of the colon: recurrence after apparently adequate segmental resection. Am. J. Surg., 103:51, 1962.

43. Littre, A., 1700. Cited by Finney, J.M.T.: Diverticulitis and its sur-gical treatment. Proc. Interstate Post-Grad. Med. Assembly North Am., 55:57, 65, 1928.

44. Lockhart-Mummery, J.P.: Late results in diverticulitis. Lancet, 2: 1401, 1938.

45. Markham, N.I., and Li, A.K.: Diverticulitis of the right colon—experience from Hong Kong. Gut, 33:547, 1992.

46. Mayefsky, E., Sicular, A. and Hodgson, W.J.: Recurrent diverticulitis after conservative surgery. Mt. Sinai J. Med., 46:556, 1979.

47. Mayo, W.J.: Diverticulitis of the large intestine. JAMA, 69:781, 1917.

48. Mayo, C.W., and Blunt, C.P.: Symposium on abdominal surgery. The surgical management of the complications of diverticulitis of the large intestine: Analysis of 202 cases. Surg. Clin. North Am., 30:1005, 1950.

49. Mayo, W.J., Wilson, L.B., and Giffin, H.Z.: Acquired diverticulitis of the large intestine. Surg. Gynecol. Obstet., 5:8, 1907.

50. McGowan, F.J., and Wolff, W.I.: Diverticulitis of the sigmoid colon. Gastroenterology, 21:119, 1952.

51. McGuire, H.H., Jr., and Haynes, B.W., Jr.: Massive hemorrhage from diverticulosis of the colon: Guidelines for therapy based on bleeding patterns observed in fifty cases. Ann. Surg., 175: 847, 1972.

52. Murray, J.J., Schoetz, D.J., Jr., Coller, J.A., et al.: Intraoperative co-lonic lavage and primary anastomosis in nonelective resection of the colon. Dis. Colon Rectum, 34:527, 1991.

53. Ouriel, K., and Schwartz, S.I.: Diverticular disease in the young patient. Surg. Gynecol. Obstet., 156:1, 1983.

54. Painter, N.S., and Burkitt, D.P.: Diverticular disease of the colon: A 20th century problem. Clin. Gastroenterol., 4:3, 1975.

55. Painter, N.S., Truelove, S.C., Ardran, G.M., et al.: Segmentation and the localization of intraluminal pressures in the human co-lon, with special reference to the pathogenesis of colonic diver-ticula. Gastroenterology, 49:169, 1965.

56. Parks, T.G.: Natural history of diverticular disease of the colon: A review of 521 cases. BMJ 4:639, 1969.

57. Parulekar, S.G.: Sonography of colonic diverticulitis. J. Ultrasound Med., 4:659, 1985.

58. Pemberton, J., Black, B.M., and Maino, C.R.: Progress in the sur-gical management of diverticulitis of the sigmoid colon. Surg. Gynecol. Obstet., 85:523, 1947.

59. Perkins, J.D., Shield, C.F., III, Chang, F.C., et al.: Acute diverticu-litis: Comparison of treatment in immunocompromised and nonimmunocompromised patients. Am. J. Surg., 148:745, 1984.

60. Ponka, J.L.: Emergency surgical operations for diverticular dis-eases. Dis. Colon Rectum, 13:235, 1970.

61. Potier, F.: Diverticulite et appendicite. Bull. Mem. Soc. Anat. Paris, 87:29, 1912.

62. Rauch, R.F.: Coexisting diverticulitis and carcinoma of the colon: Comprehensive study on survival. Arch. Surg., 73:823, 1956.

63. Ravitch, M.M.: A Century of Surgery: 1880–1980. Philadelphia, J.B. Lippincott, 1981, p. 375.

64. Ravo, B., Ali Khan, S., Ger, R., et al.: Unusual extraperitoneal pre-sentations of diverticulitis. Am. J. Gastroenterol., 80:346, 1985.

65. Reilly, M.: Sigmoidal myotomy for acute diverticulitis. Dis. Colon Rectum, 8:42, 1965.

66. Robbins, S.L., Cotran, R.S., and Kumar, V.: Pathologic Basis of Dis-ease. Philadelphia, W.B. Saunders, 1984, p. 856.

67. Rodkey, G.V., and Welch, C.E.: Changing patterns in the surgical treatment of diverticular disease. Ann. Surg., 200:466, 1984.

68. Schauer, P.R., Ramos, R., Ghiatas, A.A., et al.: Virulent diverticular disease in young obese men. Am. J. Surg., 164:443, 1992.

69. Scheff, R.T., Zuckerman, G., Harter, H., et al.: Diverticular disease in patients with chronic renal failure due to polycystic kidney disease. Ann. Intern. Med., 92(2 Pt. 1):202, 1980.

70. Schwerk, W.B., Schwarz, S., and Rothmund, M.: Sonography in acute colonic diverticulitis: A prospective study. Dis. Colon Rec-tum, 35:1077, 1992.

71. Simonowitz, D., and Paloyan, D.: Diverticular disease of the colon in patients under 40 years of age. Am. J. Gastroenterol., 67:69, 1977.

72. Slack, W.W.: The anatomy, pathology, and some clinical features of diverticulitis of the colon. Br. J. Surg., 50:185, 1962.

73. Smith, A.N. (ed.): Diverticular disease. Clin. Gastroenterol., 4:1, 1975.

74. Smithwick, R.H.: Experiences with surgical management of diver-ticulitis of sigmoid. Ann. Surg., 115:969, 1942.

75. Snape, W.J., Jr., Carson, G.M., and Cohen, S.: Colonic myoelectric activity in the irritable bowel syndrome. Gastroenterology, 70: 326, 1976.

76. Stabile, B.E., Puccio, E., vanSonnenberg, E., et al.: Preoperative percutaneous drainage of diverticular abscesses. Am. J. Surg., 159:99, 1990.

77. Starnes, H.F., Jr., Lazarus, J.M., and Vineyard, G.: Surgery for di-verticulitis in renal failure. Dis. Colon Rectum, 28:827, 1985.

78. Sugihara, K., Muto, T., Morioka, Y., et al.: Diverticular disease of the colon in Japan: A review of 615 cases. Dis. Colon Rectum, 27:531, 1984.

79. Tagart, R.E.: General peritonitis and haemorrhage complicating colonic diverticular disease. Ann. R. Coll. Surg. Engl., 55:175, 1974.

80. Tyau, E.S., Prystowsky, J.B., Joehl, R.J., et al.: Acute diverticulitis: A complicated problem in the immunocompromised patient. Arch. Surg., *126:*855, 1991.

81. Veidenheimer, M.C.: Surgical management of diverticulitis and its complications. *In* Kodner, I.F., Fry, R.D., and Roe, J.P. (eds.): Colon, Rectal, and Anal Surgery: Current Techniques and Controversies. St. Louis, C.V. Mosby, 1985, p. 117.

82. Veidenheimer, M.C., and Lawrence, D.C.: Anastomotic myotomy: An adjunct to resection for diverticular disease. Dis. Colon Rectum, *19:*310, 1976.

83. Waugh, J.M., and Walt, A.J.: Current trends in the surgical treatment of diverticulitis of the sigmoid colon. Surg. Clin. North Am., *42:*1267, 1962.

84. Welch, C.E., Allen, A.W., and Donaldson, G.A.: An appraisal of resection of the colon for diverticulitis of the sigmoid. Ann. Surg., *138:*332, 1953.

85. Whiteway, J., and Morson, B.C.: Pathology of the ageing—diverticular disease. Clin. Gastroenterol., *14:*829, 1985.

86. Wilson, L.B.: Diverticula of the lower bowel: Their development and relationship to carcinoma. Ann. Surg., *53:*223, 1911.

87. Wychulis, A.R., Beahrs, O.H., and Judd, E.S.: Surgical management of diverticulitis of the colon. Surg. Clin. North Am., *47:*961, 1967.

Chapter 10

POLYPS, POLYPOSIS, AND BENIGN TUMORS

JEROME J. DECOSSE

Nonmalignant growths in the large bowel have various causes and also vary in malignant potential, association with disorders elsewhere in the body, and association with symptoms and dysfunction. By far, the most common benign colorectal tumors are polyps. Other submucosal tumors include lipomas, endometriomas, and leiomyomas.

Estimates of the prevalence of asymptomatic polyps in the general population range from 1.6 to 12%, and in the population older than 70 years of age, the prevalence is estimated to be as high as 40%. Not all polyps have malignant potential, but given their prevalence and given the incidence of and mortality associated with colorectal cancer, a detected polyp is a "call to action."

In addition to requiring correct classification and local treatment, tumors of the large bowel in many cases require assessment of the risk of malignancy, screening for extracolonic expressions, and, in the case of inherited disorders, outreach to relatives who are at risk.

POLYPS OF THE LARGE BOWEL

Definitions and Classification

A polyp is an excrescence or elevation on a mucosal surface. The term polyp has a macroscopic connotation, but the microscopic appearance of polyps of the large bowel varies substantially, with major clinical ramifications. Polyps are conventionally classified as neoplastic or non-neoplastic (Table 10–1). Among the latter, the polyps associated with Cowden's disease and the Peutz-Jeghers syndrome are hamartomas, whereas juvenile polyps are retention polyps. The pseudopolyps of chronic ulcerative colitis are inflamed fragments of retained rectal mucosa surrounded by serpiginous ulcerations. Many patients have one or two common, harmless, small metaplastic or hyperplastic polyps.

Only neoplastic polyps, or adenomas, have malignant potential. Adenomas are conventionally classified as tubular, villous, and tubulovillous (Fig. 10–1). Of these three types, tubular adenomas are the most common, and villous adenomas have the greatest malignant potential.

The malignant potential of an adenoma varies with size, conformation, histologic character, and presence of dysplasia. Invasive malignancy is more often found in sessile (flat) than in pedunculated (long-stalked) adenomas.

Adenomatous Polyps

Pathogenesis

The natural history of colorectal adenomas is not well understood. Most adenomas of the large bowel are asymptomatic and are found only as a result of surveillance. Adenomas may result in occult rectal bleeding but rarely in hemorrhage or anemia.[1] Villous adenomas may sometimes produce a mucoid diarrhea with resultant hypokalemic alkalosis. A colonic adenoma may be the lead point for colonic intussusception.

Except in the familial polyposis syndromes, colorectal adenomas are rarely found in patients less than 40 years of age. They are most commonly found in patients older than 60 years and are found more frequently in men than in women. Patients older than age 70 years are more likely to have adenomas on the right side of the colon than are younger patients, and adenomas on the right side tend to be larger than those on the left side, while dysplastic adenomas are more frequent on the left side. The geographic variation in frequency of adenomas parallels that of colorectal carcinoma and suggests that environment plays an important role in adenoma formation.[42]

Colorectal adenomas tend to grow slowly and continuously, although some small sporadic adenomas regress spontaneously. A polyp may take 10 years to double its diameter.[25] As the polyp grows, so does the risk that cancer will develop within it. Once present within a polyp, cancer may progress through in situ and intramucosal stages, to invasive cancer within the polyp, and finally to an invasive colorectal cancer.

Identification of patients who are at high risk for co-

114

TABLE 10-1. CLASSIFICATION OF POLYPS

HAMARTOMATOUS POLYPS
  Cowden's disease
  Cronkhite-Canada syndrome
  Peutz-Jeghers syndrome
  Juvenile (retention) polyps

INFLAMMATORY POLYPS
  Benign lymphoid polyps
  Inflammatory (pseudopolyps)

METAPLASTIC OR HYPERPLASTIC POLYPS

NEOPLASTIC ADENOMAS
  Tubular
  Tubulovillous
  Villous

lorectal adenomas and cancer relies on historic, physical, and morphologic risk factors. The importance of dysplasia is recognized. Current studies of proto-oncogenes and DNA flow cytometry in adenomas may lead to new, clinically useful insights.[35,44]

Clinicians and pathologists experienced in the management of adenomas conclude that most or all large bowel cancers arise from pre-existing large bowel adenomas rather than arising spontaneously in otherwise normal mucosa. This theory of transition has been labeled the adenoma-cancer sequence. The evidence in favor of the adenoma-cancer sequence follows.

Large bowel cancer is associated with adenomas in both descriptive epidemiologic characteristics and experimental carcinogenesis. About one third of all operative specimens of large bowel cancer also have one or more adenomas. The presence of these additional adenomas doubles the risk of a subsequent or metachronous large bowel cancer. About 75% of patients with synchronous large bowel cancer also have adenomas. Indirect evidence suggests that removal of adenomas reduces the risk of large bowel cancer. Dysplasia in adenomas parallels the distribution of large bowel cancer, both being more common in the left colon (Table 10–2).[48] Large bowel cancer has a histologic association with adenoma, both commonly being identified in a single specimen. The larger the adenoma, the more likely the presence of superficial or invasive cancer (Table 10–3). Reciprocally, the larger and more invasive the cancer, the less frequently adenomatous tissue accompanies it. Small rectal cancers without adenomatous components are exceptionally rare. Finally, cells from colorectal cancers and colorectal adenomas show similar chromosomal deletions and mutations.

Diagnosis

Most colorectal adenomas can be identified and removed endoscopically. Endoscopy is more effective than air-contrast barium enema examination in revealing polyps smaller than 5 mm in diameter, and, in addition to being diagnostic, it provides a setting for therapy. Accurate assessment of an individual's risk for future development of adenomas, colorectal cancer, or both depends on the pathologic examination of all colorectal polyps present in the colon. The goal of therapeutic endoscopy should be removal and recovery of all colorec-

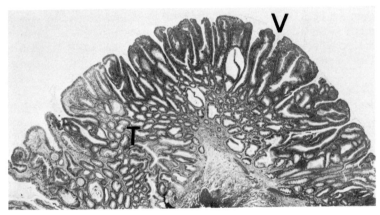

FIGURE 10-1. Tubulovillous adenoma of the colon. Both tubular (*T*) and Villous (*V*) areas are present. (Hematoxylin & eosin, ×16.) (Courtesy of Stanley Hamilton, M.D., Department of Pathology, School of Medicine, Johns Hopkins University.)

TABLE 10-2. DISTRIBUTION AND PATHOLOGIC STAGES OF ADENOMAS IN THE LARGE BOWEL*

REGION OF LARGE BOWEL	TOTAL NO.	BENIGN		DYSPLASIA		CARCINOMA IN SITU		INVASIVE CANCER	
		No.	%	No.	%	No.	%	No.	%
Rectum	418	297	6	31	5	66	8	24	7
Sigmoid colon	3,199	2,221	43	295	47	481	57	202	60
Descending colon	1,601	1,266	25	115	18	170	20	50	15
Transverse colon	824	632	12	99	16	63	7	30	9
Right colon	900	714	14	85	14	70	8	31	9
Total	6,942	5,130	100	625	100	850	100	337	100

*From Shinya, H.: Colonoscopy: Diagnosis and Treatment of Colonic Diseases. New York, Igaku-Shoin, 1982, with permission.

TABLE 10-3. CARCINOMA IN SITU AND INVASIVE CARCINOMA RELATED TO SIZE OF ADENOMA*

Size (cm)	Total No.	Carcinoma	In Situ (%)	Invasive	Carcinoma (%)
0.5–0.9	2,057	92	04.5	11	00.5
1.0–1.9	3,258	397	12.2	52	04.7
2.0–2.9	1,161	219	18.9	112	09.6
0+	466	142	30.5	62	13.3
Totals	6,942	850	08.4	337	04.9

*From Shinya, H.: Colonoscopy: Diagnosis and Treatment of Colonic Diseases. New York, Igaku-Shoin, 1982, with permission.

tal polyps. When it is not possible to remove a larger adenoma (generally, when it is sessile and >3 cm in diameter), endoscopic biopsy specimens from the lesion may be of some assistance in the histopathologic evaluation. However, information from colonoscopic biopsies must be interpreted with caution, because the specimens are small and may not be representative of the overall histopathologic condition. Carcinoma within a polyp is usually focal and can be missed if it is not present in the biopsy material.

Treatment

GENERAL PRINCIPLES. In patients with known adenomas, it is essential that the entire colon be examined because adenomas are often multiple and are associated with an increased risk of cancer elsewhere in the colon. Removal of all colorectal polyps is recommended. Even those less than 1 cm in diameter may harbor cancer.[51] Those less than 5 mm in diameter may be treated by an endoscopic method that simultaneously destroys the polyp by electrocoagulation and provides a biopsy specimen, sometimes referred to as the hot biopsy technique. Pedunculated polyps may be excised by endoscopic snare cautery. Fractionated excision of sessile adenomas is discouraged because the removed fragments, if recovered, are difficult for the histopathologist to orient properly.

Careful histopathologic assessment of all excised adenomas is therefore mandatory for proper management of patients. It is necessary to resect and retrieve all polyps and to submit these specimens promptly in the fresh state to the pathologist. Larger specimens should be oriented for proper prosection with pins or needles on a plastic block or filter paper such that the prosector can make proper vertical cuts to the diathermied base of the polyp.

A histopathologic report of in situ carcinoma describes cancer cells confined by, and superficial to, the muscularis mucosa. Superficial carcinoma, intraepithelial carcinoma, intramucosal carcinoma, or even atypia are synonyms. The main points are the absence of life-threatening risk, and, assuming complete excision, confidence that the patient has been cured.

Invasive carcinoma will be reported if cancer cells have invaded through the muscularis mucosa into the body of the adenoma (Fig. 10–2): hence the term malignant colorectal polyp. If more than 50% of the polyp

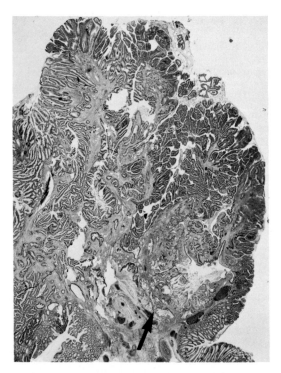

FIGURE 10-2. Pedunculated tubulovillous adenoma of the colon containing invasive adenocarcinoma that has extended into the submucosa of the stalk (*arrow*). (Hematoxylin & eosin, ×9.) (Courtesy of Stanley Hamilton, M.D., Department of Pathology, School of Medicine, Johns Hopkins University.)

is replaced by carcinoma, the specimen may be deemed a polypoid carcinoma with adenomatous elements.

In the presence of invasion, the critical issue is whether the patient has residual intramural or regional lymphatic tumor and requires operative treatment. Decisions depend upon the endoscopist's confidence of complete excision and the pathologist's assessment of risk factors in the specimen.

Depth of invasion with penetration of tumor into the submucosa (level 4) is the dominant histopathologic risk factor.[24,40] Submucosal invasion in a sessile adenoma is associated with greater risk than comparable invasion in a pedunculated adenoma. The uncommon presence of poorly differentiated (high-grade) tumor, particularly with a mucinous component, merits resection. Limited or no margin between the tumor and the cauterized base of the adenoma may lead to surgery, but is confounded by the reciprocal cautery burn left in the patient. Most such patients are cured without additional treatment. Lymphatic or venous invasion of tumor has equivocal prognostic significance.

Most malignant colorectal polyps are in the sigmoid colon or rectum. In the study by Haggitt and associates, 14 of 28 malignant colorectal polyps with level 4 invasion were located in the rectum and eight were in the sigmoid colon.[24] Level 4 invasion was more likely in large (<2.5 cm), sessile, and villous polyps. If accessible to transanal techniques, such polyps merit full-thickness, transanal excision with a margin, rather than endoscopic snare cautery.

COLONOSCOPY AND SCREENING. Efforts to visualize the

lower alimentary tract date back to ancient times. Hippocrates used a rectal speculum. In the nineteenth and early twentieth centuries, research on instrumentation resulted in the development and use of rigid sigmoidoscopes. Although rigid sigmoidoscopy remains a practical diagnostic technique for examination of the rectum, beyond the rectosigmoid junction it often causes the patient pain, and it is incomplete because of the difficulty of passing the instrument through the usual 90-degree angle between rectum and the sigmoid colon.[43] In the late 1970s, flexible fiberoptic sigmoidoscopes came into use. Flexible sigmoidoscopy has proved more acceptable to patients than rigid sigmoidoscopy[57] and also more effective in finding polyps and cancers in the sigmoid.[18]

In a series of 200 colonoscopic procedures, the average extent of colonic visualization was 93.8%. In 165 of these procedures (82.5%), visualization was complete to the cecum or terminal ileum, but in 35 procedures (17.5%), an average of less than 65% of the colon was examined.[41] Polyps are not evenly distributed throughout the large bowel; hence, the importance of incomplete observation in terms of failure to detect lesions is not a matter of strict proportionality. An estimated 49% of colorectal adenomas and 67% of invasive cancers are located in the rectosigmoid region of the large bowel (Table 10–2).[47] If colonoscopy cannot be completed, it should be followed by air-contrast barium enema examination.

The American Cancer Society recommends that asymptomatic persons at average risk initiate an annual rectal digital exam at age 40, an annual test for fecal occult blood starting at age 50, and a sigmoidoscopy, preferably flexible, at age 50, repeated at 3- to 5-year intervals. For asymptomatic but high-risk individuals, the recommendation is to perform either a total colonoscopy or sigmoidoscopy and an air-contrast barium study every 3 to 5 years starting at age 40.[11] Which technology is chosen depends on considerations of cost, patient comfort, and availability of the technology.[14]

The critical issue is whether screening does any good. The hallmark of benefit is mortality reduction. Recently, screening by sigmoidoscopy was demonstrated to reduce mortality of cancer in the rectum and rectosigmoid colon.[45] In another randomized study, annual fecal occult blood testing reduced long-term mortality from colorectal cancer by 33%.[34]

OPERATIVE TECHNIQUES. A standard cancer operation, rather than a limited colon resection or colotomy, is necessary for adenomas too large to be treated endoscopically and when endoscopic removal of a malignant colorectal adenoma is deemed inadequate according to the preceding criteria.

Be particularly wary of the villous adenoma. The risk of focal or invasive cancer is greater in a villous adenoma, and invasive cancer in that setting often has a threatening mucinous histology. Occasionally, a large villous adenoma encountered in the distal rectum is too extensive for transanal, full-thickness local excision. In this case, the first step is to perform multiple (up to five or more) representative biopsies. When there is no invasive cancer, the villous adenoma may be excised by transperineal, parasacral, or sphincter-dividing approaches, or by diathermy, which may require several sessions. If invasive cancer is detected in the specimen, an abdominal perineal resection is necessary.

It can be very difficult to identify accurately the site of removal of an endoscopically excised malignant colorectal polyp. The site of a snare cautery excision can heal in a few days and be very difficult to identify by colonoscopy or at operation. A small amount of India ink injected into the base of the polyp by the endoscopist will preserve localization. Alternatively, an air-contrast barium enema study performed prior to the excision makes it possible to locate the site of the excised polyp. If the adenoma under consideration is in the rectum or rectosigmoid, direct visualization with a rigid proctosigmoidoscope is desirable because measurement of distance on a flexible endoscope can be notoriously misleading. Accurate measurement may make the difference between a difficult low anterior resection and a relatively straightforward sigmoid resection.

Follow-Up

After removal of an adenoma, about 40% of such patients will have another adenoma at subsequent examination.[58] The likelihood of a recurrence is greater if the index adenoma was tubulovillous, villous, or a large (>1 cm) adenoma. Although many endoscopists will perform a follow-up colonoscopy 6 months to 1 year after polypectomy, the trend is toward extending that interval to 3 years or more.[3,58]

Hamartomatous Polyps

A hamartoma is a localized overgrowth of normal, mature intestinal epithelial cells. Hamartomas are pedunculated, and the stalk is lined with normal mucosa, with a submucosal core.[20] These polyps can cause intussusception, requiring an operation. Although the malignant potential of hamartomas as such appears to be small, some studies indicate that hamartomas are associated with an increased cancer risk. Intestinal hamartomas are found in the Peutz-Jeghers syndrome and Cowden's disease. These genetic disorders have extracolonic manifestations and are associated with a higher than average risk of malignancy, both in the large bowel and elsewhere.

Juvenile Polyps

Juvenile polyps are hamartomatous epithelial retentions, composed of cystically dilated glands filled with mucus and inflammatory debris (Fig. 10–3). Most juvenile polyps are pedunculated, although some are small and sessile. The peak ages for the presentation of symptomatic juvenile polyps are 4 and 5 years, but the polyps are sometimes found in infants and occasionally in adults. Typically, only one or two polyps are found; patients and the families of patients who have more than a few juvenile polyps should be evaluated for a juvenile polyposis syndrome.

The symptoms may be rectal bleeding, mucous discharge and diarrhea, and abdominal pain, or, less fre-

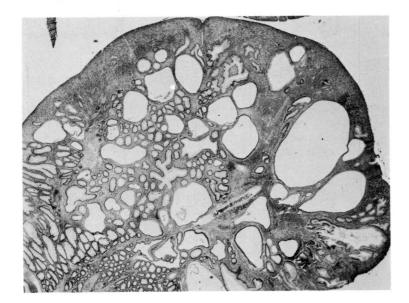

FIGURE 10-3. Juvenile polyp of the colon. Dilated glands lined by colonic type of epithelium are surrounded by inflamed, edematous stroma. (Hematoxylin & eosin, ×12.) (Courtesy of Stanley Hamilton, M.D., Department of Pathology, School of Medicine, Johns Hopkins University.)

quently, intussusception or prolapse of the polyp via the rectum.[11]

Inflammatory Polyps

Inflammatory polyps are associated with ulcerative colitis and Crohn's disease. They are almost always multiple. Most inflammatory polyps are small and sessile, but some are large enough, numerous enough, or both, to obstruct the colon or to interfere with colonoscopy. They also may be associated with bleeding that may be continuous and severe enough to cause anemia.[31] Patients with inflammatory polyps usually need no treatment apart from that for the underlying colitis condition. In a rare condition known as colitis polyposa, the large bowel mucosa of the colitic patient is carpeted with inflammatory polyps.

Hyperplastic (Metaplastic) Polyps

Hyperplastic polyps are the most common small (<3 mm), benign tumors of the large bowel. Located most often in the rectosigmoid mucosa, these polyps increase in frequency with age and are more common in men than in women.[16,55]

Hyperplastic polyps are the product of excessive cell replication. The cells themselves differentiate and mature, producing small, sessile mucosal elevations with microscopic intraluminal pleats (as a result of crowding), producing a sawtooth pattern. These polyps are almost always asymptomatic, although when they are very numerous, there may be associated rectal bleeding, diarrhea, or both. They are not believed to have malignant potential. However, a small number (<1%) of colonic polyps cannot be strictly classified as either hyperplastic or adenomatous, and 36% of hyperplastic polyps have been found to contain adenomatous elements.[23] Because of their neoplastic characteristics, these polyps should be treated, and the patients followed, as if they were adenomas.

POLYPOSIS SYNDROMES

Classification

The most prevalent and best known of the genetic multiple polyp syndromes is familial adenomatous polyposis. Several other multiple polyp conditions appear to be familial. Most, but not all, are autosomal dominant disorders. The key discriminant is histopathologic scrutiny.

Although the polyposis syndromes seem discrete and easily diagnosed, they are not. Some older patients may have 10 to 20 adenomas scattered across their large bowel, sometimes in association with cancer, but without any familial background or other associated defects. These patients do not represent the genetic trait. About 30% of polyposis patients represent new gene mutations and do not have a family history of large bowel neoplasia. A small number of cases of chronic ulcerative colitis evolve to a mucosal condition called colitis polyposa, which is not easily distinguished from adenomatous polyposis without biopsy and histologic verification. In rare cases, the first clinical expression of familial adenomatous polyposis will be periampullary carcinoma or a truncal desmoid tumor.

Because of the elevated risk of cancer and the familial nature of the polyposis syndromes, about a dozen registries have been established at medical centers across the United States, and there are an additional dozen or so around the world. These registries monitor, treat, and follow probands; develop pedigrees; provide genetic counseling; make contact with and monitor family members at risk; and collect and share data on these conditions with the other registries.

Familial Adenomatous Polyposis

Pathogenesis

Familial adenomatous polyposis (FAP) (formerly called familial polyposis, polyposis cali, adenomatosis of the colon and rectum) is conventionally characterized

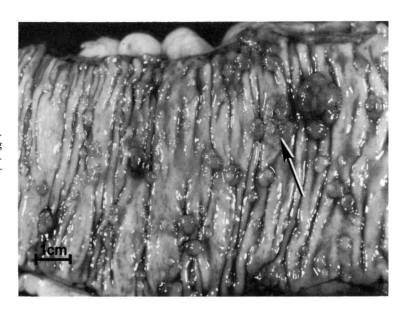

FIGURE 10-4. Adenomatous polyposis of the colon. The mucosal surface is covered with polyps of varying sizes. An early invasive adenocarcinoma (*arrow*) is present. (Courtesy of Stanley Hamilton, M.D., Department of Pathology, School of Medicine, John Hopkins University.)

by autosomal dominant inheritance, expression of numerous colorectal adenomas at adolescence, and a powerful risk for invasive colorectal cancer first appearing about 10 years later (Fig. 10-4). The presence of adenomas distinguishes FAP from the hamartomas of the Peutz-Jeghers syndrome and the retention polyps of juvenile polyposis. In contrast to texts that indicate uniform death from colorectal cancer by age 40 if untreated, about 20% of polyposis patients will not present themselves until after that age.

In patients with FAP, loss of a suppressor gene on chromosome 5q21 has been found, confirmed, and the gene has been cloned.[5,30,39] Both alleles are lost. Inheritance is dominant at a cellular level, whereas phenotypic expression is recessive at a molecular level, paralleling inheritance of congenital retinoblastoma. These findings provide a model for human carcinogenesis and have led to application of molecular genetics to screen and counsel possibly affected persons. Linkage analysis is being replaced by direct scrutiny for germ-line mutations.[2]

All patients with FAP are at risk for extracolonic expressions. These systemic expressions include desmoids (a nonmetastasizing soft tissue tumor of fibroblasts), osteomas, sebaceous cysts, soft tissue fibromas, lipomas, hamartomatous polyps of the stomach, adenomas of the duodenum, and periampullary adenomas and cancer. Most expressions are benign: periampullary carcinoma and desmoid disease are life threatening. Presence of extracolonic expressions has led to the term Gardner's syndrome. Molecular studies have shown loss of the same gene loci in both FAP and Gardner's syndrome. The custom of distinguishing FAP and Gardner's syndrome as separate entities interferes with surveillance of all patients with FAP and should be discarded.

Several eponymic designations have been created for the various modes of presentation. The Muir-Torre syndrome includes colonic polyposis with sebaceous cysts of the face and squamous cancer of the skin. Turcot's syndrome links medulloblastoma with colonic polyposis and is described as an autosomal recessive disorder.

Studies have demonstrated that these systemic expressions are diffuse and widespread. Osteomas and dental abnormalities, for example, can be found in virtually all patients with familial adenomatous polyposis or their immediate relatives.[7,10,52] Eponymic designations for subcategories of familial syndromes involving multiple adenomatous polyps are probably misleading with respect to etiology.

Desmoid tumors are a major life-threatening condition of polyposis patients. Most desmoids occur in intraperitoneal or retroperitoneal locations, and many follow operative intervention or pregnancy. A desmoid tumor may present as a solid mass that does not metastasize or as sheets of fibrous tissue in the root of the mesentery called desmoid fibroplasia. Desmoids present an important problem in the management of polyposis patients because they may grow and infiltrate surrounding viscera, causing pain, intestinal or ureteral obstruction, and fistulas.[32] They also often recur following excision. In one study of a polyposis registry, six patients died of progression of desmoids—almost as many as the eight patients who died of colorectal carcinoma.[8,46] The risk of desmoids was associated with increasing age and female sex. Of 468 polyposis registry patients, 40 had desmoids.[33] Desmoids may respond to chemotherapy with prostaglandin synthetase inhibitors and antiestrogens.[32]

Polyposis patients are at risk for cancer and polyps throughout the gastrointestinal tract, excluding the esophagus. In particular, they are at risk for adenomas in the duodenum and ampulla of Vater and also for invasive cancer at that site.[27] In addition, they are at risk for polyps in the stomach, but these polyps are usually fundic gland polyps, not adenomas. Outside geographic high-risk areas for gastric cancer, the polyposis patient has little or no risk of cancer at that site. Polyposis patients also are at greater risk than the general population for thyroid cancer, hepatoblastoma in childhood, and a host of other expressions (Table 10-4).

An apparently innocuous but interesting extracolonic expression of polyposis is congenital hypertrophy of the retinal pigment epithelium.[49] This condition is detecta-

TABLE 10-4. EXTRACOLONIC EXPRESSIONS IN FAMILIAL ADENOMATOUS POLYPOSIS

MALIGNANCY
Upper gastrointestinal neoplasia (except esophagus and perhaps stomach)
Adrenal neoplasia
Papillary thyroid cancer
Multiple endocrine neoplasia (MEN) syndrome
Hepatoblastoma
Medulloblastoma, malignant glioma

OTHER PROLIFERATIVE EXPRESSIONS
Desmoid disease
Cysts (sebaceous, pilonidal, ovarian, breast, renal, Bartholin's, bone)
Fibromas
Lipomas
Osteomas
Hypertrophy of the retinal pigment

ble in very small children and may be useful as a marker for screening in polyposis-affected families.[4]

Diagnosis

Patients with polyposis are increasingly detected through surveillance. When an affected person is identified, other members of the immediate family need to undergo evaluation. Surveillance of asymptomatic children of a proband ordinarily begins in adolescence, preferably by flexible sigmoidoscopy. If there are no rectal polyps or symptoms, a repeat study is deferred for 2 years. It is important to maintain allegiance of the young patient. Invasive colorectal cancer does not occur in the absence of rectal adenomas. A colonoscopy or barium enema is not necessary if the patient is asymptomatic and rectal adenomas are absent. If polyps are detected, a biopsy is essential to confirm the presence of adenoma, and colonoscopy is indicated.

If a diagnosis of familial adenomatous polyposis is made, total colectomy will be necessary. This procedure is deferred, when possible, to mid or late adolescence when patients are mature enough to handle the emotional aspects of the operation.

Work-up of the polyposis patient ought to include upper gastrointestinal endoscopy for gastric or duodenal polyps. A side-viewing endoscope should be used to examine the ampulla of Vater.

As increasing numbers of polyposis patients are found and treated with colectomy, the incidence of and mortality from colorectal cancer in this group is declining, increasing the importance of routine follow-up and screening for extracolonic expressions of this disorder.

Treatment

With a single exception, there is little controversy about elective management of the large bowel in the patient with FAP. Limited colon surgery is not an option, and, in the absence of invasive distal rectal cancer, a permanent ileostomy should not be necessary. Excision of the colon and rectum with ileoanal anastomosis should be the treatment for those with middle or upper

rectal cancer, or with large or confluent adenomas of the rectum, and for those who will not adhere to regular follow-up.

The exception is preservation of the rectum in the patient, usually young, with few (<10) small adenomas and no cancer in the rectum who will subscribe to long-term surveillance. The two options are a total colectomy with an ileorectal anastomosis (IRA) about 12 cm from the anal verge, or a total proctocolectomy with ileoanal anastomosis, preservation of the anal sphincters, and construction of a pelvic ileal reservoir. A temporary ileostomy is generally necessary. Although the main discriminant in decision making is the risk of cancer in the retained rectal segment, other issues include the value, unproven, of long-term surveillance and the likelihood that most patients will have some incontinence or sexual dysfunction after restorative procedures. Following total colectomy, about one third of patients who are left with 20 or fewer rectal polyps will experience spontaneous regression—complete disappearance of remaining polyps.[19] In another one third, the remaining polyps will diminish in size or number or both, and will remain stable for many years. Some fears about restorative surgery remain unfounded: anal incontinence has not worsened with aging, and cancer has not occurred in the "colonized" ileal pouch.

The argument for removal of the rectum has been based primarily on hospital-derived data about risk for rectal cancer, 42% at 20 years in a well-recognized study.[36] This estimate is at considerable variance with an estimated risk of 9.4% at 20 years in population-based data.[13] Moreover, given a prior IRA and absence of colon cancer, the risk of death from rectal cancer was 1.0% at 10 years and 2.0% at 15 years.

A rectal anastomosis at 10 to 15 cm from the anal verge is made easier if a measured rectal tube is inserted preoperatively and taped to the operating table. When that level for rectal resection is accurately identified, the rectal tube can be withdrawn slightly and, after clamping the rectum, used for irrigation of the distal rectum before the anastomosis to the distal ileum is completed. The distal ileum is clamped immediately adjacent to the ileocecal valve to preserve bile-absorbing function. In general, an end-to-end anastomosis is preferred because it eliminates the risk of blind segments intruding on subsequent visualization by endoscopy. At the time of the anastomosis, small, directly visible adenomas are cauterized, but adenomas less than 5 mm in the distal rectum are left alone.

Follow-Up

Because about two thirds of polyposis patients will have either reduction or disappearance of remaining rectal polyps, further diathermy is deferred for approximately 6 months, when residual adenomas are evaluated. We disagree with a widely held principle that *all* rectal polyps should be removed or destroyed. Small rectal polyps tend to wax and wane over long periods, and slow regression can be anticipated. Rectal polyps that exceed 5 mm in diameter probably should be removed by hot biopsy. For smaller polyps, periodic observation is warranted. These rectal polyps are the setting for nutritional and pharmacologic efforts to maintain long-term regression.[12,22]

A patient whose rectum has been retained should have a proctosigmoidoscopy at 3- to 6-month intervals for the rest of his or her life and should have adenomas larger than 5 mm removed. It also is imperative that upper gastrointestinal endoscopy be repeated, particularly if duodenal adenomas or abnormalities of the papilla are identified. As a guideline, patients who have duodenal adenomas should have endoscopy performed annually. Those who have only gastric polyps should have endoscopy performed at 3- to 5-year intervals. In addition, they should undergo routine screening for other extracolonic expressions, particularly for desmoids.

Other Polyposis Syndromes

Juvenile Polyposis

In juvenile polyposis, numerous retention polyps are present throughout the gastrointestinal tract; they may appear in infancy or as late as adulthood. This condition is believed to have an autosomal dominant mode of inheritance and is not considered premalignant. In some families, the polyps appear only in the colon; in others, they also may be present in the esophagus, stomach, and small intestine. A small number of juvenile polyposis patients have some adenomatous polyps in addition to the hamartomatous retention polyps characteristic of the syndrome. In addition, several families with juvenile polyposis have been described in which members not diagnosed with the syndrome have had a diagnosis of colon or gastric carcinoma. Biopsy verification of the polyp type is necessary, but once the diagnosis of juvenile polyposis is made, surgery is usually not necessary except to treat symptoms such as rectal bleeding, polyp prolapse, or diarrhea and protein-losing enteropathy that is so severe that total colectomy or total proctocolectomy is required.

The Cronkhite-Canada syndrome is characterized by juvenile-type polyps of the colon, small intestine, and esophagus, as well as ectodermal lesions, alopecia, and nail dystrophy. It is not reported to have malignant potential.

Peutz-Jeghers Polyposis

In the Peutz-Jeghers syndrome, numerous hamartomatous polyps are present in the gastrointestinal tract, most frequently in the small intestine but also often in the large bowel as well as the stomach. Patients with the Peutz-Jeghers syndrome also have a brownish pigmentation on the lips (most frequent site), buccal surfaces, periocular skin surface,[50] and perianal area. Fewer than 5% of patients with intestinal Peutz-Jeghers polyps have no characteristic mucocutaneous melanotic macules, and fewer than 5% of patients with the pigmentation have no Peutz-Jeghers polyps.[15]

Peutz-Jeghers polyposis is less common than familial adenomatous polyposis, but it also appears to have an autosomal dominant mode of inheritance. Although these patients may have a somewhat elevated risk of large bowel carcinoma, it is not great enough to justify prophylactic colectomy. The risk appears related to adenomatous elements in association with the hamartomatous histopathologic condition. Peutz-Jeghers polyps may be quite large, however, and require operation for bleeding or intussusception or both.

Children with Peutz-Jeghers syndrome appear to be at increased risk of unusual tumors of the reproductive system[56] and bladder.[28] In a registry study, cancer at gastrointestinal and nongastrointestinal sites was reported in 15 of 31 Peutz-Jeghers patients followed from 1973 to 1985.[21] Although selection bias is inherent in such studies, it is difficult to ascribe the high frequency of cancers in this group to chance. It seems reasonable for management of Peutz-Jeghers patients to include emphasis on screening for cancer of the gastrointestinal and reproductive systems.

Cowden's Disease

Like Peutz-Jeghers syndrome, Cowden's disease is an autosomal dominant condition involving multiple hamartomas. Although colonic polyps are found frequently enough to be considered characteristic in Cowden's disease, hyperkeratotic cutaneous and gingival lesions are equally important for diagnosis of the disease. These lesions include trichilemmomas, acral keratoses, and oral mucosal papillomas.[9] Patients with Cowden's disease are also at increased risk for cancers of the breast, thyroid, and skin.[6] Prophylactic mastectomy has been recommended for affected young women.[53]

BENIGN TUMORS

Lipoma

Among colonic lesions, lipomas run a distant second to polyps in frequency, with estimates of incidence ranging from 0.035 to 4.4%.[59] Lipomas may occur anywhere in the gastrointestinal tract but are most often found in the right colon. The most common type of lipoma is submucosal; it may be pedunculated, sessile, or polypoid and may cause obstruction, intussusception, and hemorrhage.[37] The less common subserous type, which makes up about 10% of cases, may be pedunculated or circular so that it surrounds and sometimes obstructs the colon. Lipomas are most commonly found in the cecum but appear, with diminishing frequency, in more distal sites in the colon and rectum. Lipomas are more common in women than in men and are most often symptomatic in the fifth and sixth decades of life.

Lipomas consist of adult fat cells surrounded by a fibrous layer and interspersed with fibrous septa. They may range from a few millimeters to 30 cm in diameter. They may be radiologically distinguished from cancer by radiolucency caused by their fat content and by their tendency to change from a sphere to a sausage shape with peristaltic bowel movements—a trait called the squeeze sign.[26] In recent years, computed tomography and colonoscopy have been the most favored diagnostic tools for lipomas.[59]

Many lipomas may be endoscopically excised or removed by colotomy.[29] In some instances, intussusception or twisting of the pedicle causes necrosis, in which case the lipoma is spontaneously eliminated.

Endometrioma

Endometriomas are benign tumors consisting of endometrial tissue outside the uterus. Endometriosis, the abnormal condition associated with the invasion of organs and other structures by such tissue, has been found in almost every organ and site in the female body. An estimated 8 to 15% of menstruating women have endometriosis, and of them, up to a third are estimated to have bowel involvement.[38] Although general surgeons encounter endometriosis relatively rarely, it should be considered in the differential diagnosis of masses in any area of the female body.[60]

Most bowel endometriomas are in the distal portions of the large bowel, although ileocecal and appendiceal lesions also are relatively frequent. The symptoms that should arouse suspicion of colorectal endometriosis are cyclic changes in bowel function, loose stools, rectal bleeding, crampy abdominal pain, and abdominal distention (Table 10-5).

Malignant disease is a far more common cause of bowel obstruction than is endometriosis, but endometriotic lesions are more often associated with pain and cyclic, rather than randomly intermittent, bleeding.

Endometriosis is only rarely diagnosed by endoscopy or barium enema examination because, although it may narrow the colon, it seldom affects the appearance of the mucosa. However, endometriomas that cause rectal bleeding produce recognizable lesions. When the mucosa is intact, biopsy is uninformative, and because of the obstacles to ultrasonography and radiographic diagnosis, laparascopic investigation may be warranted. Segmental colectomy is usually the treatment of choice for this condition.

TABLE 10-5. SYMPTOMS OF ENDOMETRIOSIS OF THE BOWEL (163 CASES)*

	No.	%
Endometriosis		
Dysmenorrhea	71	44
Dyspareunia	39	24
Unspecified abdominal pain	23	14
Infertility	39	24
Suggestive of Bowel Involvement		
Diarrhea, cyclic	42	26
Constipation, cyclic	19	12
Rectal bleeding, cyclic	26	16
Dyschezia	25	15
Abdominal distention, cyclic	3	2
Bowel obstruction, partial	18	11
Bowel obstruction, complete	1	1

*From Weed, J.C., and Ray, J.E.: Endometriosis of the bowel. Obstet. Gynecol., 69:727, 1987, with permission.

Leiomyoma

Leiomyoma is a smooth muscle tumor rarely found in the colon and rectum. Leiomyomas are usually small—less than 1.5 cm in diameter—and are difficult to distinguish from adenomas[47] and leiomyosarcomas.[17] Distinguishing leiomyomas from leiomyosarcomas may depend more on size and clinical features than on histologic appearance.

These tumors may be pedunculated or sessile. Sessile colonic leiomyomas require surgical resection. Some rectal and pedunculated tumors can be excised colonoscopically. Leiomyomas and leiomyosarcomas of the perianal tissues, however, often constitute very difficult management problems. These lesions are discussed in later chapters.

REFERENCES

1. Ahlquist, D.A., McGill, D.B., Schwartz, S., et al.: Fecal blood levels in health and disease: A study using Hemo-Quant. N. Engl. J. Med., 312:1422, 1985.
2. Ando, H., Miyoshi, Y., Nagase, H., et al.: Detection of 12 germ-line mutations in the adenomatous polyposis coli gene by polymerase chain reaction. Gastroenterology, 104:989, 1993.
3. Atkin, W.S., Morson, B.C., and Cuzick, J.: Long-term risk of colorectal cancer after excision of rectosigmoid adenomas. N. Engl. J. Med., 326:658, 1992.
4. Baker, R.H., Heinemann, M.-H., Miller, H.H., and DeCosse, J.J.: Hyperpigmented lesions of the retinal pigment epithelium in familial adenomatous polyposis. Am. J. Med. Genet., 31:427, 1988.
5. Bodmer, W.F., Bailey, C.J., Bodmer, J., et al.: Localization of the gene for familial adenomatous polyposis on chromosome 5. Nature, 328:614, 1987.
6. Brownstein, M.H., Wolf, M., and Bikowski, J.B.: Cowden's disease: A cutaneous marker of breast cancer. Cancer, 41:2393, 1978.
7. Bulow, S., Sondergaard, J.O., Witt, I., et al.: Mandibular osteomas in familial polyposis coli. Dis. Colon Rectum, 27:105, 1984.
8. Bussey, H.J.R., Eyers, A.A., Ritchie, S.M., and Thompson, J.P.S.: The rectum in adenomatous polyposis: The St. Mark's policy. Br. J. Surg., 72(Suppl.):29, 1985.
9. Carlson, G.J., Nivatvongs, S., and Snover, D.C.: Colorectal polyps in Cowden's disease (multiple hamartoma syndrome). Am. J. Surg. Pathol., 8:763, 1984.
10. Cohen, S.B.: Familial polyposis and its extracolonic manifestations. J. Med. Genet., 19:193, 1982.
11. DeCosse, J.J.: Early cancer detection: Colorectal cancer. Cancer, 62:1787, 1988.
12. DeCosse, J.J., Miller, H.H., and Lesser, M.L.: Effect of wheat fiber on rectal polyps in patients with familial adenomatous polyposis. J. Natl. Cancer Inst., 81:1290, 1989.
13. DeCosse, J.J., Bülow, S., Neale, K., et al.: Rectal cancer risk in patients treated for familial adenomatous polyposis. Br. J. Surg., 79:1372, 1992.
14. Eddy, D.M., Nugent, F.W., Eddy, J.F., et al.: Screening for colorectal cancer in a high-risk population. Gastroenterology, 92:682, 1987.
15. Erbe, R.W.: Current concepts in genetics. Inherited gastrointestinal-polyposis syndromes. N. Engl. J. Med., 294:1101, 1976.
16. Estrada, R.G., and Spjut, J.H.: Hyperplastic polyps of the large bowel. Am. J. Surg. Pathol., 4:127, 1980.
17. Evans, H.L.: Smooth muscle tumors of the gastrointestinal tract: A study of 56 cases followed for a minimum of 10 years. Cancer, 56:2242, 1985.
18. Farrands, P.A., Vellacott, K.D., Amar, S.S., et al.: Flexible fiberoptic sigmoidoscopy and double-contrast barium enema examination in the identification of adenomas and carcinomas of the colon. Dis. Colon Rectum, 26:727, 1983.
19. Feinberg, S.M., Jagelman, D.G., Sarre, R.G., et al.: Spontaneous resolution of rectal polyps in patients with familial polyposis fol-

lowing abdominal colectomy and ileorectal anastomosis. Dis. Colon Rectum, *31:*169, 1988.

20. Fenoglio-Preiser, C.M., and Hutter, R.V.P.: Colorectal polyps: Pathologic diagnosis and clinical significance. CA, *35:*4, 1985.

21. Giardiello, F.M., Welsh, S.B., Hamilton, S.R., et al.: Increased risk of cancer in the Peutz-Jeghers syndrome. N. Engl. J. Med., *316:*1511, 1987.

22. Giardiello, F.M., Hamilton, S.R., Krush, A.J., et al.: Treatment of colonic and rectal adenomas with sulindac in familial adenomatous polyposis. N. Engl. J. Med., *328:*1313, 1993.

23. Granqvist, S., Gabrielsson, N., and Sundelin, P.: Diminutive colonic polyps—clinical significance and management. Endoscopy, *11:*36, 1979.

24. Haggitt, R.C., Glotzbach, R.E., Soffer, E.E., and Wruble, L.D.: Prognostic factors in colorectal carcinomas arising in adenomas: Implications for lesions removed by endoscopic polypectomy. Gastroenterology, *89:*328, 1985.

25. Hoff, G., Foerster, A., Vatn, M.H., et al.: Epidemiology of polyps in the rectum and colon, recovery and evaluation of unresected polyps 2 years after detection. Scand. J. Gastroenterol., *21:*853, 1986.

26. Hurwitz, M.M., Redleaf, P.D., William, H.J., et al.: Lipomas of the gastrointestinal tract: An analysis of seventy-two tumors. Am. J. Roentgenol., *99:*84, 1967.

27. Jagelman, D.G., DeCosse, J.J., Bussey, H.J.R., et al.: Upper gastrointestinal cancer in familial adenomatous polyposis. Lancet, *1:*1149, 1988.

28. Keating, M.A., Young, R.H., Lillehei, C.W., and Retik, A.B.: Hamartoma of the bladder in a 4-year-old girl with hamartomatous polyps of the gastrointestinal tract. J. Urol., *138:*366, 1987.

29. Khawaja, F.I.: Pedunculated lipoma of the colon: Risks of endoscopic removal. Soc. Med. J., *80:*1176, 1987.

30. Kinzler, K.W., Nilbert, M.D., Li-Kuo, S., et al.: Identification of FAP locus genes from chromosome 5q21. Science, *253:*661, 1991.

31. Kirsner, J.B., and Shorter, R.G.: Diseases of the Colon, Rectum, and Anal Canal. Baltimore, Williams & Wilkins, 1988.

32. Klein, W.A., Miller, H.H., Anderson, M., and DeCosse, J.J.: The use of indomethacin, sulindac, and tamoxifen for the treatment of desmoid tumors associated with familial polyposis. Cancer, *60:*2863, 1987.

33. Klemmer, S., Pascoe, L., and DeCosse, J.: Occurrence of desmoids in patients with familial adenomatous polyposis. Am. J. Med. Genet., *28:*385, 1987.

34. Mandel, J.S., Bond, J.H., Church, T.R., et al.: Reducing mortality from colorectal cancer by screening for fecal occult blood. N. Engl. J. Med., *238:*1365, 1993.

35. Meltzer, S.J., Ahnen, D.J., Battifora, H., et al.: Protooncogene abnormalities in colon cancers and adenomatous polyps. Gastroenterology, *92:*1174, 1987.

36. Moertel, C.F., Hill, J.R., and Adson, M.A.: Management of multiple polyposis of the large bowel. Cancer, *28:*160, 1971.

37. Michowitz, M., Lazebnik, N., Noy, S., and Lazebnik, R.: Lipoma of the colon: A report of 22 cases. Am. Surg., *51:*449, 1985.

38. Myers, W.C., Kelvin, F.M., and Jones, R.S.: Diagnosis and treatment of colonic endometriosis. Arch. Surg., *114:*169, 1979.

39. Nishisho, I., Nakamura, Y., Miyoshi, Y., et al.: Mutations of chromosome 5q21 genes in FAP and colorectal cancer patients. Science, *253:*665, 1991.

40. Nivatvongs, S., Rojanasakul, A., Reiman, H.M., et al.: The risk of lymph node metastasis in colorectal polyps with invasive adenocarcinoma. Dis. Colon Rectum, *34:*323, 1991.

41. Obrecht, W.F., Wu, W.C., Gelfand, D.W., and Ott, D.J.: The extent of successful colonoscopy: A second assessment using modern equipment. Gastrointest. Radiol., *9:*161, 1984.

42. Radi, M.J., and Fenoglio-Preiser, C.M.: Colorectal polyps and polyposis syndromes: Pathological features. *In* Kirsner, J.B., and Shorter, R.G. (eds.): Diseases of the Colon, Rectum, and Anal Canal. Baltimore, Williams & Wilkins, 1988.

43. Rogers, B.H.G.: Endoscopy in diseases of the large bowel and anal canal. *In* Kirsner, J.B., and Shorter, R.G. (eds.): Diseases of the Colon, Rectum, and Anal Canal. Baltimore, Williams & Wilkins, 1988.

44. Sciallero, S., Bruno, S., Di Vinci, A., et al.: Flow cytometric DNA polidy in colorectal adenomas and family history of colorectal cancer. Cancer, *61:*114, 1988.

45. Selby, J.V., Friedman, G.D., Queensberry, C.J., and Weiss, N.S.: A case-control study of screening sigmoidoscopy and mortality from colorectal cancer. N. Engl. J. Med., *326:*653, 1992.

46. Sener, S.F., Miller, H.H., and DeCosse, J.J.: The spectrum of polyposis. Surg. Gynecol. Obstet., *159:*525, 1984.

47. Shinya, H.: Colonoscopy: Diagnosis and Treatment of Colonic Diseases. New York, Igaku-Shoin, 1982.

48. Shinya, H., and Wolff, W.I.: Morphology, anatomic distribution and cancer potential of colonic polyps: An analysis of 7,000 polyps endoscopically removed. Ann. Surg., *190:*679, 1979.

49. Traboulsi, E.K., Krush, A.J., Gardner, E.J., et al.: Prevalence and importance of pigmented ocular fundus lesions in Gardner syndrome. N. Engl. J. Med., *316:*661, 1987.

50. Traboulsi, E.I., and Maumenee, I.H.: Periocular pigmentation in the Peutz-Jeghers syndrome. Am. J. Ophthalmol., *102:*126, 1986.

51. Urbanski, S.J., Haber, G., Kortan, P., and Marcon, N.E.: Small colonic adenomas with adenocarcinoma: A retrospective analysis. Dis. Colon Rectum, *31:*58, 1983.

52. Utsonomiya, J., and Nakamura, T.: The occult osteomatous changes in the mandible in patients with familial polyposis coli. Br. J. Surg., *62:*45, 1975.

53. Walton, B.J., Morain, W.D., Baughman, R.D., et al.: Cowden's disease: A further indication for prophylactic mastectomy. Surgery, *99:*82, 1986.

54. Weed, J.C., and Ray, J.E.: Endometriosis of the bowel. Obstet. Gynecol., *69:*727, 1987.

55. Williams, G.T., Arthur, J.H., Bussey, H.J.R., and Morson, B.C.: Metaplastic polyps and polyposis of the colorectum. Histopathology, *4:*155, 1980.

56. Wilson, D.M., Pitts, W.C., Hintz, R.L., and Rosenfeld, R.G.: Testicular tumors with Peutz-Jeghers syndrome. Cancer, *57:*2238, 1986.

57. Winawer, S.J., Miller, C., Lightdale, C., et al.: Patient response to sigmoidoscopy: A randomized controlled trial of rigid and flexible sigmoidoscopy. Cancer: *60:*1905, 1987.

58. Winawer, S.J., Zauber, A.G., O'Brien, M.J., et al.: Randomized comparison of surveillance intervals after colonoscopic removal of newly diagnosed adenomatous polyps. N. Engl. J. Med., *328:*901, 1993.

59. Zamboni, W.A., Fleisher, H., Zander, J.D., and Folse, J.R.: Spontaneous exclusion of lipoma per rectum occurring with colonic intussusception. Surgery, *101:*104, 1987.

60. Ziv, Y., Waizer, A., Wolloch, Y., and Dintsman, M.: Pitfalls in the preoperative diagnosis of endometriosis. Arch. Surg., *121:*367, 1986.

Chapter 11

ADENOCARCINOMA OF THE COLON AND RECTUM

GLENN D. STEELE, JR. / ROBERT J. MAYER

INCIDENCE AND EPIDEMIOLOGIC ASSOCIATIONS

In terms of both occurrence and number of deaths, colorectal cancer is second only to lung cancer as the most common visceral malignancy in men and women in the United States. An estimated 152,000 patients will be newly diagnosed with bowel cancer during the next year, and more than 57,000 deaths will occur.[9] The probability of colorectal cancer developing from birth to age 70 years is approximately 4%.[110] In the United States, the incidence rises with age. Twice as many cancers are diagnosed in the colon as in the rectum. The incidence of colon cancer has risen among blacks, with the black and white male age-adjusted incidence being equal (rates for 1973 to 1977—white men, 36.7:100,000; black men, 36.3:100,000). Among white and black women, age-adjusted incidence rates are equal at approximately 31:100,000. Incidence rates for rectal cancer are highest among white men. Age-adjusted rates for 1973 to 1977 for white men was 19.1:100,000.

Mortality rates parallel the incidence rates of colorectal cancer. Between 1950 and 1980, mortality from colon cancer decreased slightly among white females but rose among other population groups (Fig. 11–1). Mortality from rectal cancer has declined slightly in all groups (Fig. 11–2).

Throughout the world, high rates of colorectal carcinoma predominate in the more industrialized countries. Lower rates are found in eastern Europe, Asia, Africa, and South America.[35] Studies of Japanese migration to the United States, Asiatic Jewish migration to Israel, and eastern European migration to Australia have found that the migrants acquire the high rates of colorectal cancers that are prevalent in their adopted countries. There is little question that environmental factors, most likely dietary, may be the explanation for the rise in cancer rates. This does not conflict with accumulating data on genetic predisposition, even for nonfamilial or sporadic colorectal carcinoma.[15,98]

Certain groups of patients have a predisposition to the development of cancer of the large bowel. These identifiable high-risk groups also have a greater possibility for early intervention and cancer prevention. Patients with familial polyposis (frequency estimated at 1 in 7,000 to 10,000 live births) have a lifetime risk of colorectal cancer developing that approaches 100% if they survive long enough, and these individuals will transmit this predisposition, with each of their offspring having nearly a 50% chance of developing polyposis coli.

Occasionally, patients with polyposis are found to have no affected family members. Presumably, this represents a new mutation.[49,60] Histologically, normal mucosa in patients with Gardner's syndrome is cytokinetically abnormal. Numerous molecular, biologic, and biochemical screening tests have attempted to define better predictors of mucosal transformation in such patients.[17,41,51,104] However, without a proven screening test, offspring of affected patients should have annual or biannual colonoscopy or air-contrast barium enema studies starting at age 15 years. Screening should continue until about 30 years of age. The median age at which colorectal cancer is diagnosed in polyposis patients is approximately 40 years, which is approximately 2 decades earlier than its occurrence in the general population. Since stage-specific survival of colorectal cancer appears to be the same for polyposis patients as for those who have sporadic bowel cancer, total colectomy at the time polyposis is diagnosed remains the treatment of choice, particularly since recent technical modifications have allowed the surgeon to remove all of the large bowel mucosa without sacrificing continence.[24,97,104]

Other polyposis variants have been recorded, including Turcot's syndrome and Gardner's syndrome, which feature not only multiple polyposis associated with os-

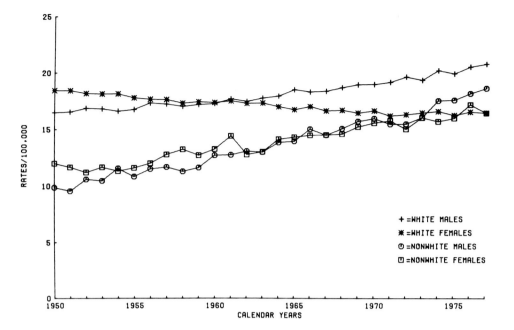

FIGURE 11-1. Mortality rates of cancer of the colon (excluding the rectum) in the United States by race and sex.

teomas of the jaw and other bones, cutaneous fibromas, and occasionally desmoids of the abdomen after operation, but also carcinoma of the ampulla of Vater and the thyroid gland. All of these syndromes, in which true polyps of the bowel proliferate, predispose to colorectal cancer.

Patients with hamartomatous polyps of the intestine, as in the dominantly inherited Peutz-Jeghers syndrome and juvenile polyposis coli,[21,47] do not have a particularly high risk of colon or rectal adenocarcinoma developing. Aggressive screening and surgical management for these inherited polyposis diseases is not necessary.

Cancer that occurs in ulcerative colitis patients can arise in any portion of the large bowel, and it carries the same prognosis as colon cancer in general.[45] Although the risk of cancer is relatively low in the first

decade after the onset of colitis, it increases to approximately 20% each decade thereafter (Figs. 11–3 and 11–4). Since all currently available screening tests (including repetitive biopsies linking dysplasia and bowel mucosa transformation to cancer) are problematic,[68] most patients with this unusually high risk for colon cancer will probably benefit at some point from prophylactic colectomy. Application of new molecular markers (such as sucrase isomaltase) may more quantitatively define risk for transformation in an individual patient, allowing a more rational recommendation for preemptive surgery.[3] When ileoproctostomy is performed, preserving the distal rectum and anus, a worrisome incidence of carcinoma has still been observed. Proctocolectomy with a Brooke ileostomy or abdominal colectomy, mucosal proctectomy, and ileoanal reconnection

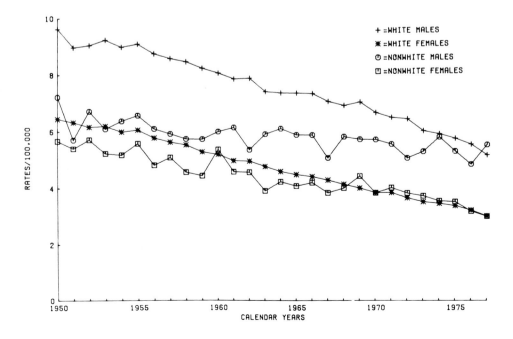

FIGURE 11-2. Mortality rates of cancer of the rectum in the United States by race and sex. (From McKay, F.W., Hanson, M.R., and Miller, R.W.: Cancer mortality in the United States: 1950–1977. Natl. Cancer Inst. Monogr., *59:*96, 1983 [NIH Publication No. 82-2435], with permission.)

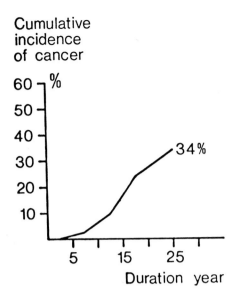

FIGURE 11-3. Patients with ulcerative colitis are at high risk for the development of colorectal cancer. (From Kewenter, J., Ahlman, H., and Hulten, L.: Cancer risk in extensive ulcerative colitis. Ann. Surg., *188*:824, 1978, with permission.)

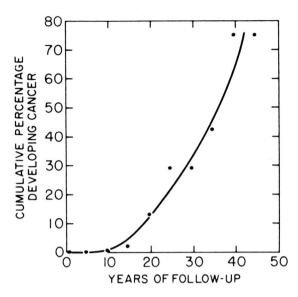

FIGURE 11-4. Risk correlates with duration of active disease, degree of involved bowel, and the development of mucosal dysplasia. (From Greenstein, A.J., Sachar, D.B., Smith, H., et al.: Cancer in universal and left-sided ulcerative colitis: Factors in determining risk. Gastroenterology, 77:290, 1979, with permission.)

with one or another of the reservoir procedures can be applied to individual patients, allowing complete freedom from subsequent cancer development and choosing the most appropriate bowel function for the patient's psychologic and functional well-being. Treatment options are discussed fully in Chapter 6.

Crohn's disease has also been found to predispose to large bowel cancer. Excess risk is probably age dependent. Overall, the probability of colorectal cancer developing may be low, but in patients who are found to have symptomatic Crohn's disease early in life, the excess risk of colon cancer may be anywhere from 3- to 20-fold that of the non–Crohn's disease cohort.[34]

Other well-known acquired conditions that predispose to colon and rectal cancer include the formation of a ureterosigmoidostomy. A 5 to 10% incidence of colon cancer has been found up to 15 to 30 years after this procedure is performed to correct congenital exstrophy of the bladder.[75] Tumors characteristically develop distal to the ureteral implant and, as has been shown in a model system, the site of transformation is the location at which colonic mucosa is chronically exposed to *both* urine and feces.[16] The association between *Streptococcus bovis* endocarditis and colon carcinoma has been generally accepted during the last several years. Confirmation of *S. bovis* bacteremia should initiate appropriate large bowel mucosal screening studies.[38]

Although several studies have reported that cholecystectomy is associated with an increased risk of bowel cancer, this association is probably due to the fact that rates of both gallstone formation and colorectal cancer are higher in industrialized countries, but they are not necessarily etiologically related. Linos and co-workers have postulated that the link between cholecystectomy and an increased risk of bowel cancer may result in part from increased medical surveillance of patients who have cholelithiasis.[48]

Regardless of the cause, the majority of colorectal cancers are thought to arise from adenomatous polyps. Throughout the entire population, therefore, the most usual premalignant phenotype of bowel cancer is the polyp. The diagnosis of a polyp, either during screening or as a response to symptoms, should initiate examination of the entire colorectal mucosa, with subsequent serial follow-up. In addition, patients diagnosed with and treated for sporadic colon or rectal cancer are at high risk for synchronous and metachronous bowel tumors (predominantly polyps). These patients benefit from routine endoscopic screening to diagnose and pre-empt progression of polypoid tumors in what is probably "initiated" but not "promoted" colonic mucosa.[61,106]

Although questions concerning the possible premalignant potential of hyperplastic polyps continue, in general, hyperplastic mucosal proliferation of the large bowel is not thought to be preneoplastic. Only adenomas are clearly premalignant, and only a minority of adenomas ever develop into cancer.[82] Adenomatous polyps are more likely to become malignant if they are sessile rather than pedunculated, villous rather than tubular, and large rather than small. Following the detection of an adenomatous polyp, the entire large bowel should be visualized endoscopically, since synchronous lesions are found 35 to 40% of the time. The frequency of subsequent colonoscopic surveillance is hard to pinpoint, since there must be a balance between the cost of the endoscopic procedure and the fact that more than 5 years is probably required for an adenomatous polyp to grow to the size that neoplastic transformation is likely.[76] It is, however, mandatory that two successive colonoscopic examinations be done to assure clearance of the entire bowel mucosa before the endoscopic interval is lengthened in patients who have already been diagnosed as having colorectal cancer or sporadic polyp formation.

Few occupations have been linked to the development of colorectal cancer. With the exception of occupational exposure to asbestos, in which an increased risk of colorectal cancer has been reported to be in the range of two- to threefold, only slight increases in colorectal cancer rates have been reported in a smattering of studies of occupational or work hazards.

The association between dietary factors and the development of colorectal cancer is extraordinarily complex. A positive association has been reported among high meat intake, high saturated fat and cholesterol diets, increased bowel anaerobic microflora, diets that increase deconjugated fecal bile acid excretion, vitamin D, and calcium content.[11,50,94,111] No distinct association has been proven between constipation or dietary fiber content and the development of large bowel cancer.[10] Undoubtedly, the complexity of the environmental factors, including diet, that relate to colon and rectal cancer is a function of the multiple factors that lead to the development of sporadic polyps, the genetics of at least a two-step process between bowel mucosa initiation and promotion before the polyps occur, the ability of the host to defend itself once polyps occur (since so few of them become cancer), and simple methodologic problems such as the difficulty of designing dietary questionnaires that reliably establish specific dietary intake histories that can be related to polyp and colorectal cancer rates.

Despite numerous empiric dietary recommendations, at present common sense provides as good a set of rules as anything else. High fat intake and high meat intake are probably not good. The eventual ability to define precise risks in first-degree relatives of patients with sporadic carcinoma may allow relatively limited populations to avoid specific foodstuffs or to supplement their diets specifically. However, the likelihood is much greater that before precise dietary manipulations will be found to prevent colon and rectal cancer, population groups at risk, defined genetically or biochemically, will undergo routine screening of the colorectal mucosa to diagnose and remove premalignant polyps.[4,74]

NATURAL HISTORY

In the recent past, most colorectal carcinomas were reported to arise in the distal bowel. The rubric that rectal examination plus rigid proctosigmoidoscopy finds 75% of all colorectal carcinomas has recently been challenged (Fig. 11-5). Although no satisfactory explanation for the change in the segmental distribution of colon and rectal carcinoma is conclusive, there are numerous possibilities. First, since the more proximal colon is currently more accessible through wider application of endoscopic techniques, and there is greater use of double-contrast barium studies, we may be diagnosing more right-sided or proximal bowel lesions that were always there but were less frequently diagnosed. Second, there may actually be multiple environmental and genetic risk factors that determine right-sided or proximal bowel lesions that are distinct from the causes of left-sided or distal bowel tumors. Numerous formalized treatment protocols of bowel cancer are beginning to demonstrate that the natural history of right-sided lesions differs from that of left-sided lesions. The natural history of sigmoid cancers differs from more proximal colonic tumors. The natural history of rectal cancer is different from that of colon cancer. These differences include responsiveness to multimodality adjuvant therapy.[23,27,109]

Regardless of the reasons for the change in segmental distribution, the effect is obvious from both the presenting symptoms and the screening techniques one devises for diagnosing colorectal carcinoma in asymptomatic patients. The patient will present with symptoms that vary with the anatomic location of the large bowel disease (Tables 11-1 through 11-3).

Screening of symptomatic patients includes routine

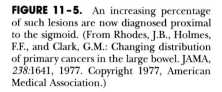

FIGURE 11-5. An increasing percentage of such lesions are now diagnosed proximal to the sigmoid. (From Rhodes, J.B., Holmes, F.F., and Clark, G.M.: Changing distribution of primary cancers in the large bowel. JAMA, 238:1641, 1977. Copyright 1977, American Medical Association.)

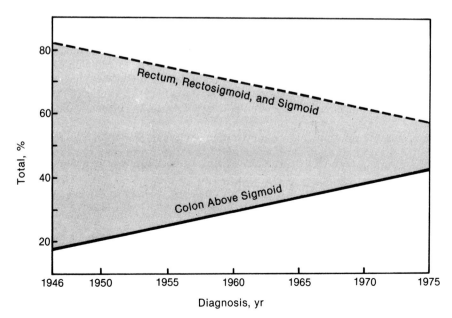

TABLE 11-1. COMPARISON OF THE FIVE MOST FREQUENT SYMPTOMS IN RECTAL, LEFT COLON, AND RIGHT COLON CANCER*

RECTUM AND RECTOSIGMOID (258) PATIENTS	LEFT COLON (99 PATIENTS)	RIGHT COLON (984 PATIENTS)
Melena (85%)	Abdominal pain (72%)	Abdominal pain (74%)
Constipation (46%)	Melena (53%)	Weakness (29%)
Tenesmus (30%)	Constipation (42%)	Melena (27%)
Diarrhea (30%)	Nausea (25%)	Nausea (24%)
Abdominal pain (26%)	Vomiting (23%)	Abdominal mass (23%)

*From Sugarbaker, P.H.: Clinical evaluation of symptomatic patients. *In* Steele, G., Jr., and Osteen, R.T. (eds.): Colorectal Cancer: Current Concepts in Diagnosis and Treatment. New York, Marcel Dekker, 1986, p. 60, with permission.

digital rectal examination, routine stool guaiac testing (Hemoccult), proctosigmoidoscopy or pancolonoscopy, and barium enema with air-contrast studies. The individual choice of test and order of test priority depends upon the precise symptoms of the patient as well as on the availability of the various endoscopic procedures in a particular practice location.

Rules for screening asymptomatic patients are empiric or dependent upon data derived from statistical modeling. Major studies attempting to determine the benefit of screening large population groups for occult blood in the stool have led to mixed results.[46,56,107] More than likely, the increased accuracy of modifications of the Hemoccult or Hemoquant tests, the new designs for testing occult blood in the stool that make application of the test more palatable to the general population and, perhaps most importantly, increased communication of the algorithms for correctly interpreting the tests and correctly studying patients who have truly positive tests will all increase the cost-effectiveness of mass screening approaches in the future. Nevertheless, at present, screening is effective only among high-risk populations and is generally felt to include mandatory testing of stool for occult blood at the time of routine history taking and physical examination.[106]

Recent data from the Strang Clinic study by Winawer and co-workers[105] have begun to show what most people would predict. Patients whose colorectal tumors (polyps as well as carcinomas) are diagnosed in the asympto-

TABLE 11-2. VARIATION IN SYMPTOMS OF RIGHT COLON, LEFT COLON, AND RECTAL CANCER*

SYMPTOM	RIGHT COLON	LEFT COLON	RECTUM
Pain	Ill-defined	Colicky[†]	Steady, gnawing
Obstruction	Infrequent[‡]	Common	Infrequent
Bleeding	Brick red	Red, mixed with stool	Bright red, coating stool
Weakness[§]	Common	Infrequent	Infrequent

*From Sugarbaker, P.H.: Clinical evaluation of symptomatic patients. *In* Steele, G., Jr., and Osteen, R.T. (eds.): Colorectal Cancer: Current Concepts in Diagnosis and Treatment, New York, Marcel Dekker, 1986, p. 61, with permission.
[†]Made worse by the ingestion of food.
[‡]If obstruction occurs, tumor often located at ileocecal valve region.
[§]Weakness secondary to anemia.

TABLE 11-3. PATHOPHYSIOLOGY OF SYMPTOMS FROM RIGHT COLON, LEFT COLON, AND RECTAL CANCER*

SYMPTOM	RIGHT COLON	LEFT COLON	RECTUM
Caliber of lumen	6–10 cm	1–2 cm	5–7 cm
Consistency of stool	Liquid	Semisolid	Firm
Proteolytic enzymes	Present[†]	Lacking	Lacking

*From Sugarbaker, P.H.: Clinical evaluation of symptomatic patients. *In* Steele, G., Jr., and Osteen, R.T. (eds.): Colorectal Cancer: Current Concepts in Diagnosis and Treatment. New York, Marcel Dekker, 1986, p. 162, with permission.
[†]Accounts for brick red color of stool and persistent, sometimes massive blood loss.

matic state have more superficial lesions than do patients who present with signs or symptoms that lead to the diagnosis of colorectal cancer. Although it will take a number of years before the mortality consequences are known, it stands to reason that Winawer and colleagues will eventually show that patients whose early lesions are removed will live longer than patients whose more invasive lesions are removed. Undoubtedly, lead time bias will be discussed. However, most thoughtful people, given the choice, would rather have colon or rectal cancer diagnosed earlier!

With the exception of certain high-risk groups, application of statistical models to "standard-risk" patients has shown that the most cost-effective application of Hemoccult testing and either colonoscopy or air-contrast barium enema studies begins at age 40 years, and when nothing is found, they should be repeated every 5 years (Fig. 11-6).[19] Which endoscope to use (colonoscope, 60-cm flexible colonoscope, flexible sigmoidoscope, rigid proctosigmoidoscope), whether double-contrast enema or endoscopy is more cost-effective, and precisely when screening should be applied to patients who are asymptomatic but are related to individuals with sporadic nonfamilial colon or rectal cancer would ideally be defined in clinical trials. These trials will never be done because they are extraordinarily difficult to design and prohibitively expensive. Therefore, we will

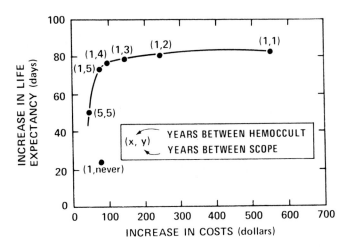

FIGURE 11-6. Cost-effectiveness—based on clinical assumptions of questionable validity applied to "standard-risk" patients. (From Eddy, D.M.: The economics of cancer prevention and detection: Getting more for less. Cancer, *47*:1200, 1981, with permission.)

TABLE 11-4. CARCINOMA OF THE COLORECTUM: STAGE CLASSIFICATION AND STAGE GROUPING*

AJCC 1982	UICC 1978 (3RD ED.)	DUKES (1932, 1936)[†]	ASTLER-COLLER[‡]
Stage 0	Stage 0		Stage 0
Carcinoma in situ T_{is}, N_0, M_0	T_{i5}, N_0, M_0		0
Stage I	Stage I	A	Stage I
1_A Tumor confined to mucosa or submucosa T_1, N_0, M_0	1_A		
1_B Tumor involves muscularis propria but not beyond T_2, N_0, M_0	T_1, N_0, M_0, 1_B	A	A
	T_2, N_0, M_0		
Stage II	Stage II	A	B_1
Involvement of all layers of bowel wall with or without invasion of immediately adjacent structures T_3, N_0, M_0	T_3, T_4, N_0, M_0 (T_{3a} with fistula) (T_{3B} without fistula)	B	Stage II B_2
Stage III	Stage III	C (1932)	Stage III
Any degree of bowel wall with regional node metastasis	Any T, N_1, M_0	C_1 (1935)	C_1
		C_2 (1935)	C_2
Any T, N_2–N_3, M_0 Extends beyond contiguous tissue or immediately adjacent organs with no regional lymph node metastases T_4, N_0, M_0			
Stage IV	Stage IV	Type 4	Stage IV
Any invasion of bowel wall with or without regional lymph node metastases but with evidence of distant metastasis Any T, any N, M_1	Any T, any M_1	(so-called D)	D

*From American Joint Committee on Cancer, Beahrs, O.H., and Myers, M.H. (eds.): Manual for Staging of Cancer, 2nd ed. Philadelphia, J.B. Lippincott, 1983, with permission.
†Dukes, A., limited to bowel wall; B, spread to extramural tissue; C, involvement of regional nodes (C_1, near primary lesion; C_2, proximal node involved at point of ligation); type 4 (so-called D), distant metastasis.
‡Astler-Coller A., limited to mucosa; B_1, same as AJCC, stage 1_B (T_{2a}); B_2, same as AJCC stage I_B (T_{2b}); C_1, limited to wall with involved nodes; C_2, through all layers of wall with involved nodes.

likely fall back on statistical modeling and common sense empiricism for future screening rules. Asymptomatic individuals in the standard-risk group who ask for screening recommendations should be told that 60-cm flexible colonoscopy should be initiated between the ages of 40 and 50 years. At present, carcinoembryonic antigen (CEA), as well as other more experimental tumor markers, is ineffective for cancer screening purposes, since no marker, including CEA, is tumor specific.

Prognosis of bowel cancer is related to the stage of disease at diagnosis, histologic differentiation, lymphatic invasion, and the extent of tumor-free surgical resection margins and is inversely related to the size of the primary tumor. Additional variables that define DNA ploidy may become important prognostic factors. Definition of subpopulations of cells in the primary tumor that have a particular predisposition to metastasize to particular sites also has exciting potential for the near future.[22,88]

Numerous staging schemes have been defined. Most, however, are derived from either the original classification of tumor penetration into the bowel wall as re-

ported by Dukes in 1932[102] or the TNM staging classification originally applied by the International Union Against Cancer (UICC) in 1978 and adopted by the American Joint Committee on Cancer (AJCC) in 1982 (Table 11–4). The influence of disease stage on prognosis during two successive 10-year intervals is depicted in Table 11–5. These data reflect the need for concurrent nontreatment controls in any primary and adjuvant treatment protocol. This has most recently been exemplified by the Gastrointestinal Tumor Study Group colon adjuvant protocol.[27] If treated groups had been compared to historic nontreatment controls, all three of the treatment arms would have been considered positive. However, with inclusion of concurrent nontreated controls, none of the adjuvant treatment arms was found to provide a significant benefit to the patients.

Although the data showing increased probability of 5-year survival, particularly for the Dukes-Kirklin A, B_1, and B_2 categories (Fig. 11–7) of primary colon and rectal cancer patients, may be interpreted as indicating more effective surgery or a change in the underlying cause or biologic features of the disease, neither explanation seems reasonable. More than likely, thorough preoperative staging and more thorough staging during abdominal exploration has led to the detection of otherwise occult metastases in patients who earlier would have been thought to have resectable primary cancer. In addition, more thorough pathologic examination of the resected specimens will tend to improve the 5-year survival rate of patients with Dukes B disease and those with Dukes C disease. In contrast to many other solid tumors, prognosis in patients with colorectal cancer is not influenced by the size of the primary lesion if data are corrected for nodal involvement and histologic dif-

TABLE 11-5. INFLUENCE OF DISEASE STAGE ON PROGNOSIS DURING TWO SUCCESSIVE 10-YEAR INTERVALS

SURGICAL STAGE	5-YEAR SURVIVAL (1940s AND 1950s)	5-YEAR SURVIVAL (1960s and 1970s)
Dukes-Kirklin A	80%	>90%
Dukes-Kirklin B_1	60%	85%
Dukes-Kirklin B_2	45%	70–75%
Dukes C	15–30%	35–65%

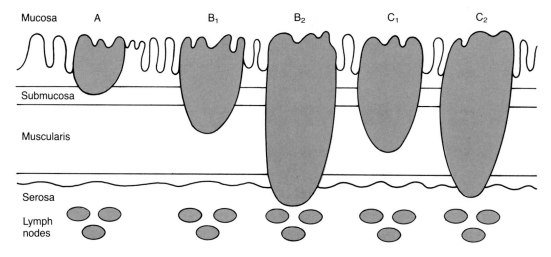

FIGURE 11-7. Kirklin modification of Dukes classification of colonic carcinomas.

ferentiation. In fact, an inverse relationship between size and prognosis may exist.[108]

Recurrence rates, determined by number of involved nodes and serosal penetration (Table 11–6), as defined by the Gastrointestinal Tumor Study Group adjuvant trial, agree with most modern single-institutional series. The median survival time from the clinical detection of metastases (so-called Dukes D) is 6 to 8 months.[39] However, larger reviews of patients with metastatic disease do not represent survival statistics applicable to smaller, more selected series. For instance, numerous single-institutional treatment series have consistently selected smaller groups of patients with either isolated liver metastases or isolated pulmonary metastases from colon and rectal carcinoma, who have been shown to have long-term survival regardless of treatment response. If patients are diagnosed with minimal metastatic disease isolated to a single organ and have no dysfunction (so-called Eastern Cooperative Study Group [ECOG] 0 performance status), median survival without any treatment at all may be between 2 and 3 years.[31,70] If these "good biology" patients are accrued to treatment protocols and compared with historic controls, whatever treatment is being examined could inappropriately be touted as effective.

TUMOR MARKERS

CEA was isolated by Gold in 1965 by using an antiserum prepared in adult rabbits against an extract of human colonic tumor that had been absorbed with an excess of normal colonic tissue to remove nonspecific antibody. CEA remains the prototypical solid tumor marker. All new markers will have to pass many of the same clinical research tests that have been formulated for CEA during the last 24 years. These tests allow us to conclude the following. First, CEA is not tumor specific. It is found in endodermally derived carcinomas, normal and fetal gut, pancreas, and liver. CEA activity is detect-

TABLE 11-6. RECURRENCE RATES BY NUMBER OF POSITIVE NODES AND SEROSAL PENETRATION*

CATEGORY	TOTAL NO. OF PATIENTS	NO. WITH RECURRENCE	RECURRENCE (%)
Serosal penetration negative nodes	232	47	20
No serosal penetration 1–4 positive nodes	33	6	18
Serosal penetration 1–4 positive nodes	205	77	38
No serosal penetration 5+ positive nodes	16	6	38
Serosal penetration 5+ positive nodes	85	55	65
Serosal penetration unknown positive nodes	1	1	100
Total patients	572	192	34

*Modified from Olson, R.M., Perencevich, N.P., Malcolm, A.W., et al.: Patterns of recurrence following curative resection of adenocarcinoma of the colon and rectum. Cancer, 45:2969, 1980, with permission.

able in the blood of patients with other than colorectal malignancies, as well as in patients with certain benign conditions, including pneumonitis, bronchitis, pancreatitis, bowel obstruction, inflammatory bowel disease with active inflammation, and extrahepatic biliary obstruction not caused by tumor. Patients who are cigarette smokers will have a mildly elevated serum CEA level.

Nevertheless, despite its lack of specificity, if used correctly, CEA determination is a valuable addition to clinical decision-making in patients who have been diagnosed with colon or rectal carcinoma. CEA is not an appropriate screening test. Whether sampled once or serially, CEA cannot be used to help in the differential diagnosis of an unknown suspected bowel problem or malignancy. When CEA concentrations are determined before primary tumor resection, they may provide additional prognostic value, particularly for patients who have nodal involvement. However, CEA should not be used to stratify patients who are undergoing primary or adjuvant colorectal cancer therapy.[30,59,80]

If once the primary tumor has been removed, morphologic examination shows predominantly or exclusively poorly differentiated tumor, histologic sections should be stained for evidence of CEA production. The more poorly differentiated tumors that have no positive CEA staining can be ruled out as producing and secreting this marker. Patients with such tumors should not have serial CEA values obtained as part of their postoperative follow-up.[31]

In patients who have been shown to have CEA elevation in blood samples drawn prior to primary tumor resection, and in patients who have predominantly moderately to well-differentiated tumors, serial CEA values obtained postoperatively offer an effective means of monitoring response to therapy. A CEA titer postoperatively serves as a measure of the completeness of tumor resection. If a preoperative elevated CEA value does not fall to normal within 2 to 3 weeks after surgery, the resection was most likely incomplete or occult metastases are present. A rising trend in serial CEA values from a normal postoperative baseline (<5 ng/nl) may predate any other clinical or laboratory evidence of recurrent disease by 6 to 9 months.[53]

Serial CEA values parallel either tumor regression or tumor progression during treatment for metastatic disease.[90] Although not quantitatively related to volume of disease, CEA titers most often are highest when either liver or lung metastases are present. The vast majority of patients who respond to treatment will demonstrate a decline in CEA levels. Rising CEA values are almost always incompatible with tumor regression.[12,64]

The controversy regarding patient benefit when second-look surgery is performed solely on the basis of a rise in serial CEA determinations is focused more on the limited options for therapy in patients found to have recurrent disease than on the efficacy of the marker itself. When CEA is monitored correctly, surprisingly few false-positive or false-negative results are found. However, the initial enthusiasm for resection of recurrent disease and claims of durable disease-free survival have evolved to the present realization that probably no more

than 10 to 15% of patients whose recurrences are defined, whether by a rise in CEA or by conventional studies, will have disease that is potentially curable by currently available surgical or nonsurgical means.[52,57,73] In more recent applications of radioimmunologic scanning techniques, using either external or intraoperative gamma-scanning,[96] the weak link will still be a lack of effective systemic therapy even when disease recurrence is found early.

Most localized recurrences represent a foreshadowing of either regional or systemic disease. This was the implication of the original Wangensteen CEA second-look surgery papers, describing patterns of initial recurrence defined in the late 1940s and 1950s[33] and updated more recently by Gunderson and Sosin.[33] The major impact of CEA and other potentially new, useful markers for colon and rectal carcinoma will be in decreasing the number of patients who need to be studied by examining only those with elevated CEA values. However, until new therapeutic options become available for all sites of recurrence, or until effective systemic therapy for colon and rectal cancer is available, no more than 10 to 15% of patients determined to have recurrence, whether early or late, will have any greater potential for cure than that described in the retrospective series of Welch and Donaldson in 1978.[101] These authors reviewed all patients at Massachusetts General Hospital with diagnosed recurrence from colon and rectal carcinoma and found that only approximately 10% were amenable to repeat surgical resection. These patients were, in fact, in exactly the same category as the patients noted in our more recent CEA-directed second-look surgery series[90] as having the highest probability of resectable recurrent disease (i.e., those patients with isolated liver or lung metastases).

When liver or lung is the first or only site of recurrence, the serial CEA rise will show the steepest slope. Specific diagnostic tests to confirm recurrence in the liver or lung are now preferable to so-called blind CEA-directed second-look procedures.[77] At present, only patients who have recurrence of colorectal carcinoma that necessitates palliation, or patients with defined isolated liver or lung metastases, should undergo surgery. Broad-based CEA second-look surgery trials are probably also unethical, since they will undoubtedly prove to be of no benefit for the large group of patients in whom recurrence may be diagnosed earlier by CEA determinations but for whom no effective therapy is yet available.

THERAPY FOR PRIMARY COLON AND RECTAL CARCINOMA

The mainstay of therapy for colon and rectal carcinoma is surgery. Despite earlier as well as recent attempts to justify more extensive surgery as leading to better cure rates for primary colon and rectal carcinomas, the accepted surgical techniques for curing colon and rectal tumors have remained unchanged over the last 3 decades.[20,87,95] Application of minimally invasive techniques by endoscopy for better staging[25] and for therapy[8] await testing in prospective randomized trials. Such multi-institutional studies are presently underway.

Surgery

Surgical treatment of primary colon and rectal cancer is based on an understanding of anatomy and the mechanisms of colorectal cancer spread. Adenocarcinomas of the colon and the rectum spread in the lymphatics of the bowel submucosa. Adequate lengths of bowel proximal and distal to the cancer must be resected to avoid cutting across tumor in these intramural lymphatics. Bowel cancer grows through the serosa into mesenteric lymphatics that run along the blood vessels draining into the portal watershed at the root of the mesentery. Resection of colon and rectal cancers therefore includes resection of the major lymphatic drainage in the mesentery. Since anatomic resections designed to include named blood vessels also include the draining lymphatics, boundaries for resecting large bowel cancer are uniform (Fig. 11–8). Right hemicolectomy, transverse colectomy, left hemicolectomy, sigmoid resection, or low anterior resection can all be done, adhering to good cancer surgery principles without permanent sacrifice of the patient's bowel function (see Chapters 17 and 18 for technical details).

An abdominoperineal resection (with sacrifice of the sphincter and permanent colostomy) is necessary only in patients with adenocarcinoma in the distal third of the rectum and only if the tumor has been shown to invade the muscularis mucosa. Thus, despite the overriding fear of most patients with bowel cancer, only 5 to 10% will need a permanent colostomy.

Treatment of superficial carcinomas or polyps will depend upon location, the depth of bowel invasion if a focus of carcinoma is found, and whether or not the entire tumor can be removed through an endoscope. For otherwise healthy patients who are found to have a focus of carcinoma invading through the muscularis mucosa, or who have an undefined or "dirty" margin after endoscopic biopsy, formal surgical resection of the bowel is the safest option.

A variety of protocols attempting to preserve the external anal sphincter necessitate transsphincteric or transsacral removal of superficial adenocarcinomas of the distal rectum and stratification of patients with T_2 or early T_3 lesions to adjuvant radiation and chemotherapy protocols. These treatments are experimental. The hope is to prove that multimodality approaches including more limited resection will give an equal chance of cure without the need for abdominoperineal resection and permanent colostomy.

Patients with bowel obstruction from colon or rectal cancer may benefit from an initial temporary colostomy,

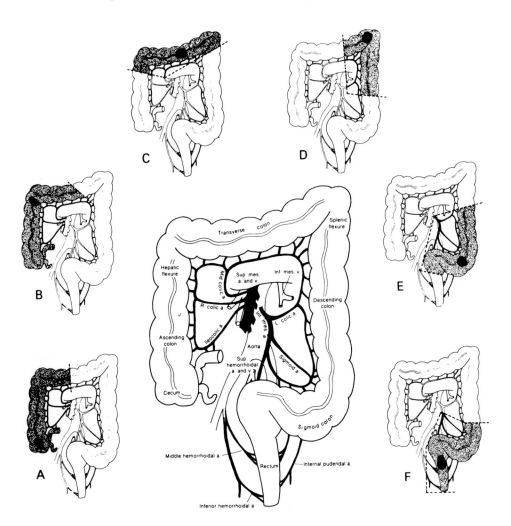

FIGURE 11–8. Anatomic segments, arterial and venous blood supply, and surgical resections of the colon and rectum. (From Steele, G., Jr., and Osteen, R.T.: Surgical treatment of colon cancer. *In* Steele, G., Jr., and Osteen, R.T. [eds.]: Colorectal Cancer. New York, Marcel Dekker, 1986, p. 137, with permission.)

subsequent mechanical preparation of the bowel, and a second-stage cancer resection under less emergent conditions. Patients with bowel cancer perforating into the peritoneal cavity or into adjacent organs, such as the stomach, small bowel, anterior abdominal wall, or bladder, should have the cancer and the adjacent involved tissue removed in continuity. Despite intuition to the contrary, there is little evidence that patients with obstructive or perforated bowel cancer do worse, stage for stage, than their counterparts with obstruction or perforation.

In patients with fixed rectal carcinoma, defined by digital examination under anesthesia, preoperative external beam radiation therapy has proved beneficial. If such patients respond to 45 cGy and are found on subsequent digital examination to have mobile tumors, they should undergo abdominoperineal resection and, if available, additional intraoperative radiation therapy to the pelvis and perineum. In several recent studies, this combination of intraoperative radiation therapy after proven response to external beam radiation therapy has significantly improved local as well as distant control.[93]

Patients with squamous cell or cloacogenic carcinomas of the anus and rectum do not have surgically curable disease. In numerous multimodality studies that have followed the initial Nigro regimen,[63] external beam radiation therapy combined with chemotherapy will cure 90 to 100% of such patients (see Chapter 28). If patients do not show a complete response, or if after a complete response therapy fails and abdominoperineal resection is performed, all these patients will ultimately die of recurrent disease. Abdominoperineal resection in such patients is strictly palliative and usually provides short-lived palliation at best.[63]

Adjuvant therapy for high-risk (Dukes-Kirklin C_1, C_2) colon carcinoma is still not widely accepted, but several multi-institutional trials show statistically significant benefit of adjuvant chemotherapy for high-risk colon cancer patients.[80,109] Despite new statistical analytic tools (meta-analysis), which allow minor benefits from separate trials to be combined to discern effect, many cancer specialists point to numerous well-done prospective trials in which chemotherapy, immunotherapy, immunochemotherapy, and radiation therapy alone or together have not increased disease-free or overall survival after curative surgery for patients with primary colon cancer.[13] Adjuvant therapy for anything other than stage III colon cancer should be given only as part of a formalized trial.

For stage III colon cancer, postoperative 5-fluorouracil (5-FU) and levamisole is now considered standard adjuvant therapy.[58]

Several well-done prospective multi-institutional trials have shown that patients with high-risk rectal adenocarcinoma (Dukes-Kirklin B_2, C_1, C_2) will benefit from external beam irradiation and chemotherapy after curative surgery. The precise timing and content of this combined adjuvant therapy is still being defined; however, adjuvant combined therapy should be considered the conventional therapy for patients with high-risk rectal carcinoma and specific contraindications.[44,109]

Although many single-institutional studies of preoperative radiation therapy have implied increased survival in irradiated versus nonirradiated patients, particularly those with rectal or sigmoid colon carcinoma, none of the results have been reproduced in randomized, controlled prospective series. Only one properly designed study[36] has shown survival benefit for a small subset of patients receiving a dose of preoperative radiation that most present-day radiotherapists would consider suboptimal. Preoperative irradiation is, therefore, applicable only for patients who are diagnosed as having fixed rectal carcinoma. There is no doubt that if patients who respond to external beam radiation are then selected for surgical resection, the addition of intraoperative radiation therapy in such patients will increase the regional, and probably the overall, disease-free survival beyond that found when external beam irradiation alone is used.[93] Outside of this setting, however, there is no justification for conventional preoperative adjuvant radiation or chemotherapy.

With the advent of surgical stapling devices, low anterior resection of mid and even distal rectal tumors has become more popular. There has been an increasing interest in defining the biologic adequacy of the distal bowel margin (Table 11–7). This question is largely moot in resection for more proximal tumors, since during any conventional abdominal colectomy, more than the necessary 6 cm or so of bowel both proximal and distal to the tumor is automatically included within the resected specimen. However, as one moves closer to the external anal sphincter, the distal margin becomes a more important matter. Wilson and Beahrs[103] have convincingly demonstrated that a 2-cm distal margin of rectum, as defined by the surgeon and pathologist, is probably adequate to encompass the probable distal intramural lymphatic spread of rectal cancer. However,

TABLE 11–7. SURVIVAL RELATED TO MARGIN BETWEEN TUMOR AND LEVEL OF RESECTION*

| Length of Margin (cm) | SURVIVAL (% MEAN ± SD)† | | | | | |
| | LOW ANTERIOR RESECTION | | | ANTERIOR RESECTION | | |
	No. of Patients	5 Yr	10 Yr	No. of Patients	5 Yr	10 Yr
<2	39	78.4 ± 6.8	56.5 ± 9.9	5	80.0 ± 20.0	80.0 ± 20.0
2 to <3	111	74.8 ± 4.1	66.3 ± 4.8	17	82.4 ± 9.2	60.0 ± 13.0
3 to <4	155	70.8 ± 3.7	49.7 ± 4.8	44	81.8 ± 5.8	61.2 ± 8.4
4 to <5	95	60.9 ± 5.0	47.2 ± 5.4	36	74.3 ± 7.4	48.7 ± 9.5
≥5	156	73.6 ± 3.5	56.1 ± 4.4	244	70.0 ± 2.9	54.3 ± 3.5

*From Beart, R.W., Jr.: Rectal and anal cancer. In Steele, G., Jr., and Osteen, R.T. (eds.): Colorectal Cancer. New York, Marcel Dekker, 1986, p. 170, with permission.
†Differences between operative groups are not significant at 5 or 10 yr.

they have also correctly pointed out that as one moves to within 5 to 6 cm of the dentate line, the most significant biologic weak link is not spread in the bowel wall distally but radial spread of the rectal cancer. Radial spread may cause surgical trespass in two ways. First, there is a natural tendency to cone down as one dissects the anterior aspect of the rectum, moving closer to the perineum. Second, the lateral bony pelvic margins quite often restrict the radial extent of the dissection as one moves toward the perineum, particularly in men. For both of these reasons, the distal margin may not be the limiting factor.

The anatomic restriction of the radial dissection margin is the reason why several nonabdominoperineal resection options are touted as appropriate alternatives for curative therapy of rectal adenocarcinoma. Sischy[84] has applied Papillon's intraluminal radiation therapy quite successfully for a selected group of patients who have T_1 and T_2 superficial rectal adenocarcinomas. Biggers and colleagues[7] at the Mayo Clinic have applied transsphincteric or transsacral local rectal cancer excision to a selected group of patients with T_1 and T_2 lesions. In the Sischy group, none of the patients has been reported to have recurrence. In the Mayo Group, up to 20% of patients have had recurrence but salvage was purportedly obtained in all of them by subsequent abdominoperineal resection.[7,84] Recent reports from M. D. Anderson Hospital have looked at possible complications in patients undergoing rectal sphincter preservation for T_1, T_2, and even early T_3 rectal adenocarcinomas. This combined retrospective and prospective series is being enlarged in order to define more formalized ground rules for selecting patients appropriate for either local surgery alone or surgery plus postoperative radiation and chemotherapy.[54]

Only patients who have superficial rectal adenocarcinoma (T_1 and T_2) with less than one third of the circumference of the bowel involved, no evidence of ulceration or involvement of the sphincter (i.e., no tenesmus), and no palpable or radiologically documented perirectal nodes should have lesions in the lowest 6 cm of the rectum approached conservatively. All other patients should undergo abdominoperineal resection unless entered in a formal trial or treatment plan.

With conventional surgery, as described for resectable colon and rectal carcinoma, approximately 50% of all colon cancer patients and approximately 45% of all rectal carcinoma patients will be alive after 5 years.[66] This expected survival has not changed for 4 decades. Recurrence patterns in these patients have also not changed. In cases of rectal cancer, there have been trials showing the possibility of increasing the patient's disease-free and overall survival when both external beam irradiation and combination chemotherapy are given after adequate surgery to patients with the highest risk cancers (Figs. 11–9 and 11–10). Initial publication by the Gastrointestinal Tumor Study Group of disease-free survival benefit in patients treated with adjuvant radiation and chemotherapy following either low anterior or abdominoperineal resection of Dukes-Kirklin B_2, C_1, and C_2 rectal cancers was subsequently extended to demonstrate overall survival benefit in the same patients. More

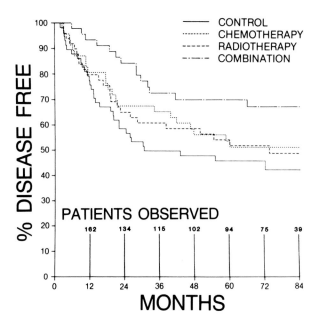

FIGURE 11-9. Time to recurrence, according to treatment. (From Gastrointestinal Tumor Study Group: Prolongation of the disease-free interval in surgically treated rectal carcinoma. N. Engl. J. Med., *312:* 1470, 1985. Reprinted by permission of the New England Journal of Medicine.)

recently, completed adjuvant therapy trials have confirmed the synergistic benefit of external beam irradiation and chemotherapy.[27] At present, the most pressing questions are the exact timing and dose of the radiation therapy, whether continuous-infusion 5-FU is better than intermittent doses with the radiation therapy, and whether levamisole or leucovorin will be an added benefit.

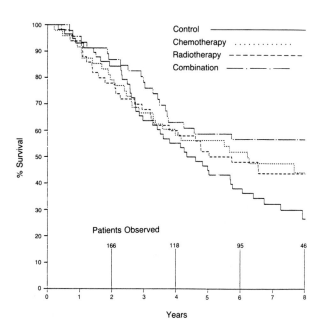

FIGURE 11-10. Survival distribution according to treatment. (From Gastrointestinal Tumor Study Group: Survival after postoperative combination treatment of rectal cancer. N. Engl. J. Med., *315:*1294, 1985. Reprinted by permission of the New England Journal of Medicine.)

Only a single multi-institutional prospective randomized trial has shown benefit of adjuvant chemotherapy alone in patients with high-risk colon carcinoma.[23] Despite the statistical significance of a relatively small survival benefit in this group of patients, advocates of statistical analysis techniques in which individual small benefits are analyzed together (so-called meta-analysis) argue that a 7 to 8% increase in disease-free and expected overall survival could save many lives, considering the prevalence of such a common tumor as colon cancer. These statisticians argue that 5-FU alone remains the only consistent adjuvant of proven effect in patients with stage II or III colon cancer. Nevertheless, follow-up studies of the original North Central Cancer Treatment and subsequent intergroup adjuvant trials are beginning to convince most practitioners in North America that standard treatment is now 5-FU and levamisole after surgical resection of stage III colon cancer.[92]

In 1979, Taylor and colleagues first reported a study of adjuvant portal vein infusion of 5-FU in patients undergoing resection for primary colon and rectal cancer. In a small group of patients, they claimed significant benefit in decreasing the chance of tumor recurrence in the liver and an overall survival benefit in patients who had adjuvant therapy compared with controls. Table 11–8 reviews the subsequent Taylor data and all additional institutional and multi-institutional trials in which one or another variation of the original adjuvant portal infusion protocol was attempted. The matter continues to be interesting, but a conclusion has not been reached. Neither the Swiss trial nor the National Surgical Adjuvant Breast and Bowel Project trials allow one to conclude whether or not this experimental approach should be applied as conventional adjuvant therapy.

Follow-Up

Of patients who have recurrences after curative resection of colon and rectal carcinomas, 80% do so within 2 years. Therefore, any follow-up plan should have a higher frequency of follow-up during these 2 years and a decreasing frequency thereafter. An additional biologic precept in designing follow-up should take into account the effectiveness of therapy once recurrent disease is found. At present, outside of the setting of experimental treatment protocols, only the rare, true suture line recurrence, or the infrequent, isolated, resectable liver or lung metastasis, or the even rarer isolated, regional recurrence are amenable to curative repeat resection. These facts dictate the schedule summarized in Table 11–9.

An additional important point in follow-up is instruction of the patient. A series of specific and nonspecific signs and symptoms that should initiate a patient's return to the physician for routine history and physical examination and appropriate diagnostic studies should be detailed if signs and symptoms of possible recurrence are confirmed. When these signs and symptoms are not present, and since palliation will be the only goal in treating most recurrences, there is little justification for attempting to define recurrence early.

The rationale for colonoscopy as part of perioperative staging and follow-up is not to define recurrent cancer. The yield in diagnosing isolated suture line recurrence either by endoscopy or guaiac testing of the stool is low. The major rationale for colonoscopy is to define synchronous or metachronous bowel tumors, usually polyps. As patients are exposed more uniformly to follow-up endoscopy subsequent to primary colorectal cancer resection, the incidence of metachronous lesions seems to be increasing.[62,65,71] Whatever the ultimate incidence of metachronous bowel lesions, there is no question that patients with sentinel colorectal carcinomas are at significant risk for the development of metachronous polyps. If these polyps are discovered and removed, the risk of colon and rectal cancer developing subsequently decreases. Quite aside from the many methodologic problems in the original University of Minnesota rigid sigmoidoscopic experience, as defined by Gilbertsen and co-workers,[29] adequate screening at the time of primary surgery or afterward to rule out synchronous lesions and serial follow-up (yearly or every 2 years) should be a mandatory part of any good postoperative surveillance program in colorectal cancer patients.

Treatment of Systemic Disease

5-FU remains the most effective chemotherapeutic agent in the management of patients with metastatic disease, achieving a response rate of about 20% when given in standard doses. This response rate has been shown to be increased when the 5-FU dose is increased; it may be increased when 5-FU is given as a continuous infusion as opposed to a standard intravenous bolus, and it is increased when 5-FU is combined with leucovorin.[67] Besides 5-FU, only mitomycin-C and experimental systemic agents have shown even marginal activity in the treatment of widespread colon and rectal carcinoma. In addition, with the exception of an extraordinarily select group of patients with resectable lung or liver metastases, response of systemic colon and rectal carcinoma to one or another of the chemotherapeutic agents is not complete and will not cure the patient.

In numerous single-institutional studies, as well as in a retrospective registry, it now becomes clear that only 2,000 to 4,000 patients each year will have resectable isolated liver metastases. These patients should undergo resection. The expected 5- and 10-year disease-free survival in these patients will be 20 to 30%.[1,14,26,40,81,86]

The key biologic question is how can this narrowly directed benefit be expanded to a much greater group of patients having only liver metastases not amenable to resection or patients having predominantly liver metastases but with known extrahepatic disease? At present, there is no conventionally accepted therapy that will benefit these patients, despite some unconventional experimental therapy that has focused either on cryosurgical ablation of multiple liver metastases[69] or on the addition of systemic chemotherapeutic or hepatic artery infusion chemotherapy at the time of liver resection (ECOG trial under way).

The benefit of hepatic artery infusion chemotherapy for patients who have predominantly liver metastases not amenable to resection is clear-cut. Both the

TABLE 11-8. PROSPECTIVE RANDOMIZED TRIALS WITH ADJUVANT PORTAL INFUSION

Institution	No. of Patients	Entry	Primaries	Treatment (versus control)	Results	
Liverpool*	257	1976–1980	C + R	1 g 5-FU + heparin/d × 7	Survival (4 yr) (Colon Dukes B)	70% versus 50% 92% versus 60%
St. Mary's	451	1978–1983	C + R	1 g 5-FU + heparin/d × 7 or 10,000 units heparin/d × 7	Liver metastases	6.5% versus 8.8% versus 15.3% (control)
Rotterdam	303	1981–1984	C + R	1 g 5-FU + heparin/d × 7 or 240,000 units urokinase/24 hr	Liver metastases at 24 months	7% versus 12% versus 15% (control)
Mayo-NCCTG	219	1980–1988	C	1 g 5-FU + heparin/d × 7	No data	
NSABP	1300	1984–1989	C	600 mg/m² 5-FU + heparin/d × 7	No data	
EORTC 40812 40871	359	1983–1987	C	500 mg/m² 5-FU + heparin/d × 7	No data	
SAKK 40/81	530	1981–1987	C + R	500 mg/m² 5-FU + heparin/d × 7	Relapses 25.1%/34.3% (control)	
				+10 mg/m² micomycin-C d 1	Survival 80% versus 72% at 36 months	
Australia	215	?	C	600 mg/m² 5-FU + heparin/d × 7 intraportal or same dose intravenously	Cancer deaths 4.5% versus 20% (intravenous) versus 22% (control)	

*From Taylor, I., Rowling, J.T., and West, C.: Adjuvant cytotoxic liver perfusion for colorectal cancer. Br. J. Surg., *66:*833, 1979, with permission. C = colon, R = rectum, 5-FU = 5-fluorouracil.

Northern California Oncology Group experience and the Memorial Hospital experience reported by Kemeny and colleagues have shown that floxuridine (FUDR) infused directly into the hepatic artery increases the probability of regression or stabilization of liver metastasis. However, this is at the risk of a dose-related sclerosing cholangitis-like toxicity developing. In addition, the benefit of regression or stabilization of liver metastasis is neutralized by an increased probability of extrahepatic disease.[37,42] Since these trials were designed with a crossover from one treatment arm to another at the time of failure, no comments can be made as to survival benefit. However, after analyzing the data, it should be obvious that survival benefit is not a function of delivery of this relatively ineffective chemotherapeutic agent through any particular portal.

Palliation is the goal of surgical, radiotherapeutic, chemotherapeutic, or multimodality therapy protocols for all sites of regional recurrence. Despite several recent trials to extend the indications for resection of recurrent carcinoma,[6,79] once recurrence has occurred, cure of patients is unlikely. The only question is whether palliation is good enough to justify the major procedures described.

A most salient point concerning treatment of recurrence is that the patient's best hope of cure is to design the best therapy for primary treatment of colon and rectal carcinoma. Even more important is the extraordinary movement in our understanding of mucosal transformation and the molecular biology techniques that in the next decade will allow us to define individuals at risk for initiation and promotion of bowel mucosa. Once a blood test or a tissue sample has identified the individual at risk, endoscopic techniques are already in hand to screen patients in this category. Premalignant tumors (i.e., polyps) can be removed, and subsequent cancer should be prevented.

REFERENCES

1. Adson, M.A., and van Heerden, J.A.: Major hepatic resections for metastatic colorectal cancer. Ann. Surg., *191:*576, 1980.
2. American Joint Committee on Cancer, Beahrs, O.H., and Myers, M.H. (eds.): Manual for Staging of Cancer, 2nd ed. Philadelphia, J.B. Lippincott, 1983.
3. Andrews, C.W., Jr., O'Hara, C.J., Goldman, H., et al.: Sucrase-isomaltase expression in chronic ulcerative colitis and dysplasia. Hum. Pathol., *23:*774, 1992.
4. Atkin, W.S., Morson, B.C., and Cuzick, J.: Long-term risk of co-

TABLE 11-9. BASIC FOLLOW-UP SCHEDULE

Schedule	History/Physical Laboratory Tests	CEA Determination	Colonoscopy or Double-Contrast Studies	Chest X-Ray Studies
Preoperative	X	X (2 successive procedures)	X	X
Postoperative, 3–4 wk		X (2 successive procedures)		
Every 2–3 mo for 5 yr		X		
3 mo			X (if not done before)	
Every 2–3 yr			X	

lorectal cancer after excision of rectosigmoid adenomas. N. Engl. J. Med., 326:658, 1992.

5. Beart, R.W., Jr.: Rectal and anal cancer. In Steele, G., Jr., and Osteen, R.T.: Colorectal Cancer: Current Concepts in Diagnosis and Treatment. New York, Marcel Dekker, 1986, p. 170.

6. Benotti, P.B., Bothe, A., Jr., Eyre, R.C., et al.: Management of recurrent pelvic tumors. Arch. Surg., 122:461, 1987.

7. Biggers, O.R., Beart, R.W., Jr., and Ilstrup, D.M.: Local excision of rectal cancer. Dis. Colon Rectum, 29:374, 1986.

8. Bleday, R., and Wong, W.D.: Recent advances in surgery for colon and rectal cancer. In Steele, G., Jr., and Kinsella, T.J. (eds.): Current Problems in Cancer. St. Louis, Mosby-Year Book, 1993, p. 1.

9. Boring, C.C., Squires, T.S., and Tong, T.: Cancer Statistics, 1993. CA Cancer J. Clin., 43:7, 1993.

10. Bowman, B.B., Kushner, R.F., Dawson, S.L., and Levin, B.: Macrobiotic diet for cancer treatment and prevention. J. Clin. Oncol., 2:702, 1984.

11. Bresalier, R.S., and Kim, Y.S.: Diet and colon cancer—putting the puzzle together. N. Engl. J. Med., 313:1413, 1984.

12. Bronstein, B.R., Steele, G., Jr., Ensminger, W., et al.: The use and limitations of serial plasma carcinoembryonic antigen (CEA) levels as a monitor of changing metastatic liver tumor volume in patients receiving chemotherapy. Cancer, 46:266, 1980.

13. Buyse, M., Zeleniuch-Jacquotte, A., and Chalmers, T.C.: Adjuvant therapy of colorectal cancer: Why we still don't know. JAMA, 259:3571, 1988.

14. Cady, B., and McDermott, W.V.: Major hepatic resection for metachronous metastases from colon cancer. Ann. Surg., 201:204, 1985.

15. Cannon-Albright, L.A., Skolnick, M.H., Bishop, T., et al: Common inheritance of susceptibility to colonic adenomatous polyps and associated colorectal cancers. N. Engl. J. Med., 319:533, 1988.

16. Crissey, M.M., Steele, G.D., Jr., and Gittes, R.F.: Rat model for carcinogenesis in ureterosigmoidostomy. Science, 207:1079, 1980.

17. Danes, B.S.: Increases in vitro tetraploidy: Tissue specific within the hereditable colorectal cancer syndromes with polyposis coli. Cancer, 41:2330, 1978.

18. Eddy, D.M.: The economics of cancer prevention and detection: Getting more for less. Cancer, 47:1200, 1981.

19. Eddy, D.M., Nugent, F.W., Eddy, J.F., et al.: Screening for colorectal cancer in a high-risk population. Results of a mathematical model. Gastroenterology, 92:682, 1987.

20. Enker, W.E., Laffer, U.T., and Block, G.E.: Enhanced survival of patients with colon and rectal cancer is based upon wide anatomic resection. Ann. Surg., 190:350, 1979.

21. Erbe, R.W.: Inherited gastrointestinal-polyposis syndromes. N. Engl. J. Med. 294:1101, 1976.

22. Fidler, I.J., Morikawa, K., Pathek, S., et al.: Development of an in vivo model to study the biology of human colorectal carcinoma metastasis. In Levin, B. (ed.): Gastrointestinal Cancer—Current Approaches to Diagnosis and Treatment. Austin, TX, University of Texas Press, 1988, p. 87.

23. Fisher, B., Wolmark, N., Rockette, H., et al.: Postoperative adjuvant chemotherapy or radiation therapy for rectal cancer: Results from NSABP protocol R-01. J. Natl. Cancer Inst., 80:21, 1988.

24. Fonklasrud, E.W.: Update on clinical experience with different surgical techniques of the endorectal pull-through operation for colitis and polyposis. Surg. Gynecol. Obstet., 165:309, 1987.

25. Forse, R.A., Babineau, T., Bleday, R., and Steele, G., Jr.: Laparoscopy/thoracoscopy for staging: I. Staging endoscopy in surgical oncology. Semin. Surg. Oncol., 9:51, 1993.

26. Foster, J.H., and Berman, M.M.: Solid liver tumor. In Ebert, P.A. (ed.): Major Problems in Clinical Surgery. Philadelphia, W.B. Saunders, 1977, p. 209.

27. Gastrointestinal Tumor Study Group: Prolongation of the disease-free interval in surgically treated rectal carcinoma. N. Engl. J. Med., 312(23):1465, 1985.

28. Gastrointestinal Tumor Study Group: Survival after postoperative combination treatment of rectal cancer. N. Engl. J. Med., 315:1294, 1985.

29. Gilbertsen, V.A., and Nelms, J.M.: The prevention of invasive cancer of the rectum. Cancer, 41:1137, 1978.

30. Goslin, R., Steele, G., Jr., MacIntyre, J., et al.: The use of preop-

erative plasma CEA levels for the stratification of patients after curative resection of colorectal cancers. Ann. Surg., 192:747, 1980.

31. Goslin, R., Steele, G., Jr., Zamcheck, N., et al.: Factors influencing survival in patients with hepatic metastases from adenocarcinoma of the colon or rectum. Dis. Colon Rectum, 25:749, 1983.

32. Greenstein, A.J., Sachar, D.B., Smith, H., et al.: Cancer in universal and left-sided ulcerative colitis: Factors in determining risk. Gastroenterology, 77:290, 1979.

33. Gunderson, L.L., and Sosin, H.: Areas of failure found at reoperation (second or symptomatic look) following "curative surgery" for adenocarcinoma of the rectum. Cancer, 34:1278, 1974.

34. Gyde, S.N., Prior, P., Macartney, J.C., et al.: Malignancy in Crohn's disease. Gut, 21:1024, 1980.

35. Haenszel, W.: Migrant studies. In Schottenfeld, D., and Fraumeni, F.J., Jr. (eds.): Cancer Epidemiology and Prevention. Philadelphia, W.B. Saunders, 1982, p. 194.

36. Higgins, G.A., Jr., Conn, J.H., Jordan, P.H., et al.: Preoperative radiotherapy for colorectal cancer. Ann. Surg., 181:624, 1975.

37. Hohn, D., Stagg, R., Friedman, M., et al.: The NCOG randomized trial of intravenous (IV) versus hepatic arterial (IA) FUDR for colorectal cancer metastatic to the liver (Abstract No. 333). Proc. Am. Soc. Clin. Oncol., 6:85, 1987.

38. Hossenbux, K., Dales, B.A.S., Walls, A.D.F., and Lawrence, J.R.: Streptococcus bovis endocarditis and colonic mucosa: A neglected association. BMJ., 287:21, 1983.

39. Hoth, D.R., and Petrucci, P.E.: Natural history and staging of colon cancer. Semin. Oncol., 3:331, 1976.

40. Hughes, K.S., Rosenstein, R.B., Steele, G., Jr., et al.: Resection of the liver for colorectal carcinoma metastases: A multi-institutional study of long-term survivors. Dis. Colon Rectum, 31:1, 1988.

41. Jessup, J.M., and Gallick, G.E.: The biology of colorectal carcinoma. In Ozols, R.F., Steele, G., Jr., Kinsella, T.J. (eds.): Current Problems in Cancer. St. Louis, Mosby-Year Book, 1992, 16(5), p. 265.

42. Kemeny, N., Daly, J., Oderman, P., et al.: Hepatic artery pump infusion: Toxicity and results in patients with metastatic colorectal carcinoma. J. Clin. Oncol., 2:595, 1984.

43. Kewenter, J., Ahlman, H., and Hulten, L.: Cancer risk in extensive ulcerative colitis. Ann. Surg., 188:824, 1978.

44. Krook, J.E., Moertel, C.G., Gunderson, L.L., et al.: Effective surgical adjuvant therapy for high-risk rectal carcinoma. N. Engl. J. Med., 324:709, 1991.

45. Lavery, I.C., Schiulli, R.A., Jagelman, D.G., et al.: Survival with carcinoma arising in mucosal ulcerative colitis. Ann. Surg., 195:508, 1982.

46. Levin, B.: Screening sigmoidoscopy for colorectal cancer. N. Engl. J. Med., 326(10):700, 1992.

47. Linos, D.A., Dozois, R.R., Dahlin, D.C., and Bartholomew, L.G.: Does Peutz-Jeghers syndrome predispose to gastrointestinal malignancy? Arch. Surg., 116:1182, 1981.

48. Linos, D.A., O'Fallon, W.M., Thistle, J.L., and Kurland, L.T.: Cholelithiasis and carcinoma of the colon. Cancer, 50:1015, 1982.

49. Lipkin, M., Blattner, W.A., Gardner, L.J., et al.: Classification and risk assignment of individuals with familial polyposis, Gardner's syndrome, and familial non-polyposis colon cancer from (^{3}H) thymidine labeling patterns in colonic epithelial cells. Cancer Res., 44:4201, 1984.

50. Lipkin, M., and Newmark, H.: Effect of added dietary calcium on colonic epithelial cell proliferation in subjects at high risk for familial colonic cancer. N. Engl. J. Med., 313:1381, 1984.

51. Luk, G.D., and Baylin, S.B.: Ornithine decarboxylase as a biological marker in familial colonic polyposis. N. Engl. J. Med., 311:80, 1984.

52. Martin, E.W., Jr., Minton, J.P., and Carey, L.C.: CEA-directed second-look surgery in the asymptomatic patient after primary resection of colorectal carcinoma. Ann. Surg., 202:310, 1985.

53. Mayer, R.J., Garnick, M.B., Steele, G.D., Jr., and Zamcheck, N.: Carcinoembryonic antigen (CEA) as a monitor of chemotherapy in disseminated colorectal cancer. Cancer, 42:1428, 1978.

54. McCready, D.R., Ota, D.M., Rich, T.A., et al.: Prospective phase I trial of conservative management of low rectal lesions. Arch. Surg., 124(1):67, 1989.

55. McKay, F.W., Hanson, M.R., and Miller, R.W.: Cancer mortality in

the United States: 1950–1977. Natl. Cancer Inst. Monogr., *59:* 96, 1983 (NIH Publication No. 82-2435).

56. Miller, M.P., and Stanley, T.V.: Result of a mass screening program for colorectal cancer. Arch. Surg., *123:*63, 1988.

57. Minton, J.P., Hoehn, J.L., Gerber, D.M., et al.: Results of a 400-patient carcinoembryonic antigen second-look colorectal cancer study. Cancer, *55:*1284, 1985.

58. Moertel, C.G., Fleming, T.R., Macdonald, J.S., et al.: Levamisole and fluorouracil for adjuvant therapy of resected colon carcinoma. N. Engl. J. Med., *322(6):*352, 1990.

59. Moertel, C.G., O'Fallon, J.R., Go, V.L.W., et al.: The preoperative carcinoembryonic antigen test in the diagnosis, staging, and prognosis of colorectal cancer. Cancer, *58:*603, 1986.

60. Mulvihill, J.J.: The frequency of hereditary large bowel cancer. *In* Ingall, J.R.F., and Mastromarino, A.J. (eds.): Prevention of Heredity Large Bowel Cancer. New York, Alan R. Liss, 1983, p. 61.

61. Nava, H., Carlsson, G., Petrelli, N., and Mittelman, A.: Follow-up of colonoscopy in patients with colorectal adenomatous polyps. *In* Steele, G., Jr., Randall, W.B., Winawer, S.J., and Karr, J.P. (eds.): Basic and Clinical Perspectives of Colorectal Polyps and Cancer. New York, Alan R. Liss, 1988, p. 79.

62. Nava, H.R., and Pagana, T.J.: Postoperative surveillance of colorectal carcinoma. Cancer, *49:*1043, 1982.

63. Nigro, N.A., Vaitkevicius, V.K., Buroker, T., et al.: Combined therapy for cancer of the anal canal. Dis. Colon Rectum, *24:*73, 1981.

64. NIH Consensus Panel: Carcinoembryonic antigen: Its role as a marker in the management of cancer. Ann. Intern. Med., *94:* 407, 1981.

65. Nivatongs, S., and Fryd, D.S.: How far does the proctosigmoidoscope reach? A prospective study of 1000 patients. N. Engl. J. Med., *303:*380, 1980.

66. Olson, R.M., Perencevich, N.P., Malcolm, A.W., et al.: Patterns of recurrence following curative resection of adenocarcinoma of the colon and rectum. Cancer, *45:*2969, 1980.

67. Petrelli, N., Herrera, L., Steele, G., Jr., et al.: A phase III study of 5-fluorouracil (5-FU) versus 5-FU + methotrexate (MTX) versus 5-FU + high dose leucovorin (CF) in metastatic colorectal adenocarcinoma (Abstract). Proc. Am. Soc. Clin. Oncol., *6:*74, 1987.

68. Ransohoff, D.F., Riddell, R.H., and Levin, B.: Ulcerative colitis and colonic cancer. Problems in assessing the diagnostic usefulness of mucosal dysplasia. Dis. Colon Rectum, *28:*383, 1985.

69. Ravikumar, T.S., Kane, R., Cady, B., et al.: Hepatic cryosurgery with intraoperative ultrasound monitoring for metastatic colon carcinoma. Arch. Surg., *122:*403, 1987.

70. Ravikumar, T.S., Olsen, C.O., and Steele, G., Jr.: Resection of pulmonary and hepatic metastasis in the management of cancer. Crit. Rev. Oncol. Hematol., *10:*111, 1990.

71. Reasbeck, P.G.: Colorectal cancer: The case for endoscopic screening. Br. J. Surg., *74:*12, 1987.

72. Rhodes, J.B., Holmes, F.F., and Clark, G.M.: Changing distribution of primary cancers in the large bowel. JAMA, *238:*1641, 1977.

73. Sandler, R.S., Freund, D.A., Herbst, C.A., Jr., and Sandler, D.P.: Cost effectiveness of post-operative carcinoembryonic antigen monitoring in colorectal cancer. Cancer, *53:*193, 1984.

74. Selby, J.V., Friedman, G.D., Quesenberry, C.P., Jr., and Weiss, N.S.: A case-control study of screening sigmoidoscopy and mortality from colorectal cancer. N. Engl. J. Med., *326:*653, 1992.

75. Sheldon, C.A., McKinley, C.R., Hartig, P.R., and Gonzalez, R.: Carcinoma at the site of the ureterosigmoidostomy. Dis. Colon Rectum, *26:*55, 1983.

76. Shinya, H., and Wolff, W.I.: Morphology, anatomic distribution and cancer potential of colonic polyps: An analysis of 7000 polyps endoscopically removed. Ann. Surg., *190:*679, 1979.

77. Staab, H.J., Anderer, F.A., Hornung, A., et al.: Doubling time of circulating CEA and its relation to survival of patients with recurrent colorectal cancer. Br. J. Cancer, *46:*773, 1982.

78. Steele, G., Jr.: Follow-up plans after "curative" resection of primary colon or rectum cancer. *In* Steele, G., Jr., and Osteen, R.T. (eds.): Colorectal Cancer: Current Concepts in Diagnosis and Treatment. New York, Marcel Dekker, 1986, p. 247.

79. Steele, G., Jr.: New surgical treatments for recurrent colorectal cancer. Cancer, *65:*723, 1990.

80. Steele, G.D., Jr., Augenlicht, L.H., Begg, C.B., et al.: National Institutes of Health Consensus Development Conference Statement—adjuvant therapy for patients with colon and rectal cancer. JAMA, *264:*1444, 1990.

81. Steele, G., Jr., Bleday, R., Mayer, R.J., et al.: A prospective evaluation of hepatic resection for colorectal carcinoma metastases to the liver: Gastrointestinal Tumor Study Group Protocol 6584. J. Clin. Oncol., *9:*1105, 1991.

82. Steele, G., Jr., Burt, R.W., Winawer, S.J., and Karr, J.P.: Basic and Clinical Perspectives of Colorectal Polyps and Cancer. New York, Alan R. Liss, 1988.

83. Steele, G.D., Jr., Ellenberg, S., Ramming, K., et al.: CEA monitoring among patients in multi-institutional adjuvant G.I. therapy protocols. Ann. Surg., *196:*162, 1982.

84. Sischy, B., Graney, M.J., and Hinson, E.J.: Endocavitary irradiation for adenocarcinoma of the rectum. CA-A, *24:*6, 1984.

85. Steele, G., Jr., and Osteen, R.T.: Surgical treatment of colon cancer. *In* Steele, G., Jr., and Osteen, R.T. (eds.): Colorectal Cancer: Current Concepts in Diagnosis and Treatment. New York, Marcel Dekker, 1986, p. 137.

86. Steele, G., Jr., Osteen, R.T., Wilson, R.E., et al.: Patterns of failure after surgical "cure" of large liver tumors—a change in the proximate cause of death and a need for effective systemic adjuvant therapy. Am. J. Surg., *147:*554, 1984.

87. Stearns, M.E., Jr., and Schottenfeld, D.: Techniques for surgical management of colon cancer. Cancer, *28:*165, 1971.

88. Steele, G., Jr., and Thomas, P.: Biologic perspectives and new treatment approaches for hepatic metastases of colorectal carcinoma. *In* Levin, B. (ed.): Gastrointestinal Cancer—Current Approaches to Diagnosis and Treatment. Austin, TX, University of Texas Press, 1988, p. 211.

89. Steele, G.D., Jr., Winchester, D.P., Menck, H.R., and Murphy, G.P.: National Cancer Data Base. Annual Review of Patient Care. American Cancer Society/American College of Surgeons Commission on Cancer, Atlanta, 1993.

90. Steele, G.D., Jr., Zamcheck, N., Wilson, R., et al.: Results of CEA-initiated second-look surgery for recurrent colorectal cancer. Am. J. Surg., *139:*544, 1980.

91. Sugarbaker, P.H.: Clinical evaluation of symptomatic patients. *In* Steele, G., Jr., and Osteen, R.T. (eds.): Colorectal Cancer: Current Concepts in Diagnosis and Treatment. New York, Marcel Dekker, 1986, p. 59.

92. Taylor, I., Rowling, J.T., and West, C.: Adjuvant cytotoxic liver perfusion for colorectal cancer. Br. J. Surg., *66:*833, 1979.

93. Tepper, J.E., Cohen, A.M., Wood, W.C., et al.: Intraoperative electron beam radiotherapy in the treatment of unresectable rectal cancer. Arch. Surg., *86:*421, 1986.

94. Tornberg, S.A., Holm, L.E., Carstenson, J.M., and Eklund, G.A.: Risks of cancer of the colon and rectum in relation to serum cholesterol and beta-lipoprotein. N. Engl. J. Med., *315:*1269, 1986.

95. Turnbull, R.B., Kyle, K., Watson, F., et al.: Cancer of the colon: The influence of the *no-touch isolation* technic on survival rates. Ann. Surg., *166:*420, 1967.

96. Tuttle, S.E., Jewell, S.D., Mojzisik, C.M., et al.: Intraoperative radioimmunolocalization of colorectal carcinoma with a hand-held gamma probe and MAb B72.3: comparison of *in vivo* gamma probe counts with *in vitro* MAb radiolocalization. Int. J. Cancer, *42:*352, 1988.

97. Utsunomiya, J., Murata, M., and Tanimura, M.: An analysis of the age distribution of colon cancer in adenomatosis coli. Cancer, *45:*198, 1980.

98. Vogelstein, B., Fearon, E.R., Hamilton, S.R., et al.: Genetic alterations during colorectal tumor development. N. Engl. J. Med., *319:*525, 1988.

99. Wangensteen, O.H.: Cancer of the colon and rectum with special reference to (1) earlier recognition of alimentary tract malignancy and (2) secondary delayed re-entry of the abdomen in patients exhibiting lymph node involvement. Wis. Med. J., *48:* 591, 1949.

100. Watne, A.L., Carrier, J.M., Durham, J.P., et al.: The occurrence of carcinoma of the rectum following ileoproctostomy for familial polyposis. Ann. Surg., *197:*550, 1983.

101. Welch, J.P., and Donaldson, G.A.: Detection and treatment of recurrent cancer of the colon and rectum. Am. J. Surg., *135:*505, 1978.

102. Wilson, R.E.: Prognostic factors and natural history. *In* Steele, G., Jr., and Osteen, R.T. (eds): Colorectal Cancer: Current Concepts in Diagnosis and Treatment. New York, Marcel Dekker, 1986, p. 121.
103. Wilson, S.M., and Beahrs, O.H.: The curative treatment of carcinoma of the sigmoid, rectosigmoid, and rectum. Ann. Surg., *183:*556, 1976.
104. Wiltz, O., O'Hara, C.J., Steele, G.D., Jr., and Mercurio, A.M.: Expression of enzymatically active sucrase isomaltase is a ubiquitous property of colon adenocarcinoma. Gastroenterology, *100:* 1266, 1991.
105. Winawer, S.J., Fleisher, M., Baldwin, M., et al.: Current status of fecal occult blood testing in screening for colorectal cancer. CA, *32:*100, 1982.
106. Winawer, S.J., Zauber, A., Diaz, B., et al., The National Polyp Study Group: The national polyp study: Overview of program and preliminary report of patient and polyp characteristics. *In* Steele, G., Jr., Randall, W.B., Winawer, S.J., and Karr, J.P. (eds.):

Basic and Clinical Perspectives of Colorectal Polyps and Cancer. New York, Alan R. Liss, 1988, p. 35.
107. Winchester, D.P., Schull, J.H., Scanlon, E.F., et al.: A mass screening program for colorectal cancer using chemical testing for occult blood in the stool. Cancer, *45:*2955, 1980.
108. Wolmark, N., Cruz, I., Redmond, C.K., et al.: Tumor size and regional lymph node metastasis in colorectal cancer. A preliminary analysis from the NSABP Clinical Trials. Cancer, *51:*1315, 1983.
109. Wolmark, N., Fisher, B., Rockette, H., et al.: Postoperative adjuvant chemotherapy or BCG for colon cancer: Results from NSABP protocol C-01. J. Natl. Cancer Inst., *80:*36, 1988.
110. Young, J.L., Jr., Percy, C.L., and Asire, A.J. (eds.): Surveillance, epidemiology, and end results (SEER): Incidence and mortality data, 1973–77. Natl. Cancer Inst. Monogr., *57:*1981 (NIH Publication No. 81-2330).
111. Zaridze, D.G.: Environmental etiology of large bowel cancer. J. Natl. Cancer Inst., *70:*389, 1983.

Chapter 12

APPENDIX

GORDON L. TELFORD / ROBERT E. CONDON

ACUTE APPENDICITIS

Acute appendicitis is one of the most common causes of an abdominal emergency and accounts for approximately 1% of all surgical operations.[19] Although rare in infants, appendicitis becomes increasingly common throughout childhood and reaches its maximal incidence between the ages of 10 and 30 years. After 30 years of age, the incidence declines, but appendicitis can occur in individuals of any age. Among teenagers and young adults, the male/female ratio is about 3:2. After age 25 years, the ratio gradually declines until the sex ratio is equal by the mid-30s.

Pathophysiology

The most commonly accepted theory of the pathogenesis of appendicitis is that it results from obstruction followed by infection.[7,31] The lumen of the appendix becomes obstructed by hyperplasia of submucosal lymphoid follicles, a fecalith, stricture, tumor, or other pathologic condition. Once the lumen of the appendix is obstructed, the sequence of events leading to acute appendicitis is probably as follows. Mucus accumulates within the lumen of the appendix, and pressure within the organ increases. Virulent bacteria convert the accumulated mucus into pus. Continued secretion combined with the relative inelasticity of the serosa leads to a further rise in pressure within the lumen. This results in obstruction of the lymphatic drainage, leading to edema of the appendix, diapedesis of bacteria, and the appearance of mucosal ulcers. At this stage, the disease is still localized to the appendix; therefore, the pain perceived by the patient is visceral and is localized to the epigastrium or periumbilical area. This pain usually is accompanied by anorexia, nausea, and, on occasion, vomiting.

Continued secretion into the lumen and increasing edema bring about a further rise in intraluminal and tissue pressure, resulting in venous obstruction and ischemia of the appendix. Bacteria spread through the wall of the appendix, and acute suppurative appendicitis ensues. Somatic pain occurs when the inflamed serosa of the appendix comes in contact with the parietal peritoneum and results in the classic shift of pain to the right lower quadrant.

As this pathologic process continues, venous and arterial thromboses occur in the wall of the appendix, resulting in gangrenous appendicitis. At this stage, small infarcts occur, permitting escape of bacteria and contamination of the peritoneal cavity. The final stage in the progression of acute appendicitis is perforation through a gangrenous infarct and the spilling of accumulated pus. Perforating appendicitis is now present, and morbidity and mortality increase.

Symptoms

The symptomatic history in acute appendicitis may vary, but the cardinal symptoms are usually present.[19,23] The history usually begins with abdominal pain that often is localized to the epigastrium or the periumbilical area, followed by anorexia and nausea. Vomiting, if it occurs, appears next. After a variable period, usually about 8 hours, the pain shifts to the right side and usually into the right lower quadrant.

PAIN. As already mentioned, the typical pain of acute appendicitis initially consists of diffuse, central, minimally severe visceral pain, which is followed by somatic pain that is more severe and usually well localized to the right lower quadrant. Failure to follow the classic visceral-somatic sequence is common in acute appendicitis, occurring in up to 45% of patients who prove to have appendicitis. Atypical pain may be somatic and localized to the right lower quadrant from its initiation. Conversely, the pain may remain diffuse and may never become localized. In older patients, atypical pain is found more frequently.

Patients with high retrocecal appendicitis may present with only diffuse pain in the right flank. Similarly, patients in whom the entire appendix is within the true pelvis may never experience somatic pain and, instead, may have tenesmus and vague discomfort in the suprapubic area.

ANOREXIA, NAUSEA, AND VOMITING. Anorexia and nausea are present in almost all cases of acute appendicitis, but they are not always followed by vomiting. The presence or absence of vomiting is not a criterion for the diagnosis of appendicitis. When vomiting does occur, it is

140

not persistent, and most patients vomit only once or twice. Vomiting occurs after the onset of pain with such regularity that if it precedes pain, the diagnosis of appendicitis should be questioned.

CONSTIPATION AND DIARRHEA. A history of the recent onset of constipation or diarrhea is not exceptionally helpful in the diagnosis of appendicitis. A greater percentage of patients with appendicitis complain of constipation, but some give a history that defecation relieves the pain.

Physical Examination

Typical physical signs of acute appendicitis include localized tenderness, muscle guarding, and rebound tenderness. Cutaneous hyperesthesia, right-sided pelvic tenderness on rectal examination, and the presence of a psoas or obturator sign occur less frequently and tend to be highly dependent on the examiner. Although often temperature is normal, fever up to 38° C occurs. In the usual case of acute appendicitis, higher fever occurs infrequently.

TENDERNESS AND MUSCLE GUARDING. On routine abdominal examination, an area of maximal tenderness often will be elicited in the area of McBurney's point, which is located two thirds of the distance along a line from the umbilicus to the right anterior superior iliac spine. It should be remembered that if the appendix is in a high retrocecal position or is entirely within the true pelvis, point tenderness and muscle spasm might not be elicited. In high retrocecal appendicitis, tenderness may occur over a large area, and there may be no signs of muscle spasm. In pelvic appendicitis, neither tenderness nor muscle guarding may be present. Both signs are often lacking or minimal in the aged population.

Signs of peritoneal inflammation or irritation in the right lower quadrant are also helpful in the diagnosis of acute appendicitis and can be demonstrated by many methods. Asking the patient to cough or to bounce up and down on the heels will elicit this type of pain. Rebound tenderness is elicited by the sudden release of abdominal palpation pressure. Rovsing's sign—pain elicited in the right lower quadrant with palpation pressure in the left lower quadrant—can be a sign of acute appendicitis. Muscle guarding, manifested as resistance to palpation, increases as the severity of inflammation of the parietal peritoneum increases. Initially, there is only voluntary guarding, but this is replaced by reflex involuntary rigidity.

ABDOMINAL MASS. As the disease process progresses, it may be possible to palpate a tender mass in the right lower quadrant. Although the mass may be caused by an abscess, it can also result from adherence of the omentum and loops of intestine to an inflamed appendix. When appendicitis becomes advanced enough that there is a large, inflamed mass and the anterior abdominal wall is involved, the patient often avoids sudden movements that can cause pain.

PSOAS SIGN. The right hip is often kept in slight flexion to keep the iliopsoas muscle relaxed. Stretching the muscle by extension of the hip or further flexion against resistance can initiate a positive psoas sign, indicating irritation of the muscle by an inflamed appendix. A psoas sign is seldom seen in early appendicitis and can be demonstrated in many patients without pathologic condition.

RECTAL EXAMINATION. Rectal examination, although essential in all patients with suspected appendicitis, is helpful in only a small percentage of them. In patients with an uncomplicated appendicitis, the finger of the examiner cannot reach high enough to elicit pain on rectal examination. Even with an early pelvic appendicitis in an anxious patient, it is often hard to elicit pure right-sided pain on rectal examination. It must be remembered, though, that in those few patients in whom the appendix lies almost wholly within the pelvis, a well-performed rectal examination may be the only way to elicit tenderness.

If the appendix ruptures, the physical examination will change. If the infection is contained, a soft, tender mass will often develop in the right lower quadrant, and the area of tenderness will now encompass the entire right lower quadrant. Involuntary guarding will become evident and rebound tenderness more marked. The patient's temperature will be more like that seen with abscess formation and may rise to 39° C with a corresponding tachycardia.

If appendiceal rupture fails to localize, signs and symptoms of diffuse peritonitis will develop. Tenderness and guarding will become generalized, the temperature will remain higher than 38° C with spikes to 40° C, and the pulse rate will increase to more than 100 beats/min.

Laboratory Tests

In the early diagnosis of acute appendicitis, laboratory tests are of little value. Up to one third of patients, particularly older patients,[14] will have a normal total leukocyte count with acute appendicitis.[3,19] Even when the total leukocyte count and the differential white cell count are abnormal, the degree of abnormality does not correlate well with the degree of appendiceal inflammation. Even when the total white cell count is normal, the differential white cell count often reveals a shift to the left with an increase in the percentage of polymorphonuclear neutrophils.[3] Less than 4% of patients will have both a normal total white cell count and a normal differential count. The most important fact to remember when considering the diagnosis of appendicitis is that the clinical findings take precedence over the white cell count when they are at variance.

Urinalysis is helpful in the differential diagnosis of patients with lower abdominal pain only when it reveals significant numbers of red cells, white cells, or bacteria. Minimal numbers of red cells, white cells, and bacteria are seen in normal patients as well as in patients with appendicitis.

Patients with advanced appendicitis and abscess formation or generalized peritonitis may have abnormalities in liver function tests that mimic obstructive jaundice, biliary stasis, or other primary liver problems.

X-Ray Examination

With rare exceptions, roentgenologic examination of the abdomen is of little help in the differential diagnosis of acute appendicitis. The exceptions are when a fecalith is demonstrated and when other diagnoses—such as acute cholecystitis, perforating duodenal ulcer, perforating colon cancer, acute diverticulitis, and pyelonephritis—are being excluded.

It is not unusual to see cecal distention or a sentinel loop of distended small intestine in the right lower quadrant in appendicitis. In late appendicitis with perforation and abscess formation, a mass can often be demonstrated that is extrinsic to the cecum. There may be scoliosis to the right, lack of the right psoas shadow, lack of small bowel gas in the right lower quadrant with abundant gas elsewhere in the small bowel, and signs of edema of the abdominal wall. With late appendicitis and generalized peritonitis, there will be an ileus pattern with generalized gas throughout the small and large intestine.

Barium enema examination, although not indicated in cases in which the diagnosis of acute appendicitis is evident on clinical grounds, can be helpful in some situations.[15,24] It can be helpful in young women in whom the diagnosis is still in question after hours of observation; lack of findings on laparotomy is high in this patient population. Also, barium enema studies are useful in patients with a debilitating systemic disease, such as leukemia, in whom the operative risk is markedly increased. The findings of significance on barium enema include lack of filling or partial filling of the appendix and an extrinsic pressure defect on the cecum (the "reverse 3" sign).[15,28]

As demonstrated in many studies, an experienced radiologist is able to diagnose acute appendicitis using ultrasonography with an accuracy of greater than 90%.[12,25,27] Appendicitis is diagnosed if the maximal cross-sectional diameter of appendix exceeds 6 mm, if it is noncompressible, if an appendolith is present, or if a complex mass is demonstrated. There are other criteria that are not universally agreed upon, such as rigidity and nonmobility, and further studies are necessary to identify the most appropriate criteria for the ultrasound diagnosis of acute appendicitis. Nonvisualization of the appendix is not a criterion for appendicitis. Ultrasonography can also be helpful in the diagnosis of perforated appendicitis with abscess formation.

Although more expensive, computed tomography (CT) has also been demonstrated to be of benefit in the diagnosis of acute appendicitis and has an accuracy of greater than 90%.[2,20] The cost can be reduced with no significant loss in diagnostic accuracy by performing a limited, unenhanced CT.[20] Appendicitis is diagnosed when the appendix is thickened with a diameter greater than 6 mm and there are inflammatory changes in the periappendiceal fat (streaking and poorly defined increased attenuation).[2,20,26] The presence of pericecal inflammation without the presence of an inflamed appendix or an appendolith without the presence of periappendiceal inflammation are both insufficient to diagnose acute appendicitis. As with ultrasonography, the specific criteria for the CT diagnosis of acute appendicitis are not universally agreed upon and further prospective studies are necessary to identify the most appropriate criteria.

Acute Appendicitis in Infants and Young Children

The diagnosis of acute appendicitis is difficult in infants and young children for many reasons. The patient is unable to give an accurate history, and although appendicitis is infrequent, acute nonspecific abdominal pain is common in infants and children. Because of such factors, the diagnosis and treatment are often delayed, and complications develop.[29]

The clinical presentation of appendicitis in children can be very similar to nonspecific gastroenteritis; thus, the suspicion of appendicitis often is not aroused until the appendix has ruptured and the child is obviously ill.[10] Two thirds of young children with appendicitis have had symptoms for more than 3 days prior to appendectomy.[29] Because children often cannot give an accurate history of their pain, the physical examination and other aspects of the history must be relied on to make the diagnosis. Vomiting, fever, irritability, flexing of the thighs, and diarrhea are likely early complaints. Abdominal distention is the most consistent physical finding. As in adults, the total leukocyte count is not a reliable test.

The incidence of perforation in infants less than 1 year of age is almost 100%, and although it decreases with age, it is still 50% at 5 years of age. The mortality rate in this age group remains as high as 5%. In one series, nearly 40% of children with complicated appendicitis had been seen previously by a physician who failed to make the diagnosis of appendicitis.[29]

Appendicitis in Young Women

Although the overall incidence of negative laparotomy in patients suspected of having appendicitis is as high as 20%, the incidence in women less than 30 years of age is as high as 45%. Pain associated with ovulation; diseases of the ovaries, fallopian tubes, and uterus; and urinary tract infections (cystitis) account for the majority of the misdiagnoses. If a young woman has atypical pain; no muscular guarding in the right lower quadrant; and no fever, leukocystosis, or leftward shift in the differential white cell count, it is best to observe the patient with frequent re-examinations. If after several hours the patient's signs and symptoms remain stable, it is appropriate to perform a barium enema examination.

Appendicitis During Pregnancy

The risk of appendicitis during pregnancy is the same as it is in nonpregnant women of the same age; the incidence is 1 in 2,000 pregnancies. Appendicitis occurs more frequently during the first two trimesters, and during this time period the symptoms of appendicitis are similar to those seen in nonpregnant women.[9] Surgery should be performed during pregnancy when appendicitis is suspected, just as it would be in a nonpregnant woman. As in the nonpregnant patient, the effects of a laparotomy that produces no findings are minor, whereas the effects of a ruptured appendicitis can be catastrophic.

During the third trimester of pregnancy, the cecum and appendix are displaced laterally and are rotated by the enlarged uterus. This results in localization of pain either more cephalad or laterally in the flank, leading to delay in diagnosis and an increased incidence of perforation. Factors such as displacement of the omentum by the uterus also impair localization of the inflamed appendix and result in diffuse peritonitis. In cases of uncomplicated appendicitis, the prognosis for the infant following appendectomy is directly related to the infant's birth weight. If peritonitis and sepsis ensue, infant mortality increases because of prematurity and the effects of sepsis.

Acute appendicitis can be confused with pyelitis and torsion of an ovarian cyst. However, it must be remembered that mortality from appendicitis during pregnancy is mainly caused by a delay in diagnosis. In the final analysis, early appendectomy is the appropriate therapy in suspected appendicitis during all stages of pregnancy.[9]

Appendicitis in the Elderly Population

Appendicitis has a much greater mortality rate among elderly persons when compared with young adults. The increased risk of mortality appears to result from both delay in seeking medical care and delay in making the diagnosis.[22,30] The presence of other diseases associated with aging contributes to mortality, but the major reason for the increased mortality of appendicitis in the aged is delay in treatment. Classic symptoms are present in elderly persons but are often less pronounced. Right lower quadrant pain localizes later and may be milder in elderly persons. On initial physical examination, the findings are often minimal, although right lower quadrant tenderness will eventually be present in most patients.[6] Distention of the abdomen and a clinical picture suggesting small bowel obstruction are commonly seen.

More than 30% of elderly patients will have a ruptured appendix at the time of operation.[6] Although other factors play a role, delay in seeking care and in making the diagnosis are the major reasons for perforation. It is imperative, therefore, that once the diagnosis of acute appendicitis is made, an urgent operation must be advised.

Differential Diagnosis

The differential diagnosis of abdominal pain is one of the most stimulating exercises in clinical medicine. When the classic symptoms of appendicitis are present, the diagnosis of appendicitis is usually easily made and is seldom missed. When the diagnosis is not obvious, knowledge of the differential diagnosis becomes very important. Most of the entities in the differential diagnosis of appendicitis also require operative therapy or are usually not made worse by an exploratory laparotomy. Therefore, it is essential that one eliminate those diseases that do not require operative therapy and can

be made worse by operation; for example, pancreatitis, myocardial infarction, and basilar pneumonia.

The diseases in young children that are most frequently mistaken for acute appendicitis are gastroenteritis, mesenteric lymphadenitis, Meckel's diverticulum, pyelitis, small-intestinal intussusception, enteric duplication, and basilar pneumonia. In mesenteric lymphadenitis, an upper respiratory infection is often present or has recently subsided. Acute gastroenteritis is usually associated with crampy abdominal pain and watery diarrhea. Intestinal intussusception occurs most frequently in children younger than the age of 2 years, an age at which appendicitis is uncommon. With intussusception, a sausage-shaped mass is frequently palpable in the right lower quadrant. The preferred diagnostic procedure is a gentle barium enema, which, in addition to making the diagnosis, will usually reduce the intussusception.

In teenagers and young adults, the differential diagnosis is different in men and women. In young women, the differential diagnosis includes diseases of the ovaries and fallopian tubes, including ruptured ectopic pregnancy, mittelschmerz, endometriosis, and salpingitis.[4] Chronic constipation also needs to be considered in young women. The symptoms that accompany the acute onset of regional enteritis can mimic acute appendicitis, but a history of cramps and diarrhea, and the lack of an appropriate history for appendicitis, are hints that the diagnosis is regional enteritis.

In young men, the potential list of differential diagnoses is smaller and includes the acute onset of regional enteritis, right-sided renal or ureteral calculus, torsion of the testes, and acute epididymitis.

In older patients, the differential diagnosis of acute appendicitis includes diverticulitis, a perforated peptic ulcer, acute cholecystitis, acute pancreatitis, intestinal obstruction, perforated cecal carcinoma, mesenteric vascular occlusion, rupturing aortic aneurysm, and the disease entities already mentioned for young adults.

Treatment

PREOPERATIVE PREPARATION. It is not necessary to rush a patient with a presumed diagnosis of acute appendicitis directly to the operating room. All patients, especially those with a presumed diagnosis of peritonitis, should be adequately prepared before being taken to the operating room. It should be remembered that selected patients with a palpable right lower quadrant mass may be initially managed without operation.[13]

Intravenous fluid replacement should be initiated and the patient resuscitated as rapidly as possible, especially when peritonitis is suspected. Once the patient has a good urinary output, it can be assumed that resuscitation is complete. Nasogastric suction is especially helpful in patients with peritonitis and profound ileus. If the patient's body temperature is higher than 39° C, appropriate measures should be taken to reduce fever prior to beginning an operation.

A broad-spectrum antibiotic, such as cefoxitin, should be administered preoperatively to help control sepsis and to reduce the incidence of postoperative wound infections. If, at the time of operation, the patient has early appendicitis, antibiotic administration can be stopped after one postoperative dose. Antibiotics should be continued as clinically indicated in patients who have gangrenous or ruptured appendicitis with localized or generalized peritonitis.

EXAMINATION UNDER ANESTHESIA. After the induction of anesthesia, the patient's abdomen should be systematically palpated. Such an examination may, on occasion, demonstrate another pathologic condition to be the cause of the patient's symptoms, such as acute cholecystitis. It also may be possible to palpate an appendiceal mass that will confirm the suspected diagnosis.

UNCOMPLICATED APPENDICITIS WITHOUT A PALPABLE MASS. In this circumstance, when the diagnosis of acute appendicitis has been made and there is no reason to suspect that the appendix has ruptured, an appendectomy should be performed. The earlier the diagnosis is made and the sooner the appendectomy is performed, the better the prognosis. As stated earlier, if there is any doubt about whether the appendix has ruptured, the operation should be performed at once, because the morbidity of a perforated appendix is greater than that of an uncomplicated appendectomy. The latter procedure should have a surgical mortality rate of less than 0.1%. In contrast, the mortality rate of a ruptured appendix can be as high as 10%.

The recommended incision for a routine appendectomy is a transverse incision (Rockey-Davis incision, Fowler-Weir-Mitchell incision). The incision is made in a transverse direction, 1 to 3 cm below the umbilicus, and is centered on the midclavicular line. The length of the incision should be approximately 1 cm longer than the breadth of the surgeon's hand. The aponeurosis and muscles of the abdominal wall are split or incised in the direction of the incision (Fig. 12–1). Exposure of the appendix through this incision is much better when compared with that obtained through the classic McBurney incision, particularly in patients with a retrocecal appendix and in those who are obese.

As an alternative, the gridiron, or muscle-splitting incision (McBurney incision) can be used. This is the most widely used incision in uncomplicated appendicitis, largely reflecting surgical tradition rather than utility. The skin incision is made through a point one third of the way along a line from the anterior superior spine of the ileum to the umbilicus. The incision is made obliquely, beginning inferiorly and medially, and extending laterally and superiorly. It should be 8 to 10 cm in length, with its most medial extent being the lateral edge of the rectus muscle. The aponeurosis and muscles of the abdominal wall are split or incised in the direction of their fibers in such a manner that the entire skin incision can be used for exposure. After entering the peritoneum, the appendix is found as described for the transverse incision. The exposure through a McBurney incision, especially for a retrocecal appendix, can be awkward unless the appendix lies immediately below the incision. If necessary, the incision can be extended medially, partially transecting the rectus sheath, but this maneuver is usually helpful only in a pelvic appendicitis.

If there is doubt about the diagnosis of acute appendicitis and an exploratory laparotomy is indicated, a vertical midline incision is appropriate. An appendectomy can be performed with little difficulty through such an incision, and if an appendiceal mass is encountered, the midline incision can be closed and a more direct approach can be made through another incision.

After the peritoneum is opened, the appendix is identified by following the anterior cecal taenia to the base of the appendix. The inflamed appendix is coaxed into the wound by gentle traction and the transection of adhesions, if present. If the appendix is retrocecal or retroperitoneal, or if the local inflammation and edema are intense, exposure is improved by dividing the lateral peritoneal reflection of the cecum. At the end of this maneuver, the cecum should lie within the wound and the appendix should be at the level of the anterior abdominal wall so that continuing vigorous retraction is unnecessary while removing the appendix (Fig. 12–1).

After the cecum has been identified, it is rolled upward into the operative field and the longitudinal taenia followed downward to the base of the appendix. If the appendix is not adherent, its base can be easily identified because the entire appendix often pops into the operative field. If the appendix is adherent, however, its base may be difficult to recognize. Aids in recognition include the following: (1) all three taeniae lead to and end at the base of the appendix and (2) the ileocecal junction can usually be identified, just below which is the base of the appendix. If the appendix does not come into the wound but the base has been identified, an Allis clamp can be placed around but not on the appendix for traction. An effort is made to deliver the tip of the appendix into the operative field. If the appendix is not adherent to surrounding tissues, traction on the Allis clamp is usually successful in delivering the appendix.

Once the appendix has been freed up, the mesoappendix is transected beginning at its free border, taking small bites of the mesoappendix between pairs of hemostats placed approximately 1 cm from and parallel to the appendix. This process should be repeated until the base of the appendix is reached. A suture is passed through the mesoappendix and through the wall of the cecum close to the base of the appendix in order to secure the intramural accessory branch of the posterior cecal artery. If exposure of a long, adherent appendix is difficult, the mesoappendix can be transected in a retrograde manner beginning at the base of the appendix.

There are three ways to handle the appendiceal stump: simple ligation, inversion, and a combination of ligation and inversion. Either simple ligation or inversion are acceptable and have a comparable incidence of complications. The combination of ligation and inversion is not recommended, since it does not reduce the risk of septic complications,[16] but it does create conditions conducive to the development of an intramural abscess or mucocele. Also, the ligated and inverted appendiceal stump may later appear on a subsequent barium enema as a cecal "tumor" and be a source of diagnostic difficulties.[21]

Simple ligature of the appendiceal stump is accomplished by crushing the appendix at its base with a hemostat, then moving the hemostat and replacing it on

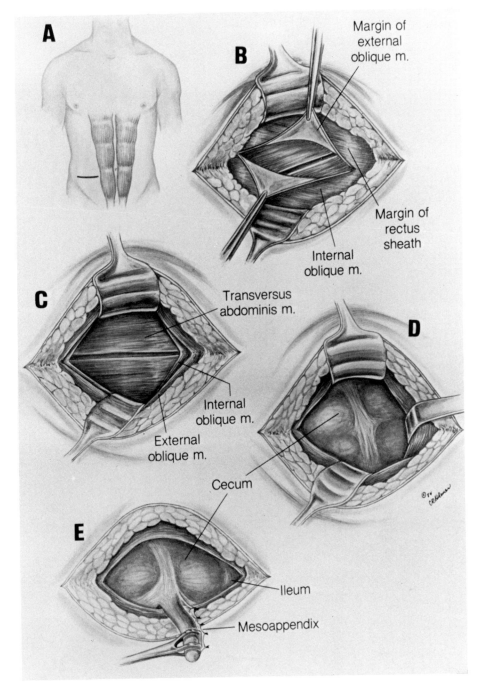

FIGURE 12-1. Steps in performing an appendectomy through a transverse incision. *A,* Placement of the skin incision. *B* and *C,* External and internal oblique and transversus abdominis muscles are divided in the direction of their fibers. *D,* After incising the peritoneum, the cecum is exposed and the appendix is located by following the anterior cecal taenia inferiorly. *E,* The cecum is mobilized into the wound by incising its lateral peritoneal reflections. (Reproduced with permission from Moody, F.G., Carey, L., Jones, R.S., et al.: Surgical Treatment of Digestive Diseases. Copyright © 1986, Year Book Medical Publishers, Chicago.)

the appendix just distal to the crushed line. A ligature of monofilament suture is placed in the groove caused by the crushing clamp and is tied tightly (Fig. 12–2). The appendix is transected just proximal to the hemostat and removed. Inversion of an unligated stump using a Z stitch (Fig. 12–3), rather than the more conventional pursestring suture, is preferred. The upper level of the Z stitch is placed as a Lembert suture in the cecum, just distal to the base of the appendix. The suture is then brought around the base of the appendix and continued as a second Lembert suture beneath the base of the appendix. The appendix is then transected between clamps, the stump is inverted into the cecum, the proximal clamp is removed, and the ends of the Z stitch

are tied over the stump of the appendix. The appendiceal stump is not ligated. If the appendiceal stump is unsuitable for inversion because of edema, it should simply be ligated and not inverted.

LAPAROSCOPIC APPENDECTOMY. Laparoscopy is rapidly gaining acceptance in the diagnosis and treatment of acute appendicitis (see Chapter 14). If uncomplicated appendicitis is encountered at the time of laparoscopy, an appendectomy can be performed with relative ease. If a normal appendix is encountered, the abdomen can easily be examined with the laparoscope, thus avoiding a large abdominal incision. Details of the technique are presented in the chapter on laparoscopic techniques.

PERFORATED OR GANGRENOUS APPENDICITIS WITH A PERIAPPEN-

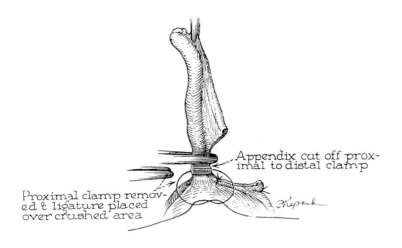

Appendix cut off prox-
imal to distal clamp

Proximal clamp remov-
ed & ligature placed
over crushed area

FIGURE 12-2. Ligation of the stump of the appendix in the groove formed by a crushing clamp. (From Partipilo, A.V.: Surgical Technique and Principles of Operative Surgery, 4th ed. Philadelphia, Lea & Febiger, 1949, with permission.)

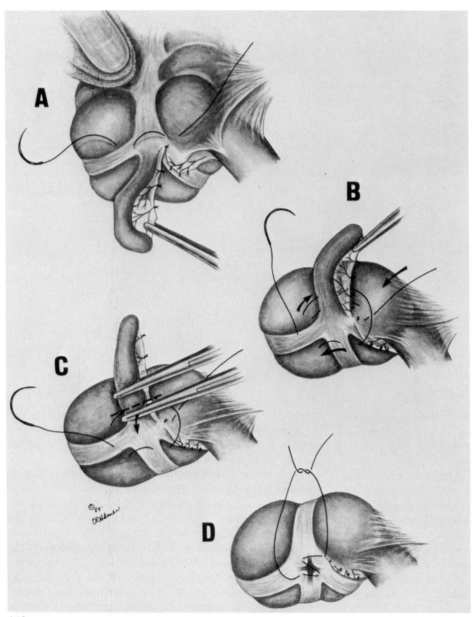

FIGURE 12-3. Use of a Z stitch to invert the unligated appendiceal stump. *A,* Two bites of the suture are placed in the cecum 1 cm distal to the base of the appendix. *B,* The suture is then brought around the appendix medially and two additional bites are placed beneath the base of the appendix. *C,* The appendix is then transected. *D,* The stump of the appendix is inverted into the cecum and the clamp is removed as the suture is tightened. (From Adams, J.T.: Z-Stitch suture for inversion of the appendiceal stump. Surg. Gynecol. Obstet., *127:*1321, 1968, with permission.)

DICEAL MASS. When a mass is detected by examination under anesthesia, a transverse incision is made over the most prominent portion of the mass. The muscles and aponeuroses are split along their lines of cleavage in gridiron fashion. After entering the peritoneal cavity, the wound should be packed immediately to prevent contamination of the abdominal cavity. Any fluid or pus is aspirated, and a specimen is sent for culture and sensitivity studies. As mentioned earlier, the mass may be made up of omentum and loops of small intestine adherent to the inflamed appendix, and an abscess may not be present. If feasible, an appendectomy is then performed; usually it will not be possible to invert the stump, so simple ligation is preferred.

It is not necessary to place a subfascial drain in a patient with a gangrenous appendix and minimal or no periappendiceal pus. If there is a periappendiceal abscess and the tissues are fixed so as to create a dead space, the cavity should be drained with one or more closed suction drains brought out through a separate stab incision.

Prior to fascial closure, the right iliac fossa and the wound should be liberally irrigated. Muscles and aponeuroses should be closed with interrupted nonabsorbable sutures. The skin should be left open, to be closed with adhesive paper tapes on the fifth or sixth postoperative day. Parenteral antibiotics should be continued for 5 days after operation or until clinical signs indicate no infection. A rectal examination is performed daily to detect the presence of a pelvic abscess.

PERFORATED APPENDICITIS WITH LOCALIZED ABSCESS FORMATION. If, at the time of initial physical examination, a well-localized periappendiceal mass is found and the patient's symptoms are improving, it is acceptable in healthy adults to initiate parenteral antibiotic treatment and to follow the patient expectantly. This form of therapy is not appropriate in children, pregnant women, or elderly patients. In these groups, an emergency operation is indicated. In two thirds of patients, expectant treatment of an appendiceal mass will succeed, and an interval appendectomy can be performed at a later date. In one third of patients, symptoms will not subside and an emergency operation should be performed.

The skin incision for drainage of a periappendiceal abscess is made just medial to the crest of the ilium at the level of the abscess. Using a muscle-splitting technique, the lateral edge of the peritoneum is exposed and pushed medially so that the abscess is approached from its lateral aspect. Once the abscess is entered, a finger should be used to break up the loculations. If the appendix can be freed up without breaking down adhesions, an appendectomy should be performed. If an appendectomy is not performed, an interval appendectomy should be done 6 to 8 weeks after drainage from the abscess has ceased and the wound has completely healed.

After the wound has been thoroughly irrigated with normal saline, a closed suction drain should be inserted into the abscess cavity and brought out through a separate stab wound in the flank. The muscles and aponeuroses are closed with interrupted nonabsorbable sutures, and the skin and subcutaneous tissues are packed open with saline-soaked gauze. The drain should be left in place until it is draining less than 50 ml/day and then advanced progressively until removed.

Systemic antibiotics should be continued for 5 days postoperatively or until signs of sepsis have cleared. A daily rectal examination should be done to detect pelvic abscess. The patient may be discharged from the hospital when there is no fever 48 hours after the discontinuation of antibiotic therapy.

PERFORATED APPENDICITIS WITH DIFFUSE PERITONITIS. The major cause of mortality from appendicitis is generalized peritonitis. Therefore, immediate exploration is indicated in a patient with a diagnosis of acute appendicitis in whom the physical findings are consistent with diffuse peritonitis. If a perforated appendix and diffuse peritonitis are documented at operation, an appendectomy should be performed and the abdomen thoroughly irrigated. The use of drains in diffuse peritonitis is not recommended unless there are localized abscesses requiring drainage.[11] The wound and postoperative care should be handled as described in a patient with a periappendiceal abscess.

NORMAL APPENDIX WHEN APPENDICITIS IS SUSPECTED. If a patient undergoes exploratory laparotomy (especially through a right lower quadrant incision) for suspected acute appendicitis, and a normal appendix is subsequently found, a careful search for another pathologic condition should be made and an appendectomy performed. The abdomen should not be closed until the cause of the symptoms has been identified and treated or the surgeon is sure that no lesion requiring treatment is present. The normal appendix is removed to obviate diagnostic confusion in the future.

If the history and physical examination were appropriate for the diagnosis of acute appendicitis, it is not an error to perform an exploratory laparotomy and remove what appears to be a normal appendix. A policy of early surgical intervention on the basis of clinical suspicion has been demonstrated overall to reduce both the morbidity and mortality of acute appendicitis.

COMPLICATIONS. Postoperative complications occur in 5% of patients with an unperforated appendix but in more than 30% of patients with a gangrenous or perforated appendix. The most frequent complications after appendectomy are wound infection, intra-abdominal abscess, fecal fistula, pylephlebitis, and intestinal obstruction.

Subcutaneous tissue infection is the most common complication after appendectomy. The organisms most frequently cultured are anaerobic *Bacteroides* species and the aerobes *Klebsiella, Enterobacter,* and *Escherichia coli.*[18] When early signs of wound infection (undue pain and edema) are present, the skin and subcutaneous tissue should be opened. The wound should be packed with saline-soaked gauze and reclosed with Steri-strips in 4 to 5 days.

Pelvic, subphrenic, or other intra-abdominal abscesses occur in up to 20% of patients with a gangrenous or perforated appendicitis. They are accompanied by recurrent fever, malaise, and anorexia of insidious onset. CT scanning is of great help in making the diagnosis of intra-abdominal abscess. When an abscess is diagnosed, it should be drained either operatively or percutaneously.

Some fecal fistulas will close spontaneously, provided that there is no anatomic reason for the fistula remaining open. Those that do not close spontaneously obviously require operation. Pylephlebitis, or portal pyemia, is characterized by jaundice, chills, and high fever. It is a serious illness that frequently leads to multiple liver abscesses. The infecting organism is usually *E. coli*. This complication has become rare with the routine use of antibiotics in complicated appendicitis. Although not frequent, true mechanical bowel obstruction may occur as a complication of acute appendicitis. As with any other mechanical small bowel obstruction, operative therapy is indicated.

CHRONIC AND RECURRENT APPENDICITIS

There are occasional patients who have had one or more attacks of what appears to be acute appendicitis. Between attacks, these patients are free of symptoms and the physical examination is normal. In such patients, if a fecalith is present on abdominal x-ray film, if a barium enema demonstrates no filling of the appendix, or if repeated examinations during an attack provide evidence of recurrent appendicitis, elective appendectomy should be undertaken.[17] To sustain a diagnosis of chronic appendicitis, the resected appendix must demonstrate fibrosis in the appendiceal wall, partial to complete obstruction of the lumen, evidence of old mucosal ulceration and scarring, and infiltration of the wall of the appendix with chronic inflammatory cells.

MUCOCELE

Mucocele of the appendix occurs in benign and malignant forms. In the benign form, there is obstruction of the lumen of the appendix and the accumulation of mucus distal to the obstruction. The classic clinical features of mucocele of the appendix include lower right quadrant discomfort, a palpable mass in the lower right quadrant, and the x-ray findings of a filling defect in the cecum with nonvisualization of the appendix. When this lesion is discovered at the time of exploratory laparotomy for suspected acute appendicitis, a simple appendectomy should be performed.[5]

The malignant variety of mucocele occurs from distention of the lumen of the appendix by the mucus secreted by proliferating tumor cells. The tumor is more properly termed a mucous cystadenocarcinoma of the appendix. If this lesion is suspected, right hemicolectomy should be performed, since appendectomy is not curative in the usual circumstance. When there are numerous peritoneal implants of a mucinous-like substance, a diagnosis of pseudomyxoma peritonei is appropriate. Within these gelatinous masses are nests of tumor cells attached to the peritoneum.

TUMORS OF THE APPENDIX

Neoplasms of the appendix are rare. The two most frequently observed are argentaffinoma, or carcinoid tumor, and adenocarcinoma. The appendix is the most common site of carcinoid tumor, and carcinoid is the most common neoplasm of the appendix. It is found in approximately 0.1% of all surgically removed appendices. Such a tumor can be found incidentally at the time of operation or while performing an exploratory operation for suspected acute appendicitis or for a diagnosis of chronic, recurrent appendicitis. The only setting in which the diagnosis is suspected preoperatively is in the very rare patient with symptoms of the carcinoid syndrome. This syndrome is characterized by flushing, diarrhea, and asthma-like symptoms. If a carcinoid tumor is, without question, localized to the appendix, a simple appendectomy is adequate therapy. If the tumor is greater than 1 cm in diameter or if there is evidence of nodal metastases, a right hemicolectomy is recommended.[8]

Adenocarcinoma of the appendix may appear as either a well-differentiated mucus-producing tumor, referred to as a malignant mucocele, or as a poorly differentiated adenocarcinoma that appears as a solid mass. Both types of adenocarcinoma of the appendix have been reported to metastasize to regional lymph nodes, although malignant mucocele has been considered clinically to be less virulent. If an adenocarcinoma of the appendix is confined to the mucosa (carcinoma in situ), there is no difference in survival between simple appendectomy and appendectomy combined with right hemicolectomy. If the tumor is invasive, however, the prognosis is improved by right hemicolectomy, so the more extensive operation is recommended for most cases.[1]

REFERENCES

1. Andersson, A., Bergdahl, L., and Boquist, L.: Primary carcinoma of the appendix. Ann. Surg., *183*:53, 1976.
2. Balthazar, E.J., Megiban, A.J., Siegel, S.E., and Birnbaum, B.A.: Appendicitis: Prospective evaluation with high-resolution CT. Radiology, *180*:21, 1991.
3. Bolton, J.P., Craven, E.R., Croft, R.J., and Menzies-Gow, N.: An assessment of the value of the white cell count in the management of suspected acute appendicitis. Br. J. Surg., *62*:906, 1975.
4. Bongard, F., Landers, D.V., and Lewis, F.: Differential diagnosis of appendicitis and pelvic inflammatory disease. A prospective analysis. Am. J. Surg., *150*:90, 1985.
5. Broders, C.W., and Miranda, R.: Mucocele of the appendix: Review of eleven cases and report of two cases. Am. Surg., *37*:434, 1971.
6. Burns, R.P., Cochran, J.L., Russell, W.L., and Bard, R.M.: Appendicitis in mature patients. Ann. Surg., *201*:695, 1985.
7. Dennis, C.: Physiologic behavior of the human appendix and the problem of appendicitis: Reaction of the appendix to drugs. Arch. Surg., *43*:1021, 1941.
8. Dent, T.L., Batsakis, J.G., and Lindenauer, S.M.: Carcinoid tumors of the appendix. Surgery, *73*:828, 1973.
9. Gomez, A., and Wood, M.: Acute appendicitis during pregnancy. Am. J. Surg., *137*:180, 1979.
10. Graham, J.M., Pokorny, W.J., and Harberg, F.J.: Acute appendicitis in preschool age children. Am. J. Surg., *139*:247, 1980.
11. Haller, J.A., Shaker, I.J., Donahoo, J.S., et al.: Peritoneal drainage versus non-drainage for generalized peritonitis from ruptured appendicitis in children. Ann. Surg., *177*:595, 1973.
12. Hayden, C.K., Kuchelmeister, J., and Lipscomb, T.S.: Sonography of acute appendicitis in childhood: Perforation versus nonperforation. J. Ultrasound Med., *11*:209, 1992.
13. Hoffman, J., Lindhard, A., and Jensen, H-E.: Appendix mass: Conservative management without interval appendectomy. Am. J. Surg., *148*:379, 1984.

14. Hubbell, D.S., Barton, W.K., and Soloman, O.D.: Leukocytosis in appendicitis in older patients. JAMA, *175*:139, 1961.
15. Jona, J.Z., Belin, R.P., and Selke, A.C.: Barium enema as a diagnostic aid in children with abdominal pain. Surg. Gynecol. Obstet., *144*:351, 1977.
16. Kingsley, D.P.E.: Some observations on appendectomy with particular reference to technique. Br. J. Surg., *56*:491, 1969.
17. Lee, A.W., Bell, R.M., Griffen, W.O., and Hagihara, P.F.: Recurrent appendiceal colic. Surg. Gynecol. Obstet., *161*:21, 1985.
18. Leigh, D.A., Simmons, K., and Norman, E.: Bacteria flora of the appendix fossa in appendicitis and postoperative wound infection. J. Clin. Pathol., *27*:997, 1974.
19. Lewis, F.R., Holcroft, J.W., Boey, J., and Dunphy, J.E.: Appendicitis: A critical review of diagnosis and treatment in 1,000 cases. Arch. Surg., *110*:677, 1975.
20. Malone, A.J., Wolf, C.R., Malmed, A.S., and Melliere, B.F.: Diagnosis of acute appendicitis: Value of unenhanced CT. Am. J. Radiol., *160*:763, 1993.
21. Myllariemi, H., Perttala, Y., and Peltokallio, P.: Tumor-like lesions of the cecum following inversion of the appendix. Dig. Dis., *19*:547, 1974.
22. Owens, B.J., III, and Hamit, H.F.: Appendicitis in the elderly. Ann. Surg., *187*:392, 1978.
23. Pieper, R., Kager, L., and Nasman, P.: Acute appendicitis: A clinical study of 1018 cases of emergency appendectomy. Acta. Chir. Scand., *148*:51, 1982.
24. Rajagopalan, A.E., Mason, J.H., Kennedy, M., and Pawlikowski, J.: The value of the barium enema in the diagnosis of acute appendicitis. Arch. Surg., *112*:531, 1977.
25. Rioux, M.: Sonographic detection of the normal and abnormal appendix. Am. J. Radiol., *158*:773, 1992.
26. Shapiro, M.P., Gale, M.E., and Gerzof, S.G.: CT of appendicitis: Diagnosis and treatment. Radiol. Clin. North Am., *27*:753, 1989.
27. Sivit, C.J., Newman, K.D., Boenning, D.A., et al.: Appendicitis: Usefulness of US in diagnosis in a pediatric population. Radiology, *185*:549, 1992.
28. Smith, D.E., Kirchmer, N.A., and Stewart, D.R.: Use of the barium enema in the diagnosis of acute appendicitis and its complications. Am. J. Surg., *138*:829, 1979.
29. Stone, H.H., Sanders, S.L., and Martin, J.D.: Perforated appendicitis in children. Surgery, *69*:673, 1971.
30. Thorbjarnarson, B., and Loehr, W.J.: Acute appendicitis in patients over the age of sixty. Surg. Gynecol. Obstet., *125*:1277, 1967.
31. Wangensteen, O.H., and Dennis, C.: Experimental proof of obstructive origin of appendicitis in man. Ann. Surg., *110*:629, 1939.

Chapter 13

ANTIBIOTICS IN COLON SURGERY

RONALD LEE NICHOLS / JAMES WM.C. HOLMES

We collectively reviewed many of the important historical aspects of preoperative bowel preparation over 20 years ago.[75] It was apparent at that time that surgeons knew that the colon contained a luxuriant aerobic bacterial flora that was excluded from the rest of the body by the normal mucous membrane barrier. If this barrier was disturbed by disease or trauma or if the colon was opened to the peritoneal cavity, bacteria escaped and invaded adjacent tissues, often producing serious infection. Since the colonic lumen must be opened during many operations and since such operations are associated with some infectious morbidity, a reliable method of sterilizing colonic content has been the objective of surgeons throughout this century. During the last 20 years, great advances have been made in preoperative intestinal antisepsis due primarily to the fact that the bacteriologic techniques developed allowed for the isolation of the predominant anaerobic microflora, including *Bacteroides fragilis*. This in turn resulted in major modifications of our approaches to preoperative colon preparation and a much-improved reduction of postoperative infections.

HISTORICAL REVIEW

Early attempts at intestinal antisepsis made use of charcoal, chlorine, naphthalene, iodoform, and salicylates.[99] These agents did not reduce the incidence of infection and were often responsible for toxic complications. The introduction of sulfonamides in the late 1930s, however, offered hope for effective preoperative intestinal antisepsis. Garlock and Seley[36] published a preliminary report which revealed that only one wound infection occurred among 21 patients given oral sulfanilamide prior to elective operations of the colon. The authors concluded that preoperative administration of sulfanilamide resulted in a reduction in postoperative morbidity. Unfortunately, a definitive study on this subject was never published by the authors.

During the ensuing 3 decades, numerous clinical studies of various antibiotic preparations used for intestinal antisepsis were reported. Most of these studies were retrospective in nature and inadequately controlled. All of the antibiotic regimens studied were chosen to be effective against the aerobic colonic microflora that was thought at the time to be the major cause of postoperative infections. These reports fueled a debate regarding the value of various schemes of preoperative antibiotic preparation but failed to reach any clear conclusions about the ideal antibiotic regimen or whether the chosen antibiotics were better than mechanical preparation alone.[110]

It is worthwhile to review some of the major studies that investigated mechanical cleansing, oral antibiotics, and the complications of the various colon preparations that resulted in the confusion which existed until the mid 1970s.

Early Attempts at Preoperative Intraluminal Antibiotic Preparation

Most early studies of nonabsorbable oral antibiotics also utilized some form of mechanical cleansing. Antibiotics alone had been noted to have a minimal effect on suppressing the colonic aerobes unless the bulk of fecal material had also been removed.[9] Poth[93] was the first to characterize the ideal oral antiseptic for the intestine as having the properties of broad bacterial spectrum, low toxicity, stability in the presence of digestive enzymes, capacity to prevent development or overgrowth of resistant bacteria, and rapidity of action. Other important characteristics mentioned were limited absorption, activity in the presence of food (thereby permitting continued dietary intake in the preoperative period), capacity to aid in mechanical cleansing of the intestine without inducing dehydration, lack of tendency to irritate the gastrointestinal mucosa, and lack of interference with normal tissue growth and repair. Qualities such as low dosage requirement, solubility in water, palatability, inhibition of excessive fungal growth, and administration restricted to use only as an intestinal antiseptic were also included.

Cohn[16] later indicated that it would be difficult for

any single agent to fulfill these formidable characteristics. He stressed that the three major requirements for an effective intestinal antiseptic were rapid, highly bactericidal activity against pathogenic organisms in the gastrointestinal tract; ability to prevent development or overgrowth of pathogenic organisms; and low toxicity, local as well as systemic, together with limited absorption from the intestine. He also reported on the efficacy of 48 different intestinal regimens, given usually for 72 hours, on suppressing the human aerobic and anaerobic colonic microfloras.[16] Once again, it should be noted that before the acceptance in the mid 1970s of *Bacteroides fragilis* as the predominant fecal constituent and frequent cause of postoperative infection after colon surgery, the antibiotic agents chosen as intestinal antiseptics were primarily effective against the aerobic colonic flora.

Sulfonamides

Garlock and Seley,[36] in 1939, administered preoperative doses of sulfanilamide of up to 15 g/day to 21 patients having operations of the colon and rectum. A peculiar cyanosis was common among these patients, but no other toxic manifestations were seen, and the postoperative course was uncomplicated, morbidity was slight (one wound infection), and peritonitis was nonexistent.

This work stimulated the development of other sulfonamide agents that exhibited less systemic absorption and toxicity after oral intake and which were thought to have enhanced bacteriostatic activity against fecal microorganisms. Firor and Jonas[32] reported in 1941 on the use of sulfanilylguanidine in 12 patients. Although their initial clinical experience was favorable, further studies done the same year showed that sulfanilylguanidine had an erratic effect on the stool flora and little activity at all in the presence of an ulcerating lesion.[33]

Succinylsulfathiazole (Sulfasuxidine) was introduced in 1942 as an intestinal antiseptic agent by Poth and Knotts.[97] Administered in doses of 3 g every 4 hours for 5 to 10 days, it was found to be associated with low systemic absorption and to decrease markedly the numbers of aerobic coliform organisms in stool.[97,94] Diarrhea, which most frequently accompanied the use of this drug, was thought to be a positive adjunct to mechanical cleansing. The effect of this agent on the anaerobic flora was not studied.

Poth and Ross[98] reported in 1943 on their experience with phthalylsulfathiazole (Sulfathalidine). This agent, administered in a dose of 1.5 g every 4 hours, had twice the bacteriostatic activity of succinylsulfathiazole. If administration was continued for 5 to 10 days, the number of coliforms was reduced in most patients from 10^7 to 10^2 organisms/g of feces. The effect of this drug on fecal bacteria other than coliforms was not investigated. Unlike succinylsulfathiazole, phthalylsulfathiazole caused the stool to become tenacious and stringy, with a tendency for feces to adhere to the intestine mucosa.

The incidence of sensitivity reactions after use of either succinylsulfathiazole or phthalylsulfathiazole was reported to be low. The most frequent side effect was nausea and vomiting. Because of low systemic absorption, crystalluria did not occur unless the urine was unusually acidic.

Despite earlier clinical and experimental reports of the effectiveness of sulfonamides in suppressing the aerobic fecal flora, current studies have indicated that these agents have a variable effect on colon aerobes and are ineffective in controlling the anaerobic bacterial flora of the colon. These findings make the sulfonamide agents unsatisfactory for routine preoperative preparation of the colon.[75]

Tetracyclines

The tetracyclines were the first of the broad-spectrum antibiotics to be used extensively as intestinal antiseptics. Chlortetracycline, introduced in 1948, was noted to be bacteriostatic and absorbed partially from the gastrointestinal tract, and acted systemically as well as locally within the lumen of the intestine.[93,99]

Dearing and Heilman[23] reported that oral administration of chlortetracycline in doses of 250 or 500 mg four times daily was not effective in suppressing the fecal flora. A dose of 750 mg administered four times daily resulted in elimination of most colonic bacteria in 75 or 91 patients; only proteus and pseudomonas persisted. In the remaining 16 patients, *Escherichia coli*, *Aerobacter* (*Enterobacter*) *aerogenes*, or *Streptococcus faecalis* also persisted. After the third day of therapy, an increase in numbers of resistant organisms was noted, and these authors recommended limiting preoperative chlortetracycline preparation to 3 days. Other reports revealed that anaerobes such as *Bacteroides fragilis* were regularly suppressed, but the frequent finding (10%) of diarrhea due usually to *Staphylococcus aureus* greatly inhibited the use of this agent as well as the other tetracyclines from use as bowel antiseptics.[31] It should be noted, however, that formulations of both oral and parenteral tetracyclines have been utilized successfully in later reported clinical studies of preoperative bowel preparation.[80]

In 1974, Washington and colleagues[115] reported a blinded prospective clinical trial comparing mechanical cleansing alone and mechanical cleansing with either oral neomycin alone or a combination of neomycin and tetracycline. The results in 196 patients revealed a high postoperative infection rate in those patients treated with preoperative mechanical cleansing alone (43%) or with mechanical cleansing and oral neomycin alone (41%). A significantly reduced infection rate of 5% was noted in the group of patients receiving both mechanical cleansing and a combination of oral neomycin and tetracycline. The success of this study, in our opinion, was due to the choice of antibiotic agents that suppress both the colonic aerobes and anaerobes, and which were given for a proper time period along with adequate mechanical cleansing.

Aminoglycosides

Streptomycin, in 1945, was the first bactericidal antibiotic recommended for use as an intestinal antiseptic.[117] Inactivation of streptomycin was not noted to occur in the gastrointestinal tract, little was absorbed, and systemic toxicity after oral administration was not observed.[75] A marked and sustained reduction of coliforms, enterococci, and clostridia appeared to occur 24 to 48 hours after oral administration.[75] However, Lockwood and associates[62] reported that bacterial resistance developed rapidly after oral streptomycin therapy, and they cautioned against the use of this agent. Their observation was confirmed by Dearing and Heilman,[23] who found resistant strains of bacteria developing after only 1 day of dihydrostreptomycin therapy. Although streptomycin suppressed growth of the aerobic coliforms, its effectiveness in controlling other major constituents of the stool flora was irregular. In addition, as noted in most studies, the rapid development of resistant bacteria has led to abandonment of oral streptomycin as an intestinal antiseptic.

The next aminoglycoside agent to be studied as an oral intestinal antiseptic was neomycin.[95] Poth and colleagues[96] reported that neomycin, administered 1 g orally every 4 hours for 3 days, was effective in eliminating nearly all easily cultured bacteria from the stool. Dearing and Needham[24] studied 37 patients who received neomycin orally in varying doses for 3 to 7 days. Neomycin effectively eliminated the aerobic bacteria, including *Escherichia coli, Aerobacter aerogenes, Streptococcus faecalis, Proteus* spp., and *Pseudomonas* spp., from the intestinal tract but did not alter appreciably the numbers of anaerobic species such as *Bacteroides* and *Clostridium*. No serious toxic effects of neomycin or emergence of resistant organisms were observed in this study. Mann and associates,[65] Plumley,[89] and Rowlands and Scorer[101] found that a loading dose of neomycin (1 g hourly for four doses) followed by 1 g every 4 hours for the remainder of the preoperative day achieved a better clinical and bacteriologic effect. No resistant organisms were encountered.

Although bacterial resistance to neomycin is a relatively uncommon event, occasional strains of *A. aerogenes* are not inhibited by this drug and may overgrow in large numbers. Poth and associates,[95,96] reported emergence of resistant *A. aerogenes* in approximately 10% of patients receiving neomycin and recommended that this drug not be used alone as an intestinal antiseptic.

In summary, because of its rapid effect when used in preoperative preparation of the colon, neomycin should be given for no more than 24 hours. This drug readily suppresses growth of all colon aerobes but is not effective against the predominant anaerobic flora. Resistant organisms, usually *A. aerogenes*, may appear with prolonged therapy. Because of its failure to control growth of anaerobes, neomycin should not be used as a single agent in regimens of antibiotic preparation of the intestine.

As will be mentioned later in the section dealing with current practices of oral intestinal antisepsis, neomycin is most frequently combined with an oral antianaerobic agent such as erythromycin base, tetracycline, or metronidazole.[80] Historically, the agents most frequently combined with neomycin included phthalylsulfathiazole or bacitracin.[75] This was done to assure good aerobic activity, and the short duration of usage (24 hours) was utilized to prevent resistance.

The last aminoglycoside agent to be recommended for intestinal antisepsis was kanamycin. Cohn reported that 72 hours of oral administration produced significant reduction of all stool bacteria, except bacteroides. Since Cohn thought bacteroides rarely were associated with major surgical infections, he believed that lack of control of bacteroides was not a significant disadvantage to the use of kanamycin as an intestinal antiseptic.[17] Mann[64] also found that bacteroides frequently were unaffected by 72 hours of therapy with kanamycin.

Major Complications of Early Attempts at Antibiotic Preparation of the Colon

The complications that were reported or predicted to follow early attempts at intestinal antisepsis, as well as the failure of early approaches to suppress the complete colonic flora, greatly dulled the luster concerning the use of oral antibiotics in preparation for colon surgery.[75]

Overgrowth of Staphylococci and Yeasts

The long duration of early preoperative antibiotic bowel preparation (≥72 hours) frequently resulted in the overgrowth of resistant micro-organisms that were reported to cause an increased incidence of postoperative diarrhea, enteritis, and postoperative infections.[75] As the duration of antibiotic intake was reduced to 24 hours or less, the associated overgrowth of micro-organisms was essentially eliminated.

Metabolic Effects of Preoperative Preparation of the Colon

Patients receiving preoperative preparation of the colon frequently are malnourished or chronically ill and poorly tolerate additional metabolic insults. Trinkle and associates[109] studied patients during a 5-day preoperative preparation of the intestine that included both mechanical cleansing, such as enemas and cathartics, and administration of neomycin and succinylsulfathiazole. Iatrogenically induced metabolic abnormalities were significant and included negative nitrogen balance; weight loss; decreased serum electrolyte concentrations; a relative excess of total body water; and decreased total body potassium, magnesium, calcium, and phosphorus levels.

Mikal[69] also reported metabolic abnormalities after preparation of the colon which, he believed, were due to decreased caloric intake and gastrointestinal absorption, decreased colonic transit time, and a loss of water and electrolytes as the result of repeated enemas. He recommended that patients undergoing preoperative preparation, particularly those with carcinoma or chronic inflammatory disorders, be given appropriate parenteral fluid and electrolyte replacement during the period of colonic preparation.

The time-honored approach to preoperative colon preparation lasting 5 or more days has been appropriately long abandoned. Modern approaches last less than 24 hours, with both the mechanical and antibiotic parts usually being accomplished in the outpatient setting.

Intestinal Antibiotics and Tumor Implantation

Buinauskas and co-workers[12] emphasized the clinical importance of implantation of tumor cells into the anastomotic suture line in patients undergoing resection of the colon for carcinoma. Although factors such as operative trauma and suture technique were thought to influence the frequency of anastomotic suture line recurrence, the single factor that received widespread attention in the 1950s was the possibility of frequent tumor implantation following antibiotic preparation of the intestine.

This hypothesis was investigated in experimental animals by Vink,[113] who injected a suspension of Brown-Pearce carcinoma cells into the colonic lumen of rabbits. The colon then was transected distal to the point of tumor injection and an anastomosis performed. Suture line tumor implants developed in 12 of 27 (44%) rabbits treated preoperatively with a bowel preparation of sulfonamide and streptomycin. In untreated control rabbits, tumor in the anastomosis developed in only 3 of 23 (12%).

These experiments were repeated with more elegant bacteriologic techniques by Cohn and Atik.[18] Brown-Pearce carcinoma was injected into segments of rabbit colon isolated between noncrushing clamps. The colon then was transected and anastomosed. Suture line implantation of tumor occurred in 18 of 44 control rabbits (40%), in 16 of 30 rabbits (53%) having saline irrigation of the colonic segments, and in 29 of 40 rabbits (72%) having the colon irrigated with neomycin-tetracycline solution. There was no difference between untreated controls and rabbits in which the colon was irrigated with the saline solution, but the increase in tumor implantation in the group treated with antibiotics was significant.

A similar study utilizing both Brown-Pearce carcinoma and V-2 carcinoma was conducted by Herter and his associates.[44] In their experiments, tumor implants in the colonic suture line developed in 10 of 31 animals (32%) receiving neomycin preparation of the colon, as compared with 8 of 39 untreated controls (20%). Similarly, anastomotic implants of tumor developed in 15 of 24 animals (62%) prepared with phthalylsulfathiazole, as compared with 14 of 25 untreated controls (56%). In contrast to earlier studies, these experiments did not demonstrate any significant difference between control animals and animals receiving antibiotic preparation of the intestine. The authors properly pointed out the difficulties of extrapolation of experimental data from tumor systems of animals to a comparable situation in man.

In a retrospective clinical study, Herter and Slanetz[46] reported experiences with 790 patients who underwent various types of resection of the colon for carcinoma. The differences in suture line recurrence of carcinoma between antibiotic-prepared and unprepared patients who underwent intra-abdominal colectomy were slight. However, patients who underwent anterior resection with an extraperitoneal anastomosis demonstrated a 9.5% incidence of suture line recurrence if preoperative antibiotic preparation of the intestine had been carried out, while in patients not receiving antibiotics, a suture line recurrence developed in only 1.6%. The incidence of anastomotic leak after anterior resection was considerably lower in antibiotic-prepared patients and there was no evidence that other variables, such as details of surgical technique, accounted for the observed differences. The authors concluded that effective suppression of colonic bacterial flora appeared to enhance implantation of tumor at suture line. They stated, however:

We are, therefore, faced with the choice of either leaving the bacterial flora undisturbed, thereby lowering the risk of anastomotic implantation but increasing the likelihood of significant infection, or continuing the practice of antibiotic preparation of the intestine but concomitantly adopting specific mechanical and chemical measures to minimize the chances of cell implantation to the suture line.[46]

Since the 1960s, no study has been directed to gain further insight into this subject. Based on the failure of the experimentally employed regimens to suppress the total colonic flora, it is doubtful that the use of intestinal antisepsis had any influence on tumor cell reimplantation.

BACTERIOLOGY OF THE GASTROINTESTINAL TRACT

The human gastrointestinal tract in utero is sterile.[75] Within a few hours of birth, the oral and anal orifices are colonized, and organisms can be cultured from the rectum. The intestinal flora at this time is variable and is derived from the environment of the infant. A few days after birth, a more stable gastrointestinal flora begins to establish itself. The bacteria that colonize the colon at this time depend on whether the newborn infant is formula-fed or breast-fed. The stool of the breast-fed infant is characterized by large concentrations of gram-positive organisms, predominantly *Lactobacillus bifidus*. The stool flora of formula-fed infants is more complex, with a predominance of gram-negative aerobic and anaerobic organisms, and resembles the stool of children eating a mixed diet.

Smith and Crabb[105] studied the stool flora of a variety of newborn animals and human infants. During the early weeks of life the flora was similar in all species, but as the animals grew older, differences developed. Bacteroides and lactobacilli were the most common organisms found in the stool of human infants, and clostridia, coliforms, or streptococci predominated in the feces of lower animals. *Staphylococcus aureus* was never isolated from animals and appeared only in human stool. Because of such differences in fecal flora between animals and man, the results of antibiotic preparation of the colon studies in lower animals must be applied with considerable caution to humans.

During the last 20 years, many thoughtfully designed and scientifically accurate studies have outlined the gastrointestinal flora in both healthy and diseased colons.[81,82] These reports have demonstrated that anaerobic, nonsporulating, gram-negative rods, predominantly *Bacteroides*, are the most prevalent bacteria in the colon. These anaerobic micro-organisms are 1,000 to 100,000 times more numerous than aerobic coliforms. Stool specimens usually contain 10^{10} to 10^{11} anaerobic bacteroides/g, and aerobic coliforms number 10^6 to 10^8 organisms/g. Other major fecal organisms are aerobic lactobacilli, anaerobic lactobacilli or bifidobacilli, and streptococci. The minor bacterial constituents of human stool include proteus, pseudomonas, clostridia, and staphylococci.

Most recently, emphasis has been placed on studying both the luminal and mucosa-associated colonic flora.[61,104] These qualitatively and quantitatively different populations of colonic bacteria appear to have varying degrees of importance concerning bacterial translocation, anastomotic healing, and the development of wound and intra-abdominal infections.

RISK FOR INFECTION IN COLON SURGERY

Many clinical studies of risk factors for infection in specific operative procedures have been published during the 1980s. Knowledge of the presence or absence of these risk factors in the perioperative period may allow for alterations of infection control techniques in the studies conducted during the 1990s.[83]

Kaiser and associates,[55] studying elective colon resection and different approaches to preoperative antibiotic prophylaxis, have shown a direct correlation between the duration of the operation and the postoperative infection rate. In operations lasting less than 3 hours, no infections were identified when the antibiotic prophylaxis was with a parenteral agent alone or a combination of oral and parenteral agents. However, in operations lasting more than 4 hours, a significant reduction of infection was observed in those patients receiving the combination prophylactic regimen. Coppa and Eng[21] in a similar study of elective colon resection have stressed that postoperative wound infections are associated with the length of operation and location of the colonic resection (intraperitoneal colon resection versus rectal resection). These authors showed that the wound infection rate in high-risk patients with long operations (>215 minutes) and rectal resection could significantly benefit from the use of a combination of oral and parenteral prophylactic antibiotics. Whether to primarily repair the injured colon or to do a colostomy has been the subject of a recent prospective study of colonic injuries after penetrating abdominal trauma.[38] The authors, utilizing logistic regression analysis, have identified that transfusion with 4 or more units, more than two associated injuries, significant intraperitoneal contamination, and increasing colon injury severity score significantly correlate with postoperative wound and intra-abdominal infection. The authors concluded that nearly all penetrating colon wounds can be repaired primarily regardless of risk factors. It should be noted that finding a colonic perforation and performance of a colostomy during exploration for penetrating abdominal trauma have been identified to be the prime risk factors for postoperative infections.[78,79]

MECHANICAL PREPARATION BEFORE COLON SURGERY

Historical Aspects

Historically, mechanical preparation by means of purgation, enemas, and dietary restriction was utilized in nearly all patients undergoing elective operations on the colon. Clinical experience long ago demonstrated that mechanical removal of gross feces from the colon was associated with decreased morbidity and mortality in patients undergoing operations on the colon.

Although there was no universally accepted regimen for mechanical preparation of the colon, in most schemes preparation in hospitalized patients with a nonobstructed colon was carried out during a 48- to 72-hour period. It included a low-residue diet for 1 or 2 days and, often, a clear liquid diet on the day immediately preceding operation. Daily use of cathartics and enemas in various combinations were common components. Saline enemas were preferred by some surgeons to reduce the electrolyte loss that accompanies repeated enemas. Altemeier and colleagues[1] recommended that enemas not be given if antibiotics are utilized in preoperative preparation of the intestine due to the possibility of introducing staphylococci or other pathogenic organisms into the colon during the conduct of the enema.

Did mechanical preparation influence the numbers and composition of the colonic flora? What evidence was available? Gliedman and associates[40] studied the effect of saline irrigation on closed loops of canine colon. Saline irrigation resulted in a progressive reduction of total bacterial count that was related linearly to the volume of saline irrigation. Tyson and Spaulding[111] showed that mechanical preparation of the colon decreased the fecal bacterial population from 10^8 or 10^9 to 10^6 or 10^7 organisms/g of stool. This decrease was shown to persist for 12 to 18 hours after completion of the mechanical preparation. Bornside and Cohn,[9] on the other hand, found that 72 hours of mechanical preparation did not result in any decrease in numbers of fecal microorganisms. Our study of 12 patients undergoing a vigorous 72-hour mechanical bowel preparation with dietary restriction, cathartics, and enemas showed a significant reduction only in the mean concentration of coliforms within standardized segments of the colonic lumen and stool.[77] Obligate anaerobes, the major constituents of the colonic microflora, and other aerobic and microaerophilic bacteria were not significantly altered. Our conclusion was that vigorous mechanical cleansing reduces total fecal mass, but that the residual bowel contents harbor microflora, a potential source of wound infection following colonic resections.

Early studies of the efficacy of mechanical cleansing alone compared with mechanical cleansing and preoperative oral antibiotics provided insight into the lack of efficacy of the often-utilized prolonged course of effective antibiotics.[37,43,45,90] Gaylor and co-workers[37] compared patients receiving mechanical preparation alone with patients receiving various antibiotics and mechanical preparation. In those receiving only mechanical preparation, the postoperative infection rate was lower than in patients receiving antibiotics. Coagulase-positive *S. aureus* was recovered from stool during the postoperative period in 30% of patients treated with antibiotics; no staphylococci were recovered from patients receiving only mechanical preparation. Although this study indicated that mechanical preparation without antibiotics might be preferable, it must be pointed out that the antibiotic doses used were lower than were recommended at the time for adequate suppression of fecal flora.

Grand and Barbara[43] reported a lower incidence of wound infections and anastomotic leaks when only preoperative mechanical preparation of the colon was used, as compared with the incidence in patients who also received preoperative antibiotics. Other observers also have reported a lower incidence of infective complications in patients receiving only mechanical preparation.[90]

In a retrospective study of 1,042 patients who underwent colon resection, Herter and Slanetz[45] compared the effects of mechanical preparation alone and in combination with nonabsorbable antibiotics. There was no difference in the incidence of wound infections between the two groups of patients. However, there was a marked increase in the incidence of anastomotic disruption and leakage in patients who underwent anterior resection with only mechanical preparation.

Modern Approaches

The modern approaches to mechanical cleansing still vary considerably.[80] In comparison to 1979, when a survey of surgeons' preferences for preoperative colon preparation indicated that 5 to 16% relied solely on mechanical cleansing,[20] a 1990 survey of active board-certified colorectal surgeons revealed that all who answered the survey (72%) utilized antibiotics in addition to mechanical cleansing.[106]

Modern approaches in the nonobstructive elective procedure fall into two general categories: (1) whole-gut lavage with either an electrolyte solution, 10% mannitol, or polyethylene glycol on the day before operation; and (2) standard mechanical cleansing that utilizes dietary resection, cathartics, and enemas for a 2-day period. In most patients, the majority of the preparation is accomplished on an outpatient basis.[35] Our approach to the two alternative techniques of mechanical cleansing as well as antibiotic coverage is offered in Table 13–1.

The choice of mechanical cleansing technique depends primarily on the surgeon's preference. Traditional bowel preparation including dietary restriction, cathartics, and enemas, if carried out for an unnecessarily long period of time (3 to 5 days), will be associated with less patient acceptability, greater patient fatigue, and other related complications than other cleansing techniques. Similarly, whole-gut irrigation techniques previously recommended using large amounts of fluid (10 to 15 L) should be discouraged. The use of mannitol in varying concentrations has been recommended in lavage solutions.[50] Other studies[7,8] have warned about the possibility of developing clinical dehydration when 15% mannitol is used and also of colonic explosions with the use of electrocautery when mannitol was used without oral antibiotics. The use of polyethylene glycol–electrolyte lavage solutions appears today to be the preferred cleansing method before elective colorectal surgery.[8,34]

In patients presenting with partially obstructing lesions of the large bowel, surgery is more often urgent than elective. These individuals often will not tolerate a rapid mechanical preoperative bowel preparation as shown in Table 13–1 due to the potential of impacting stool proximal to the obstructing lesion and thereby converting a partial to a complete obstruction. Fortunately, these patients will most often tolerate decelerated mechanical bowel preparation. Such a partially obstructed patient who is stable and in good clinical condition is admitted to the hospital while undergoing preoperative bowel preparation. Resuscitation with parenteral fluids and their continuation at maintenance rate is usually necessary, although many patients will tolerate clear liquids by mouth. Fleets phosphosoda is also given orally in 10-ml aliquots at hourly intervals for 6 doses on day 2 preoperatively and is repeated starting at 6 A.M. on the preoperative day. If the patient develops worsening abdominal distention or signs of complete obstruction, the oral mechanism bowel preparation is stopped and the patient is prepared for urgent surgery using an appropriate perioperative parenteral antimicrobial agent or agents. In the patient who tolerates the decelerated mechanical bowel preparation, oral preoperative antibiotic prophylaxis is given and surgery is done the following morning utilizing additional perioperative parenteral antibiotic coverage (Table 13–2).

Emergency situations often require immediate surgical intervention, precluding preoperative mechanical and oral antibiotic bowel preparation. In selected patients with limited intra-abdominal disease and without

---

TABLE 13-1. SUGGESTED APPROACH TO PREOPERATIVE PREPARATION FOR ELECTIVE COLON RESECTION

2 DAYS BEFORE SURGERY (At home)
Dietary restriction: low residue or liquid diet.
Magnesium sulfate, 30 ml of 50% solution (15 g) p.o. at 10 A.M., 2 P.M., and 6 P.M.
Fleet enemas until diarrhea effluent clear in the evening.

DAY BEFORE SURGERY (At home or in hospital if necessary)
Admit in morning (if necessary).
Clear liquid diet, IV fluids as needed.
Magnesium sulfate, in dosage given above, at 10 A.M. and 2 P.M.
or
Whole-gut lavage with Golytely (1 L/hr for 2–3 hr until diarrhea effluent clear) before administration of oral antibiotic, starting at 9 A.M. and ending at the latest at noon.
No enemas.
All patients receive neomycin–erythromycin base, 1 g each p.o. at 1 P.M., 2 P.M., and 11 P.M.

DAY OF SURGERY
Operation at 8 A.M.
A single dose of antibiotic with broad-spectrum aerobic/anaerobic activity given IV by anesthesia personnel in the operating room just before incision. Repeat dosage if operation lasts over 2 hours.

IV = intravenous.

TABLE 13-2. SELECTED SINGLE AND COMBINATION PARENTERALLY ADMINISTERED ANTIBIOTIC AGENTS THAT COVER FACULTATIVE/ANAEROBIC COLONIC MICROFLORA

FACULTATIVE COVERAGE (To be combined with a drug having anaerobic activity)

Amikacin
Aztreonam
Cefotaxime
Ceftriaxone
Ciprofloxacin
Gentamicin
Tobramycin

ANAEROBIC COVERAGE (To be combined with a drug having facultative activity)

Chloramphenicol
Clindamycin
Metronidazole

FACULTATIVE—ANAEROBIC COVERAGE—SINGLE AGENTS

Ampicillin (sulbactam)
Cefotetan
Cefoxitin
Ceftizoxime
Imipenem (cilastatin)
Piperacillin (tazobactam)
Ticarcillin (clavulanic acid)

peritonitis or free pus, resection of the diseased segment of large bowel with primary anastomosis is possible. This is routinely done without the benefit of preoperative mechanical bowel preparation in patients with lesions of the right colon. Under identical clinical settings, emergency surgery for distal colonic lesions presents a greater challenge. Intraoperative antegrade colonic lavage following resection of the diseased distal segment of colon or rectum will facilitate primary anastomosis in many cases. Although this technique has a place in the surgeon's armamentarium, it is not recommended for the surgeon operating alone; it is most often useful

when adequate assistance is available allowing a group effort to prevent loss of control of either the proximal or distal ends of the lavage circuit, which would result in gross fecal contamination of the abdominal cavity with disastrous results in the postoperative course of the patient.[70,71] Perioperative coverage with parenteral antibiotic agents with aerobic and anaerobic activity are indicated in these emergency procedures (Table 13–2).

It should be emphasized that all modern prospective clinical studies utilizing appropriate orally or parenterally administered antibiotics have shown a benefit over mechanical cleansing alone (Table 13–3). The use of placebo-controlled studies in clinical trials of antibiotic prophylaxis in colon surgery has been abandoned since the early 1980s.[6]

CURRENT ALTERNATIVES OF ANTIBIOTIC PREPARATION BEFORE COLON SURGERY

The use of antibiotics in addition to mechanical cleansing is currently the standard of care before colon surgery.[42] It is also generally agreed that the antibiotics chosen for usage should be able to suppress both the colonic aerobes and anaerobes.[42,80,106] However, some disagreement continues concerning which route of administration is preferred.[15,55,76] Advocates of oral administration typically emphasize the importance of reducing the number of micro-organisms in the colonic lumen before opening the colon, while those who advocate parenteral administration emphasize the importance of adequate tissue levels of antibiotic. It appears today that the great majority of surgeons prefer to use a combination of both oral and parenteral antibiotic agents before elective colon resection.[86,106]

Oral Antibiotic Usage

As reviewed in our previous section dealing with historical aspects of antibiotic intestinal antisepsis, early

TABLE 13-3. PROSPECTIVE CLINICAL TRIALS COMPARING THE USE OF MECHANICAL CLEANSING ALONE WITH MECHANICAL CLEANSING AND ANTIBIOTICS IN ELECTIVE COLON RESECTION

Year	No. of Patients	Antibiotic	Route	INFECTION RATE (%) Mechanical Cleansing Alone	INFECTION RATE (%) Mechanical Cleansing and Antibiotics
1973[27]	87	Cephaloridine	Parenteral	44	34*
1973[73]	20	Neomycin-erythromycin	Oral	30	0*
1974[115]	196	Neomycin	Oral	43	41*
		Neomycin-tetracycline	Oral	43	5†
1975[14]	80	Gentamicin	Parenteral	31	34*
1975[41]	50	Kanamycin-metronidazole	Oral	44	8†
1976[11]	67	Cephalothin	Parenteral	27	24*
1977[58]	87	Cephalothin	Parenteral	59	17†
1977[13]	75	Cephalothin	Parenteral	21	19*
1977[15]	116	Neomycin-erythromycin	Oral	43	9†
1978[47]	118	Doxycycline	Parenteral	42	9†
1978[39]	71	Kanamycin-metronidazole	Oral	46	12†
1978[66]	110	Neomycin-metronidazole	Oral	42	18†
1979[28]	83	Metronidazole	Parenteral	77	34†

*Not significant.
†Significant at $P < .05$.

studies did not greatly consider the predominant role of the obligate anaerobes in the human colonic microflora or their frequent isolation from postoperative infections when appropriate anaerobic collection and culturing were exercised.[82] The fact that many anaerobes were resistant to antimicrobial agents commonly employed for bowel preparation made it likely that regimens previously recommended had been pharmacologically inadequate.[76] Therefore, it became apparent that employment of effective antimicrobial agents for oral bowel preparation required knowledge of the normal bowel flora, the capacity of various fecal bacteria to produce infections, the frequency with which each species of micro-organisms is involved in infection, and the patterns of antimicrobial sensitivity of these pathogens. On the basis of these questions we organized a series of prospective, randomized clinical trials. The combination of neomycin and erythromycin base was chosen for trial because these drugs were likely to be effective in controlling both aerobic and anaerobic fecal pathogens and at that time were not generally used for treatment of surgical infections. In addition, these antibiotic agents were well tolerated by patients and were relatively inexpensive.

The objective of our first study was to determine the effectiveness of neomycin–erythromycin base as compared with antibiotic regimens recommended for bowel preparation by other recognized experts. The results of this study indicated that although most of the recommended antibiotic regimens reduced the concentration of aerobes in the colon, the preparation with neomycin–erythromycin base was most effective in reducing the numbers of both aerobic and anaerobic fecal pathogens.[76]

We next turned to a prospective, randomized clinical trial of the effectiveness of preparation with neomycin-erythromycin base in controlling wound infections in patients with disease of the colon.[73] By the time 20 patients had been entered in this trial, the rate of septic complications among patients who did not receive antibiotics was 30%. No septic complications had occurred among ten antibiotic-treated patients, but there had been three serious wound infections and one death among ten control patients. Clinically, the difference seemed quite clear to our colleagues, especially to our surgical residents, and the study was stopped. Unfortunately, because of the small numbers involved, the difference was not statistically significant.

Over the next 5 years, data were collected from two Veterans Administration Cooperative Studies. These prospective, randomized, double-blind studies were conducted with patients undergoing elective colonic resection.[20,15] In the first study, the effectiveness was proven of short-term, low-dose, preoperative, oral neomycin-erythromycin base combined with vigorous purgation compared with placebo and the same mechanical preparation.[15] The overall rate of directly related septic complications was 43% in the group given a placebo and 9% in the group given neomycin–erythromycin base.

The second Veterans Administration Cooperative Study was designed to compare the commonly advocated parenteral use of cephalothin with oral neomycin–erythromycin base as preoperative preparation prior to elective colonic resection.[20] In this prospective, randomized, double-blind study, three groups receiving the following regimens were compared: intravenous (IV) cephalothin, oral neomycin–erythromycin base, or a combination of the IV and oral antibiotics. All groups received the same mechanical preparation. The addition of patients to the group given IV cephalothin was stopped after 10 months because sequential analysis of the data indicated that this method of prophylaxis resulted in significantly higher numbers of septic complications. The incidence of wound infections was 30%, and the overall incidence of septic complications was 39% in patients receiving only IV cephalothin combined with mechanical cleansing. The incidence of septic complications was only 6% in the groups receiving the oral neomycin–erythromycin base.

Other oral antibiotic combinations that usually included combinations of neomycin or kanamycin with either metronidazole or tetracycline have been used successfully compared to either mechanical preparation alone (Table 13–3) or to parenteral antibiotic agents (Table 13–4).

The three oral regimens now most frequently in use are: (1) an aminoglycoside with erythromycin base, (2) an aminoglycoside with metronidazole, and (3) an aminoglycoside with tetracycline. The regimen most often chosen in the United States is neomycin–erythromycin base, which was introduced in 1972.[76] In Europe and Australia, physicians often prefer kanamycin-metronidazole or neomycin-metronidazole.[80]

The timing of the administration of these oral agents appears to be critical.[74,25] It is recommended that 1 g each of neomycin and erythromycin base be given at 1:00 P.M., 2:00 P.M., and 11:00 P.M. on the day before surgery (6 g total) (see Table 13–1). Surgery should then be scheduled for about 8:00 A.M. the next day. If the operation must be scheduled for later in the day, the times at which the oral agents are administered should be changed accordingly to preserve the 19 hours of preparation time. Giving more than three doses of oral antibiotics as prophylaxis is unwarranted and may induce the emergence of resistant flora.[54] Authoritative reviews of antibiotic prophylaxis in colon surgery confirm the value of the oral neomycin–erythromycin base preparation in preventing infection after elective colon resection[2,42]; however, there appears to be no convincing evidence to suggest that erythromycin base is superior to metronidazole in this clinical setting, or vice versa. The pharmacokinetics of the oral neomycin–erythromycin base preparation have been studied in healthy volunteers[74] and in patients undergoing elective colon resection.[25] The findings suggest that when adequate mechanical preparation is also carried out, significant intraluminal (local) and serum (systemic) levels of erythromycin and significant local levels of neomycin are present and that both techniques may help prevent infection after colon operation.

Parenteral Antibiotic Usage

In 1969 the first prospective, randomized, double-blind study published on parenteral antibiotic prophy-

TABLE 13-4. PROSPECTIVE STUDIES OF ORAL AND PARENTERAL ANTIBIOTIC REGIMENS IN PATIENTS RECEIVING MECHANICAL CLEANSING

Year	No. of Patients	Neomycin-Erythromycin Base Given to All Patients	Antibiotic	Route	Infection Rate (%)
1976[107]	144	Yes	Cefazolin	Parenteral	6
			Placebo		
1978[60]	79	No	Neomycin-erythromycin	Oral	12
			Cephaloridine	Parenteral	13†
1978[10]	79	No	Neomycin-erythromycin	Oral	25
			Neomycin-metronidazole	Oral	5*
1979[56]	93	No	Metronidazole-kanamycin	Oral	32
			Metronidazole-kanamycin	Parenteral	7*
1979[20]	193	No	Neomycin-erythromycin	Oral	6
			Cephalothin	Parenteral	30*
1979[114]	77	No	Kanamycin	Oral	46
			Kanamycin-erythromycin	Oral	13*
1979[108]	126	No	Thalazole	Oral	49
			Metronidazole-thalazole	Oral	13*
1979[5]	59	Yes	Placebo	Parenteral	4
			Clindamycin-gentamicin	Parenteral	7†
1979[103]	34	No	Cephalothin	Parenteral	31
			Cefamandole	Parenteral	33†
1982[63]	92	Yes	Cefazolin	Parenteral	13
			Ceftizoxime	Parenteral	7†
			Cefoxitin	Parenteral	3†
1982[48]	102	No	Doxycycline	Parenteral	13
			Cefoxitin	Parenteral	18†
1982[85]	74	No	Cephalothin	Parenteral	25
			Cefoxitin	Parenteral	4†
			Metronidazole	Parenteral	4†
1983[26]	123	No	Neomycin-erythromycin	Oral	2
			Cephaloridine	Parenteral	12*
1983[92]	104	Yes	Placebo	Parenteral	35
			Cefazolin	Parenteral	7*
			Ticarcillin	Parenteral	5*
1983[55]	119	No	Neomycin-erythromycin plus cefazolin	Oral Parenteral	3
			Cefoxitin	Parenteral	12†
1983[22]	241	Yes	No additional antibiotics		18
			Cefoxitin	Parenteral	7*
1983[68]	100	No	Cefoxitin	Parenteral	12
			Metronidazole-gentamicin	Parenteral	12†
1983[19]	1,082	Yes	Placebo	Parenteral	8
			Cephalothin	Parenteral	6†
1984[29]	57	Yes	Cefonicid	Parenteral	6
			Cefoxitin	Parenteral	10†
1984[30]	93	No	Neomycin-erythromycin	Oral	9
			Metronidazole-gentamicin	Parenteral	27*
1985[84]	267	No	Tinidazole-doxycycline	Parenteral	3
			Tinidazole	Parenteral	10*
1986[67]	86	No	Moxalactam	Parenteral	12
			Metronidazole-gentamicin	Parenteral	13†
1986[116]	60	No	Neomycin-erythromycin	Oral	41
			Metronidazole-ceftriaxone	Parenteral	10*
1987[52]	100	Yes	Cefazolin	Parenteral	3†
			Cefoxitin	Parenteral	3†
			Cefotaxime	Parenteral	14
1987[112]	167	No	Ticarcillin-clavulanic acid	Parenteral	2
			Tinidazole	Oral	14*
1988[49]	239	Variable	Cefotetan	Parenteral	12
			Cefoxitin	Parenteral	8†
1988[88]	119	No	Neomycin-metronidazole plus metronidazole	Oral Parenteral	14
			Metronidazole	Parenteral	28*
1988[21]	310	No	Neomycin-erythromycin plus cefoxitin	Oral Parenteral	5
			Cefoxitin	Parenteral	18*
1989[57]	102	No	Neomycin-erythromycin plus cefazolin	Oral Parenteral	11
			Metronidazole	Parenteral	32*
1989[87]	403	No	Cefoxitin	Parenteral	11
			Cefotetan	Parenteral	9†
1989[59]	54	No	Neomycin-erythromycin	Oral	4†
			Metronidazole-ceftriaxone	Parenteral	7

*Significant at $P > .05$.
†Not significant.

laxis in elective colon resection used cephaloridine administered intramuscularly during the perioperative period.[91] This study revealed a significant reduction of postoperative infections (from 30% to 7%) in the group of patients receiving antibiotics and mechanical preparation when compared to patients who received mechanical preparation alone. Other clinical studies using the same or similar first-generation cephalosporins for prophylaxis failed, however, to show efficacy of this approach when compared to placebo (mechanical preparation alone)[27] or to oral neomycin–erythromycin base.[20,26] However, Kaiser and associates[55] did not observe differences in postoperative infectious complications in operations of less than 4 hours when parenteral first-generation cefazolin (1.8-hour half-life) was compared to oral neomycin and erythromycin and parenteral cefazolin. Other clinical studies comparing parenteral cephalosporin alone showed lack of efficacy unless the antibiotic agent possessed aerobic and anaerobic activity (Table 13–4).

Parenteral agents that have shown efficacy alone or in combination with an aminoglycoside include cefoxitin, cefotetan, metronidazole, and doxycycline. Most investigators recommend the perioperative use of one to five doses of parenteral agents during the 24-hour period shortly before and after operation. A recent multicenter study showed that a single dose of cefotetan was equal in efficacy to multiple-dose cefoxitin in preventing infection after colon resection.[49]

The worst result ever published using neomycin–erythromycin base reported a 41% infection rate compared to a 10% rate with parenteral metronidazole and ceftriaxone.[116] To add to the confusion and cast a cloud of doubt on this report, the other center in this two-center trial has recently reported a 3.7% infection rate with the oral agents compared to 7.4% rate with the parenteral agents.[59] It is up to responsible surgeons to read these two very different studies and reach their own conclusions. Parenteral antibiotics are currently utilized alone for preoperative colon by less than 10% of actively involved colon and rectal surgeons who were surveyed in 1990.[106]

Combination Oral and Parenteral Antibiotics

Most surgeons presently use both oral and parenteral antibiotic agents in addition to mechanical cleansing as preoperative preparation before elective colon resection in hopes of further reducing the postoperative infection rate.[86,106] In a survey of over 500 surgeons reported in 1979, only 8% used systemic antibiotics alone, 37% used oral antibiotics alone, and 49% used oral plus systemic antibiotics before colon surgery.[20] Recently, a survey of over 360 colon and rectal surgeons revealed that over 88% used both oral and systemic antibiotic agents before elective colon resection.[106] The most commonly used agents were oral neomycin and erythromycin and a parenterally administered second-generation cephalosporin having aerobic and anaerobic activity.

Condon and associates[19] reported the results of a 5-year cooperative Veterans Administration study of over 1,000 patients undergoing elective colon surgery, com-

paring oral neomycin–erythromycin base with and without parenteral perioperative cephalothin. In this study the infection rate was not significantly different and was below 9% in both groups.

Studies using newer systemic agents with both aerobic and anaerobic coverage such as cefoxitin, cefotetan, or ceftizoxime, along with oral neomycin–erythromycin base, have shown a low incidence of infection.[49,63] It appears at this time, with somewhat conflicting evidence, that the addition of one dose of parenteral cephalosporin with aerobic and anaerobic activity given intravenously within 15 minutes of incision may be beneficial when added to mechanical and oral antibiotic bowel preparation. The use of the parenteral antibiotic may provide a fail-safe mechanism in cases when the oral agents have been administered in an inappropriate time sequence or in cases when the time of operation has been delayed.

Topical Prophylaxis

Another possible approach to the prevention of wound infection in colon surgery is the use of topically administered antibiotics such as ampicillin, which was first shown to be effective in 1967.[72] Although this study is difficult to evaluate because other routes of antibiotic administration were used and some patients undergoing emergency colon procedures without mechanical bowel preparation were included, it should be pointed out that only 1 of 36 patients (3%) receiving topical ampicillin experienced wound infection. Many other studies have suggested the value of topically administered antibiotics, but almost always the concomitant use of additional parenteral antibiotic agents has confused the strength of the message. In recent studies no advantage was gained by adding topical ampicillin when adequate oral or parenteral regimens were employed.[53,102] The use of so-called instant preparation of the colon, in which povidone-iodine solutions are instilled or injected into the colonic lumen, has been studied experimentally and clinically, but has not been generally adopted.[3,4,51] Two experimental studies have shown that povidone-iodine irrigation of the colon markedly reduced luminal bacteria but did not significantly reduce the colonic mucosal populations.[61,100]

PREOPERATIVE BOWEL PREPARATION FOR EMERGENCY COLON SURGERY

Some aspects of this topic have been discussed briefly above in the section dealing with mechanical cleansing.

Antibiotics

Among the clinical conditions that most often necessitate emergency colon surgery are acute bleeding, perforated diverticulum or perforated carcinoma, ischemic intestinal disease, obstructing lesions, and trauma involving the colon. Under emergency conditions, the operation must be performed without any bowel preparation because oral antibiotic prophylaxis and mechanical cleansing are either impossible or potentially harmful.

Prevention of infectious complications after emergency colon surgery depends on proper operative technique, sound judgment, and appropriate choice and administration of parenteral antibiotics. As in elective surgery, the antibiotics chosen should be active against both aerobic and anaerobic colonic microflora. They should be given intravenously in appropriate doses, starting shortly before the operation and continued postoperatively for 1 to 7 days. The duration of administration is governed by the operative findings and by whether the antibiotic regimen is intended to be *prophylactic* (in which case the antibiotics are given for 1 day) or *therapeutic* to manage the intra-abdominal infection for which the surgery is being performed (in which case antibiotics are given for 2 days or more). Many single agents and combinations appear to be equally efficacious, and our current recommended choices are listed in Table 13–2. The actual choice from this list depends largely on local hospital prices, bacterial sensitivity, and the surgeon's familiarity with the agents.

Intraoperative Colonic Lavage

One-stage resection and anastomosis is currently an accepted technique in emergency surgery of the right side of the colon in a patient given appropriate parenteral antibiotics. For lesions of the left side of the colon requiring rapid or immediate surgical intervention, intraoperative lavage is a useful supplement to a surgeon's armamentarium. We have performed the lavage successfully in many patients in the following manner. A ring-type plastic wound protector is inserted at the time of laparotomy in all patients. The large bowel is initially transected proximally and distally with a linear stapling device. The obstructed segment is resected and removed from the operative field. The splenic and hepatic flexures are mobilized, allowing easy mechanical manipulation of the large bowel.

The abdominal cavity is then protected from the proximal colon with laparotomy pads, towels, and plastic barrier drapes. Following mobilization of the hepatic and splenic flexures, laparotomy pads are used to isolate the distal ileum and colon from other abdominal contents and the operating field. The distal colonic segment is brought out of the field through a sterile, sticky, small-aperture plastic rape. A Steridrape irrigation pouch is placed over the small aperture drape to contain the distal stapled end of the colon. A pursestring suture is placed in the antimesenteric border of the ileum approximately 5 cm proximal to the ileocecal valve. A No. 18 Foley catheter with a 5-ml balloon is inserted through an ileotomy in the center of the pursestring suture. The Foley catheter is passed through the ileocecal valve so that the inflated balloon lies within the cecum snugly against the valve. The pursestring suture is then tightened and tied with a bow onto the shaft of the catheter. An alternative method is to perform an appendectomy and introduce the catheter through the stump, which is ducked as the pursestring suture is tied when the catheter is withdrawn at the end of the irrigation.

The distal stapled end of the colon is held off the field over a sterile receptacle as the staple line is resected, thus opening the bowel. We do not use a sterile conduit tube for outflow but rely on direct manual control of the open end. The cecum is held by the surgeon, and an assistant holds the transected distal colonic end securely. The stool present in patients with chronic obstruction has often undergone liquefaction, resulting in a pasty to fluid consistency that is easier to remove with lavage. The irrigation is performed with warm saline solution. The distal stapled end of colon is excised and inspissated stool is manually expressed. Small amounts of saline solution are instilled proximally to soften it if necessary. Once evacuation of gross stool is complete, the irrigation fluid is administered as rapidly as possible while the colon is manually agitated. It is more efficient to administer the saline solution from bags, each containing 3,000 ml. A circulator is assigned to control the inflow of saline solution. Colonic lavage is continued until the effluent is clear, which usually requires 6 to 9 L warm saline solution. The distal contaminated colon is then excised and closed with a linear stapling device and handed off field. The Foley ligature is untied, the balloon is deflated, and the catheter is withdrawn as the pursestring suture is tied. A sterile laparotomy pad is held around the catheter as it is withdrawn to minimize fecal contamination. The ileotomy site is closed transversely with Lembert sutures.

The rectal stump is washed out from below with sterile saline solution. Gloves and instruments are changed before performing a primary anastomosis. The distal rectal washout device can be saved to test the anastomosis for leakage (water- or airtight) following its completion. An intraoperative lavage takes approximately 30 minutes; therefore, only low-risk, stable patients should be selected for this procedure. The intraoperative lavage requires a group effort and is therefore not recommended for use by a solitary surgeon. The use of antimicrobial or antiseptic solutions for lavage or peritoneal irrigation is not recommended because they are frequently absorbed with possibly increased toxicity and they lack definite evidence of improved efficacy.

SUMMARY

The busy colon and rectal surgeon deals daily with a sea of bacteria. Using good surgical judgment as well as time-honored techniques and innovative equipment, the postoperative results are generally good. The role that appropriately administered efficacious antibiotics play in this scenario should not be underestimated and can only be realized when historic controls are evaluated.

The results of studies of antibiotic bowel preparation suggest that many different approaches may be equally effective in reducing infection after elective colonic resection. Certain features, however, appear to be common to most of the studies:

1. Oral antibiotic regimens with both aerobic and anaerobic activity (e.g., neomycin–erythromycin base) were utilized.

2. The oral agents were given in limited doses the day before operation.

3. Addition of systemic antibiotic agents without broad-spectrum coverage to the oral generally did not improve the results.

4. Use of broad-spectrum parenteral antibiotic agents alone was associated with a lower infection rate than the use of systemic agents having only limited coverage.

5. Addition of a broad-spectrum parenteral antibiotic to the oral antibiotics may further reduce the postoperative infection rate.

6. Parenteral or oral antibiotics should be administered only for a short time during the perioperative period.

REFERENCES

1. Altemeier, W.A., Hummel, R.P., and Hill, E.O.: Prevention of infection in colon surgery. Arch. Surg., 93:226, 1966.
2. Antimicrobial prophylaxis in surgery. Med. Lett. Drugs Ther., 34: 5, 1992.
3. Arrango, A., Lester, L., Martinez, O., et al.: Bacteriologic and systemic effects of intraoperative segmental bowel preparation with povidone iodine. Arch. Surg., 114:154, 1979.
4. Banich, F.E., and Mendak, S.J., Jr.: Intraoperative colonic irrigation with povidone iodine—an excellent method of wound sepsis prevention. Dis. Colon Rectum, 32:219, 1989.
5. Barber, M.S., Hirschberg, B.C., Rice, C.L., et al.: Parenteral antibiotics in elective colon surgery? A prospective, controlled clinical study. Surgery, 86:23, 1979.
6. Baum, M.L., Anish, D.S., Chalmers, T.C., et al.: A survey of clinical trials of antibiotic prophylaxis in colon surgery: Evidence against further use of no-treatment controls. N. Engl. J. Med., 305:795, 1981.
7. Beck, D.E., Harford, F.J., and DiPalma, J.A.: Comparison of cleansing method in preparation for colonic surgery. Dis. Colon Rectum, 28:491, 1985.
8. Beck, D.E., Harford, F.J., DiPalma, J.A., et al.: Bowel cleansing with polyethylene glycolelectrolyte lavage solution. South. Med. J., 78:1414, 1985.
9. Bornside, G.H., and Cohn, I., Jr.: Intestinal antisepsis; stability of fecal flora during mechanical cleansing. Gastroenterology, 57: 569, 1969.
10. Brass, C., Richards, G.K., Ruedy, J., et al.: The effect of metronidazole on the incidence of postoperative wound infection in elective colon surgery. Am. J. Surg., 135:91, 1978.
11. Brote, I., Gillquist, J., and Hojer, H.: Prophylactic cephalothin in gastrointestinal surgery. Acta. Chir. Scand., 142:238, 1976.
12. Buinauskas, P., McDonald, G.O., and Cole, W.H.: Role of operative stress on the resistance of the experimental animal to inoculated cancer cells. Ann. Surg., 148:642, 1958.
13. Burdon, J.G.W., Morris, I.J., Hunt, P., et al.: A trial of cephalothin sodium in colon surgery to prevent wound infection. Arch. Surg., 112:1169, 1977.
14. Burton, R.C., Hughes, E.S.R., and Cuthbertson, A.M.: Prophylactic use of gentamicin in colonic and rectal surgery. Med. J. Aust., 2:846, 1975.
15. Clarke, J.S., Condon, R.E., Bartlett, J.G., et al.: Preoperative oral antibiotics reduce septic complications of colon operations: Results of a prospective, randomized, double-blind clinical study. Ann. Surg., 186:251, 1977.
16. Cohn, I., Jr.: Intestinal Antisepsis. Springfield, Charles C. Thomas, 1968.
17. Cohn, I., Jr.: Kanamycin for bowel sterilization. Ann. N.Y. Acad. Sci., 76:212, 1958.
18. Cohn, I., Jr., and Atik, M.: The influence of antibiotics on the spread of tumors of the colon: An experimental study. Ann. Surg., 151:917, 1960.
19. Condon, R.E., Bartlett, J.G., Greenlee, H., et al.: Efficacy of oral and systemic antibiotic prophylaxis in colorectal operations. Arch. Surg., 118:496, 1983.
20. Condon, R.E., Bartlett, J.G., Nichols, R.L., et al.: Preoperative prophylactic cephalothin fails to control septic complications of colorectal operations: Results of controlled clinical trial—a Veterans Administration Cooperative Study. Am. J. Surg., 137: 68, 1979.
21. Coopa, G.F., and Eng, K.: Factors involved in antibiotic selection in elective colon and rectal surgery. Surgery, 104:853, 1988.
22. Coppa, G.E., Eng, K., Gouge, T.H., et al.: Parenteral and oral antibiotics in elective colon and rectal surgery: A prospective and randomized trial. Am. J. Surg., 145:62, 1983.
23. Dearing, W.H., and Heilman, F.R.: The effect of antibacterial agents on the intestinal flora of patients; the use of aureomycin, chloromycetin, dihydrostreptomycin, sulfasuxidine and sulfathalidine. Gastroenterology, 16:12, 1950.
24. Dearing, W.H., and Needham, G.M.: Effect of oral administration of neomycin and the intestinal bacterial flora of man. Proc. Mayo Clin., 28:502, 1953.
25. DiPiro, J.T., Patrias, J.M., Townsend, R.J., et al.: Oral neomycin sulfate and erythromycin base before colon surgery: A comparison of serum and tissue concentrations. Pharmacotherapy, 5:91, 1985.
26. Edmondson, H.T., and Rissing, J.P.: Prophylactic antibiotics in colon surgery. Arch. Surg., 118:227, 1983.
27. Evans, C., and Pollack, A.V.: The reduction of surgical wound infection by prophylactic parenteral cephaloridine: A controlled clinical trial. Br. J. Surg., 60:434, 1973.
28. Eykyn, S.J., Jackson, B.T., Lockhart-Mummery, H.E., et al.: Prophylactic perioperative intravenous metronidazole in elective colorectal surgery. Lancet, 2:761, 1979.
29. Fabian, T.C., Mangiante, E.C., and Boldreghini, S.J.: Prophylactic antibiotics for elective colorectal surgery or operation for obstruction of the small bowel: A comparison of cefonicid and cefoxitin. Rev. Infect. Dis., 6(Suppl.4):S896, 1984.
30. Figueras-Felip, J., Basilio-Bonet, E., Lara-Eisman, F., et al.: Oral is superior to systemic antibiotic prophylaxis in operations upon the colon and rectum. Surg. Gynecol. Obstet., 158:359, 1984.
31. Finland, M., Grigsby, M.E., and Haight, T.H.: Efficacy and toxicity of oxytetracycline (terramycin) and chlortetracycline (aureomycin) with reference to use of doses of 250 mgm every 4–6 hours and to occurrence of staphylococcal diarrhea. Arch. Intern. Med., 93:23, 1954.
32. Firor, W.M., and Jonas, A.F.: The use of sulfanilylguanidine in surgical patients. Ann. Surg., 114:19, 1941.
33. Firor, W.M., and Poth, E.J.: Intestinal antisepsis with special reference to sulfanilylguanidine. Ann. Surg., 114:663, 1941.
34. Fleites, R.A., Marshall, J.B., Eckhauser, M.L., et al.: The efficacy of polyethylene glycol-electrolyte lavage solution versus traditional mechanical bowel preparation for elective colonic surgery: A randomized prospective, blinded clinical trial. Surgery, 98:708, 1985.
35. Frazee, R.C., Roberts, J., Symmonds, R., et al.: Prospective randomized trial of inpatient vs. outpatient bowel preparation for elective colorectal surgery. Dis. Colon Rectum, 35:223, 1992.
36. Garlock, J.H., and Seley, G.P.: The use of sulfanilamide in surgery of the colon and rectum; preliminary report. Surgery, 5:787, 1939.
37. Gaylor, D.W., Clarke, J.S., Kudinoff, Z., et al.: Preoperative bowel "sterilization"; a double blind study comparing kanamycin, neomycin, and placebo. In Gray, P., et al. (eds.): Antimicrobial Agents Annual: Proceedings. Conference on Antimicrobial Agents. New York, Plenum Publishing Corporation, 1960, p. 392.
38. George, S.M., Jr., Fabian, T.C., Voeller, G.R., et al.: Primary repair of colon wounds: A prospective trial in nonselected patients. Ann. Surg., 209:728, 1989.
39. Gillespie, G., and McNaught, W.: Prophylactic oral metronidazole in intestinal surgery. J. Antimicrob. Chemother., 4(Suppl.):29, 1978.
40. Gliedman, M.L., Grant, R.N., Vestal, B.L., et al.: Impromptu bowel cleansing and sterilization. Surgery, 43:282, 1958.
41. Goldring, J., McNaught, W., Scott, A., et al.: Prophylactic oral antimicrobial agents in elective colon surgery: A controlled trial. Lancet, 2:7943, 1975.
42. Gorbach, S.L., Condon, R.E., Conte, J.E., Jr., et al.: General guide-

lines for the evaluations of new anti-infective drugs for prophylaxis of surgical infections—evaluations of new anti-infective drugs for surgical prophylaxis. Clin. Infect. Dis., *15*(Suppl. 1):S313, 1992.

43. Grant, R.B., and Barbara, A.C.: Preoperative and postoperative antibiotic therapy in surgery of the colon. Am. J. Surg., *107:*810, 1964.

44. Herter, F.P., Santulli, T.V., Terry, S., et al.: An experimental study of the influence of the intestinal bacterial flora on suture line recurrence following resection for carcinoma of the colon. Surg. Gynecol. Obstet., *114:*267, 1962.

45. Herter, F.P., and Slanetz, C.A.: Influence of antibiotic preparation of the bowel on complications after colon resection. Am. J. Surg., *113:*165, 1967.

46. Herter, F.P., and Slanetz, C.A.: Preoperative intestinal preparation in relation to the subsequent development of cancer at the suture line. Surg. Gynecol. Obstet., *127:*49, 1968.

47. Hojer, H., and Wetterfors, J.: Systemic prophylaxis with doxycycline in surgery of the colon and rectum. Ann. Surg., *187:*362, 1978.

48. Ivarsson, L., Darle, N., Kewenter, J.G., et al.: Short-term systemic prophylaxis with cefoxitin and doxycycline in colorectal surgery—a prospective, randomized study. Am. J. Surg., *144:*257, 1982.

49. Jagelman, D.G., Fabian, T.C., Nichols, R.L., et al.: Single dose cefotetan versus multiple dose cefoxitin as prophylaxis in colorectal surgery. Am. J. Surg., *155*(Suppl. 5A):71, 1988.

50. Jagelman, D.G., Fazio, V.W., Lavery, I.C., et al.: A prospective, randomized, double-blind study of 10% mannitol mechanical bowel preparation combined with oral neomycin and short-term, perioperative intravenous Flagyl as prophylaxis in elective colorectal resections. Surgery, *98:*861, 1985.

51. Jones, F.E., DeCosse, J.J., and Condon, R.E.: Evaluation of "instant" preparation of the colon with povidone-iodine. Ann. Surg., *184:*74, 1976.

52. Jones, R.N., Wojeski, W., Bakke, J., et al.: Antibiotic prophylaxis of 1,036 patients undergoing elective surgical procedures. Am. J. Surg., *153:*341, 1987.

53. Juul, P., Merrild, U., and Kronbord, O.: Topical ampicillin in addition to a systemic antibiotic prophylaxis in elective colorectal surgery: A prospective randomized study. Dis. Colon Rectum, *28:*800, 1985.

54. Kaiser, A.B.: Antimicrobial prophylaxis in surgery. N. Engl. J. Med., *315:*1129, 1986.

55. Kaiser, A.B., Herrington, J.L., Jr., Jacobs, J.K., et al.: Cefoxitin versus erythromycin, neomycin, and cefazolin in colorectal operations. Ann. Surg., *198:*525, 1983.

56. Keighley, M.R.B., Arabi, Y., and Alexander-Williams, J.: Comparison between systemic and oral antimicrobial prophylaxis in colorectal surgery. Lancet, *1:*894, 1979.

57. Khubchandani, I.T., Karamchandani, M.C., Sheets, J.A., et al.: Metronidazole vs. erythromycin, neomycin and cefazolin in prophylaxis for colon surgery. Dis. Colon Rectum, *32:*17, 1989.

58. Kjellgren, K., and Sellstrom, H.: Effect of prophylactic systemic administration of cephalothin in colorectal surgery. Acta. Chir. Scand., *143:*437, 1977.

59. Kling, P.A., and Dahlgren, S.: Oral prophylaxis with neomycin and erythromycin in colorectal surgery—more proof for efficacy than failure. Arch. Surg., *124:*705, 1989.

60. Lewis, R.T., Allan, C.M., Goodall, R.G., et al.: Antibiotics in surgery of the colon. Can. J. Surg., *21:*339, 1978.

61. Lindsey, J.T., Smith, J.W., McClugage, S.G., Jr., et al.: Effects of commonly used bowel preparations on the large bowel mucosal-associated and luminal microflora in the rat model. Dis. Colon Rectum, *33:*554, 1990.

62. Lockwood, J.S., Young, A.D., Bouchelle, M., et al.: Appraisal on oral streptomycin as an intestinal antiseptic with observation on rapid development of resistance of *E. coli* to streptomycin. Ann. Surg., *129:*14, 1949.

63. Maki, D.G., and Aughey, D.R.: Comparative study of cefazolin, cefoxitin and ceftizoxime for surgical prophylaxis in colo-rectal surgery. J. Antimicrob. Chemother., *10*(Suppl. C):281, 1982.

64. Mann, C.V.: Kanamycin in preoperative bowel sterilization. Postgrad. Med. J., *43:*22, 1967.

65. Mann, L.S., Schumer, W., and Tomusk, A.: Twenty-four hour neomycin preparation for intestinal operations. J. Int. Coll. Surg., *22:*602, 1954.

66. Matheson, D.M., Arabi, Y., Baxter-Smith, D., et al.: Randomized multicentre trial of oral bowel preparation and antimicrobials for elective colorectal operations. Br. J. Surg., *65:*597, 1978.

67. McCulloch, P.G., Blamey, S.L., Finlay, I.G., et al.: A prospective comparison of gentamicin and metronidazole and moxalactam in the prevention of septic complications associated with elective operations of the colon and rectum. Surg. Gynecol. Obstet., *162:*521, 1986.

68. McDonald, P.J., and Karran, S.J.: A comparison of intravenous cefoxitin and a combination of gentamicin and metronidazole as prophylaxis in colorectal surgery. Dis. Colon Rectum, *26:*661, 1983.

69. Mikal, S.: Metabolic effects of preoperative intestinal preparation. Am. J. Proctol., *16:*437, 1965.

70. Muir, E.G.: Safety in colonic resection. Proc. R. Soc. Med., *61:*401, 1968.

71. Murray, J.J., Schoetz, D.J., Jr., Coller, J.A., et al.: Intraoperative colonic lavage and primary anastomosis in nonelective colon resection. Dis. Colon Rectum, *34:*527, 1991.

72. Nash, A.G., and Hugh, T.B.: Topical ampicillin and wound infection in colon surgery. BMJ, *1:*147, 1967.

73. Nichols, R.L., Broido, P., Condon, R.E., et al.: Effect of preoperative neomycin-erythromycin intestinal preparation on the incidence of infectious complications following colon surgery. Ann. Surg., *178:*453, 1973.

74. Nichols, R.L., Condon, R.E., and DiSanto, A.R.: Preoperative bowel preparation: Erythromycin base serum and fecal levels following oral administration. Arch. Surg., *112:*493, 1977.

75. Nichols, R.L., and Condon, R.E.: Preoperative preparation of the colon. Surg. Gynecol. Obstet., *132:*323, 1971.

76. Nichols, R.L., Condon, R.E., Gorbach, S.L., et al.: Efficacy of preoperative antimicrobial preparation of the bowel. Ann. Surg., *176:*227, 1972.

77. Nichols, R.L., Gorbach, S.L., and Condon, R.E.: Alteration of intestinal microflora following preoperative mechanical preparation of the colon. Dis. Colon Rectum, *14:*123, 1971.

78. Nichols, R.L., Smith, J.W., Klein, D.B., et al.: Risk of infection after penetrating abdominal trauma. N. Engl. J. Med., *311:*1065, 1984.

79. Nichols, R.L., Smith, J.W., Robertson, G.D., et al.: Prospective alterations in therapy for penetrating abdominal trauma. Arch. Surg., *128:*55, 1993.

80. Nichols, R.L.: Bowel preparations. *In* Wilmore, D.W., Brennan, M.F., Harken, A.H., et al. (eds.): Care of the Surgical Patient. VI Preoperative Care, 2nd ed. New York, Scientific American, *1:*10, 1990.

81. Nichols, R.L.: Prophylaxis for surgical infections. *In* Gorbach, S.L., Bartlett, J.G., and Blacklow, N.R. (eds.): Infectious Diseases. Philadelphia, W.B. Saunders, 1992, p. 393.

82. Nichols, R.L.: Surgical bacteriology: An overview. *In* Nyhus, L.M. (ed.): Surgery Annual. East Norwalk, CT, Appleton & Lange, *13:*205, 1981.

83. Nichols, R.L.: Surgical wound infection. Am. J. Med., *91*(S3B): 54s, 1991.

84. Norwegian Study Group for Colorectal Surgery: Should antimicrobial prophylaxis in colorectal surgery include agents effective against both anaerobic and aerobic microorganisms? A double-blind, multicenter study. Surgery, *97:*402, 1985.

85. Panichi, G., Pantosti, A., Giunchi, G., et al.: Cephalothin, cefoxitin or metronidazole in elective colon surgery? A single blind randomized trial. Dis. Colon Rectum, *25:*783, 1982.

86. Peck, J.J., Fuchs, P.C., and Gustafson, M.E.: Antimicrobial prophylaxis in elective colon surgery—experience of 1035 operations in a community hospital. Am. J. Surg., *147:*633, 1984.

87. Periti, P., Mazzei, T., Tonelli, F., et al.: Single dose cefotetan versus multiple dose cefoxitin—antimicrobial prophylaxis in colorectal surgery. Dis. Colon Rectum, *32:*121, 1989.

88. Playforth, M.J., Smith, G.M.R., Evans, M., et al.: Antimicrobial bowel preparation—oral, parenteral or both? Dis. Colon Rectum, *31:*90, 1988.

89. Plumley, P.F.: A simple regimen for preparation of colon before large bowel surgery. Br. J. Surg., *53:*413, 1966.

90. Polacek, M.A., and Sanfelippo, P.: Oral antibiotic bowel prepa-

ration and complications in colon surgery. Arch. Surg., *97*:412, 1968.

91. Polk, H.C., Jr., and Lopez-Mayor, J.F.: Postoperative wound infections. A prospective study of determinant factors and prevention. Surgery, *66*:97, 1969.

92. Portnoy, J., Kagan, E., Gordon, P.H., et al.: Prophylactic antibiotics in elective colorectal surgery. Dis. Colon Rectum, *26*:310, 1983.

93. Poth, E.J.: Intestinal antisepsis in surgery. JAMA, *153*:1516, 1953.

94. Poth, E.J.: Succinylsulfathiazole (sulfasuxidine). JAMA, *120*:265, 1942.

95. Poth, E.J., Fromm, S.M., Martin, R.G., et al.: Neomycin: An adjunct in abdominal surgery. South. Med. J., *44*:226, 1951.

96. Poth, E.J., Fromm, S.M., Wise, R.I., et al.: Neomycin, a new intestinal antiseptic. Tex. Rep. Biol. Med., *8*:353, 1950.

97. Poth, E.J., and Knotts, F.L.: Clinical use of succinylsulfathiazole. Arch. Surg., *44*:208, 1942.

98. Poth, E.J., and Ross, C.A.: Bacteriostatic properties of sulfanilamide and some of its derivates — II, phthalylsulfathiazole, a new chemotherapeutic agent locally active in the gastroenteric tract. Tex. Rep. Biol. Med., *1*:345, 1943.

99. Riddell, M.I.: A review of the literature on preoperative prophylaxis of the bowel with antibacterial agents. Am. J. Med. Sci., *223*:301, 1952.

100. Rotstein, O.D., Wells, C.U., Pruett, T.L., et al.: Reevaluation of the "instant" colon preparation with povidone-iodine. Surg. Forum, *35*:70, 1985.

101. Rowlands, B.C., and Scorer, E.M.C.: Preoperative preparation of the bowel with neomycin. Lancet, *2*:950, 1955.

102. Salvati, E.P., Rubin, J., Eisenstat, T.E., et al.: Value of subcutaneous and intraperitoneal antibiotics in reducing infection in clean contaminated operations of the colon. Surg. Gynecol. Obstet., *167*:315, 1988.

103. Slama, T.G., Carey, L.C., and Fass, R.J.: Comparative efficacy of prophylactic cephalothin and cefamandole for elective colon surgery: Results of a prospective, randomized, double-blind study. Am. J. Surg., *137*:593, 1979.

104. Smith, M.B., Goradia, V.K., Holmes, J.W., et al.: Suppression of the human mucosal-related colonic microflora with prophylactic parenteral and/or oral antibiotics. World J. Surg., *14*:636, 1990.

105. Smith, W.H., and Crabb, W.E.: The fecal-bacterial flora of animals and man; its development in the young. J. Pathol. Bacteriol., *82*:53, 1961.

106. Solla, J.A., and Rothenberger, D.A.: Preoperative bowel preparation. A survey of colon and rectal surgeons. Dis. Colon Rectum, *33*:154, 1990.

107. Stone, H.H., Hooper, C.A., Kolb, L.D., et al.: Antibiotic prophylaxis in gastric, biliary and colonic surgery. Ann. Surg., *184*: 443, 1976.

108. Taylor, S.A., Gawdery, H.M., and Smith, J.: The use of metronidazole in the preparation of bowel for surgery. Br. J. Surg., *66*: 191, 1979.

109. Trinkle, J.K., Fisher, L.J., Ketcham, A.S., et al.: The metabolic effects of preoperative intestinal preparation. Surg. Gynecol. Obstet., *118*:739, 1964.

110. Tyson, R.R., and Spaulding, E.H.: Antibiotic preparation of the bowel-a chimera. *In* Finland, M., Ingelfinger, F.J., and Relman, A.S. (eds.): Controversies in Internal Medicine. Philadelphia, W.B. Saunders, 1966, p. 615.

111. Tyson, R.R., and Spaulding, E.H.: Should antibiotics be used in large bowel preparations? Surg. Gynecol. Obstet., *108*:623, 1959.

112. University of Melbourne Colorectal Group: Systemic Trimentin is superior to oral tinidazale for antibiotic prophylaxis in elective colorectal surgery. Dis. Colon Rectum, *30*:786, 1987.

113. Vink, M.: Local recurrence of cancer in the large bowel. Br. J. Surg., *41*:431, 1954.

114. Wapnick, S., Guinto, R., Reizis, I., et al.: Reduction of postoperative infection in elective colon surgery with preoperative administration of kanamycin and erythromycin. Surgery, *85*:317, 1979.

115. Washington, J.A., II, Dearing, W.H., Judd, E.S., et al.: Effect of preoperative antibiotic regimen on development of infection after intestinal surgery: Prospective, randomized, double-blind study. Ann. Surg., *180*:567, 1974.

116. Weaver, M., Burdon, D.W., Youngs, D.J., et al.: Oral neomycin and erythromycin compared with single-dose systemic metronidazole and ceftriaxone prophylaxis in elective colorectal surgery. Am. J. Surg., *151*:437, 1986.

117. Zintel, H.A., Flippin, H.F., Nichols, A.C., et al.: Studies on streptomycin in man. Am. J. Med. Sci., *210*:421, 1945.

Chapter 14

LAPAROSCOPIC APPENDECTOMY AND COLECTOMY

STEVEN D. WEXNER / STEPHEN M. COHEN

During the past 5 years a tremendous increase in the use of the laparoscope has occurred. It has gone from a simple instrument utilized by the gynecologist for the evaluation of pelvic disorders to a leading tool applied to therapeutic intervention in all fields of surgery. Much of the demand for this "minimally invasive surgery" has been both patient and market driven. The thought of less pain and shorter hospitalization may be just as persuasive as the promise of an improved long-term cosmetic result. As this patient demand increases, the natural progression is to evaluate more complex intra-abdominal conditions in which the laparoscope can be effectively utilized. Laparoscopic herniorrhaphy, fundoplication, nephrectomy, splenectomy, and adrenalectomy have all been reported.

HISTORY

Georg Kelling is given credit for the origins of laparoscopy, the description of which was published in 1901.[39] He successfully introduced air through a needle puncture into the abdomen of a live dog to produce a pneumoperitoneum. A cystoscope was then inserted through a large trocar. The feasibility of directly observing the abdominal cavity was established and he later reported his experience in humans. Kelling called the procedure "Koelioskopie." The first major series to be reported in man is attributed to H.C. Jacobaeus. He initially examined patients with ascites. He also used this technique to explore the thorax and coined the term "Laparothorakoskopie." Identification of tuberculosis, malignancy, cirrhosis, and syphilis were reported in his clinical publication.

The entry of laparoscopy into the United States was established in 1911 by Bertram M. Bernheim from Johns Hopkins University.[10] He reported his experience with two patients. In the first case, he confirmed the subsequent celiotomy findings in a patient with obstructing pancreatic cancer. In the second case, he diagnosed chronic appendicitis. Two additional studies were published from the United States in 1924.[90,91] In the following year, Nadeau and Kampmeier[51] reported on three of their own patients; however, they also gave a detailed historical summary of laparoscopy with 42 references. Furthermore, they evaluated the instruments available at the time and reported on an experiment they performed in dogs in which they studied the absorption of air in the pneumoperitoneum.

A landmark paper was published in *Surgery, Gynecology and Obstetrics* in 1937.[75] John C. Ruddock, an internist, reported his personal experience of 500 cases, 39 of which were biopsies. In this same year, E.T. Anderson published a report entitled "Peritoneoscopy."[4] He discussed a method for performing a tubal ligation in addition to a description of transillumination of the walls of several structures in combination with laparoscopy for better visualization.

Janos Veress in 1938 developed the spring-loaded needle, similar to the present-day instrument, used for creating a pneumoperitoneum.[98] Kurt Semm, in the 1960s, developed the instrumentation for controlled, automatic insufflation.[86] The next several decades brought optical lens systems, video transmission, and computer-chip television cameras with improved resolution and contrast. The first laparoscopic cholecystectomy was performed by Moruet in 1987.[21] The exponential increase in acceptance of the technology is attested to by the fact that, in 1991 alone, seven papers were published on laparoscopic-assisted colon resections. As we continue to embark on this new technology and look for additional applications, it remains of paramount importance that we do not forsake essential surgical tenets to facilitate inadequate technology.

APPENDECTOMY

The gynecologist's use of the laparoscope predates the general surgeon's. In 1983, Kurt Semm reported the first case of an incidental laparoscopic appendectomy.[85] He advised against attempting the removal of an inflamed appendix. However, several years later, Schreiber reported a series of 70 patients in whom he performed a laparoscopic appendectomy, 24% of whom had acute appendicitis.[79]

Appendicitis is one of the more common surgical conditions, occurring in 500,000 patients hospitalized for over 1 million days per year in the United States.[1] The actual role of laparoscopic appendectomy is still in evolution, as a simple appendectomy through a muscle-splitting McBurney's incision is arguably associated with little morbidity and a short hospitalization. In fact, the statistics above suggest that the mean length of stay after "standard" appendectomy in the United States is 2 days. Certainly it would be difficult to fathom a statistically significantly shorter stay after laparoscopic appendectomy. More common, however, is the case in which there is suspected appendicitis or the diagnosis is in doubt. The laparoscope permits adequate exploration if a normal appendix is encountered.

There have been two large recent reports that demonstrate the safety and feasibility of laparoscopic appendectomy. Pier and associates reported on a series of 625 laparoscopic appendectomies performed mostly for acute appendicitis.[64] The procedure was aborted in 14 patients (2.2%). Three patients had serious postoperative complications; one had a stump leak and two required re-exploration for an intra-abdominal abscess. Their wound infection rate was less than 2%. Valla and co-workers reported a similar series of 465 pediatric patients.[96] In five patients (1%), the appendix could not be removed under laparoscopic guidance and the procedure was converted to a laparotomy. There were 17 (3.6%) intraoperative problems such as omental emphysema, visceral injury, and appendiceal rupture. A total of 14 (3%) postoperative complications were identified, including three intra-abdominal abscesses; four patients required a laparotomy and two underwent a second laparoscopy.

Advantages

One of the advantages of a laparoscopic appendectomy is the potential for less postoperative pain. When compared to a standard "open" procedure, the sum length of the fascial incisions is equal to a standard McBurney incision. Do several 5- to 10-mm incisions cause less pain than one 2-cm incision? Advocates of the laparoscopic procedure state that there is less pain because there is less traction on both the abdominal organs and the peritoneum.[41]

Another potential advantage of the laparoscopic procedure is a decrease in wound infection rate. Wound infection is the most common complication reported following standard appendectomy, occurring in 1.2 to 5.7% of patients.[6,67,111] Gotz and associates[28] reported no port infections after 388 laparoscopic appendectomies despite the omission of prophylactic antibiotics. They did, however, report 14 cases of "slight omphalitis," which did not prolong hospitalization. They felt that they had eliminated the problem by using a more thorough cleaning and disinfecting procedure. Furthermore, Valla and colleagues[96] had no wound infections after 465 pediatric laparoscopic appendectomies.

One theory that supports the decrease in wound infection rate is the absence of contact between the inflamed appendix and the skin. The inflamed appendix can either be pulled into one of the trocars or placed into a plastic bag prior to removal.

Another potential advantage of a laparoscopic appendectomy is faster recovery.[72] As seen by the U.S. statistics, patients after open appendectomy are usually discharged from the hospital on the second postoperative day and return to work 1 or more weeks after the operation.[111] Following laparoscopic appendectomy, patients are able to return to normal activity in 3 to 4 days.[78] However, interpretation of these data is fraught with problems. One must be cognizant of the tremendous variability in patient response to pain and motivation to work. Even after standard operations we have all seen some patients linger while others eagerly and quickly cease analgesic use and resume full preoperative activity.

The diagnosis of acute appendicitis remains a clinical challenge even to the most astute surgeon. Until only recently, when the decision was made to operate on a patient with right lower quadrant pain, the patient was committed to an incision with removal of the appendix. With laparoscopy now a part of the surgeon's armamentarium, a diagnostic laparoscopy can be undertaken to confirm the diagnosis. This feature is one of the clearest advantages of laparoscopic surgery. Since the negative appendectomy rate can be as high as 15 to 20%,[46] an exploratory laparoscopy can significantly decrease the rate of misdiagnosis. If acute appendicitis is confirmed, a laparoscopic appendectomy is performed. If another reason for the previously undiagnosed right lower quadrant pain is found, such as Crohn's disease, pelvic inflammatory disease, diverticulitis, or endometriosis, a decision regarding removal of the appendix and additional appropriate treatment of the primary pathology can be expeditiously instituted.

It has been well documented that the rate of diagnostic error is highest for young women of reproductive age.[55] This rate of 31 to 46% is presumably due to the high incidence of gynecologic diseases that may mimic acute appendicitis. Ragland and associates,[70] through a retrospective audit, found the incidence of removing a normal appendix in this patient population to be 42%. After instituting laparoscopy in this group of 21 patients, they were able to reduce their rate of removal of normal appendices to 15%. Acute appendicitis was confirmed in 12 of their 21 cases (57%). Tubo-ovarian abscess was found in five patients and no pathology was found in four patients. There were no serious complications associated with laparoscopy. They concluded that diagnostic laparoscopy should be liberally employed in women of reproductive age with suspected appendicitis.

Whitworth and associates[101] prospectively evaluated

the usefulness of laparoscopy in improving diagnostic accuracy in young women with possible appendicitis. Thirty-one of 51 women had initial laparoscopy. The appendix was found to be inflamed in five patients, while another disease was diagnosed in 15 and no diagnostic abnormalities were seen in six; five patients had a normal appendix removed. Twenty patients who had classic history and physical findings underwent standard appendectomy without laparoscopy; 5 of the 20 (25%) appendices removed were normal. The authors concluded that preliminary diagnostic laparoscopy should be considered for all young women with suspected appendicitis, even when classic signs and symptoms are present.

Controversies

Since a standard appendectomy is generally well tolerated by patients of all ages with minimal morbidity, the laparoscopic form of this operation has not reached the same acceptance and popularity as laparoscopic cholecystectomy. Moreover, since the traditional incisional appendectomy is still considered the gold standard, there are few data to advocate the laparoscopic approach.

One area of controversy is the perforated appendix. If one is suspicious of a perforated appendix, one may reasonably elect a traditional incisional appendectomy. A simple mid or distal perforation can be handled in the usual fashion with or without the placement of a drain. A perforated base of the appendix or inflammation that extends to the base of the cecum is more difficult to manage. Again, even the skilled laparoscopic surgeon may elect to perform an open procedure in order to ensure the proper placement of Lembert sutures or a Z stitch to close the defect. However, as surgeons become more and more facile with intracorporeal suturing, the laparoscopic method may become the standard of care.

Another area of controversy is in the management of an intra-abdominal abscess. If an abscess is encountered during laparoscopic exploration, many surgeons convert the procedure to an open operation in order to ensure thorough irrigation and drainage of all potential regions of infection. Indeed, in some series the finding of an intra-abdominal abscess was the reason for conversion to an open procedure.[28] Drainage of a pelvic abscess can be more effectively performed via the open technique. Moreover, there is always the possibility of spreading the infection to other regions of the abdomen during the exploration or attempted drainage via the laparoscope.

Another area of controversy for some surgeons is action to be taken on finding a normal appendix. During an open exploration, the current teaching is to remove the appendix for two reasons: (1) the patient will always have a right iliac fossa incision, and if the patient has future abdominal pain, or more specifically right lower quadrant pain, no confusion will exist in making the diagnosis; and (2) chronic appendicitis is a well-known entity with microscopic changes that could be the cause of pain even despite a normal-appearing gross appendix. Since tactile sensation is lost during laparoscopy, what may appear normal through the laparoscope may

in fact be chronic inflammation; therefore, the current recommendation is the removal of the appendix.

Similarly, a question arises as to what to do with the appendix when performing another laparoscopic procedure. Since the incidence of appendicitis is low in the older age group, the potential risks of incidental appendectomy outweighs the benefits of this procedure. This knowledge is controversial because gynecologists frequently operate for chronic pelvic pain and in doing so remove the appendix in order to simplify future diagnosis. In fact, there is a variable rate of pathology noted when removing an "incidental" appendix. Ikard[33] performed 47 incidental appendectomies on patients undergoing elective cholecystectomies and found appendiceal pathology in 6% of the cases. In contrast, von Rechenberg[100] reported abnormal appendices in 82.9% of 113 incidental appendectomies among 627 gynecologic laparotomies.

Technique

It is important to emphasize that the indications for performing a laparoscopic appendectomy should not be different from those for an incisional appendectomy.

As surgeons become more familiar with this minimally invasive technology, more and more difficult cases will be encountered. Currently, the only absolute contraindication for performing a laparoscopic procedure is generalized peritonitis. Previous abdominal procedures, abscesses, and obesity are relative contraindications for the novice. However, experienced laparoscopic surgeons are more aggressive.

Preoperative preparation is similar to that used for an open procedure. Patients are given intravenous antibiotics prior to the operation. Regardless of the individual surgeon's experience or skill, all patients must give consent for a formal laparotomy. After the induction of general endotracheal anesthesia, a nasogastric tube and an indwelling bladder catheter are placed to minimize the risk of trocar injury to the stomach and bladder, respectively. The patient is placed in the supine modified lithotomy position in Allen stirrups (Allen Medical, Bedford Heights, OH). The hips and knees should each be flexed no more than 15 degrees; greater flexion will hamper instrument movement. This position allows more flexibility for the surgeon, assistant, and designated camera operator.

The abdomen is prepared and draped in standard fashion to provide wide exposure. The patient is then placed in steep Trendelenburg position and a 1-cm transverse incision is made below the umbilicus. The Verres needle is introduced and correct placement is verified in four ways. First, the surgeon should have a manual tactile sense that the needle has entered the peritoneal cavity. Second, an audible noise should be appreciated as the needle enters the abdominal cavity. Third, a few milliliters of sterile water is placed on top of the vertically held needle conus. By lifting the anterior abdominal wall, negative intra-abdominal pressure is created and the liquid is drawn into the abdominal cavity. Fourth, high-flow insufflation should result in a gradual rise in intra-abdominal pressure. A rapid rise in pressure or the appearance of subcutaneous crepitus indicates preperitoneal needle placement. After pneumoperitoneum is established with carbon dioxide to a pressure of 15 mm Hg, the Verres needle is removed and a 10/12-mm trocar is placed through this infraumbilical port site. The camera is then introduced through the port and all subsequent work is undertaken under direct endoscopic visualization.

In general, the surgeon and assistant should be on the side opposite the pathology. Thus the left side is utilized for a laparoscopic appendectomy (Fig. 14–1). Furthermore, monitors can be placed either on the right side or between the legs. The surgeon will often stand between the legs if mobilization of the right colon is necessary.

Port placement may vary depending on the angle of the appendix (Fig. 14–1). Initially, a 10/12-mm trocar is placed through the periumbilical incision and a thorough visual exploration of the entire abdominal cavity and pelvis is undertaken. If the diagnosis of acute appendicitis is confirmed, additional trocars can be placed. The second 10/12-mm trocar should be placed in a suprapubic position, below the hairline just cephaled to the symphysis pubis. A grasping instrument, scissors, or endoscopic stapler can be used through this port and the camera can also be moved to that position prior to extraction of the appendix through the umbilical portal. A third trocar (5 mm) should be placed in the right upper quadrant lateral to the rectus muscle. A grasping instrument is used in this port in order to elevate the cecum. If an additional port is necessary for retraction, it should be 5 mm and placed in the right lower quadrant. If the patient has a mobile cecum, an additional port can also be placed in the midline between the first two trocars.

The dissection is begun by elevating the cecum and identifying the appendix. Complete visualization of the entire appendix from base to tip is mandatory to exclude the diagnosis of acute appendicitis. If only a part of the appendix is visualized it may be necessary to mobilize the peritoneal reflection of the right colon and cecum to properly expose a retrocecal appendix. If difficulty or excessive bleeding are encountered, the procedure should be converted to an open appendectomy. Conversion to laparotomy must be regarded as good judgment instead of a failure of laparoscopy. The word "failure" is inappropriate, as it connotes the inability of the surgeon to achieve the optimal result. However, ultimately the optimal goal is not a technical triumph for the surgeon but a safe operation for the patient.

Once the mesoappendix is in view, removal of the appendix can be performed. The distal end of the appendix is retracted laterally and a "window" is made between the vessels in the mesoappendix. Either clips, ligatures, staples, or electrocoagulation can be used for securing these vessels (Fig. 14–2). The appendiceal artery should be either doubly clipped proximally or divided with an endoscopic linear cutter stapler.

The stump of the appendix can be managed in a number of ways (Fig. 14–3). Pretied endoloops can be placed proximally and distally or large hemoclips can be utilized. Usually two clips are placed at the base and the third about 2 cm distally to prevent spillage of intraluminal contents. The appendix is then divided with scissors. A more popular method is an endoscopic linear cutter stapler instrument. Preliminary experience has demonstrated these instruments to effect a safe, easy, and rapid method of excision.[47] However, the staplers also add expense to the operation.

Inversion of the appendiceal stump can be performed if desired; however, most surgeons find a pursestring suture or a Z-stitch placement difficult. This change represents abandonment of well-elucidated surgical doctrine because of technical difficulty and not due to scientific data. Data to support this step have been shown in a prospective, randomized study of traditional appendectomies.[22] However, laparoscopy continues to

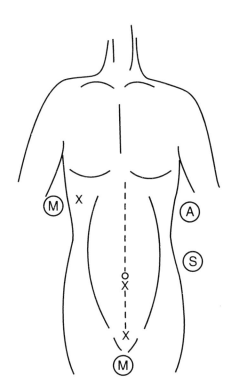

FIGURE 14-1. Port placement for appendectomy. (S = surgeon, A = assistant, M = monitor, X = port sites.)

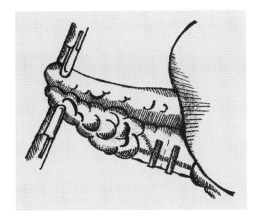

FIGURE 14-2. Ligation of appendiceal artery and mesoappendix.

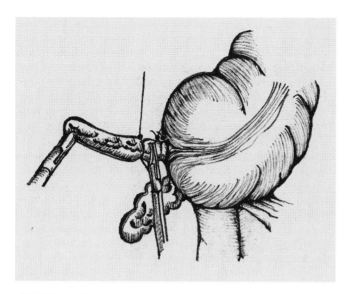

FIGURE 14-3. Ligation of the base of the appendix.

advance ahead of the studies that prove its merit. Only after widespread acceptance of the laparoscopic methods do the results, sometimes serendipitously, appear in support of the practices. However, one advantage in this ever-accelerating industry- and patient-driven quest to increase the scope of laparoscopic applications is that some traditional teachings can be proven to be in error. The issue of inverting the appendiceal stump may well be one such area. Through the technical challenge of laparoscopy, an unnecessary routine open surgical practice may be abandoned in open cases as well as in laparoscopic ones. However, in the absence of a prospective randomized trial, one's own practice and methods must be guided by beliefs more than by facts.

If marked inflammation of the distal appendix is noted or difficulty is encountered in mobilization, retrograde dissection can be performed as initially described by Schultz and associates.[81] Hemoclips or a stapling device can be placed across the base of the appendix followed by skeletonization of the appendix with ligation of the mesoappendix in the manner already described. The free base of the appendix can then be grasped, pulled medially or laterally, and the remaining appendix can be dissected from the retroperitoneum.

Removal of the appendix can be performed in several ways. If the appendix is small and noninflamed, it can be drawn within one of the 10/12-mm trocars and the entire organ and trocar can be removed together. If the appendix is long and thickened from inflammation, a commercially available bag can be placed intraperitoneally and the appendix inserted within this bag prior to removal (Fig. 14–3, *inset*). This maneuver should potentially lessen the chance of wound contamination and appendiceal rupture. Some surgeons use the finger of a sterile surgical glove for this purpose. Since the bag containing the inflamed appendix is too big to be brought into the trocar, the trocar is removed and the bag is grasped with clamps and manually removed. The camera should be moved to the supraumbilical portal and the extraction done through the umbilical trocar, as a

cosmetically superior result will occur from a slightly enlarged umbilical portal as compared to the suprapubic site. Inspection and irrigation of the abdominal cavity can be performed and hemostasis obtained either after the appendix is removed or just prior to extraction. The decision to use an intraperitoneal drain should not be dependent on the use of the laparoscope. In general, drains are utilized only for the evacuation of an abscess cavity and not to drain the peritoneal cavity after routine appendectomy.

The trocars should be removed under direct vision to ensure that there is no bleeding or hematoma formation from the port sites. The final umbilical trocar is removed and the incisions are closed. Many surgeons close the fascia of the 10/12-mm trocar sites because of reports of small bowel herniation through these defects.[73] The skin can be closed in any manner desired.

Postoperatively, the nasogastric tube and Foley catheter are removed; also, the patient should ambulate the evening of surgery. Antibiotic and pain management is the same as after incisional appendectomy. Diet can be advanced depending on how the patient progresses clinically, with hospital discharge anticipated generally 2 to 3 days after surgery.

Results

Laparoscopic surgeons have espoused that laparoscopic appendectomy confers many advantages over the standard incisional appendectomy. Diagnosis, intraoperative decision making, and postoperative care are claimed to be simplified, with a better cosmetic result and more rapid return of normal activity. Most of these claims, however, have been made without properly designed large, randomized, prospective studies. There are, however, a few published trials.

Atwood and co-workers[5] prospectively randomized 62 consecutive patients. Thirty were randomized to laparoscopy and 32 to a classical open appendectomy. All patients had signs and symptoms of acute appendicitis. The laparoscopy group was discharged home earlier (2.5 versus 3.8 days, $P < .01$). Postoperative complications were more frequent after open appendectomy. Follow-up showed less pain, shorter bed stay at home, and a faster return to work and athletic activities after laparoscopic appendectomy. They concluded that in terms of patient comfort, complications, and early and late recovery, the laparoscopic approach is superior to open appendectomy. They further recommended that laparoscopy be the approach of choice in all patients with suspected acute appendicitis.

In a similar study by McAnena and colleagues,[48] 65 patients with signs and symptoms of acute appendicitis necessitating surgery were assigned to open ($n = 36$) or laparoscopic ($n = 29$) appendectomy. The mean postoperative stay was shorter for the laparoscopy group (2.2 versus 4.8 days, $P < .05$). Wound infection was more frequent for the open group (11% versus 4%, $P < .05$), and there was a higher number of intramuscular injections of analgesia for the open group (median 5 versus 1, $P < .05$). They concluded that laparoscopic appendectomy resulted in a shortened hospital stay and a significantly diminished wound infection rate. Patients were quite satisfied with the cosmetic result. However, they stated that prospective randomized trials with greater numbers are required to ascertain the true role of laparoscopic surgery in acute appendicitis.

In addition, Kum and associates,[41] assessed 137 patients diagnosed with acute appendicitis. They were prospectively randomized to either open or laparoscopic appendectomy. Patients with either perforated appendicitis or histologically normal appendices were excluded from comparison. The length of time for the operation was similar as was the amount of pain medicine in the immediate postoperative period. There was no difference in the delay before tolerating fluids or diet, or in the length of hospital stay between the two groups. There were five (8.8%) wound infections in the conventional group compared with none in the laparoscopy group ($P < .01$). Although the authors claimed that patients were able to return to full activities after laparoscopy sooner than after open surgery, the difference was not statistically significant.

In general, these prospective randomized trials clearly show a benefit in selected cases of laparoscopic appendectomy. However, further properly constructed studies will be necessary in order for this procedure to become the standard of care. Moreover, the potential for translation of these results from a high-volume specialty practice setting to the average surgical practice is unknown.

Another issue in the minds of every surgeon today is cost. Sosa and colleagues[89] retrospectively reviewed 41 consecutive laparoscopic appendectomies performed over an 18-month period and compared them with 41 randomly selected open cases. Time from surgery to discharge was considerably shorter for patients who underwent laparoscopic appendectomy, for both nonperforated (45.3 versus 74.6 hours) and perforated appendicitis (137.7 versus 183.3 hours). The two groups were similar as regards age, sex, pathologic diagnoses and perforation rates. There were no complications unique to the laparoscopic group. Operative time was longer for the laparoscopic appendectomy group with nonperforated acute appendicitis. The authors attributed this fact to the learning curve of the residents performing the procedure.

In the only direct comparison of total hospital cost, Cohen and Dangleis[15] prospectively compared their first 26 laparoscopic appendectomies with age- and sex-matched controls. Although there was a 1-day reduction in hospital stay, it did not compensate for the increased operating room costs. This expense caused an overall higher hospital cost for the laparoscopic appendectomy group. However, they concluded that the overall cost-effectiveness was superior for the laparoscopic group, since the time to full recovery was significantly shorter (11.1 versus 23.7) days.

As also stated earlier in this chapter, certain "advantages" of laparoscopy may not be strictly attributable to the laparoscope. For instance, could the rate of wound infection after standard appendectomy be decreased by the routine use of an impervious wound protector to keep the appendix away from cut tissue surfaces? Could feeding and discharge from the hospital be accelerated after standard appendectomy? Such applications of laparoscopic methods to standard surgery may improve the results of surgery in all patients regardless of the method.

COLECTOMY

The use of the laparoscope in the field of colon and rectal surgery is still in its nascent stages in terms of the ease, efficacy, and safety of colonic mobilization, resection, and anastomosis. Not only should laparoscopic colectomy be regarded as a new technique but its role in the staging and treatment of colorectal carcinoma has yet to be defined. In May 1991, the American Society of Colon and Rectal Surgeons (ASCRS) stated that laparoscopic colorectal surgery should only be undertaken in a setting in which properly constructed prospective data retrieval will occur.[65] The Society of American Gastrointestinal Endoscopic Surgeons (SAGES) published similar guidelines.[77] Because of these statements, many centers began to prospectively assess the safety and efficacy of laparoscopic colon and rectal surgery.[23,109]

The collection of prospective data will serve two important purposes. First, it will enable the precise definition of any advantages and disadvantages as well as indications and contraindications for laparoscopic colectomy. Second, by these specific definitions, it is hoped that the problem seen in New York will be obviated.[42] As reported in the *New York Times* on June 14, 1992, because of the multitude of "serious or life-threatening complications," the legislators of that state have removed from surgeons the ability to credential each other. Subsequently, SAGES proposed specific training and credentialing guidelines. The establishment of a ubiquitous statewide policy that refuses to acknowledge differences in individual skills or practice settings is a dangerous and sobering prospect. It is hoped that by the application of sound surgical principles as well as common sense, a parallel situation will not develop in laparoscopic colectomy.

In order to facilitate these goals, several precepts are of paramount importance. First, never forsake fundamental tenets of surgery to facilitate inadequate technology. The different manufacturing companies are continuing to develop a spectrum of instruments that enable safe application of basic surgical principles. Second, accept only those maneuvers during a laparoscopic procedure that would be acceptable during an open procedure. This statement applies to handling of the bowel, manipulation of the tumor, fashioning of the anastomosis, management of the mesenteric defect, and all other steps in the procedure. If a given technique violates the accepted principles, an alternate technique should be applied. If an alternate technique is not available or not suitable, the laparoscopic phase should be terminated. Third, conversion to a laparotomy should not be considered failure but good surgical judgment. Willingness to increase the morbidity and mortality are unacceptable. Fourth, never favor a triumph of technology over sound common sense. A case in point is the laparoscopic right colectomy with intracorporeal anastomosis. Since a small incision is necessary for removal of the specimen, an extracorporeal anastomosis can save much time and money and may result in less contamination relative to an intracorporeal anastomosis. Surgeons have described successful intracorporeal right hemicolectomy utilizing two cameras, two surgeons, up to 14 ports, up to 11 applications of an endoscopic stapler, and requiring double the time and triple the cost needed for a standard right hemicolectomy. In addition to these disadvantages, an incision is still required to remove the specimen.[109] Even though there have been some encouraging preliminary results, there have been no prospective randomized trials or other statistically valid data to prove the superiority or even the equivalence of laparoscopic colectomy as compared to standard laparotomy.

Laparoscopic colorectal surgery is markedly different from all of the other laparoscopic procedures being performed. In fact, all of the other attempted procedures have several common denominators. First, all of these other procedures are performed in a relatively fixed intra-abdominal location. From a practical point of view, this feature is of paramount importance, as there is virtually no need for intraoperative repositioning of instruments, monitors, ports, and personnel. The pathology is always in the anticipated position.

Second, the other operations include either no vascular division (herniorrhaphy or fundoplication) or limited vascular division (cholecystectomy, appendectomy). Thus, vascular control can be rapidly and inexpensively undertaken. Conversely, the colonic mesentery includes numerous, large vessels. Thus, vascular control requires considerably more time and quite often considerably more cost than in the other procedures.

Third, in none of these procedures is an anastomosis fashioned. The dissection, mobilization and mere harvesting of an organ or suturing a defect in situ requires certain skills and instrumentation. However, the advanced skills and equipment necessary for a tension-free, well-vascularized anastomosis are obviously different. Furthermore, although the failure of sutures or staples after laparoscopic hernia or fundoplication may or may not result in recurrence, this complication may be asymptomatic. Conversely, the failure of a bowel anastomosis is a potentially lethal complication associated with significant increases in morbidity, length of hospitalization, cost, and mortality.

Fourth, the other procedures entail either removal of a small specimen, or no retrieval at all. There is no specimen removal in either laparoscopic herniorrhaphy or laparoscopic fundoplication. The specimens removed during laparoscopic appendectomy and cholecystectomy can be easily delivered via one of the 10-mm trocars or stab wounds, thus allowing surgery without an incision. Removal of a properly resected segment of colon with its attendant mesentery requires either a very large port or a small incision.

Fifth, none of the other currently performed laparoscopic procedures includes the cure of a malignancy. Again, there is a marked difference in clinical sequelae between an asymptomatic hernia recurrence and an early pelvic recurrence after resection of a rectal carcinoma. The major morbidity after laparoscopic cholecystectomy, appendectomy, herniorrhaphy, or fundoplication is usually seen in the intraoperative or immediate postoperative period. However, recurrent neoplasia may not be discerned for 2 to 5 years. Furthermore, if such recurrences are initially asymptomatic, and appropriate prospective randomized trials are not utilized, laparoscopic recurrence rates reported will be erroneously low in the absence of diligent routine long-term postoperative assessment.

These major differences demand a different approach to laparoscopic colorectal surgery as compared to other procedures. Surgeons throughout the world are clearly cognizant of these differences as noted by the paucity of laparoscopic colorectal literature as compared with the abundance of publications regarding other procedures.

The need to convert any laparoscopic procedure to an open operation should not be considered a failure; conversely, it must be considered good judgment. For the reasons enumerated above, most of the colorectal procedures are, at least technically, amenable to the laparoscopic or laparoscopic-assisted approach. Such procedures include segmental or total colectomy, small bowel resection, anastomosis of a Brooke ileostomy or an end-descending colostomy to a Hartmann's pouch, and creation of an ileostomy or a colostomy. All of these procedures can be undertaken either completely laparoscopically or as assisted procedures.

One of the major concerns for the colorectal surgeon is the proposal that the colon be transanally delivered. Physiologic data have confirmed that even appropriate use of the transanal circular stapling device results in decreased resting pressures.[31] This injury pattern is due to the detrimental effect of internal anal sphincter dilation. Even in a well-controlled setting, limited sphincter dilation results in at least transient, and possibly permanent, decreased resting internal anal sphincter pressure that can translate into varying degrees of anal incontinence.[8] Given the unphysiologic effects of rapid but gentle controlled introduction and removal of a 3-cm diameter circular stapling device, it is easy to understand that forcible uncontrolled transanal delivery of the sigmoid colon and its mesentery would not be beneficial to the anal sphincter mechanism. Advocates of this particular technique of specimen removal have yet to demonstrate either objective manometric or subjective functional data to prove the physiologic acceptability of this technique.

Since there is no proof of the acceptability of transanal specimen removal, and given the published reports that refute the advisability of this type of approach,[105] there is no question that presently the specimen must be transcutaneously extracted. Specifically, both segmental and total colectomy specimens must either be delivered through a small incision or retrieved through a large port.

Indications and Contraindications

Current universally accepted indications for laparoscopic bowel resection include only benign conditions, and palliation for malignancy. It has been suggested by the ASCRS that laparoscopic colorectal cancer resections should only be performed in prospective randomized trials. This guideline resulted from the problems that will be discussed later in this chapter.

Essentially any of the commonly performed colorectal operations that can be performed open have the potential for being done laparoscopically. In theory, all colorectal conditions could be successfully treated by the laparoscopic approach. It would seem prudent, however, to limit laparoscopic bowel resections to elective situations in which the bowel is not compromised and has been properly prepared with mechanical cleansing. Similarly, there are no absolute contraindications except for gross fecal peritonitis. Obesity, previous abdominal incisions, and a large abscess or phlegmon may require more skill and can be very frustrating for the novice. In general, common sense should dictate patient selection. However, although the laparoscope will not make a marginal surgeon into an excellent one, it may unfortunately cloud the judgment and hamper the skills of the latter. No laparoscopy course or textbook chapter can impart to the surgeon the requisite common sense to help ensure good results.

The instruments available for laparoscopic colon resections are changing daily. Initial products were too small, as they were designed specifically for laparoscopic cholecystectomy and not laparoscopic bowel surgery. Present enthusiasm for the application of this technology for diseases of the colon and rectum, however, have led to the rapid development of larger and more appropriate instruments for intestinal surgery.

Preoperative Preparation and the Initiation of Laparoscopic Surgery

The most important facet of preoperative preparation is the decision to perform laparoscopy. The patient must be counseled as to the potential risks, benefits, alternatives, and complications. The patient must be aware of the surgeon's experience and whether or not data are being scrutinized. All patients must also give consent for a laparotomy. Preoperative preparation for laparoscopic colon and rectal surgery is the same as for open procedures.[103] All patients undergo a standard mechanical cathartic bowel preparation on the day prior to surgery. In addition, both oral and broad-spectrum parenteral antibiotics are administered.

As for appendectomy, after the induction of general endotracheal anesthesia, a nasogastric tube and an indwelling bladder catheter are placed to minimize the risk of trocar injury to the stomach and bladder, respectively. All patients are placed in the supine modified lithotomy position in Allen stirrups (Allen Medical, Bedford Heights, OH). The hips and knees should each be flexed no more than 15 degrees; greater flexion will hamper instrument movement. This position allows transanal colonic access should colonoscopic identification of the site of a small lesion be required. This maneuver is more important in a laparoscopic colectomy than in a laparotomy situation, as tactile sensation is lost in the former condition.

Current technological constraints demand either the often prohibitively expensive use of multiple staples or force a compromise in basic surgical tenets. Exercise of this latter option requires leaving open ends of bowel within the peritoneal cavity during at least part of the anastomotic procedure. The sequelae of fecal contamination are potentially disastrous. Moreover, anecdotal cases of postoperative intraperitoneal abscess and even death have been reported after such cavalier, misguided adventures. In addition, multiple tales of inadvertent and even unrecognized enterotomies during dissection have been reported. All patients with polyps or other localized pathology should be prepared to undergo intraoperative colonoscopy. The equipment should be prepared and available in the operating room during all laparoscopic colectomies. The surgeon performing the resection or one of the assistants must be capable of safely and rapidly performing the colonoscopic exam. The ability to use the colonoscope for intraoperative intracolonic lavage and verification of bowel preparation is an added advantage of the supine modified lithotomy position.

The abdomen is prepared and draped in standard fashion to provide wide exposure. The patient is then placed in steep Trendelenburg position, and placement of the Verres needle and insufflation of the abdominal cavity is performed as previously described in this chapter for appendectomy.

Regardless of the type of resection contemplated, there must be adequate exposure of the intraperitoneal structures allowing the surgeon and assistants good visualization. Thus, as in open procedures where both incision location and length are crucial to facilitate these important goals, port placement for laparoscopic colon and rectal surgery assumes an equally important role. Furthermore, the objective that some surgeons can accomplish with six or more ports may in reality, with good traction and countertraction, be reached with only three or four ports.

The selection of port sites depends on both the patient's body habitus and the type of resection. In general, it is important that ports be close enough to one another so that instruments can reach the operative field with ease and aid in traction, yet not so close as to cause intracorporeal clashing of the instruments ("swordfighting"). If future incisions are planned, such as for a drain, stoma, or for specimen removal and anastomosis, attempts should be made to place the ports in these locations. The previously placed port sites can be either enlarged or several can be incorporated within the incision.

It is important to note that all ports should be at least 10 mm in diameter for laparoscopic intestinal surgery for two reasons. First, unlike the gallbladder, the target organ is not fixed or localized and thus the camera and all instruments must be able to be used in all ports. In laparoscopic intestinal surgery, there is frequent need for repositioning both the camera and instruments in order to ensure adequate visualization around the colon and rectum. Hence, the use of 10-mm ports ensures maximal surgical flexibility. Second, in order to markedly decrease the size of a Kocher cholecystectomy incision, the ports utilized for laparoscopic cholecystectomy must be as few in number and as small in diameter as possible. This feature is critical, since a Kocher incision is often only 8 to 10 cm in length. However, an appreciable reduction from a standard 25- to 30-cm midline incision can be realized even after the introduction of five or more 10/12-mm ports.

For right colectomy, two monitors are used, each positioned at a 45-degree angle, one near the head of the bed, the other near the foot (Fig. 14–4). The surgeon and assistant stand on the left side of the patient. After the initial umbilical port is placed, subsequent ports are placed under direct vision, one suprapubic to the left of the rectus muscle and the other adjacent to the umbilicus to the left of the left rectus muscle. A fourth trocar may be needed in the right iliac fossa to fully mobilize the hepatic flexure. However, this fourth port is initially omitted and is inserted only as needed.

For sigmoid colectomy, both the surgeon and assistant stand to the right side of the patient, while the monitors are being placed to the patient's left and at the foot of the bed at 45-degree angles (Fig. 14–5). After the initial umbilical port is placed, a second trocar is placed in the suprapubic position, slightly to the right of the right rectus muscle, while a third port is placed at the same level as the infraumbilical port in the midclavicular line.

For a loop ileostomy or sigmoid colostomy, the Veress needle should be placed above the umbilicus to allow adequate distance between the camera and stoma site. After exploration, the second trocar should be placed under direct vision through the previously marked stoma site. Once it has been determined that the small bowel will reach beyond the abdominal wall with no tension, an 18-mm port is used to replace the lateral trocar

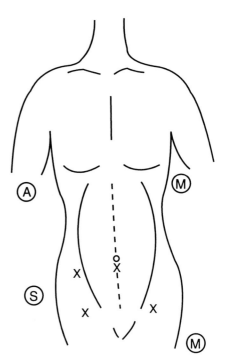

FIGURE 14–5. Port placement for sigmoid colectomy. (S = surgeon, A = assistant, M = monitor, X = port site.)

(Fig. 14–6). The bowel is gently grasped, the abdomen desufflated and the trocar with the attached bowel delivered, the fascia scored, and the stoma primarily matured. It is also of paramount importance to laparoscopically reinspect both the bowel and mesentery to ensure viability, hemostasis, and proper rotational alignment. Similar principles are utilized for the creation of a sigmoid colostomy. The 18-mm port also can be used for insertion of a linear stapling device.

The port placement for a total abdominal colectomy is a combination of the two segmental colectomies (Figs. 14–4 and 14–5). Both the camera and surgeon must be moved in order to facilitate the proper angle for safe mobilization.

It should be noted that optimal port placement for various bowel resections is still evolving as experience is being gained with laparoscopic colon and rectal surgery. Certainly, "ideal" port placements will vary depending on the body habitus of the individual patient and disease entity. For example, for a thin patient with a chronic ileocecal volvulus, three properly placed ports could complete the laparoscopic mobilization. Both the resection and anastomosis could be performed through one of the port sites after enlargement. For this reason, we prefer not to place all ports prior to beginning of the dissection, but to add ports as needed after the initial exploration to assess the location of the pathology.

Dissection and Mobilization

Prior to attempting mobilization, a thorough and complete inspection of the abdominal cavity should be performed as in open surgery. All abdominal wall adhesions are lysed in order to allow safe placement of

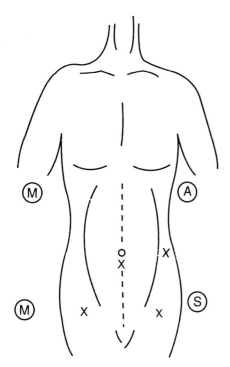

FIGURE 14–4. Port placement for right colectomy. (S = surgeon, A = assistant, M = monitor, X = port site.)

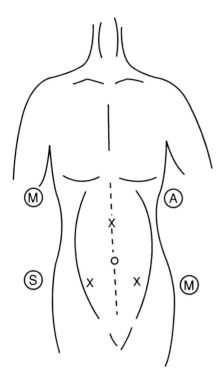

FIGURE 14-6. Port placement for ileostomy. The camera is inserted through a supraumbilical port. The working port is placed within the right rectus muscle at the future ileostomy site. For sigmoid colostomy, the set-up is a mirror-image of that illustrated, the working port being inserted through the left rectus muscle at the site of the colostomy. (S = surgeon, A = assistant, M = monitor, X = port site.)

subsequent trocars. Adhesiolysis is best accomplished by a combination of traction and division with the monopolar electrocautery. There are many advantages of the monopolar cautery as compared to laser for laparoscopic colectomy, including greater operator familiarity with cautery, much lower overall costs, and less equipment in an already crowded operating room. Furthermore, the potential for inadvertent injury to adjacent organs is a major disadvantage of the laser.

It is of paramount importance to remember that table positioning can facilitate the retraction of loops of bowel from the operative field. For example, when mobilizing the sigmoid colon, placing the table in Trendelenburg position with a tilt to the right can help to keep the small bowel loops away from the pelvis. Similarly, when mobilizing the hepatic flexure, reverse Trendelenburg and a table tilt to the left can be most helpful. If further retraction is needed, an assistant can insert a laparoscopic retractor through one of the previously placed ports. It also may be necessary to add additional ports to aid in retraction.

Mobilization of the colon from the retroperitoneum is accomplished by grasping the colon with specially designed noncrushing intestinal clamps and retracting in a medial direction, thus exposing the white line of Toldt. This avascular plane can then be divided with a combination of blunt and sharp dissection; electrocautery is used for both dissection and hemostasis. If larger vessels are encountered at the flexures, ligation with either surgical clips or endoloops can be performed.

Once full mobilization is accomplished, the mesenteric vascular supply can be divided. If an extracorporeal anastomosis is planned, this vascular ligation can also be done in an extracorporeal fashion. However, intracorporeal vascular division is necessary if an intracorporeal anastomosis is planned and can also be performed prior to exteriorization for an extracorporeal anastomosis. Vascular division is best facilitated by careful skeletonization of the larger vessels and ligation with either clips or suture material. Most vessels are either double ligated or triple clipped. Alternatively, an endoscopic linear cutter stapler with a 30- or 35-mm vascular cartridge can be used for mesenteric division. Once the mesentery is divided and the lines of resection are free of mesentery, the bowel is ready for transection.

Segmental Resection and Intracorporeal Anastomosis

The technique used for dividing the bowel will be determined in part by the planned subsequent anastomosis. The endoscopic linear cutter stapling instrument creates two stapled ends of bowel, thereby minimizing spillage of intraluminal contents. This method is certainly preferred to the potential spillage that can easily occur if the bowel is transected and left opened within the peritoneal cavity. Despite diligent preoperative bowel preparation and the use of atraumatic occlusive bowel clamps, fecal contamination is always possible, and its consequences are potentially disastrous. Furthermore, if both the proximal and distal limbs of the bowel are occluded with clamps, two additional ports would be necessary for subsequent manipulation and anastomosis. Detachable alligator clamps may solve this problem. Therefore, the endoscopic stapler is a very valuable instrument for both anastomotic construction and preliminary bowel transection. With the newer, longer staplers available for this purpose, intracorporeal anastomosis is a viable option.

After each end of the bowel segment to be resected is divided, the bowel ends are grasped with Babcock clamps and the antimesenteric corners of each staple line are excised. A side-to-side (functional end-to-end) anastomosis is then created with one or more additional applications of the endoscopic stapler in the same manner as in an open operation. The cut edges of the bowel are then grasped with Babcock clamps and the anastomosis is inspected for hemostasis. The lumen can be irrigated with saline, povidone-iodine, or both. The opposing cut edges of the bowel are held with clamps and the enterotomy is closed with one or more additional firings of the stapler. The bowel to be excised is then removed through one of the large ports. The mesenteric defect can either be closed with a suture or a series of EMS hernia clips (Ethicon Endosurgery, Cincinnati, OH).[14]

One of the controversies surrounding laparoscopic colon surgery is the need for preoperative marking or localization of lesions. Because of the loss of tactile sensation with the use of this technology, small lesions or inflammatory masses may be missed. In point of fact, there have already been two case reports of the wrong segment of colon removed during laparoscopic segmental resection secondary to the inability to feel and confirm the lesion.[43,51] There have also been three cases in which postoperative bowel obstruction required laparotomy for an unrecognized synchronous proximal lesion.[24,49] Either preoperative marking or intraoperative localization may aid in alleviating this major complication. However, such maneuvers add significant cost and time and have their own possible complications.

If the decision is made to retrieve the specimen through an abdominal incision, an extracorporeal anastomosis is appropriate. If desired, intracorporeal mesenteric vascular ligation can still be undertaken. The bowel can even be divided to allow extirpation of the specimen within a bag. However, one must be cautious as pre-exteriorization bowel division predisposes to a 180- to 360-degree rotation of one or both limbs prior to anastomosis.[105] Alternatively, after full intracorporeal mobilization, a small incision is made in the abdominal wall, usually by enlarging one of the laparoscopic ports, through which the mobilized colon is then delivered. The bowel is divided, and either a handsewn or a stapled anastomosis is created. This technique takes advantage of the ability to laparoscopically mobilize, thereby permitting a reduction in the size of the incision required to remove the specimen and create the anastomosis. The resection and anastomosis can be accomplished in the more familiar inexpensive, safe, rapid fashion. In addition, performance of an extracorporeal anastomosis allows for suture reinforcement of any nonhemostatic portions of the staple line. Furthermore, imbrication of the closed apical enterotomy and placement of a stitch to remove tension from the end of the staple line can be undertaken.

Because of the technical difficulty of intracorporeal mesenteric defect closure, some surgeons have not closed the mesentery, creating the possibility of an internal hernia. Cases of postoperative bowel obstruction requiring open repair of the defect have been reported.[7] Extracorporeal anastomosis permits rapid and technically facile mesenteric defect closure. Compromise of this accepted surgical principle is an invitation for complications. Table 14–1 delineates the definition of laparoscopic, laparoscopic-assisted, and converted procedures.

Anterior Resection

An intracorporeal stapled anastomosis is appealing due to the avoidance of the tedious laparoscopic suturing demanded to effect a hand-sewn anastomosis. Transanal circular stapler introduction is a procedure already familiar to all surgeons. After laparoscopic mobilization of the sigmoid colon, its vascular supply is interrupted. There are then a number of options available to create the end-to-end anastomosis.

The rectum is mobilized to a point sufficiently distal to the lesion to permit endoscopic linear cutter stapler application through either a suprapubic, right iliac fossa, or left upper quadrant port. Sigmoidoscopic verification of stapler position and sigmoidoscopic rectal washout prior to stapler application are useful adjuncts.

TABLE 14-1. LAPAROSCOPIC, LAPAROSCOPIC-ASSISTED, AND CONVERTED PROCEDURES

LAPAROSCOPIC COLECTOMY
All of the following critical phases are performed through ports:
Mobilization
Vascular division/ligation
Bowel division
Anastomosis creation
Specimen retrieval

LAPAROSCOPIC-ASSISTED COLECTOMY
One or more of the following critical phases are performed through an incision:
Mobilization
Vascular division/ligation
Bowel division
Anastomosis creation
Specimen retrieval

CONVERTED PROCEDURE
Any unplanned incision
or
Any planned incision made either sooner than planned
or
Any incision >10 cm

A noncrushing bowel clamp can be applied distal to the lesion prior to washout and stapler application. This point again highlights the value of the supine modified lithotomy position.

The left upper quadrant port is then exchanged for an 18- or 33-mm (Ethicon Endosurgery, Cincinnati, OH) port to permit extracorporeal delivery of the sigmoid colon for resection. The proximal pursestring can then be applied in any manner desired after the specimen is removed. Subsequently, the anvil from a circular stapler is introduced into the proximal bowel and the bowel is then returned to the peritoneal cavity. The port site is then occluded. After re-establishment of pneumoperitoneum, the circular stapler is introduced transanally.

The trocar of the circular stapler is then used to pierce the rectal staple line. The anvil is fitted onto the receptacle post with the aid of a special modified Allis anvil grasping clamp. The ECS/CDH stapler (Ethicon Endosurgery, Cincinnati, OH) is preferred to the C-EEA (US Surgical, Norwalk, CT) because the trocar is fixed to the stapler handle. The C-EEA requires removal of a very sharp small piece of plastic, a potentially hazardous extra step in our opinion. Regardless of the stapler selected, the anastomosis is created in standard fashion including inspection of the donuts and either air or povidone-iodine verification of anastomotic integrity.[45]

Although not aesthetically pleasing, the bowel can be intracorporeally transected and a distal hand-sewn pursestring suture applied. This maneuver, however, requires infinite patience and has the potential for pelvic contamination. Alternatively, the rectum can be everted through the anus to permit cross-stapling with a standard linear stapler. The stapled rectum is then reduced into the pelvis with the circular stapler with the trocar recessed within the cartridge. The trocar can then be made to protrude through the staple line as described above.

Another potential technique is triple stapling. In this modification, the detachable head of the circular stapler is transanally inserted to a level above the proximal line of resection. The bowel is transected at proximal and distal ends with a linear stapling instrument. The shaft of the proximal cartridge is then delivered through the linear staple line. The stapling instrument is then transanally introduced, and an anastomosis is performed in the same fashion as described above for the double-stapled technique. This triple-stapled anastomosis has the advantage of obviating the need for a proximal or distal pursestring, but has the disadvantage of technical difficulties in positioning the cartridge above the proximal resection line and potentially seeding malignant cells at the proximal resection line.

Hartmann Reversal

The initial step is the mobilization of the stoma and introduction of the anvil of the circular stapling device. The stoma is then placed inside the abdomen. As much enterolysis as possible is performed through the stoma site, after which one or more ports are introduced under direct vision. Grasping the fascia at the stoma site allows lifting and safe insertion of one or more 10-mm ports without the need for either a preliminary Verres needle or for subsequent "blind" trocar insertion. The stoma site is then closed with appropriate suture material or occluded with an 18- or 33-mm port and pneumoperitoneum is established. All subsequent ports are 10 mm and are inserted under direct vision. The Hartmann pouch is mobilized after complete enterolysis. In order to facilitate this procedure, the entire sigmoid colon should always be removed at the initial operation. Complete sigmoid colectomy allows for easier transanal insertion of the circular stapling device. The rest of the steps are the same as for anterior resection or sigmoid colectomy with coloproctostomy.

Abdominoperineal Resection

This operation is, in many ways, ideally suited to the laparoscope. The camera's visualization of the pelvic structures such as the sympathetic nerves, the ureter, and levator muscles is probably superior to the human eye. Thus, the dissection and the need for low rectal placement of the linear stapler is obviated. Instead, after complete pelvic dissection, the sigmoid-descending junction is transected. The proximal bowel is then delivered, as described above, to create the stoma that should be delivered through a previously marked stoma site. Since all trocars are designed to spread the fascia and not cut this tissue, it is necessary to incise the fascia prior to maturing the colostomy. This maneuver will obviate the potential for obstruction due to normal postoperative stomal swelling.[94] The perineal phase is then completed in the usual open fashion. Furthermore, because of several reports of postoperative herniation at 10-mm port sites,[59,73,92] we routinely close all sites of 10 mm or larger. Port sites can be closed either under direct vision or with commercially available closure devices.[71]

PRESENT POSITION OF LAPAROSCOPIC COLECTOMY

No prospective randomized trials have been published to demonstrate the superiority or even the equivalence of laparoscopic colectomy. These data will only become available if qualified surgeons learn, develop, and apply these new techniques in a responsible fashion. At present, the steep part of the learning curve is still being collectively ascended. As our skills develop in tandem with improved instrumentation, it is hoped results too will improve. When prospective randomized trials are initiated, therefore, equivalent skills will be compared.

Currently, it is inappropriate to compare the results of standard colectomy in the hands of a skilled specialist with the results in the hands of a laparoscopic beginner. To test this issue we compared the results of laparoscopic-assisted colectomy (LAC) to open laparotomy (OC) in 71 patients. From August 1991 to September 1992, 36 patients underwent LAC and were prospectively evaluated. Thirty-five age-, sex-, diagnosis-, and procedure-matched OC controls were reviewed for comparison. Procedures and indications in these 71 patients included: right hemicolectomy for carcinoma ($n = 12$), total colectomy with end ileostomy for toxic colitis ($n = 2$), sigmoid colectomy for diverticulitis ($n = 2$) or carcinoma ($n = 2$), abdominoperineal resection for carcinoma ($n = 2$), low anterior resection ($n = 8$), total abdominal colectomy with ileorectal anastomosis for Crohn's disease ($n = 3$) or colonic inertia ($n = 5$), ileocecectomy for Crohn's disease ($n = 4$), and restorative proctocolectomy with ileoanal reservoir for ulcerative colitis ($n = 22$) or familial adenomatous polyposis ($n = 9$). Oral intake was begun on postoperative day (POD) 0 through 9 (mean, 3.7) after LAC and on POD 2 through 7 (mean 4.1) after OC. The patients were discharged home on POD 5 through 16 (mean, 7.7) after LAC and on POD 5 through 18 (mean, 8.2) after OC.

Similar results were noted after updating the ileoanal reservoir series. Sixteen patients underwent LAC, and 15 age-, sex-, and diagnosis-matched controls underwent OC. Ileus resolved after LAC on POD 0 through 5 (mean, 4.1) and after OC on POD 2 through 7 (mean, 4.3). Hospital discharge was on POD 6 through 13 (mean, 8.4) after LAC and on POD 7 through 18 (mean, 8.9) after OC. Thus, neither of our comparative studies confirmed the "inherent" advantages that are commonly espoused by laparoscopic enthusiasts.

However, advocates of laparoscopic colon and rectal surgery claim markedly different results. For instance, Geis[26] has claimed that benefits of laparoscopic colorectal surgery are real rather than theoretical. These benefits include (1) less fluid loss and fluid shift due to peritoneal exposure to the atmosphere, (2) less postoperative pain due to a small laparotomy incision, (3) less likelihood of adynamic ileus, and (4) shorter postoperative hospitalization. Jacobs and co-workers,[36] in a nonrandomized, noncomparative, preliminary pilot study, claimed that clear fluids "were tolerated" in 18 of 20 patients on POD 1. Fourteen of the 20 patients were discharged within 4 days of surgery. The problem with some of these results is that the rules were changed to accommodate this new technology. For example, Uddo[95] reported that his patients are also discharged on the fourth postoperative day. However, he noted that patients were discharged home taking only clear fluids before they had moved their bowels. Patients in whom he performed a standard open colectomy, however, remained in the hospital until they moved their bowels and tolerated a regular diet. The disparity in results is accounted for by application of different criteria to the two patient populations.

To assess whether altered management may have any effect on standard laparotomy patients, we performed a prospective randomized study to evaluate whether or not early postoperative feeding can be solely claimed as a benefit unique to laparoscopic surgery.[11] Sixty-four consecutive patients over a 3-month period underwent standard laparotomy with either a colonic or an ileal resection. In all cases the nasogastric tube was removed immediately after the operation. Group I consisted of 32 patients (age range, 15 to 81; mean, 52 years) who received a regular diet on the first postoperative morning. Group II consisted of 32 patients (age range, 15 to 87; mean, 52 years) who were fed in a traditional manner: regular food was permitted after resolution of ileus as defined by resumption of bowel movements in the absence of abdominal distention, nausea, or vomiting. The rate of nasogastric tube reinsertion for distention with vomiting was 18.7% (six patients) in group I and 12.5% (four patients) in group II (P = NS). In the 26 patients from group I who did not require nasogastric tube reinsertion, there was a shorter hospitalization (6.7 versus 8.0 days, respectively). A second, much larger prospective randomized study (n = 162) utilized clear fluids rather than a regular diet in the early oral feeding group (n = 81).[74] The difference resulted in a mean day of discharge of 6.2 days after laparotomy. Thus, laparoscopic surgeons' claim of shorter hospitalization and earlier tolerated oral intake may not be unique to laparoscopy.

When developing laparoscopic skills, it is both unwise and illogical to immediately attempt a completely intracorporeal procedure. Laparoscopic mobilization should be the initial step, followed by laparoscopic mesenteric division and bowel transection followed eventually by anastomosis. Ideal initial procedures include laparoscopic fecal diversion (either loop ileostomy or colostomy creation), closure of an end ileostomy as an ileoproctostomy or of an end colostomy as a coloproctostomy, and right hemicolectomy for benign disease.

While it may be technically feasible to perform more surgery laparoscopically, logic and good surgical judgment must prevail. There should never be a triumph of technology over reason. Specifically, one should endeavor to perform the laparoscopic phase of the procedure for a reasonable length of time. That length may vary from a few minutes after exploration to several hours. Progress must be monitored throughout the procedure and preparation should be immediately available for conversion to an open operation.

To reiterate, early or unplanned conversion is indicative of good, sound surgical judgment and not failure.

At every step in the procedure one must query as to whether or not that particular phase of the procedure would be acceptable in an open operation. This reasoning applies to ligation of the vessels, manipulation of the bowel, treatment of the pathology, creation of the anastomosis, and all other steps of the operation. If a given laparoscopic maneuver is not acceptable, an alternative acceptable one needs to be attempted. If one is not readily available, then the laparoscopic phase should be terminated and a laparotomy should be undertaken.

Failure to adhere to these basic surgical principles will have detrimental sequelae. A recent front page *New York Times* article recounted the graphic details of forsaken logic to facilitate inadequate technology.[3] The article recounted that during laparoscopic cholecystectomy, "some patients have bled to death, others have needed several additional operations to repair and reconstruct organs and tissues damaged in the surgery." In total, seven deaths and 185 serious or life-threatening complications were reported at 99 hospitals in New York State. This problem led to a precedent ruling that regardless of an individual surgeon's stature, skill, or practice setting, they must be supervised in the performance of at least 15 laparoscopic cholecystectomies prior to eligibility for credentialing. This dangerous precedent removes surgical credentialing from the medical arena and places it into the bureaucratic political one. See and colleagues reached a similar conclusion about laparoscopic urologic procedures.[84] To avoid similar problems emanating from laparoscopic colectomy, surgeons must adopt the uniform voice of caution. Slow measured progress with continuous critical prospective assessment is crucial. Lastly, benefits must be proven with well-designed prospective randomized trials rather than extrapolated from anecdotal reports.

Another area in which benefit is unproven is cost. Falk, Thorson, and co-workers at Creighton University independently received data from Wexner and Jagelman at Cleveland Clinic Florida, Lavery at Cleveland Clinic Foundation, and Beart at Mayo Clinic Scottsdale.[23] These four surgeons sent the medical records, videos, and hospital bills of 66 consecutive laparoscopic procedures to Thorson's group for review. The mean postoperative stay for laparoscopically completed sigmoid or right hemicolectomy was significantly less than that after standard sigmoid or right hemicolectomy (P<.02). However, the laparoscopic procedures were statistically significantly more costly than were the open ones (P<.05). Therefore the total hospital cost was identical for both procedures when the two groups were compared. Moreover, none of the procedures included the use and expense of intracorporeal staplers, which are very costly. Had staplers been used, the cost assessment would have favored the open procedures. The only studies that have shown any cost savings by laparoscopy have done so by subgrouping "converted procedures" to eliminate the "costly" procedures from the laparoscopic financial analysis.[29,53,87]

Again, however, one must assess the balance between technologic feasibility and sound logic. Kmiot[40] and co-workers prospectively compared the effect of laparoscopic-assisted colectomy (n = 40) and open procedures

(n = 40) with respect to the length of hospitalization, cost, and morbidity. The two groups were age, sex, diagnosis, and operation matched. There were no significant differences in operating time, duration of ileus, length of hospitalization, or total cost. There was also a trend towards decreased morbidity in the laparoscopic-assisted group. This was the first such study to clearly demonstrate that there may not be such a difference between laparoscopic-assisted colectomies and open operations.

A basic question of paramount importance is the appropriateness of this technology for the treatment of colorectal carcinoma. The current standard of care for the treatment of colorectal carcinoma is an abundant excision of lymph node–bearing tissue. However, no study has been able to demonstrate that patients will have longer survival rates when more positive lymph nodes are removed. Olson and associates retrospectively reviewed 572 patients and concluded that there is a significant rate of recurrence that is determined both by the number of involved lymph nodes and by the presence or absence of serosal penetration.[58] Also, there are a number of studies that have demonstrated a decrease in survival rate once five or more lymph nodes are involved with tumor.[30]

The major problem in quantifying the lymph nodes identified in each resected specimen is the enormous variability among institutions.[12] Various centers around the world have assessed different methods for detecting lymph nodes other than the traditional step-sectioning.[27,32] In an attempt to improve the harvest of lymph nodes from resected specimens, a technique of fat clearance using xylene and alcohol has been developed.[13,37] Cawthorn and colleagues,[13] in a trial of adjuvant preoperative radiotherapy for rectal cancer, used this technique. They identified a significantly greater number of lymph nodes (mean, 23.1) in the mesorectum than did the pathologist at either St. Mark's Hospital or the seven other centers in the same study that did not use the clearance technique (mean, 10.5). Their study also identified a greater number of lymph nodes with metastases in cleared compared with noncleared specimens (mean, 3.7 versus 1.9, respectively). In addition, in 41 cases of rectal carcinoma, Scott and Grace[82] found an average of 6.1 nodes per specimen identified by traditional step-sectioning of the mesorectum, while following fat clearance a total of 18.9 nodes per specimen was found. Chemical lymph node clearance has been used at the Ferguson Hospital since 1977. They reported a retrospective review of 864 cases of colon and rectal cancer and found a mean of 27 lymph nodes.[32] The problem is that they used only this technique and compared their results with other centers using a similar clearance technique, not with traditional step-sectioning. In contrast, Jass and co-workers,[37] found no significant difference in the number of lymph nodes harvested when traditional dissection and fat clearance methods were compared.

Because of this confusion in the literature we prospectively assessed the effectiveness of mesenteric lymph node assessment utilizing the traditional manual step-sectioning method as compared with a xylene fat-clearance technique.[17] In the first 41 consecutive colectomies, manual clearance of mesenteric lymph nodes was the only method of staging utilized. For segmental colectomies, the range was 1 to 98 (mean, 21.2) nodes and for total colectomies, the range was 76 to 101 (mean, 88.5) nodes. After the method of xylene clearance was established, all specimens first underwent traditional step-sectioning followed by xylene clearance. For subtotal colectomy and total colectomy, the mean number of lymph nodes harvested was 13.3 and 53, respectively. After xylene clearance, the additional number of nodes found was 3.9 and 14.5 for segmental and total colectomies, respectively. Only two of the lymph nodes harvested by the xylene clearance technique changed the disease stage. This clearance technique may be of added value if the pathologist does not routinely perform meticulous step-sectioning of the resected specimen.

In our 13 laparoscopic-assisted resections for cancer, standard step-sectioning revealed a mean of 19 (range, 3 to 84) lymph nodes.[104] This number is certainly reasonable when compared with any of the previously mentioned studies, regardless of the potential merit of clearance techniques. There were two patients with C lesions but the majority were Dukes A and Dukes B lesions.

In the multicenter study by Falk and associates, 66 patients who underwent laparoscopic or laparoscopic-assisted colon resections were analyzed.[23] One of the parameters detailed was the number of lymph nodes removed. The authors demonstrated that in both their sigmoid and right colectomy specimens for carcinoma there was no statistically significant difference among laparoscopic, converted, or historical control patients.

Jacobs[35] compared the number of lymph nodes harvested by laparoscopic right colectomy or rectosigmoid resections with traditional open surgery. The average number detected when a laparoscopic resection took place was actually more than with standard right colectomy (17 versus 14, P=NS); but the reverse was true with rectosigmoid resections (6 versus 10). Dodson and associates[20] reported on their experience with three laparoscopic-assisted abdominoperineal resections. Comparable node harvesting was demonstrated between their laparoscopic-assisted cases and traditional controls (4.2 versus 7.2, respectively). However, one might reasonably argue that neither 7.2 nor 4.2 nodes are appropriate after a curative abdominoperineal resection.

These reviews clearly emphasize the fact that in the majority of cases the pathologist has control over the number of lymph nodes found in any given specimen. The impact of the pathologist on the number of evaluated lymph nodes cannot be overlooked. There is no incentive for the pathologist to find more lymph nodes. The CPT code and thus reimbursement is the same if the pathologist finds 4 or 104 lymph nodes. Reality is such that there are undoubtedly many lymph nodes that go undetected. Another problem arises from the growing enthusiasm to prove the merits of laparoscopic colectomy for cancer. There may be more enthusiasm on the part of the pathologist to help their surgical friends by searching more diligently when reviewing laparoscopic specimens.

Another variable may be the location rather than the absolute number of lymph nodes. Shida and co-workers[88] recently evaluated the prognostic value of the stage of lymph node metastases in 357 patients who underwent curative resection for colorectal cancer. There was no significant difference in the 5-year disease-free survival (5DFS) between patients with one to three nodes and those with four or more nodes. Since the Japanese classify all lymph nodes only by their location, nodal status is defined by the location of positive nodes instead of the absolute number harvested. In this way, the classification system is simply based on their location and not contingent upon the operative procedure (i.e., the level of vessel ligation). This study demonstrated a 5DFS of 70% in those who had only local node metastasis (N_1) compared with 40% in those who had distant node metastases along the major vessels (N_2). More importantly, 12 of 38 (32%) patients with N_2 disease had only one distant node metastasis with no local node involvement (skip metastasis). When these same patients with skip metastasis were compared with the group of patients with N_1 patterns involving three or more positive lymph nodes, they too had a lower 5DFS (35% versus 57%, respectively).

Thus, if one examines the resected lymph nodes in terms of their location instead of the absolute number, more emphasis is placed upon the length and size of the resected mesentery than the absolute number of nodes. Specifically, review of 15 paracolic nodes may not be as accurate a prognosticator as study of 14 nodes well distributed along the inferior mesenteric artery. This would be especially true if none of the paracolic nodes have tumor but a single highest mesenteric node is involved. Thus, one must be critical of reports emanating from laparoscopy enthusiasts who justify oncologic radicality and acceptability based strictly upon the number of lymph nodes. Distal resection margins are another prognosticator of care.[38,110] The 2-cm distal margin is well accepted as the minimum level needed for curative rectal excision. Tate and co-workers, in a nonprospectively randomized study, assessed distal margins.[93] After laparotomy and anterior resection (mean tumor 15 cm from dentate line) in 14 patients, the minimum distal margin was 2.0 cm. After laparoscopic sigmoidectomy in 11 patients (mean tumor 20 cm from dentate line), the minimum distal margin was 5 mm. Although the authors concluded that the laparoscopic sigmoidectomies were as curative as were the open high anterior resections, their data refute their conclusion.

The adverse effects of pneumoperitoneum have been well documented.[9] These effects can be classified as either pressure effects from the gas or the nature of the gas used. Some of these adverse effects include decreased return of blood from the legs and a commensurate increased risk of deep venous thrombosis. Additional problems include interference with ventilation and cardiac function causing hypotension or hypertension in addition to dysrhythmia; absorption of carbon dioxide, which can cause acidosis and hypercapnia; and the risk of air embolism. Furthermore, it has been determined that upon release of the pneumoperitoneum, the gas may contain particulate matter such as viruses.[76]

If air under pressure enters the bloodstream, is it possible for tumor cells to do the same? The 15- to 16-mm Hg sustained intraperitoneal pressure exceeds both capillary and lymphatic pressure and may also surpass pressure in the terminal venules. If tumor cells are forced into lymphatics and possibly veins, the potential for distant dissemination exists. Such a problem translates into increased distant recurrence. This complication would not be recognized in the perioperative period and therefore has been ignored by staunch laparoscopy proponents. This theoretical adverse sequela may become apparent after appropriate long-term prospectively randomized assessment is completed.

Another potential problem that has recently been recognized is one of local wound recurrence of tumor cells in port sites of patients undergoing laparoscopic or laparoscopic-assisted colectomy for cancer. The Paul-Mikulicz operation, popularized in the early part of this century, involves resection of loops of large bowel by an extracorporeal technique.[99] Although initially popular because of a reduction in operative mortality, this procedure lost its appeal due to the high incidence of local recurrence, with recurrence in the wound being the most common.

Alexander and co-workers, in a letter to the editor of *The Lancet*, reported a 67-year-old female who 3 months after a curative laparoscopic-assisted right hemicolectomy for a Dukes C adenocarcinoma, presented with a wound recurrence of her tumor.[2] There have also been numerous additional cases of port-site recurrences.[7,24,56,57,107] The real concern is not only wound recurrence in patients with Dukes C disease—some of these patients had Dukes A and B lesions. O'Rourke and co-workers described an 82-year-old woman who 10 weeks postoperatively presented with two port-site recurrences. Her initial lesion was moderately well-differentiated with no lymph node involvement (Dukes B).[60] Furthermore, not all port-site recurrences have occurred in the port of retrieval of the specimen. Fusco and co-workers reported a trocar site abdominal wall recurrence 10 months after a laparoscopic-assisted right hemicolectomy.[25] At colonoscopy, the patient was felt to have an early cancer. The final pathology revealed a T_3,N_1,M_0 lesion, with 4 of 11 resected lymph nodes positive for metastatic carcinoma. They concluded that the questions surrounding the efficacy of laparoscopic colectomy in the eradication of colorectal carcinoma support the need for prospectively randomized trials.

The best evidence for isolated port-site recurrence was presented by Wade and co-workers.[40] They reported a 59-year-old female who underwent a laparoscopic cholecystectomy for chronic calculous cholecystitis. The pathology specimen revealed an unsuspected polypoid carcinoma. Twenty-one days later, at the time of elective re-exploration, several isolated 4- to 6-mm fibrotic inflammatory nodules were palpable in the peritoneum of the umbilical port site. Frozen section revealed a nidus of metastatic gallbladder carcinoma approximately ten cells in diameter in one of the nodules. The authors postulated that the umbilical recurrence was a single-cell implantation at the time of initial laparoscopy. They used a doubling-time model for a sphere to confirm the

21-day growth spurt. These authors concluded that "this demonstration of cancer recurrence in laparoscopic port sites may limit the application of laparoscopy to elective cancer resection." Similarly, Jacobi and associates reported a 73-year-old female who underwent a laparoscopic cholecystectomy for symptomatic cholelithiasis. The procedure was converted to a laparotomy for "technical reasons." The pathologist identified a microscopic adenocarcinoma. Two months after surgery, the patient presented with implants at two port sites but not at the laparotomy incision. Thus, the implantation preferentially sought the port sites and avoided the laparotomy incision.[41] Because of these multiple concerns, the American Society of Colon and Rectal Surgeons does not condone or endorse laparoscopic colectomy for care of malignancy outside the confines of a prospective randomized trial.[69]

RESULTS OF CLINICAL EXPERIENCE

Recently, there have been several studies to document the potential advantages of laparoscopic and laparoscopic-assisted colon and rectal surgery. Phillips and associates[63] reported 51 laparoscopic colectomies performed by several surgeons at two different institutions in two states. Seven cases (14%) were converted to laparoscopic-assisted cases and four (8%) were converted to open procedures; thus, the total conversion rate was 22%. Indications included cancer, diverticulitis, endometriosis, regional enteritis, villous adenoma, and polyps. One concern was that the circular stapled anastomosis was incomplete in five cases (18%). Most series of open surgery report incomplete donuts in only 2 to 3%.[45] Thus, in the rush to prove the benefits of the completely laparoscopic coloproctostomy, the authors have instead beautifully illustrated a compromise in surgical technique to facilitate a technology. Operative time averaged 2.3 hours and one patient required blood transfusion. Clear liquids were administered until the third postoperative day. No patient required parenteral narcotics after the second postoperative day. Discharge from the hospital ranged from 1 to 30 (mean, 4.6; SD ± 4.1) days. Four patients had postoperative complications (8%), and one patient died from pneumonia. Patients who were working were able to return to work 1 week after the operation. They concluded that laparoscopic colectomy can be performed safely, but that a surgeon's awareness of his or her limitations and capabilities will be the difference between reckless or safe surgery.

One concern obviously is the six- to ninefold increase in the incidence of incomplete anastomosis. Although Phillips and co-workers recognized and treated this problem, such technical imperfections are fodder for postoperative disaster in the hands of the laparoscopic neophyte. It is also important to note that 8 of 51 patients (16%) underwent colotomy and wedge resection for polyps. This procedure has been shown to increase the rate of local recurrence[52] as compared to standard resection. Colotomy is not the standard of care. It represents another departure from accepted surgical practice to facilitate utilization of an otherwise difficult technology. Its use in laparoscopy has been proven to be associated with early local wound recurrence after "curative" resection of Dukes A lesions.[44] Nonetheless, such a compromise may account for shorter hospitalization.

Corbitt[19] was able to complete 15 of 18 attempted laparoscopic-assisted colectomies. In three patients the colonic lesion could not be laparoscopically identified and conversion was performed. Indications for colon resection were adenocarcinoma in 15 patients (five left-sided and ten right sided), two large adenomas in the ascending colon, and one perforated diverticulum of the sigmoid colon. Five patients had undergone prior abdominal surgery. All intestinal anastomoses were performed extracorporeally using a stapling instrument. No operative complications or mortality were reported. The length of the operative procedure ranged from 45 to 90 (mean, 68) minutes. Some patients were able to begin oral intake as soon as the first postoperative day, whereas others had no oral intake for 72 hours. Nonetheless, the average length of hospitalization was still 4 (range, 3 to 6) days. Although not quantified, the authors stated there was a "marked reduction" in postoperative pain and discomfort reported by the patients.

Jacobs[36] performed, laparoscopic-assisted colon resections on 20 patients. Indications for surgery were large villous adenomas or adenocarcinoma in 12, diverticular disease in five, sigmoid endometrioma in one, cecal volvulus in one, and inflammatory bowel disease in one. The mean length of operative procedures was 170 (range, 95 to 255) minutes for sigmoid colectomies and 155 (range, 110 to 260) minutes for right colectomies. There were no reported intraoperative complications, clear liquids were tolerated in 18 of the 20 patients on postoperative day 1, and 14 patients were discharged by day 4. Three patients developed a postoperative complication: hemorrhage requiring transfusion, edema of a rectosigmoid anastomosis requiring a decompressing rectal tube, and a mechanical small bowel obstruction requiring a second operation. The authors concluded that although this procedure is considered in evolution, it "will become as accepted as laparoscopic cholecystectomy."

Quattlebaum and associates[68] reported on 40 laparoscopic-assisted colon resections. Indications included cancer, diverticulitis, and a variety of other benign conditions. Procedures were generally completed in 30 to 90 minutes. There was no reported intraoperative mortality or morbidity. Gastrointestinal function, defined as intake of solid food with flatus or bowel movements, returned an average of 2.5 days after surgery. The average hospital stay for patients with benign colonic lesions was 4.2 (range, 3 to 12) days and was 4.6 (range, 2 to 6) days for those patients with malignant conditions. Postoperative complications occurred in six patients, the most severe being a transient late anastomotic obstruction that resolved spontaneously and a persistent abdominal wall hemorrhage at a trocar insertion site. They also report one patient with a Dukes C splenic flexure carcinoma who developed a local recurrence at 1 year. They concluded that this approach is a cost-effective alternative in the therapy of most colon lesions. However, no cost data were included in the study. Moreover, the oncologic merit of their approach must be questioned in light of a local recurrence after resection of a *colonic* neoplasm. Ultimately, we must question which data represent the better result for the patient—rapid discharge from the hospital or rapid recurrence of carcinoma. Again, one must be honest and detailed during the informed consent procedure.

Scoggin and colleagues[82] also reported shorter hospitalization and less patient discomfort. Twenty patients underwent laparoscopic-assisted large and small bowel surgery. Indications for surgery included polyps (ten), carcinoma (two), arteriovenous malformations (two), endoscopic perforation (one), and inflammatory bowel disease (five). Operative time ranged from 40 to 280 (mean, 178) minutes. Vessel ligation was performed intracorporeally while all anastomoses were hand sewn extracorporeally. There was no reported intraoperative morbidity or mortality. Average time for return of bowel function as marked by the patient reporting flatus was 1.9 days and oral feeding 2.3 days. However, the median postoperative hospital stay was five days. There was no mortality and morbidity was 20%, including a urinary tract infection, urinary retention, a postoperative blood transfusion, and a small bowel obstruction that required laparotomy for an internal hernia.

All of the above studies were performed on unselected groups of patients without comparison to standard open operations. Peters and associates[62] reviewed their experience with 28 attempted laparoscopic and laparoscopic-assisted colectomies and compared them to 33 patients who underwent similar procedures at the same institution by the same surgeon (OC). The two groups were similar with respect to age, weight, and the types of procedures performed. Twenty-four were successfully completed. Conversion was due to intraoperative bleeding, invasive carcinoma, or an ileosigmoid fistula. The operative times for the LAC group were significantly longer than for the OC group. However, patients also regained bowel function significantly earlier (2.7 versus 4.0 days), tolerated a regular diet earlier (2.3 versus 4.6 days), and had a markedly diminished length of stay (4.8 versus 8.2 days). Postoperative complications were noted in three (13%) patients, including a wound infection, urinary retention, and a urinary tract infection. Many surgeons claim a subjective decrease in blood loss after laparoscopic as compared to standard colectomy.[87] Peters,[62] however, measured both preoperative and 24-hour postoperative hemoglobin levels as an indirect indicator of operative blood loss. They demonstrated no statistically significant difference between the two groups, although there was a trend towards a greater fall in the laparoscopic group (more intraoperative blood loss using the laparoscope). We recently reviewed 808 cases of laparoscopic or laparoscopic-assisted colectomy published in the English language literature.[102,108] The mean length of hospitalization was 7.1 (range, 1 to 40) days. Without the laparoscope, Rajagoad and co-workers reported a mean stay of 6.3 days during 1993, decreased from 9.4 days during 1984.[69]

Similarly, Senagore and co-workers[87] assessed 140 colonic resections which included 102 OL and 38 LAC

cases. There were no significant differences with respect to surgical indications, age, or perioperative morbidity. However, the LAC group required significantly more operative time as compared to the OC group. Only one conversion was performed secondary to uncontrolled bleeding and one enterotomy was created by a laparoscopic instrument that was successfully repaired laparoscopically. Bowel function returned quicker (3.0 versus 4.9 days) and hospital stay was significantly shorter in the LAC group (6.0 versus 9.0 days). The authors demonstrated that the cost for patients who received laparoscopic colon resections was less than that for patients who underwent a standard laparotomy ($2,300; P = NS). The modest increase in operating room cost (approximately $1,000) was offset by reductions in postoperative care. Savings came not only from a reduction in hospital stay but also from administration of fewer pharmaceutical agents, intramuscular injections, and intravenous infusions.

Vayer and associates[97] examined the cost-effectiveness of laparoscopic-assisted colectomy versus open resection. Despite the higher cost of operating room time and equipment, the total cost of laparoscopic-assisted colectomy was not statistically different from open resection. They claimed that the cost savings were due to a shortened hospital stay.

Not all laparoscopic colectomy trials have been so favorable in terms of patient benefit. Monson and colleagues[51] prospectively evaluated laparoscopic-assisted colectomy in 40 patients who required elective colonic excision mainly for malignant disease. Operations included right colectomy (n = 19), left hemicolectomy (n = 11), anterior resection (n = 6), abdominoperineal resection (n = 2), and subtotal colectomy (n = 2). A total of seven procedures were converted to open operations due to either anatomic uncertainty, tumor fixation to nearby organs, or removal of the wrong segment of colon. Another patient was converted to a standard subtotal colectomy with ileorectal anastomosis after a laparoscopic right colectomy revealed unsuspected multiple adenomatous polyps. The overall completion rate was 82.5%. The time taken to finish the procedure depended on the nature of the operation; mean time for a right colectomy was 210 (range, 120 to 310) minutes while for a left-sided resection it was 240 (range, 150 to 330) minutes. Among the 40 patients in whom laparoscopic resection was attempted, one patient died of a myocardial infarct 24 hours after surgery. There were two anastomotic leaks, one after a right colectomy and the other after an anterior resection. Both resolved without an operation. Two patients developed pneumonia and there were two urinary tract infections. Excluding the single death, the mean postoperative hospital stay was 8 (range, 5 to 14) days. All patients were discharged when normal bowel function returned. When the authors assessed their previous 30 open colectomies, they found the mean postoperative stay was 14 days (range, 7 to 31), however, no information was given with respect to the nature of these operations and a mean hospital stay of 14 days is quite prolonged.

Schmitt and co-workers[80] prospectively compared the time to oral intake and to subsequent discharge from the hospital after LAC and OC. Forty-eight patients were prospectively evaluated and 45 age-, sex-, and procedure-matched OC controls were randomly selected and reviewed for comparison. Diagnoses were matched wherever possible. Oral intake was begun on postoperative day 0 to 7 (mean, 3.4) after LAC, and on postoperative day 0 to 8 (mean, 4) for OC. The patients were discharged from the hospital on postoperative day 5 to 16 (mean, 8.2) for LAC and on postoperative day 5 to 18 (mean, 8.1) for OC. The authors concluded that LAC did not appear to confer any advantage over OC in the time to oral intake or length of hospitalization. Similarly, this same group stratified their patients and individually assessed patients undergoing laparoscopic-assisted ileal pouch anal anastomosis (LAC) and prospectively compared them to age-, sex-, and diagnosis-matched controls (SC).[16] There were 22 and 20 patients in the LAC and SC groups, respectively. Ileus resolved on the fourth postoperative day in both groups (LAC mean, 4.1 [range, 0 to 5] days; SC mean, 4.3 [range, 2 to 7] days). Hospital discharge was on the eighth postoperative day in both groups (LAC mean, 8.4 [range, 6 to 13] days; SC mean, 8.9 [range, 7 to 18] days). Neither the length of time for ileus resolution nor the length of hospitalization was reduced in the LAC group.

Milsom and colleagues[50] reported their initial experience with laparoscopic-assisted ileocolectomy in patients with terminal ileal Crohn's disease. Nine patients underwent operation; there was no reported morbidity or mortality. The median time of operation was 170 (range, 150 to 210) minutes. All patients did well in the postoperative period and the median time interval to the first bowel movement was 5 (range, 4 to 6) days. The median postoperative hospital stay was 7 (range, 5 to 12) days. Although laparoscopic-assisted surgery is feasible in Crohn's disease, the authors noted no apparent differences compared with conventional surgery with respect to resumption of bowel function or length of hospital stay.

Similarly, Larach and co-workers[43] recently described their early experience with laparoscopic-assisted colectomy. Eighteen patients underwent laparoscopic procedures for benign and malignant colorectal pathology. In three of these cases, resections were not carried out secondary to abdominal wall bleeding, tumor infiltrating the abdominal wall, or diagnostic intervention alone. Seven patients (39%) had nine complications directly related to the laparoscopic procedure: two enterotomies, a partial ureteral obstruction, and resection of the wrong bowel segment. The mean length of operative procedures was 3 hours and 32 minutes (range, 1 hour to 8 hours and 35 minutes). There was one postoperative death. The mean length of hospital stay was 7.2 (range, 4 to 14) days. They concluded that laparoscopic-assisted colectomy will take more time to be assimilated into the armamentarium of surgeons than did laparoscopic cholecystectomy because of the greater technical difficulties. Furthermore, they stated that as instrumentation improves and the technique evolves, both the surgical results and operative time will likewise improve and they predict "wide acceptance" in the near future.

There still remain many unanswered questions in the laparoscopic management of diseases of the colon and rectum. Current resident training programs are teaching laparoscopy. The number of laparoscopic colon and rectal resections necessary to complete the learning curve has not yet been established. Certainly, a 1-day course does not constitute adequate knowledge and safety to perform all types of resections. The "significant cost savings" analyses in the literature never include the costs of the expensive instruments including cameras, video monitors, insufflator, recorders, printers, and cables. Nor do cost analyses ever include the expensive extra operating room time needed during the setup and takedown of the equipment necessary to perform cost-effective minimally invasive surgery. The cost effectiveness of both reusable and disposable instruments must be assessed.

CONCLUSION

It is important that science prevail and adequate prospective randomized trials be performed in order to answer the question of acceptability of laparoscopic technology for the cure of cancer.

Laparoscopy is a good tool that should be a part of every surgeon's armamentarium. There is no question that laparoscopic cholecystectomy has changed abdominal surgery forever. However, we must approach laparoscopic colon and rectal surgery with cautious enthusiasm in order to live up to the most important part of the Hippocratic oath: Primum non nocere—First, do no harm.

It is of paramount importance that the surgeon tell the patient honestly, whether if he or she personally required the same operation for the same pathology it would be undertaken with a laparoscope. A recent survey of the members of the American Society of Colon and Rectal Surgeons revealed that 47% of members perform laparoscopic colorectal surgery.[18] However, only 6% use the laparoscope in over 50% of resections. If the preoperative diagnosis is known to be cancer, 71% would use the laparoscope. However, only 6% of surgeons would have their own rectal carcinoma laparoscopically resected. We must not in our enthusiasm create a dual standard of acceptability—one for our patients and a different one for us.

REFERENCES

1. Addiss, D.G., Schaffer, N., Fowler, B.S., et al.: The epidemiology of appendicitis in the United States. Am. J. Epidemiol., 132: 910, 1990.
2. Alexander, R.J.T., Jaques, B.C., and Mitchell, K.G.: Laparoscopically assisted colectomy and wound recurrence (letter). Lancet, 341:249, 1993.
3. Altman, L.K.: Surgical injuries lead to new rule. New York Times, page 1, June 14, 1992.
4. Anderson, E.T.: Peritoneoscopy. Am. J. Surg., 35:136, 1937.
5. Attwood, S.E.A., Hill, A.D.K., Murphy, P.G., et al.: A prospective randomized trial of laparoscopic versus open appendectomy. Surgery, 112:497, 1992.
6. Bastien, J., Leconte, P., and Leconte, D.: Reflexions sur une série homogène de 5000 appendicectomies. Semin. Hop., 63:285, 1987.

7. Beart, R.W.: Presented at the Annual Meeting of the American Society of Colon and Rectal Surgeons. Orlando, May 8–13, 1994.

8. Beck, D.E., and Wexner, S.D.: Fundamentals of Anorectal Surgery. New York, McGraw-Hill, 1992.

9. Berci, G., and Cushieri, A.: Practical Laparoscopy. Baillière-Tindall, 1986.

10. Bernheim, B.M.: Organoscopy: Cystoscopy of the abdominal cavity. Ann. Surg., 53:764, 1911.

11. Binderow, S.R., Cohen, S.M., Wexner, S.D., et al.: Must early postoperative oral intake be limited to laparoscopy? Dis. Colon Rectum, 37:584, 1994.

12. Blenkinsopp, W.K., Stewart-Brown, S., Blesovsky, L., et al.: Histopathology reporting in large bowel cancer. J. Clin. Pathol., 34: 509, 1988.

13. Cawthorn, S.J., Gibbs, N.M., and Marks, C.G.: Clearance technique for the detection of lymph nodes in colorectal cancer. Br. J. Surg., 73:58, 1986.

14. Cohen, S.M., Clem, M.F., Wexner, S.D., and Jagelman, D.G.: An initial comparative study of two techniques of laparoscopic colonic anastomosis and mesenteric defect closure. Surg. Endosc., 8:130, 1994.

15. Cohen, M.M., and Dangleis, K.: The cost-effectiveness of laparoscopic appendectomy. J. Laparoendosc. Surg., 3:93, 1993.

16. Cohen, S.M., Nogueras, J.J., and Wexner, S.D.: Laparoscopic colorectal surgery: Ascending the learning curve (Abstract). Dis. Colon Rectum, 37(4):79, 1994.

17. Cohen, S.M., Wexner, S.D., Schmidt, S.L., et al.: Does xylene mesenteric fat clearance improve lymph node harvest after colon resection? Eur. J. Surg. (in press).

18. Cohen, S.M., and Wexner, S.D.: Laparoscopic colorectal surgery: Are we being honest with our patients? (Abstract). Dis. Colon Rectum, 37(4):21, 1994.

19. Corbit, J.D.: Preliminary experience with laparoscopic-guided colectomy. Surg. Laprosc. Endosc., 2(1):79, 1992.

20. Dodson, R.W., Cullado, M.J., Tangen, L.E., and Bonello, J.C.: Laparoscopic-assisted abdominoperineal resection. Contemp. Surg., 42:(1)42, 1993.

21. Dubois, F.: Laparoscopic cholecystectomy: Historical perspective and personal experience. Surg. Laparosc. Endosc., 1:52, 1991.

22. Engstrom, L., and Fenyo, G.: Appendectomy: Assessment of stump invagination versus simple ligation: A prospective randomized trial. Br. J. Surg., 72:971, 1985.

23. Falk, P.M., Beart, R.W., Wexner, S.D., et al.: Laparoscopic colectomy: A critical appraisal. Dis. Colon Rectum, 36:28, 1993.

24. Fingerhut, A.: Laparoscopic assisted colonic resection. In Jager, R., and Wexner, S.D. (eds.): Laparoscopic Colorectal Surgery. New York, Churchill Livingstone (in press).

25. Fusco, M.A., and Paluzzi, M.W.: Abdominal wall recurrence after laparoscopic-assisted colectomy for adenocarcinoma of the colon. Dis. Colon Rectum, 36:858, 1993.

26. Geis, W.P.: Laparoscopic right hemicolectomy (minimally invasive). Laparoscopic Colon and Rectal Seminar Syllabus; Ethicon Endosurgery, 1992.

27. Gilchrest, R.K., and David, V.C.: Lymphatic spread of carcinoma of the rectum. Ann. Surg., 108:621, 1938.

28. Gotz, F., Pier, A., and Bacher, C.: Modified laparoscopic appendectomy in surgery. A report of 388 operations. Surg. Endosc., 4:6, 1990.

29. Hoffman, G.C., Baker, J.W., Fitchett, C.W., and Vansant, J.H.: Laparoscopic assisted colectomy: An initial experience. Ann. Surg., 219(6):732, 1994.

30. Hojo, K., Koyama, Y., and Moriya, Y.: Lymphatic spread and its prognostic value in patients with rectal cancer. Am. J. Surg., 144:350, 1982.

31. Horgan, P.G., O'Connell, P.R., Shinkain, L.A., and Kirwan, W.O.: Effect of anterior resection on anal sphincter function. Br. J. Surg., 76:783, 1989.

32. Hyder, J.W., Talbot, T.M., and Maycroft, T.C.: A critical review of chemical lymph node clearance and staging of colon and rectal cancer at Ferguson Hospital, 1977–1982. Dis. Colon Rectum, 33:923, 1980.

33. Ikard, R.W.: Prospective analysis of the effect of incidental appendectomy on infection rate after cholecystectomy. South. Med. J., 80:292, 1987.

34. Jacobaeus, H.C.: Übersicht uber meine erfahrungen mit der Laparothorakoskopie. Munch. Med. Wochenschr., 57:2017, 1911.

35. Jacobs, M.: Laparoscopic colon resection: The Miami experience. Laparoscopic Colon and Rectal Seminar Syllabus. Ethicon Endosurgery, 1992.

36. Jacobs, M., Verdeja, J.C., and Goldstein, M.S.: Minimally invasive colon resection (laparoscopic colectomy). Surg. Laparosc. Endosc., 1(3):144, 1991.

37. Jass, J.R., Miller, K., and Northover, J.M.A.: Fat clearance method versus manual dissection of lymph nodes in specimens of rectal cancer. Int. J. Colorectal Dis., 1:155, 1986.

38. Karanjia, N.D., Schache, D.J., North, W.R., and Heald, R.J.: 'Close shave' in anterior resection. Br. J. Surg., 77(5):570, 1990.

39. Kelling, G.: Über oesophagoskopie, gastroskopie und koelioskopie. Münch. Med. Wochenschr., 49:21, 1901.

40. Kmiot, W.A., Reiver, D., Cohen, S.M., et al.: A prospective comparison of laparoscopic versus open procedures in colorectal surgery (Abstract). Dis. Colon Rectum, 37(4):22, 1994.

41. Kum, C.K., Ngoi, S.S., and Goh, P.M.Y.: Randomized control trial comparing laparoscopic appendectomy to open appendectomy. Presented at the Annual Meeting of the American Society of Colon and Rectal Surgeons, Chicago, May 2–7, 1993.

42. Laparoscopic Surgery: New York State Department of Health Memorandum—series 92–20. Albany, New York, June 12, 1992.

43. Larach, S.W., Salomen, M.C., Williamson, P.R., and Goldstein, E.: Laparoscopic assisted colectomy: Experience during the learning curve. Coloproctology, 1:38, 1993.

44. Lauroy, J., Champault, G., Risk, N., and Boutelier, P.: Metastatic recurrence at the cannula site: Should digestive carcinomas still be managed by laparoscopy (Abstract). Br. J. Surg., 81(Suppl.): 31, 1994.

45. Lazorthes, F., and Chiotassol, P.: Stapled colorectal anastomosis: Properative integrity of the anastomosis and risk of postoperative leakage. Int. J. Colorectal. Dis., 1:96, 1986.

46. Lewis, F.R., Holcroft, J.W., and Boey, J.: A critical review of diagnosis and treatment in 1000 cases of appendicitis. Arch. Surg., 110:677, 1975.

47. Ludwig, K.A., Cattey, R.P., and Henry, L.G.: Initial experience with laparoscopic appendectomy. Dis. Colon Rectum, 36:463, 1993.

48. McAnena, O.J., Austin, O., O'Connel, P.R., et al.: Laparoscopic versus open appendicectomy: A prospective evaluation. Br. J. Surg., 79:818, 1992.

49. McDermott, J.P., and Devereaux, D.A.: Pitfall of laparoscopic colectomy: An unrecognized synchronous cancer. Dis. Colon Rectum, 37(6):602, 1994.

50. Milsom, J.W., Lavery, I.C., Böhm, B., and Fazio, V.W.: Laparoscopic-assisted ileocolectomy in Crohn's disease. Surg. Laparosc. Endosc., 3(2):77, 1993.

51. Monson, J.R.T., Darzi, A., Carey, P.D., and Guillou, P.J.: Prospective evaluation of laparoscopic-assisted colectomy in an unselected group of patients. Lancet, 340:831, 1992.

52. Morson, B.C., Whiteway, J.E., Jones, E.A., et al.: Histopathology and prognosis of malignant colorectal polyps treated by endoscopic polypectomy. Gut, 25:437, 1984.

53. Musser, D.J., Boorse, R.C., Madera, F., and Reed, J.F., III: Laparoscopic colectomy: At what cost? Surg. Laparosc. Endosc., 4(1): 1, 1994.

54. Nadeau, O.E., and Kampmeier, O.F.: Endoscopy of the abdomen. Abdominoscopy: A preliminary study, including a summary of the literature and a description of the technique. Surg. Gynecol. Obstet., 41:259, 1925.

55. Nakhegivany, K.B., and Clarke, L.E.: Acute appendicitis in women of childbearing age. Arch. Surg., 121:1053, 1986.

56. Ngoi, S.S.: Laparoscopic colorectal surgery. Presented at the International Society of University Colon and Rectal Surgeons, 15th Biennial Congress. Singapore, July 2–6, 1994.

57. Nduka, C.C., Monson, J.R.T., Menzies-Gow, N., and Darzi, A.: Abdominal wall metastases following laparoscopy. Br. J. Surg., 81: 648, 1994.

58. Olson, R.M., Perencevich, N.P., Malcolm, A.W., et al.: Patterns of recurrence following curative resection of adenocarcinoma of the colon and rectum. Cancer, 45:2969, 1980.

59. O'Donovan, S.C., and Larach, S.W.: Postoperative herniation of

small bowel through a laparoscopy port site. Coloproct, *16*(2): 98, 1994.

60. O'Rourke, N., Price, P.M., Kelly, S., and Sikora, K.: Tomour inoculation during laparoscopy (letter). Lancet, *342*:368, 1993.

61. Pahlman, L., and Glimelius, B.: Local recurrences after surgical treatment for rectal carcinoma. Acta Chir. Scand., *150*:331, 1984.

62. Peters, W.R., and Bartels, T.L.: Minimally invasive colectomy: Are the potential benefits realized? Dis. Colon Rectum, *36*:751, 1993.

63. Phillips, F.H., Franklin, M., Carroll, B.J., et al.: Laparoscopic colectomy. Ann. Surg., *216*(6):703, 1992.

64. Pier, A., Gotz, F., and Bacher, C.: Laparoscopic appendectomy in 625 cases: From innovation to routine. Surg. Laparosc. Endosc., *1*:8, 1991.

65. Policy statement, American Society of Colon and Rectal Surgeons: Dis. Colon Rectum, *35*(1):5A, 1992.

66. Policy Statement, American Society of Colon and Rectal Surgeons. Dis. Colon Rectum, July 1994.

67. Putman, C., Gagaliano, N., and Emmens, R.W.: Appendicitis in children. Surg. Gynecol. Obstet., *170*:527, 1990.

68. Quattlebaum, J.K., Flanders, H.D., and Usher, C.H.: Laparoscopic assisted colectomy. Surg. Laparosc. Endosc., *3*(2):81, 1993.

69. Rajagopol, A.S., Thorson, A.G., Sentovitch, S.M., et al.: Decade trends in length of postoperative stay following abdominal colectomy (Abstract). Dis. Colon Rectum, *37*(4):26, 1994.

70. Ragland, J., Garza, J., and Mckenny, J.: Peritoneoscopy for the diagnosis of acute appendicitis in females of reproductive age. Surg. Endosc., *2*:36, 1988.

71. Reissman, P., Bernstein, M., Verzaro, R., and Wexner, S.D.: Port site fascia closure in laparoscopic assisted colectomy: A simple technique. Br. J. Surg. (submitted).

72. Reissman, P., Durst, A.L., Rivkind, A., et al.: Elective laparoscopic appendectomy in patients with familial Mediterranean fever (FMF). World J. Surg., *18*:139, 1994.

73. Reissman, P., Shiloni, E., Gofrit, O., et al.: Incarcerated hernia in a lateral trocar site — an unusual early postoperative complication of laparoscopic surgery. Eur. J. Surg., (in press).

74. Reismann, P., Teoh, T.A., Weiss, E.G., et al.: Is early oral feeding safe after elective colorectal surgery? Ann. Surg. (in press).

75. Ruddock, J.C.: Peritoneoscopy. Surg. Gynecol. Obstet., *65*:623, 1937.

76. Sackier, J.M.: The pneumoperitoneum. Laparoscopic Colon and Rectal Seminar Syllabus. Ethicon Endosurgery, 1991.

77. SAGES: Granting of privileges for laparoscopic general surgery. Am. J. Surg., *161*:324, 1991.

78. Saye, W.B., Rives, D.A., and Cochran, E.B.: Laparoscopic appendectomy: Three years' experience. Surg. Laparosc. Endosc., *1*(2):109, 1991.

79. Schreiber, J.: Experience with laparoscopic appendectomy in women. Surg. Endosc., *1*:211, 1987.

80. Schmitt, S.L., Cohen, S.M., Wexner, S.D., et al.: Does laparoscopic-assisted ileal pouch anal anastomosis reduce the length of hospitalization? Int. J. Colorectal Dis., *9*:134, 1994.

81. Schultz, L.S., Pietrafitta, J.J., Graber, J.N., and Hickok, D.F.: Retrograde laparoscopic appendectomy: Report of a case. J. Laparoendosc. Surg., *1*(2):111, 1991.

82. Scoggin, S.D., Frazee, R.C., Snyder, S.K., et al.: Laparoscopic-assisted bowel surgery. Dis. Colon Rectum, *36*:747, 1993.

83. Scott, K.W.M., and Grace, R.H.: Detection of lymph node metastases in colorectal carcinoma before and after fat clearance. Br. J. Surg., *76*:1165, 1989.

84. See, W.A., Cooper, C.S., and Fisher, R.J.: Predictors of laparoscopic complications after formal training in laparoscopic surgery. JAMA, *73*:2689, 1993.

85. Semm, K.: Endoscopic appendectomy. Endoscopy, *15*:59, 1983.

86. Semm, K.: Operative Manual for Endoscopic Abdominal Surgery. Chicago, Year Book Medical Publishers, 1987.

87. Senagore, A.J., Luchtefeld, M.A., Macheigan, J.M., and Mazier, W.P.: Open colectomy versus laparoscopic colectomy: Are there differences? Am. Surg., *59*(8):549, 1993.

88. Shida, H., Ban, K., Matsumoto, M., et al.: Prognostic significance of location of lymph nodal metastases in colorectal cancer. Dis. Colon Rectum, *35*:1046, 1992.

89. Sosa, J.L., Sleeman, D., Mckenney, M.G., et al.: A comparison of laparoscopic and traditional appendectomy. J. Laparoendosc. Surg., *3*:129, 1993.

90. Steiner, O.P.: Abdominoscopy. Surg. Gynecol. Obstet., *38*:266, 1924.

91. Stone, W.E.: Intraabdominal examination by the aid of the peritoneoscope. J. Kans. Med. Soc., *24*:63, 1924.

92. Storms, P., Stuyven, G., Vanhemelen, G., and Sebrechts, R.: Incarcerated trocar wound hernia after laparoscopic hysterectomy. Surg. Endosc., *8*:901, 1994.

93. Tate, J.J.T., Kwok, S., Dawson, J.W., Lau, W.Y., and Li, A.K.G.: Prospective comparison of laparoscopic and conventional anterior resection. Br. J. Surg., *80*:1396, 1993.

94. Teoh, T.A., Reissman, P., Cohen, S.M., Weiss, E.G., and Wexner, S.D.: Laparoscopic loop ileostomy (letter). Dis. Colon Rectum, *37*(5):514, 1994.

95. Uddo, J.: Laparoscopic colectomy. Presented at the University of Minnesota Postgraduate course. September 23–26, 1992.

96. Valla, J.S., Limonne, B., Valla, V., et al.: Laparoscopic appendectomy in children: Report of 465 cases. Surg. Laparosc. Endosc., *1*:166, 1991.

97. Vayer, A.J., Larach, S.W., Williamson, P.R., et al.: Cost effectiveness of laparoscopic colectomy. Dis. Colon Rectum, *36*:P34, 1993.

98. Veress, J.: Neves instrument zur ausführung von brust-oder bauehpunktionen und pneumothoraxbehandlung. Dtsch. Med. Wochenschr., *41*:1480, 1938.

99. Von Mikulicz, J.: Small contributions to the surgery of the intestinal tract. Boston Med. Surg. J., *148*:608, 1903.

100. von Rechenberg, K.N.: Die histopathologischen befunde bei gelegenheits appendektomien im rhamt gunakologisher laparotomient und ihre bedeutung fur die patientin. Geburtschilfe Frauenheilkd, *43*:273, 1980.

101. Whitworth, C.M., Whitmorth, P.W., Sanfillipo, J., and Polk, H.C.: Value of diagnostic laparoscopy in young women with possible appendicitis. Surg. Gynecol. Obstet., *67*:187, 1994.

102. Wexner, S.D.: Restorative proctocolectomy. *In* Jager, R., and Wexner, S.D. (eds.): Laparoscopic Colorectal Surgery. New York, Churchill Livingstone (in press).

103. Wexner, S.D., and Beck, S.D.: Sepsis prevention in colorectal surgery. *In* Fielding, L.P., and Goldberg, S.M. (eds.): Operative Surgery: Colon, Rectum, and Anus, 5th ed. London, Butterworth Heinemann, 1992.

104. Wexner, S.D., Cohen, S.M., Nogueras, J.J., et al.: Laparoscopic colorectal surgery: A prospective assessment and current perspective. Br. J. Surg., *80*:1602, 1993.

105. Wexner, S.D., James, K., and Jagelman, D.G.: The double-stapled ileal reservoir and anastomosis: A prospective review of sphincter function and clinical outcome. Dis. Colon Rectum, *34*:487, 1991.

106. Wexner, S.D., and Teoh, T.A.: Laparoscopic surgery in colorectal cancer. *In* Williams, N. (ed.): Colorectal Cancer. London, Churchill Livingstone (in press).

107. Wexner, S.D., and Cohen, S.M.: Port site metastases after laparoscopic surgery for cure of malignancy: A plea for caution. Br. J. Surg. (in press).

108. Wexner, S.D., and Reissman, P.: Laparoscopic colorectal surgery: A provocative critique. Int. Surg., *79*:235, 1994.

109. Wexner, S.D., and Johansen, O.B.: Laparoscopic bowel resection: Advantages and limitations. Ann. Med., *24*:105, 1992.

110. Williams, N.S., Dixon, M.F., and Johnston, D.: Reappraisal of the 5-cm rule of distal excision for carcinoma of the rectum. A study of distal intramural spread and of patients' survival. Br. J. Surg., *70*:150, 1983.

111. Zaaf, M., Roger, B., Vaur, J.L., et al.: Progrès diagnostique et mortalité de' une série de 1400 appendicectomies. Lyon Chir., *79*: 251, 1983.

Chapter 15

OSTOMY MANAGEMENT

LEE E. SMITH / GERALDINE M. HENEGHAN / LISA LINDBERG

Stomas are standard procedures in the practice of gastrointestinal surgery, and approximately 100,000 are performed annually in the United States.[30] In previous decades, the patient who received a stoma was often left to his or her own devices to determine how to best manage the stoma. Since the 1960s, a "visitor program," developed by the United Ostomy Association (UOA), has helped make rehabilitation easier, allowing a patient to witness that another person with the same condition has returned to being independent and well. A professional group, enterostomal therapy (ET) nurses, now plays an invaluable role in counseling and teaching patients both before and after surgery. Many ostomy supply companies have developed appliances that are flatter, lighter, odor-proof, and more adherent. Education is the key to success, and an informed patient becomes an ally. Thus, it would seem that there would be few problems with this consortium of help. However, the surgeon must select the proper patient and construct the ostomy in the correct site, with attention to details of technique, to achieve a good long-term result. Furthermore, the surgeon should know all the steps and problems of rehabilitation, even though this new cadre of assistants is available.

INDICATIONS

Generally, a permanent colostomy is performed for cancer of the rectum. Although lower anterior resections with a less extensive distal margin, and proctectomy with coloanal anastomosis, are decreasing the need for colostomy in cancer of the middle and upper thirds of the rectum, most cancers of the distal third of the rectum cannot be managed by transanal excision, and en block resection requires removal of the sphincter. Hence, a permanent stoma is necessary.

A permanent ileostomy is most often created after total proctocolectomy for inflammatory bowel disease. The number of permanent ileostomies is decreasing because of the innovative use of small bowel pouches, which serve as a "neorectum" when anastomosed to the anal sphincter. However, many people choose a permanent ileostomy because this is the fastest way back to health and work in single operation or because the pouch procedure fails and an ileostomy is necessary.

Temporary ostomies are usually performed to protect a distal site in the gut that is inflamed, infected, traumatized, obstructed, or tenuously closed. Generally, the site selected is the most distal bowel segment that will reach a suitable site on the abdominal wall without tension. These ostomies may be either loop or end type. A loop is usually faster to perform, but establishment of a good seal by an appliance is more difficult. The end ostomy reaches the skin surface more easily and can be made completely diverting if the concomitant mucous fistula is brought out through a separate opening in the abdominal wall or if the distal lumen is closed. Controversy still exists about whether a loop or end ostomy is preferable.

INTESTINAL CONTENTS

After ingestion, food passes down the esophagus into the stomach. Softening, early digestion, and liquefaction begin in the stomach. The pH in this organ is acid; however, across the pylorus, the pH becomes markedly basic because of pancreatic and biliary secretions and the succus entericus. This alkaline small bowel fluid is extremely corrosive to the skin. The liquid presented to the cecum is composed of nonabsorbed foods and secretions from the small bowel. As this material traverses the colon, water is resorbed and the stool becomes formed (Fig. 15–1).

PREOPERATIVE CARE

Counseling

Both the patient and the family will have fears about ostomy surgery. Questions regarding survival, prognosis,

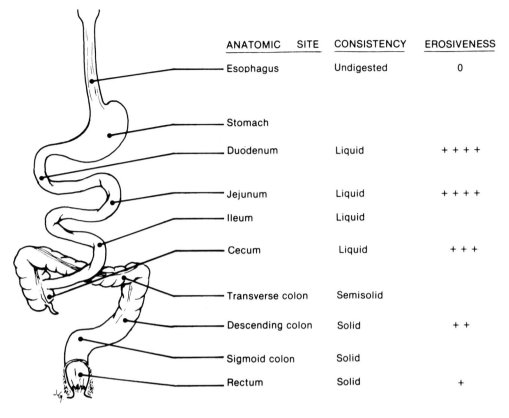

ANATOMIC SITE	CONSISTENCY	EROSIVENESS
Esophagus	Undigested	0
Stomach		
Duodenum	Liquid	+ + + +
Jejunum	Liquid	+ + + +
Ileum	Liquid	
Cecum	Liquid	+ + +
Transverse colon	Semisolid	
Descending colon	Solid	+ +
Sigmoid colon	Solid	
Rectum	Solid	+

FIGURE 15-1. Intestinal consistency and erosiveness. The stool becomes more solid as it progresses through the gastrointestinal tract. A stoma from the colon rather than the small bowel emits stool far less injurious to the skin.

and life with an ostomy need to be addressed. Rehabilitation for patients and their families begins with preoperative counseling. Some studies have examined the impact of preoperative teaching and counseling on patient outcome.[15,25,34] Decreased anxiety, a reduction in anesthesia, fewer complications, and a shorter hospital stay are some of the documented benefits associated with preoperative counseling.

Watson presents a model for meeting the needs of patients undergoing ostomy surgery.[57] Patient needs can be divided into three categories: information, technical skills, and emotional support. During the preoperative period, the greatest need is to understand the upcoming surgery. The physician should explain in lay terms the diagnosis, the surgical procedure that will be done, expectations after surgery, and the ostomy (i.e., the creation of an opening in the abdominal wall through which feces will pass).

Emotional support during the preoperative period is a critical component of patient care to allay concerns about survival, fear of pain, and a variety of individual issues. Discussion of these concerns with health care providers helps both patients and families. Patients who have a history of emotional problems should be referred for psychologic intervention throughout the period around surgery.[57]

Stoma Site Marking

The proper anatomic location of a stoma plays a major role in the quality of life after surgery. Selection of the appropriate site for the stoma maximizes comfort, improves appearance and appliance fit, and decreases

peristomal skin problems. The optimal stoma site meets the following location criteria: (1) it is within the rectus muscle and within the patient's visual field and; (2) it is away from the costal margin, the iliac crest, the umbilicus, the abdominal folds and creases, scars, and the natural beltline.[58]

A flat area approximately 8 cm in diameter must be sought (Fig. 15–2). The patient must be evaluated in the supine, standing, and sitting positions. With the patient in the supine position, several stoma sites may be selected overlying the rectus muscle, avoiding bones,

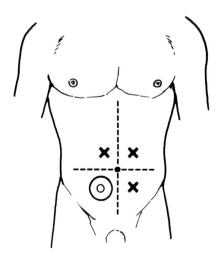

FIGURE 15-2. Stoma site selection. A round ostomy disk can be used to locate a flat site overlying the rectus muscle. An "X" indicates appropriate sites in each quadrant.

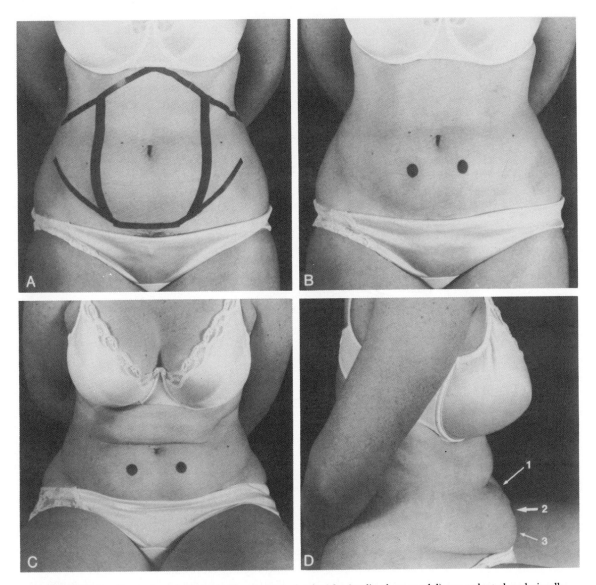

FIGURE 15-3. Stoma site selection. *A*, The anatomic landmarks (outlined on model) are palpated and visually identified. The costal margin, rectus muscle margin, symphysis, and iliac crest lines are drawn. *B*, Sites appropriate for a colostomy (the patient's left) and ileostomy (the patient's right) are marked on the model. *C*, Stoma sites are evaluated with the patient sitting upright to ensure a 6-cm flat pouching surface around the stoma. In the sitting position, abdominal fat folds and creases become visible. *D*, Stoma sites are evaluated from a lateral view for proper placement on the fat fold. *Arrow #1* indicates placement too close to a fold. *Arrow #2* indicates placement on the apex of the fat fold that is the optimal location. *Arrow #3* indicates placement out of the patient's visual field.

umbilicus, and scars (Figs. 15–2 and 15–3*A* through *C*). The patient is then seated in a chair and instructed to lean forward (Fig. 15–3*C*). If the preliminary sites selected while the patient was in the supine position are located within folds or creases, another site is chosen (Fig. 15–3*D*). When a stoma must be located on an abdominal fat fold, it should be placed on the apex of the fat fold to allow direct visualization of the stoma for pouch application (Fig. 15–4). Finally, the patient should be evaluated in the standing position and also with the hips flexed. Abdominal contours during movement and hip flexion may create folds or creases that might impair the pouch seal.

A skin barrier wafer or ostomy disk can be placed on the abdomen to select a flat site. When the best site is

found, a mark is made. Intradermal injection of methylene blue makes a tattoo that cannot be washed off, or a standard surgical marking pen makes a mark that can be sealed on the skin with a skin barrier film.

OPERATING ROOM CARE

At operation, proper site selection, adequate blood supply, and lack of tension on the stoma are the basic principles for success. The stoma is matured primarily and everted, creating a protruding "nipple" that is better for stool collection.[6] A new stoma should have a temporary appliance placed over it in the operating room. There will be little or no stool for the first day or two

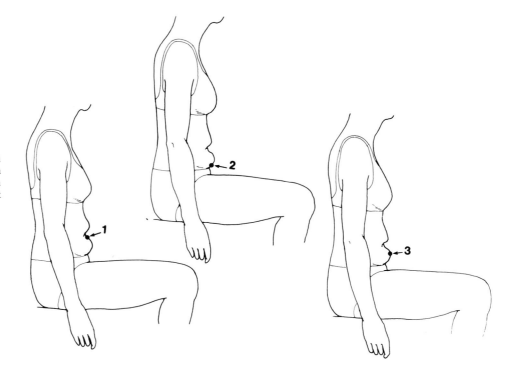

FIGURE 15-4. Stoma location on a fat fold. (*1*) Stoma site too high on the fat fold. (*2*) Site too low on the fat fold. (*3*) Site on the apex, at the optimal location.

while ileus resolves, but there is usually a small amount of blood and serous fluid to collect. The skin barrier wafer can be cut with at least a 2-mm margin around the stoma to allow for edema, which frequently follows operation. The postoperative pouch should be of a transparent material so that the stoma color can be monitored. For the first few days after surgery, the tip of the appliance should be draped laterally, so that it is dependent while the patient is at bed rest.

POSTOPERATIVE OSTOMY CARE

In the immediate postoperative period, the stoma is inspected frequently for color, condition of the mucocutaneous suture line, and drainage. A two-piece transparent drainable ostomy appliance offers ease of observation and allows access to the stoma for irrigation, if appropriate. Generally, the first pouch does not need to be removed until about the fourth postoperative day. By this time, patients are less tender and are able to participate in caring for their new ostomy.

Pouches

In the past, reusable or semireusable appliances were standard. Today, most patients are fitted with light-weight, odor-proof, disposable pouches (Fig. 15–5). The factors to consider when choosing a pouching system include the following: the type of ostomy; nature of the effluent; location of the stoma; firmness of the abdomen; presence of folds, scars, or creases; and the patient's age, functional abilities, dexterity, vision, and lifestyle. Often the patient tries different pouching systems to find the one that is most comfortable and reliable.

In the immediate postoperative period, a pouch is kept in place at all times. Later, some patients with a colostomy choose to irrigate to achieve regular, predictable bowel evacuation. If there is minimal spillage between irrigations, only a small disposable security cap is needed. One-piece security caps are available that adhere directly to the skin, or they are available in two pieces with a skin barrier, faceplate, and snap-on cap.

Patients who do not irrigate wear a drainable ostomy pouch. Because stool from the left colon is generally formed, a skin barrier is not usually necessary. With right-sided or transverse ostomies, the effluent is liquid: thus, protection with a skin barrier is necessary. For people with ileostomies, the erosive, frequent ileostomy effluent demands a secure fit by use of skin sealants and gelatin-pectin or synthetic skin barriers. If an acceptable fit cannot be achieved with disposable equipment, a reusable system may be better. If the ileostomy stoma is recessed or flush with the skin, a faceplate with convexity may be needed to achieve a seal. A variety of cements, belts, and supports are available to design a personal pouching system that permits cleanliness, security, and minimal changes each week.

Pouch Application

Before pouch removal, all equipment for the change —including the skin barrier, pouch, measuring guide or paper towel, tape, belt (optional), toilet paper, washcloth, and disposal bag—are assembled. The pouch is gently teased off the skin. The peristomal skin and the stoma can be cleansed with warm water (soap is not necessary) and dried well. The stoma is measured with a pattern, which should be 2 mm larger than the stoma to prevent pressure on the stoma during body movement or peristalsis. The chosen pattern is used to cut a hole in the skin barrier or pouch. As an alternative, there are a variety of disposable appliances with a precut opening in the skin barrier. With an ileostomy, a skin

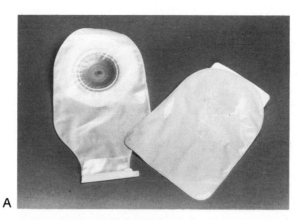

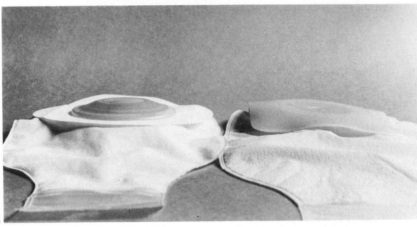

FIGURE 15-5. Ostomy supplies. *A,* On the left is a drainable pouch with a clip closing the end. On the right is a closed bag, which must be disposed of after a single use. *B,* On the left a convex faceplate is contrasted to the flat skin barrier on the right. *Illustration continued on opposite page*

sealant and skin barrier wafer are always used for skin protection. For a colostomy, a skin barrier or a karaya ring pouch may be sufficient.

The pouch should be emptied when it is one third full to avoid having the weight pull and break the seal. Pouch emptying is a simple procedure but requires practice. The patient sits on the toilet with the ostomy pouch hanging down between the legs. The pouch clamp is opened and the effluent drains out of the pouch. For cleaning, the pouch may be rinsed out with a cup of tap water.

Colostomy Irrigation

Descending and sigmoid colostomies may be irrigated to regulate stool elimination.[31,53] Tap water irrigation can be equated with an enema (Fig. 15–6). Cone tips are safer and easier to insert into the colostomy than a catheter. Only 500 ml of tap water is used initially to stimulate evacuation, but later, as needed, the volume may be increased to 1,000 ml.[39]

Irrigation is practical for patients with adequate bowel length, no diarrhea, a history of regular bowel movements, mental competency, and manual dexterity. Unless contraindicated, the decision to irrigate is a personal one. Some patients feel that irrigation offers freedom, whereas others feel that it takes too much time. When successful, irrigation offers a regular, predictable elimination pattern, and only a small stoma covering is needed for security between irrigations. A 1992 study by Sanada and associates[48] reported that ostomates who irrigate have fewer anxieties than those who use natural evacuation. Of 214 ostomates studied, those using natural evacuation experienced more trouble in daily activities and had more evacuation-related concerns than the irrigation group.

An ileostomy is never irrigated for regulation. In the case of a food blockage, 100 to 200 ml of water may be instilled through a catheter to break the blockage; this may be repeated several times, and the catheter may be repositioned for different flow (Fig. 15–7).

Psychologic Effects

Even with an uncomplicated postoperative surgical course, the emotional impact of an ostomy can be quite negative.[30,32] The patient is faced with a profound change in the body, and feelings of inadequacy and depression are common. How well the patient adjusts to an altered body image has an impact on the ability to enter interpersonal relationships, experience and express sexuality, and move through the process of rehabilitation.

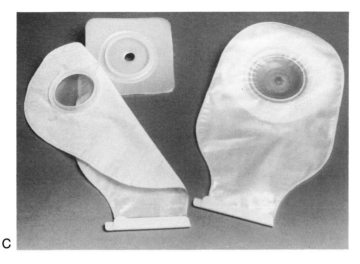

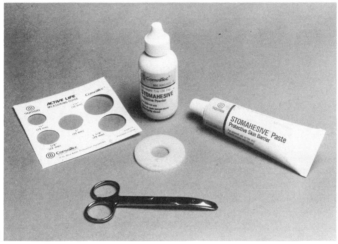

FIGURE 15-5. *Continued. C,* A two-piece appliance is shown on the left. The skin barrier can be left on the skin while the pouch can be unsnapped and removed for cleaning. The one-piece appliance on the right must be pulled off the skin in order to change the appliance. *D,* Typical supplies for managing an ostomy: a template for measuring the ostomy size, curved scissors, gelatin and pectin powder, skin barrier paste, and an adhesive sealing ring.

The diagnosis and prognosis of the disease requiring surgery are critical factors that determine psychologic effects of ostomy surgery. For example, the patient with a long history of inflammatory bowel disease will have a different reaction to ostomy surgery than will the patient with a newly diagnosed rectal cancer who must immediately have an unexpected ostomy. Fear of recurrent disease and death are primary concerns for the patient with cancer, whereas the patient with inflammatory bowel disease can look forward to improved health after surgery. Whether the ostomy is temporary or permanent influences the patient's emotional response. The concept of a temporary ostomy is easier to accept. However, if an individual focuses on the temporary nature of the ostomy as a critical component of acceptance, it may be very difficult to accept the ostomy as a permanent condition at a later date.

Adaptation to an ostomy is a lengthy process that begins before surgery and continues after wounds have healed. After a major change, or in this case the loss of a "perfect" body image, there is a normal grieving process that occurs. To adapt to the change, the patient will first experience a period of shock or disbelief. During this period, decision making and problem solving are difficult. A positive approach in a climate of support is begun with simple, clear information and education, which often needs to be repeated and reinforced.

Following initial disbelief, patients may experience a period of reactive depression. Caregivers help by accepting and acknowledging the normalcy of these feelings. Nonjudgmental opportunities to express feelings about the situation can strengthen the therapeutic relationship and assist the patient through the process of rehabilitation.

The acknowledgment and acceptance phase represents the time when patients begin to reintegrate their lives and accept the implications of their ostomy. During this phase of the adaptation process, the patient will frequently ask more specific questions and begin to make some positive moves toward self-help.

The last stage is adaptation or resolution. Patients resolve their loss of perfect body image, accept their modified situation, adapt it to their previous functional level, and begin to look ahead to the future.

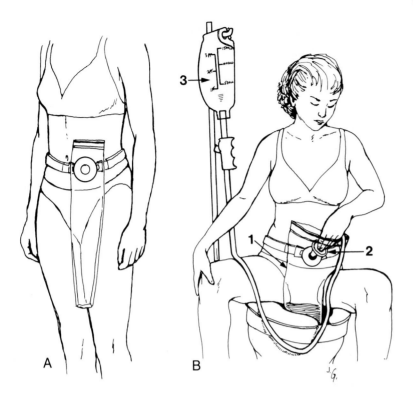

FIGURE 15-6. *A*, Irrigation equipment. An irrigation sleeve is secured by a belt. It is worn for one half hour after the irrigation to collect residual water and feces. *B*, Colostomy irrigation. The irrigation sleeve (*1*) is directed into the toilet. The cone-tip (*2*) is brought through the top of the irrigation sleeve and gently inserted into the stoma. The irrigation bag (*3*) is hung at shoulder level for gravity flow.

Body Image

A major component of a patient's concept of self and self-worth is the image of an intact body. Gillies defines body image as "the mental picture one has of his physical being, together with a heavy overlay of feelings about that structure."[17] Much of what becomes integrated into body image comes from messages the person receives from others. The reaction to the stoma by health care personnel and family and friends can facilitate or impede the patient's acceptance of his or her altered body. For example, patients are attentive to the

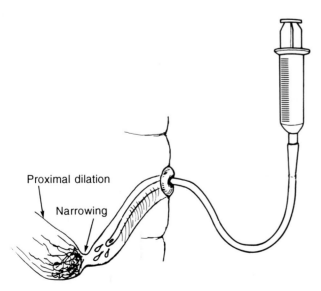

FIGURE 15-7. A catheter is inserted into the stoma and a small amount of water is injected in retrograde fashion to dislodge a food blockage.

facial expressions by which health care providers and others communicate.

Most healthy people are not consciously aware of the image of the body. Illness or injury stimulates the conscious awareness of body image.[35] Although alteration of any body structure will have an impact on body image, certain structures, such as the face and genitals, are of such importance to the individual that injury to these structures is particularly damaging to body image and self-esteem.[17]

Body image problems are frequent following the creation of an abdominal stoma. Female patients have reported equating their protruding red stomas with the phallus.[13] Both homosexual and heterosexual men have perceived their stomas as an outlet for sexual gratification.

Sexuality

Ostomy surgery is perceived by most patients as a threat to a satisfying sexual life. Prior to ostomy surgery, issues and questions regarding sexuality should be openly discussed with the patient and the patient's partner.

For men undergoing proctectomy for benign disease, the chance of impotence is 0 to 20%.[2,9,37,41,60] Conversely, abdominoperineal resection for cancer results in impotence in 33 to 95% of men.[60] Erectile dysfunction frequently results from damage to the parasympathetic nerves that control blood flow to the penis when the rectum is dissected from the prostate.[46,50] Although erection may be impaired, genital sensation is normal. Ejaculation, which is controlled by sympathetic nerves, may not be impaired, or there may be retrograde ejaculation.

A man's anxiety about sexual performance and acceptance also is associated with erectile dysfunction.[8] Surgical and nonsurgical methods are now available for men to aid erectile function. External erective devices as well as penile implants can be employed to improve the quality of sexual function.

Interruption of autonomic nerves in women may be related to decreased vaginal lubrication.[46,50] A water-soluble lubricant may be helpful to prevent dyspareunia. Sensation upon penile penetration may be different postoperatively because of "dead space" behind the posterior vaginal wall. Changing positions during intercourse, along with lubrication, may contribute to comfort and satisfaction. Women are often concerned about acceptance by their partner.[8] Specific suggestions regarding management of the pouch during sexual activity will help patients feel more confident. The pouch should be emptied and sealed before sexual activity. A pouch deodorant masks odors, and gas is prevented by avoidance of foods that cause gas and loose stool for 6 to 12 hours before sexual activity. An ostomy pouch cover, opaque pouches, or mini pouches aid in directing the focus away from the ostomy during sex.[49]

In previous years, physicians have had the misconception that pregnancy is inadvisable for women who have an ostomy. Recent questionnaires to patients and colon and rectal surgeons suggest that there are few problems with conception or delivery in these individuals.[20,38]

Postoperative Counseling

The counseling and teaching methods change during the postoperative period. At that time, the patient needs to hear again about the surgical outcome and the anticipated recovery. Patients initially are preoccupied with overcoming pain and getting well. Once the patient is stabilized, a visitor from the UOA can be helpful. Information about life with an ostomy is sometimes more believable when told by someone who has shared the experience.

Technical skills need to be learned for the patient to care for the ostomy independently. Teaching sessions with an ET nurse are an efficient way to prepare for taking care of the ostomy. When feeling better, the patient begins to participate in ostomy care, but emotional support still needs emphasis. The patient begins to look at the stoma and integrate this new body part into an established body image. Feelings about sexuality and unattractiveness may need to be verbalized.

Before discharge, the patient's knowledge of ostomy management should be assessed. Understanding can be evaluated by posing hypothetical situations and asking how the patient would manage the situation at home. The technical skills learned in the hospital must be transferred to the home environment for successful rehabilitation. Because hospital stays have become shorter over recent years, a visiting nurse (preferably an ET nurse) referral provides continuity of care. Having begun to learn about and take care of the ostomy independently, the patient needs to know about community resources to continue rehabilitation. The UOA is a self-help group that lends support by providing trained vis-

TABLE 15-1. RESOURCES

AMERICAN CANCER SOCIETY
1599 Clifton Road, N.E.
Atlanta, GA 30329
1-800-ACS-2345
The American Cancer Society is a national voluntary organization that sponsors educational programs, patient services and rehabilitation programs.

UNITED OSTOMY ASSOCIATION
36 Executive Park, Suite 120
Irvine, CA 92714
1-714-660-8624
The United Ostomy Association (UOA) is a volunteer organization for people who have ostomies and related surgeries. The UOA provides information, supportive peer visitors, and a community network. Professionals serve as advisors to the organization.

WOUND, OSTOMY, CONTINENCE NURSE'S SOCIETY (FORMERLY IAE)
2755 Bristol Street, Suite 110
Costa Mesa, CA 92626
1-714-476-0268
Professional organization for nurses who practice enterostomal therapy. The WOCN maintains an international directory of members.

AMERICAN SOCIETY OF COLON AND RECTAL SURGEONS
800 East Northwest Highway, #1080
Palatine, IL 60067
1-708-359-9184

itors, educational sessions, and social functions. For details about resources, see Table 15–1.

SPECIAL INSTRUCTIONS

Care Before Barium Studies and Colonoscopy

Twenty-four hours before a procedure such as a barium enema or colonoscopy, the patient with a colostomy should begin a clear liquid diet. Irrigation of the colostomy with 1 liter of warm water should be performed the night before and the morning of the procedure.[50] During barium enemas, an irrigation sleeve over the ostomy maintains cleanliness. Thereafter, the barium must be evacuated before it hardens and causes an impaction. Four 240-ml glasses of water should be drunk in the 8 hours after the procedure. At bedtime, a mild laxative such as milk of magnesia should be taken and a 1,000-ml irrigation performed. If the stool has barium in it the following day, the laxative and irrigation should be repeated.

For ileostomy patients, a clear liquid diet for 24 hours before a radiologic procedure or surgery is adequate preparation. Laxatives and irrigation are contraindicated.[5] Table 15–2 contains the general approach to preparation and aftercare for special procedures on ostomates.

Medication

Patients with a left-sided colostomy have no problem with medication absorption. In contrast, when a patient has a transverse or ascending colostomy, time-release

TABLE 15-2. RADIOLOGIC/ENDOSCOPIC/SURGICAL BOWEL PREPARATIONS

PROCEDURE	BEFORE PROCEDURE	EQUIPMENT	AFTER STUDY
1. Endoscopy Via colostomy	Clear liquids for 24 hours prior to procedure. One 500–1,000 ml tap water irrigation on the night before and morning of procedure until no solid is left.	A two-piece appliance with a detachable irrigation sleeve.	
Via ileostomy	Clear liquids for 24 hours prior to procedure.		
2. Barium enema Via colostomy	One 500–1000 ml tap water irrigation on the night before and morning of procedure until no solid is left.	A two-piece appliance with detachable irrigation sleeve.	Four 240-ml glasses of water in 8 hours. 30 ml MOM at bedtime. 500 ml tap water irrigation
Via ileostomy	Clear liquids for 24 hours.	A two-piece appliance with detachable irrigation sleeve.	
3. Colostomy closure Right-sided or transverse	Clear liquids for 24 hours before procedure. *Two quarts* of oral electrolyte lavage solution within 24 hours before surgery. Oral antibiotics.	Irrigation sleeve.	
Sigmoid or left Colon	Clear liquids for 24 hours before procedure. *One gallon* of oral electrolyte lavage solution within 24 hours before surgery. Laxatives, such as bisacodyl and magnesium citrate may be substituted. Oral antibiotics.	Irrigation sleeve.	
4. Ileostomy closure	Clear liquids for 24 hours before procedure.		

MOM = milk of magnesia.

medications may not be effective because of rapid excretion resulting from the shortened colon.

Likewise, enteric-coated tablets and time-release medications are not effective for the ileostomy patient. Chewable or liquid medications enhance proper absorption. Antibiotics may promote diarrhea, which in ileostomates may result in dehydration. Fluid and electrolyte replacement with clear liquids is necessary. In the case of diarrhea, patients may slow the small bowel with attapulgite (Kaopectate), loperamide (Imodium), diphenoxylate (Lomotil), or codeine.[40] For ileostomy patients, diarrhea is defined as output greater than 1,000 ml/day. In general, laxatives are contraindicated for ileostomates. When stools are liquid, bulking agents such as bran or powdered psyllium preparations may be prescribed to aid in solidification.

Bismuth subgallate is sometimes used to control odors associated with ostomies. This medication should be discontinued for 24 to 48 hours before radiologic studies because it may be visualized on roentgenograms.

Diet

The diet for ostomy patients is unrestricted, but many studies show that ostomy management is easier with some adjustment in food intake.[3,18,27,33,43,55] Perceived problems with ostomy management include high effluent output, diarrhea, odor, excess gas production, and

TABLE 15-3. FOODS AFFECTING BOWEL FUNCTION

INCREASE EFFLUENT OUTPUT
  Prune juice
  Tokay grapes
  Raw fruits (strawberries, peaches, and grapes)
  Concentrated simple sugars (syrup, cakes, candy, fruit)
  Caffeine-containing drinks (tea, coffee, cola, cocoa)
  High-fat foods (fried foods, sauces made with oils or cream, high-fat dairy products)

DECREASE EFFLUENT OUTPUT
  Well-cooked legumes
  White and whole wheat bread products
  Soft cooked brown or white rice
  Applesauce
  Tapioca
  Creamy peanut butter
  Bananas

INCREASE GASEOUS OUTPUT
  Carbonated beverages
  Onions
  Cruciferous vegetables (broccoli, cabbage, cauliflower, Brussells sprouts)
  Legumes
  Cucumbers
  Beer
  Green peppers
  Dairy products

PRODUCE OFFENSIVE ODORS
  Fish
  Eggs
  Asparagus
  Onions
  Garlic
  Cruciferous vegetables (above)

MAY CAUSE OBSTRUCTION
  Nuts
  Seeds found in fruits and vegetables
  Bean sprouts
  Bamboo shoots
  Celery
  Popcorn
  Coleslaw
  Any partially cooked vegetables that inherently contain woody stalks or undigestible fibers*
  Coconut

*Membranes between grapefruit and orange sections, unpeeled apples, stems of broccoli and asparagus, celery, unpeeled cucumbers and zucchini, oriental vegetables.

food blockages. The goal of dietary intervention is to prevent dehydration, which may occur with high ostomy output, and to minimize the incidence of blockage. Patients should be counseled on how to manipulate their diets to achieve these goals prior to leaving the hospital. Table 15-3 lists specific foods that may contribute to these problems.

High effluent output is common but manageable. Liquid diphenoxylate hydrochloride with atropine sulfate or psyllium mucilage (Metamucil) may be prescribed to slow diarrhea. Prior to discharge, patients are instructed to consume 1 liter of fluid each day and to keep an electrolyte replacement drink (e.g., Gatorade or 10-K) accessible at all times. Electrolyte drinks as a primary fluid replacement offset electrolyte imbalances that occur with large intestinal losses. An increased use of salt is encouraged to help replace lost electrolytes.

Ostomates often suffer with blockages. Decreased or no output associated with colicky pain signals this dis-

order. Many blockages resolve spontaneously, but if one persists for 3 to 4 hours, a gentle 100-ml irrigation may help to relieve it (Fig. 15-7). While in the hospital, patients who have a new ileostomy are given a low-fiber or low-residue diet and are instructed to avoid foods with large amounts of insoluble fiber. Soluble fiber is encouraged to promote a more solid, paste-like consistency. Patients progress toward a regular diet after 2 to 4 weeks on low-residue foods, but they are instructed to limit foods known to cause stoma blockage[18,27,43,55] as listed in Table 15-3. Patients who have new colostomies are given a regular, high-fiber diet with instruction to increase fluid intake.

In general, patients are advised to chew their food well and eat at regular mealtimes to promote regular bowel function.[18,43,55] Food and fluid should not be restricted to minimize ostomy output and the frequency of ileostomy emptying, because this can lead to malnutrition and dehydration. Foods that were not well tolerated prior to surgery will not be any better tolerated after surgery. Diet management in patients who have ostomies should be based upon the prevention of these problems.

Activity

In general, activity and exercise are limited initially, avoiding lifting and strenuous exercise for about 6 weeks after ostomy surgery. Thereafter when exercising, smaller pouches may be worn for ease and appearance. Contact sports that might cause trauma to the stoma (i.e., football, wrestling) should be discouraged. A gradual program of walking or swimming is excellent to regain muscle strength and endurance. Physical therapists can provide assistance with a program of muscle strengthening and endurance to prepare individuals to return to preoperative activity.

People with ostomies may bathe or shower as often as they like. Bathing or showering with the pouch off is not harmful to the stoma. If the patient prefers to keep the pouch on during bathing, paper or waterproof tape can be used to cover the edges of the skin barrier wafer.

When traveling, extra ostomy supplies should always be carried along. If irrigations are performed, distilled or bottled water should be used. Water that is not fit for drinking should not be used for irrigation. Liquid diphenoxylate hydrochloride with atropine sulfate should be carried along for the diarrhea that is frequently experienced when traveling.

COMPLICATIONS OF OSTOMY SURGERY

Although the creation of an ostomy is believed to be a relatively minor procedure, complications are frequent. For example, up to 30% of colostomy procedures have morbidity.[4,10,29,36,42] The following section enumerates many of the complications.

Ischemia

Major early complications of ostomy surgery may be the result of improper surgical technique. A small abdominal wall stoma site may constrict and obstruct the bowel vessels. Two fingers must pass easily through the prepared abdominal wall stoma site in order for it to be deemed of an adequate size. Blood flow may be compromised at the skin or fascia levels if this aperture is not adequate. Tension may also occlude the blood supply. The compromised colon will first be pale and edematous or dusky. If the blood flow is not resumed, the stoma becomes duskier until it is black. In an everted stoma, bowel death often extends from the apex of the stoma to the skin level because the fat-laden mesentery over which the bowel is everted causes kinking of the blood vessels.[1]

If the ischemia becomes apparent later, the depth of necrosis into the abdominal wall must be determined in order to decide whether there is an impending intra-abdominal perforation. A simple technique to examine blood flow at the skin level is to place a test tube into the stoma and shine a flashlight down within it. The pink color of viable bowel usually shows just below the skin level. A pediatric sigmoidoscope inserted gently can better define the limits of stomal necrosis. Emergency surgery is warranted if the level of necrosis is found to extend into the peritoneal cavity.

Stricture

Ischemic necrosis is a frequent source of late stricture. Serositis ensues at the distal necrotic margin at which a circumferential scar forms and progressively tightens, narrowing the ostomy. Other sources of serositis and scar are sepsis in the subcutaneous tissue and disruption of the mucocutaneous anastomosis. Dilation rarely corrects the problem of stricture permanently. If the scar is at skin level only, and there is some redundant colon in the subcutaneous space, local skin excision and reanastomosis under local anesthesia can open the outlet.

Infection

Infection of the wound or stoma is usually a function of technique. The bowel must be secondarily isolated to catch potential spillage; then it is cut and closed prior to drawing it through the abdominal wall. Pulling an open lumen through the abdominal wall is a source of contamination. Between the time the abdominal wound is closed and the ostomy is matured, the open bowel may retract and spill fecal matter into the stoma site or the abdomen. Infection of peristomal tissue is unusual unless the patient is obese or diabetic or has a compromised immune system. Disruption of the mucocutaneous anastomosis may lead to a local abscess. Peristomal abscess may also represent an infected hematoma. Drainage is the treatment of choice. Fistula is the result of a primary disease (such as Crohn's disease), an unrecognized enterotomy, or full-thickness suture through the bowel.

Ulcers

For no apparent reason, patients with inflammatory bowel disease, especially those with Crohn's disease, experience ulcers adjacent to the stoma. The ulcers may be small, but sometimes they are deep and almost circumferential. They will heal if local débridement is accomplished and wound care is properly instituted. Inventiveness is needed to keep an appliance sealed around the stoma when a peristomal ulcer is present. The ulcer must be covered or filled with a skin barrier substance to obtain a seal. The seal breaks frequently. Each time, the wound must be cleansed and a new pouch applied. Consultation with an ET nurse will help in developing an approach to complex wound care and pouching.

Granulomas

Granulomas due to local inflammation may form on the ostomy at the mucocutaneous junction. They are not harmful but bleed readily if abraded. If local bleeding is a problem, topical silver nitrate may arrest it; failing this, they may be excised or electrocoagulated.

Hemorrhage

Minor bleeding is common at the mucocutaneous anastomosis. An appliance may irritate the margin and incite bleeding. Usually this problem is self-limited, but suture ligation or electrocoagulation sometimes is necessary. Major bleeding requires formal investigation by endoscopy, barium studies and, perhaps, an arteriogram. A diagnosis of recurrent disease, such as neoplasm or Crohn's disease, should be entertained.

Patients with portal hypertension may form peristomal venous collateral complexes (caput medusa). Veins progressively enlarge and extend out under the skin, creating a purple hue around the stoma. These veins may bleed briskly. To stop an acute bleeding episode, the margin of the stoma may be oversewn.[14,22,23,44,59] Taking the stoma down and resuturing also may control bleeding for a short time. Relocating the stoma does not prevent recurrence of this process.

Recession

Acute recession may occur during the first postoperative day. The bowel can be everted again by reaching down into the stoma with a clamp and grasping and teasing the ileum out to an everted condition. The stoma can again be fixed by suture.

Chronic recession may result in fixation of the ileum back into the abdomen or abdominal wall. If it is in the abdomen, laparotomy must be performed and the mesentery and bowel can be refixed from within. If the recession is simply in the abdominal wall, the mucocutaneous anastomosis can be taken down and resutured. By placing sutures through the cut edge of the bowel, then through the serosa at the level at which it exits the opening in the abdominal wall, and finally to the skin edge, the stoma will be held up and will protrude.

A convex faceplate may fit around the receding stoma to create a good seal. If leak is prevented and the appliance application is not difficult, a surgical procedure may be averted.

Hernia

Peristomal hernias are frequent but not always symptomatic. Many patients do not like the appearance and want repair. Obesity and high intra-abdominal pressure contribute to the formation of these hernias. However, bringing the ostomy through the rectus muscle and carefully sizing the stoma wound prevents hernia.[24] If pain ensues or the appliance cannot be kept on, the stoma must be relocated.[19,52] Unfortunately, local repairs frequently fail. The use of mesh to reinforce the abdominal wall around the stoma is sometimes useful. At one point in history, an extraperitoneal tunnel was advocated to prevent the complication of hernia; however, the extraperitoneal stoma may also herniate.[21]

Prolapse

Ostomy prolapse is a product of abdominal pressure, obesity, placement lateral to the rectus, or poor fixation. Often this is a small protrusion that will not require revision. Conversely, in a colostomy, a hernia that extends out onto the abdominal wall may respond to excision of the redundant bowel and tightening of the opening. If there is a loop ostomy, conversion to an end ostomy usually solves the problem. With a loop ostomy, the distal end of the loop is the usual point of prolapse that pushes out of the abdominal cavity in a retrograde fashion. Intraperitoneal fixation prevents this problem. In the case of the colon, excision of redundant bowel leaves it taut to the skin surface. However, in the case of an ileostomy, ileum should never be excised to repair the prolapse; usually relocation and fixation are necessary.

Obstruction

The signs and symptoms of vomiting, distention, colic, and decreased output herald a bowel obstruction. As after any abdominal operation, adhesions or volvulus may be the source. Volvulus, prolapse, and hernia may be minimized by fixation of the bowel intraperitoneally.[16] Either the space around the stoma inside the abdomen must be left wide open to prevent obstruction or the lateral gutter must be completely closed to prevent volvulus or internal hernia. Narrowed segments of bowel predispose to obstruction secondary to boluses of undigested food particles. Often, food-related blockages will resolve spontaneously; however, the event can be very uncomfortable and frightening to the patient. It may help to review the foods associated with obstruction. Encourage thorough cooking of vegetables, complete chewing, and slow eating habits. Such obstructions may be broken up by retrograde irrigation through a catheter as shown in Figure 15–7. Normal digestion and softening of the blocking food is ongoing, and by waiting a short time, fragmentation and easy removal can be expected.

High Output

Prior to 1952, the ileal margin was not sewn to the skin edge in the standard ileostomy technique. Circumferential serositis occurred over the exposed serosa, stenosing the stoma.[12] This obstruction causes symptoms of profuse diarrhea, pain, vomiting, abdominal distention, and eventually dehydration and is termed ileal dysfunction.[56] The normal ileostomy output is 500 to 1,000 ml/day.[54] If the small bowel is resected to the point that it is a short bowel, the volume may increase tenfold.[28] The main losses in the ileal effluent are water and isotonic sodium chloride, so normal saline can be used to replace losses, along with smaller amounts of potassium, calcium, and magnesium. Dehydration is manifested in an ileostomate as diminished weight and exchangeable sodium.[11] As in other dehydration conditions, urinary calculi subsequently may form in 8% of patients.[45] Gallstones may form after ileostomy if there has been extensive resection of the ileum.[28]

High output may be caused by any of the sources of diarrhea that a nonstomate suffers; dehydration may ensue quickly. Symptomatic relief by using antidiarrheal agents, such as loperamide or diphenoxylate, and oral fluid replacement is usually adequate. Sometimes, if vomiting is also present, intravenous support for a short time may be necessary.

Trauma

The stoma is subject to trauma when the faceplate is fixed tightly with a belt and force is exerted on the side of the appliance, resulting in a shearing action. Those sports that have body contact as part of play put the stoma in the most jeopardy. Earlier generations of appliances were made of hard plastic and were held on by belts. Even walking with such a prosthesis might cause a sawing action, resulting in a cut into the side of the stoma.

Perforation

Perforation is not common, but the mortality risk is 50%.[47,51] The most frequent reason in former years was puncture of the colon wall by a catheter during irrigation. Perforation causes acute peritonitis and emergency surgery is necessary. Usually a new ostomy must be fashioned at a point proximal to the perforation and the perforated distal segment excised.[51] The use of a soft, pliable cone tip to introduce water for irrigation negates the danger of catheter-related perforation.

Skin Problems

Skin problems were found in 79% of ileostomates and 37% of colostomates by Hellman.[26] Skin irritation and inflammation occur in two situations. First, some patients are allergic to a particular skin barrier, adhesive, solvent, or pouch material used on the skin as part of the appliance system (Fig. 15–8). The patient can be tested by applying a small portion of the suspected offending skin contact substance elsewhere on the body as a "patch test." If that site also becomes inflamed, that particular product must be avoided in the future. Noting the point at which the eruption occurs and the configuration of the eruption often makes the diagnosis

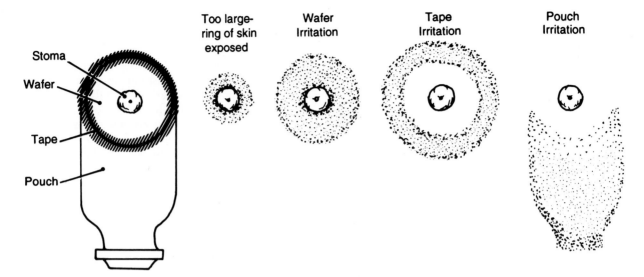

FIGURE 15-8. The various parts of the appliance in contact with the skin may be the source of skin excoriation.

(Fig. 15–8). If the hole in the skin barrier is cut too large, the exposed skin will break down directly adjacent to the stoma.

Second, the seal of the faceplate will not hold if the stoma is situated at sites near scars, the umbilicus, bone prominence, or skin folds. Even though the stool in the colon is not as corrosive as ileostomy effluent, a leak with stool trapped beneath the faceplate may macerate and inflame the skin. Ileostomy output left in contact with the skin produces ulceration. Further contact with the skin must be prevented. Coating the skin with a thin layer of an absorptive powder such as karaya and applying a sealant creates a barrier. The protective wafer should fit closely to the stoma with no exposed skin. Only a few days of protection allows the skin to heal.[7]

The faceplate of the ileostomy appliance should ordinarily be changed at 3- to 4-day intervals. Extending this time frame may be possible, but the seal may begin to loosen. If this happens on a regular basis, a more frequent change in the routine should be instituted. Conversely, changing too frequently may pull off the superficial skin cells, and ulceration will follow. An ileostomy flush to the skin surface will need revision in approximately 12% of patients.[19] An eruption conforming to the shape of the skin barrier, often with patches of *Candida*, may indicate an adverse reaction to the barrier plate material. *Candida* rashes are red in the center with maculopapular satellite lesions and may have superficial epidermal loss. The patient may complain of local pruritus. Treatment consists of application of mycostatin powder, which is fixed to the skin with a sealant prior to pouch placement.

Hernia, prolapse, and recession are obvious contributing factors to appliance failure because they break the seal. Inspection and questioning the patient allow diagnosis of one of these underlying mechanical problems.

REFERENCES

1. Babcock, G., Bivins, B.A., and Sachatella, C.R.: Technical complications of ileostomy. South. Med. J., *73*:329, 1980.

2. Bierman, H.J., Tocker, A.M., and Tocker, L.R.: Statistical survey of problems in patients with colostomy or ileostomy. Am. J. Surg., *112*:7647, 1966.
3. Bingham, S., Cummings, J.H., and McNeil, N.I.: Diet and health of people with an ileostomy. Br. J. Surg., *47*:399, 1982.
4. Birnbaum, W., and Ferrier, P.: Complications of abdominal colostomy. Am. J. Surg., *83*:64, 1952.
5. Broadwell, D., and Sorrells, S.: Ileostomy Care. Plainfield, NJ, Patient Education Press, 1989.
6. Brooke, B.N.: The management of ileostomy. Lancet, 2:102, 1952.
7. Brooke, B.N., Jeter, K., and Berk, J. (eds.): Gastroenterology. Philadelphia, W.B. Saunders, 1985, p. 2371.
8. Brouillette, J.N., Pryor, E., and Fox, T.A.: Evaluation of sexual dysfunction in the female following rectal resection and intestinal stoma. Dis. Colon Rectum, *24*:98, 1981.
9. Burnham, W.R., Lennard-Jones, J.E., and Brooke, B.N.: Sexual problems among married ileostomates. Gut, *18*:673, 1977.
10. Burns, F.J.: Complications of colostomy. Dis. Colon Rectum, *13*: 448, 1970.
11. Clarke, A.M., Chirnside, A., Hill, G.L., et al.: Chronic dehydration and sodium depletion in patients with established ileostomies. Lancet, 2:740, 1967.
12. Crile, G.W., Jr., and Turnbull, R.B.: Mechanism and prevention of ileostomy dysfunction. Ann. Surg., *14*:459, 1954.
13. Dlin, B., and Fisher, H.: Psychiatric aspects of colostomy and ileostomy. *In* Howells, J. (ed.): Modern Perspectives in the Psychiatric Aspects of Surgery. New York, Brunner Mazel, 1976, p. 321.
14. Eckhauser, F.E., Sonda, L.P., Strodel, W.E., et al.: Parastomal ileal conduit hemorrhage and portal hypertension. Ann. Surg., *192*: 620, 1980.
15. Egbert, L.D., Battit, G.E., Welch, C.E., and Bartlett, M.K.: Reduction of postoperative pain by encouragement and instruction to patients. N. Engl. J. Med., *270*:825, 1964.
16. Fazio, V.W., and Turnbull, R.B.: Ulcerative colitis and Crohn's disease of the colon: A review of surgical options. Med. Clin. North Am., *64*:1135, 1980.
17. Gillies, D.: Body image changes following illness and injury. J. Enterost. Ther., *11*:186, 1984.
18. Guinchi, F., Cacciaguerra, G., Borlotti, M.L., et al.: Bowel movement and diet in patients with stomas. Br. J. Surg., *75*:722, 1988.
19. Goldblatt, M.S., Corman, M.L., Haggitt, R.C., et al.: Ileostomy complications requiring revision—the Lahey Clinic experience. Dis. Colon Rectum, *20*:209, 1977.
20. Gopal, K.A., Amshel, A.L., Shonberg, I.L., et al.: Ostomy and pregnancy. Dis. Colon Rectum, *28*:912, 1985.
21. Goligher, J.C.: Diseases of Anus, Rectum, and Colon, 4th ed. London, Balliere Tindall, 1980.
22. Graeber, G.M., Ratner, M.H., Ackerman, N.B., et al.: Massive hemorrhage from ileostomy and colostomy stomas due to mucocu-

taneous varices in patients with coexisting cirrhosis. Surgery, *79:*107, 1976.

23. Grundfest, S., and Fazio, F.: Conservative treatment of bleeding stomal varices. Arch. Surg., *118:*981, 1983.
24. Hawley, P.R., and Ritchie, J.K.: Complications of ileostomy and colostomy following excisional surgery. Clin. Gastroenterol., *8:*403, 1979.
25. Healy, M.K.: Does preop instruction make a difference? Am. J. Nurs., *68:*62, 1968.
26. Hellman, J., and Lago, C.P.: Dermatologic complications in colostomy and ileostomy patients. Int. J. Dermatol., *29:*129, 1990.
27. Higham, S.E.: Effect of ingestion of fat on ileostomy effluent. Gut, *31:*435, 1990.
28. Hill, G.L., Maier, W.S.J., and Goligher, J.C.: Cause and management of high volume output self-depleting ileostomy. Br. J. Surg., *62:*720, 1975.
29. Hines, J.R., and Harris, G.D.: Colostomy and colostomy closure. Surg. Clin. North Am., *57:*279, 1977.
30. Hurney, C., and Holland, J.: Psychosocial sequelae of ostomies in cancer patients. CA, *35:*170, 1985.
31. Jao, S., Beart, R.W., Wendorf, L.J., and Ilstrup, D.M.: Irrigation management of sigmoid colostomy. Arch. Surg., *120:*916,
32. Kelly, M.P.: Coping with an ileostomy. Soc. Sci. Med. *33:*115, 1990.
33. Kramer, P.: Effect of specific foods, beverages and spices on amount of ileostomy output in human subjects. Am. J. Gastroenterol., *82:*327, 1987.
34. Lindeman, C., and Van Aernan, B.: Nursing interventions with the presurgical patient: The effects of structured and unstructured preoperative teaching. Nurs. Res., *20:*319, 1971.
35. McGuire, P.: The psychological and social sequelae of mastectomy. *In* Howells, J. (ed.): Modern perspectives in the psychiatric aspects of surgery. New York, Brunner Mazel, 1976, p. 390.
36. Mollitt, D.L., Malangoni, M.A., Ballantine, T.V.N., and Grosfeld, J.L.: Colostomy complications in children. Arch. Surg., *115:*455, 1980.
37. May, R.E.: Sexual dysfunction following rectal excision for ulcerative colitis. Br. J. Surg., *59:*29, 1972.
38. Metcalf, A.M., Dozois, R.R., and Kelly, K.A.: Sexual function after proctocolectomy. Ann. Surg., *206:*624, 1986.
39. Meyhoff, H.H., Anderson, B., and Nielson, S.L.: Colostomy irrigation and clinical and scintigraphic comparison between three different irrigation volumes. Br. J. Surg., *77:*1185, 1990.
40. Newton, C.R.: Effect of codeine, Lomotil, and Isogel on ileostomy function. Gut, *19:*377, 1978.
41. Nilsson, L.O., Kock, N.G., Kylberg, F., et al.: Sexual adjustment in

ileostomy patients before and after conversion to continent ileostomy. Dis. Colon Rectum, *24:*287, 1981.
42. Pearl, R.K., Prasad, M.L., Orsay, C.P., et al.: Complications of intestinal stomas. Contemp. Surg., *24:*17, 1984.
43. Raymond, J.L., and Becker, J.M.: Ileonal pull-through: A new surgical alternative to ileostomy and a new challenge in diet therapy. J. Am. Diet Assoc., *86:*663, 1986.
44. Roberts, P., Martin, F.M., Schoetz, D.J., et al.: Bleeding stomal varices. Dis. Colon Rectum, *33:*547, 1990.
45. Roy, P.R., Saver, W.G., Beahrs, O.H., et al.: Experience with ileostomies. Evaluation of 497 patients. Am. J. Surg., *119:*77, 1970.
46. Rubin, G.P., and Devlin, B.: The quality of life with a stoma. Br. J. Hosp. Med., *38:*300, 1987.
47. Salim, I., and Quan, S.H.: Colostomy perforation. Dis. Colon Rectum, *21:*92, 1977.
48. Sanata, H., Kawashima, K., and Tsuda, M.: Natural evacuation versus irrigation. Ostomy and Wound Management. *38:*24, 1992.
49. Shell, J.A.: The psychosexual impact of ostomy surgery. Progressions, *4:*3, 1992.
50. Smith, D., and Johnson, D.: Ostomy Care and the Cancer Patient. New York, Grune & Stratton, 1986.
51. Spiro, R.H., and Hertz, R.E.: Colostomy perforation. Surgery, *60:*590, 1966.
52. Taylor, R.L., Rombeau, J.L., and Turnbull, R.B.: Transperitoneal relocation of the ileal stoma without formal laparotomy. Surg. Gynecol. Obstet., *146:*953, 1978.
53. Terranova, O., Sandei, F., Rebuffat, C., et al.: Irrigation vs natural evacuation of left colostomy. Dis. Colon Rectum, *22:*31, 1979.
54. Todd, I.P.: Complications of ileostomy. *In* Todd, I.P. (ed.): Intestinal stomas. London, William Heinemann, 1978, p. 79.
55. Tyus, F.J., Austof, S.I., Chima, C.S., et al.: Diet tolerance and stool frequency in patients with ileoanal reservoirs. J. Am. Diet Assoc., *92:*861, 1992.
56. Warren, R., and McKittrick, L.S.: Ileostomy for ulcerative colitis: Technique, complications, and management. Surg. Gynecol. Obstet., *93:*555, 1951.
57. Watson, P.: Meeting the needs of patients undergoing ostomy surgery. J. Enterost. Ther., *12:*121, 1985.
58. Watt, R.: Challenging stoma placement. J. Enterost. Ther., *13:*20, 1986.
59. Weisner, R.H., LaRusso, N.F., Dozois, R.R., et al.: Peristomal varices after proctocolectomy in patients with primary sclerosing cholangitis. Gastroenterology, *90:*316, 1986.
60. Yeager, E., and Heerden, J.: Sexual dysfunction following proctocolectomy and abdominoperineal resection. Ann. Surg., *191:*169, 1980.

Chapter 16

ILEOSTOMY AND ITS ALTERNATIVES

PHILLIP R. FLESHNER / ROBERT W. BEART, JR.

An ileostomy is traditionally performed when the entire colon must be removed or when it is not capable of being used. Typical conditions in which the entire colon is frequently removed include familial polyposis (FP) and ulcerative colitis (UC). If the rectum can be preserved, the ileum can be reattached to the rectum and intestinal continuity preserved. If, however, the rectum must also be removed, fecal diversion has usually been necessary. Increased experience with anal sphincter manipulation and preservation has demonstrated that sphincter function can be preserved while still removing all diseased colon. As a result, in addition to the continent ileostomy, Brooke ileostomy, and loop ileostomy, the ileoanal procedure can now be offered to those people who have previously required a stoma. This chapter considers the surgical alternatives, decision making, and techniques surrounding these procedures.

GENERAL CONSIDERATIONS

Familial polyposis, inherited in an autosomal dominant pattern, is characterized by the development of a hundred to several thousand colorectal adenomas. The natural history of this disease and pathologic characteristics of its associated cancers have important surgical implications.[5] The most feared complication of FP is malignant degeneration of a colorectal adenoma into carcinoma. Although the development of colorectal cancer is inevitable, the cancers rarely develop before patients reach 15 years of age. Periodic endoscopic evaluation should begin at this age in potential gene carriers. Once the diagnosis is made, surgical treatment is necessary and should be instituted while the disease is still curable. Most surgeons advocate immediate operation in these patients. Pathologically, these tumors have a propensity to multicentricity, so that approximately 20% of patients develop synchronous cancers. Total extirpation of the colorectal mucosa is desirable. However, many surgeons, including the authors, believe that abdominal colectomy and an ileorectal anastomosis is an acceptable alterna-

tive in those FP patients who have a small number of rectal polyps. The rational application of ileorectal anastomosis in these patients rests on three principles: (1) removal of the majority of the large bowel mucosa should markedly reduce the chance of developing cancer, (2) in the event that rectal polyps or carcinoma develop, they could be detected early and removed, and (3) retention of the rectum and anal sphincter apparatus maximizes continence.

In contrast to FP, most patients with UC can be medically treated. Approximately 10% of UC patients will come to surgery for very specific reasons: an acute flare unresponsive to medical measures, development of a life-threatening complication (e.g., toxic megacolon, perforation, or hemorrhage), medical intractability, and the risk of malignancy. During an episode of acute colitis, the patient should be treated with intravenous steroids and bowel rest. The role of parenteral hyperalimentation in this situation is controversial. Although encouraging early results have been reported with the use of cyclosporin A in acute colitis,[19] long-term effectiveness of this treatment modality remains undefined. Patients with life-threatening complications are generally easy to recognize and define. However, these patients are frequently taking large doses of steroids and may appear deceptively well to the physician. The appreciation of the severity of the disease and the timing of operation are of paramount importance. Medical intractability may seem difficult to define. In fact, there is probably no strict definition that a physician can uniformly apply. It is important to perceive that medical intractability is a problem the patient identifies, not the physician. Although a physician may feel that 12 months of steroid or other immunosuppressive management without complete resolution of symptoms is an adequate trial, the patient must be convinced that surgery is indicated. Only the patient can decide when he or she feels so tired, has missed much work or school, or is unable to do things he or she would like to do because of fatigue. If the surgeon waits until the patient has come to the conclusion that the disease is not satisfac-

198

torily treated medically, the patient will graciously accept the alternatives the surgeon has to offer. We feel this is a particularly important strategy for the surgeon to employ if the patient is going to be satisfied.

Patients with UC are prone to the development of colorectal cancer. Certainly, with an established carcinoma, surgical treatment is inevitable. More controversial, however, is the management of patients with dysplasia. It is our belief that identification of high grade dysplasia by an experienced pathologist is an indication for colectomy.

Operative management of UC largely depends on whether the surgery is elective or emergent. Under elective conditions, the four available surgical options are: (1) total proctocolectomy and Brooke ileostomy, (2) total proctocolectomy and continent ileostomy, (3) rectal mucosectomy and endorectal ileoanal anastomosis, and (4) abdominal colectomy with ileorectal anastomosis. Total proctocolectomy and Brooke ileostomy has been traditionally regarded as the optimal surgical approach. The technique has been well described and the immediate and late results are very satisfactory. Furthermore, patients avoid any risk for cancer, steroid medications are eliminated, and physician visits and reoperations are kept to a minimum. Although many quality-of-life studies have demonstrated excellent results, the loss of fecal continence and its attendant physical and psychological sequelae continue to be significant drawbacks of the procedure. In addition, problems with nonhealing of the perineal wound, and the high incidence of small bowel obstruction and ileostomy revision, are not to be minimized.[22]

Total proctocolectomy and continent ileostomy couples the benefits of complete large bowel excision with a reduction in some of the untoward aspects of an ileostomy, since no external appliance is needed and the stoma can be placed in a less conspicuous area. In addition, the continent ileostomy can be performed in UC patients having undergone total proctocolectomy and Brooke ileostomy at anytime if they find a standard ileostomy unsatisfactory. Due to increased surgical experience and improved surgical technique, pouch morbidity has decreased markedly since its initial clinical use. Most patients are happy with the results of the operation. Nonetheless, troublesome complications leading to incontinence continue to plague the postoperative course of a significant number of patients.[8]

Mucosectomy and ileoanal pouch anastomosis have the attractive features of complete excision of the colorectal mucosa, avoidance of a permanent intestinal stoma, continence via a normal route of defecation, and no chance for a troublesome perineal wound. Continence is usually preserved and the frequency of defecation is diminished with incorporation of a pelvic pouch into the operative procedure. Although the operation is associated with minimal mortality, the morbidity of this complex procedure is relatively high, and problems such as small bowel obstruction and pouchitis continue to be cause for concern.[16]

There are many attractive features of colectomy and ileorectal anastomosis. The procedure avoids the perineal complications of total proctocolectomy, is technically easy to perform, may provide perfect control of feces and flatus, and is well accepted by most patients. However, unlike the three previously discussed surgical options, ileorectostomy does not achieve total excision of colorectal mucosa. Many surgeons have not used this operation for UC, arguing that in excess of 25% of patients wil require subsequent rectal excision for persistent proctitis, a small percentage of patients may develop cancer in the rectal remnant, and only one-half of the patients have satisfactory functional results.[7] While we concur that this operation should not be advised in most UC patients, ileorectal anastomosis does have a role in certain clinical situations. For example, an elderly patient with a long history of UC who develops a transverse colon cancer may be well served with an ileorectal anastomosis in lieu of total proctocolectomy.

Under emergent conditions, surgical alternatives available to a patient are limited. If the patient is septic, the diseased or perforated bowel should be removed. If the colon is bleeding, the colon should be removed. Traditionally, it has been taught that the rectum should also be removed. However, with the sphincter-saving alternatives that are currently available, we favor careful preoperative proctoscopic evaluation to rule out a rectal etiology for the bleeding and then abdominal colectomy. A subsequent procedure can restore intestinal continuity. Similarly, with a toxic megacolon, it is seldom necessary to carry out a proctectomy at the time of colectomy. In general, concerns over healing of the perineal wound in these frequently malnourished patients who are on high-dose steroids should restrict surgeons from doing a proctectomy in the emergent setting. We have not found it necessary to use the blow-hole technique of Turnbull, but this is a philosophically acceptable approach in that it does not preclude subsequent continence-preserving alternatives.[31]

A few technical issues regarding subtotal colectomy in these patients must be stressed. Mesenteric dissection in the vicinity of the ileocecal valve should be flush with the colon in order to preserve ileal branches of the ileocolic artery and vein. These branches are necessary to facilitate subsequent construction of an ileoanal pouch.[3] Distally, it is unnecessary to mobilize the rectum within the pelvis. In fact, a sigmoidostomy and a Hartmann procedure are recommended. This has been shown to decrease the incidence of pelvic sepsis and facilitate subsequent pelvic surgery.[25] A transanal rectal drain may prevent leakage from the diseased Hartmann pouch closure site.

There is a trend to avoid subjecting patients to multiple surgical procedures and to perform a definitive procedure at the time of emergent surgery. Although ileoanal procedures have been successfully performed in patients undergoing surgery for emergent complications, we feel this is generally not a safe approach. These patients are usually on high doses of steroids and are nutritionally depleted. From a practical standpoint, surgical options are limited in emergent situations. Salvage of the patients should be the primary concern. Colectomy does not preclude any of the other surgical alternatives in the future. Additionally, the patient is able to live with an ileostomy and assess its impact on his or her life, thus allowing for an informed decision regarding subsequent continence-preserving surgery.

SURGICAL ALTERNATIVES

Brooke Ileostomy

The preoperative period should include effective patient education. A patient must be fully informed of the effects of an ileostomy on his or her quality of life. An ileostomy visitor, preferably age and sex matched and who has completely recovered from surgery, is invaluable during this period. Resistance to a permanent ileostomy can be tempered by stressing the beneficial aspects of this operation (e.g., curing the disease). It is also beneficial to select the stoma site preoperatively with the help of an enterostomal therapist. The stoma should be clearly visible to the patient; must traverse the rectus muscle; and should be placed in a flat area away from bony prominences, scars, and significant skin creases. Attention to these details will ensure a well-functioning ileostomy.

At the preselected stoma site, a 2-cm circular piece of skin is excised and a two-finger–wide aperture made through the lateral one third of the rectus muscle. It is most important that this opening be of correct size to avoid chronic stomal obstruction or parastomal hernia. The mesentery of the ileum should be well mobilized to allow at least 5 to 6 cm of the ileum to protrude through the abdominal wall defect. The ileum may be anchored to the abdominal wall fascia with nonabsorbable sutures to prevent retraction of the stoma in the postoperative period. Some claim the sutures also help prevent parastomal herniation, but there is no proof that they are effective in preventing this complication. After the bowel is brought through the abdominal wall, a defect remains lateral to the small bowel mesentery. It is unclear whether this defect needs to be routinely closed. We tend to close it either by eliminating the defect laterally or by suturing the mesentery to the anterior abdominal wall. If the stoma is thought to be temporary, closing this mesenteric defect may complicate subsequent small bowel mobilization.

The technical contribution of Brooke was primary maturation of the ileostomy. Previously, the immature protruding ileostomy was left to hang from the abdominal wall. Exposure of the serosa resulted in ileitis characterized by symptoms of small bowel obstruction. By folding the ileum back on itself, one covers the serosa and minimizes these symptoms. The stoma is routinely matured by removing 3 to 5 cm of mesentery from the end of the ileum and folding the edge of the bowel upon itself. To anchor the edge of the bowel, we use the "three-bite" suture that includes the full thickness of the bowel and the dermis of the skin (Fig. 16–1). It seems to be important to avoid placing a suture through the epidermis, in which mucosal cells can be implanted and cause difficulty with appliance security. An appliance is then placed over the stoma. Bowel function is expected in 4 to 6 days.

In some situations, the end of the ileum does not

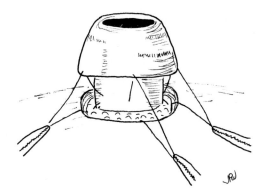

FIGURE 16-1. The "three-bite" eversion suture through bowel end, seromuscular layer, and deep dermis, demonstrating that the epidermis is not included.

reach far enough through the abdominal wall to allow primary maturation. In these situations, the mesentery is usually the limiting factor and selection of a more proximal site in the bowel may allow more mobilization. Alternatively, a loop ileostomy rather than an end ileostomy may reach more easily.[32] In these unusual situations, a segment of intact bowel is brought through the abdominal wall defect. Some prefer to suture the bowel to the fascia with nonabsorbable sutures rather than to use a glass rod to hold the bowel in place. Regardless of how the bowel is secured, the stoma also should be primarily matured. This is done by dividing the bowel distally through 85% of its circumference. The bowel is then folded back upon the proximal bowel and primarily sutured with the three-bite technique already described (Fig. 16–2).

Brooke ileostomy is a safe procedure with a predictable long-term outcome. It is, however, not entirely free of complications. Although problems from the ileostomy have diminished markedly with the use of modern appliances and the Brooke modification, skin irritation,

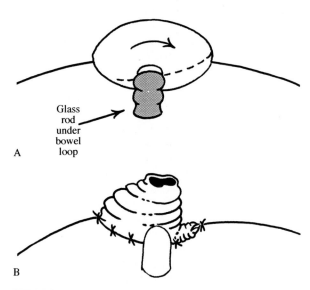

Glass rod under bowel loop

A

B

FIGURE 16-2. Loop ileostomy. A, Incision (*dotted line*) involves four fifths of the bowel circumference. B, The uneven eversion creates a "protruding spigot" configuration.

stomal stenosis, prolapse, and herniation remain significant causes of postoperative morbidity. Treatment of these disorders can be as simple as re-educating a patient about the proper maintenance of the ileostomy. However, one third of these patients ultimately require operative revision. Patients' perception of their quality of life after operation has been generally good. Over 90% of patients are happy with their current lifestyle. However, significant problems do remain. Almost 25% of patients are restricted in their social and recreation activities, and nearly 15% of patients knowledgeable of alternative procedures would consider conversion. In short, the Brooke ileostomy is generally well accepted, although a number of patients experience significant psychosocial and mechanical difficulties.[22]

CONTINENT ILEOSTOMY

Physicians involved with patients requiring an ileostomy should be aware of the continent ileostomy. Although this procedure is less commonly performed today, it remains a viable alternative in patients who have discrete problems with appliances. We rarely advise this procedure primarily after a proctocolectomy. We believe that the continent ileostomy should be reserved for patients who have failed a Brooke ileostomy or those who are candidates for an ileoanal pouch but cannot have a pouch because of rectal cancer, perianal fistulas, poor anal sphincter function, or occupations that preclude frequent visits to the toilet.

Preoperatively, a search for Crohn's disease (CD) using barium examination of the stomach and small intestine is important. Suspicion of CD contraindicates construction of a continent ileostomy, since recurrent disease in the pouch is increased and could necessitate resection of 45 cm of valuable small bowel and render the patient unable to maintain nutrition. Obesity and age over 40 years are associated with an increased risk of pouch dysfunction and represent relative contraindications to the continent ileostomy.[6,8]

The period before surgery must also include an open discussion with the patient, stressing that although continence is likely, major complications can occur. These setbacks may have to be corrected surgically, sometimes leading to pouch excision and creation of a standard Brooke ileostomy. The patient must comprehend that by learning to care for and intubate the reservoir, he or she plays an important role in its functional outcome. Only highly motivated, emotionally stable individuals should undergo this procedure.

Patients undergoing combined total proctocolectomy/continent ileostomy have a proctocolectomy performed in the usual fashion. Excision of a very short segment of terminal ileum and a diligent search for CD during the procedure are essential. The specimen should be immediately examined by a pathologist to confirm the diagnosis of UC. In patients with a standard ileostomy undergoing conversion to continent ileostomy, the stoma is mobilized from the abdominal wall. Construction of the reservoir in these two patient groups is then performed in an identical fashion.

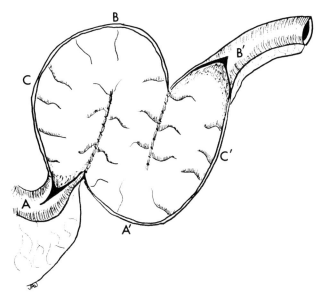

FIGURE 16-3. An alternate method of pouch construction that has longer suture lines but less line tension. After valve construction, points A, B, and C are joined to points A', B', and C', closing the pouch as a cylinder. Relatively little experience has been accrued with this pouch.

The technique of constructing a continent ileostomy is conceptually difficult. Using the terminal 45 cm of the ileum, an aperistaltic reservoir is created by making an S pouch (Fig. 16-3) or a pouch as originally described by Kock.[17] In the classic technique, two 15-cm limbs of ileum are sutured together with continuous absorbable sutures to form a pouch. The antimesenteric border is incised and then folded over to form a reservoir. The ileum immediately distal to the reservoir is then scarified with electrocautery and 5 cm of adjacent mesentery is removed and intussusception of this terminal 15 cm of ileum into the pouch is performed (Fig. 16-4). The

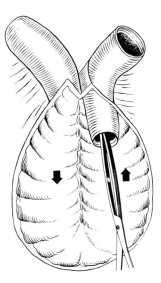

FIGURE 16-4. Intussusception of the distal limb into the pouch creating the "nipple valve." Various techniques are utilized to maintain the intussusception. (From Kretschmer, K.P.: The Intestinal Stoma. Philadelphia, W.B. Saunders, 1978, with permission.)

intussusceptum is secured with multiple nonabsorbable sutures and staples. The end of the ileum is then brought through the abdominal wall at the preoperatively identified site just above the escutcheon. The stoma is sutured flush with the skin and the pouch firmly anchored to the posterior rectus sheath. A No. 24 French tube with large openings is placed into the pouch to allow drainage of the pouch in the postoperative period. This tube is removed for progressively longer periods beginning 10 days after surgery until it can be removed for 8 hours without distress. At this point, the pouch is significantly expanded, the tube is removed, and drainage is achieved by intubating the pouch three times a day.

Postoperative complications that occur with sufficient frequency are nipple valve slippage, pouchitis, intestinal obstruction, and fistula.[8] Nipple valve slippage occurs because of the tendency of the intussuscepted segment to slide and extrude on its mesenteric aspect. Difficult pouch catheterization, chronic outflow tract obstruction, and incontinence ensue. Many techniques other than surgical stapling have been described to stabilize the valve. Wrapping the valve with prosthetic materials does prevent valve bowel slippage but also is associated with an unacceptably high incidence of parastomal abscess and fistula formation.[9] Others advocate using the small bowel itself as a collar around the base of the nipple.[2] However, the efficacy of this procedure has not been well documented. Despite these technical modifications, nipple valve slippage remains the most common complication after continent ileostomy, occurring in almost 25% of patients. Although nonoperative approaches have been tried to correct this problem, surgical correction is inevitable. Repair of the existing malfunctioning valve or creation of a new valve from the afferent ileal limb is performed.

Pouchitis is recognized in 15% of patients, making this the second most common postoperative complication after continent ileostomy. Pouchitis refers to nonspecific inflammation that develops in the reservoir, and is thought to result from stasis and overgrowth of anaerobic bacteria. Patients present with increased ileostomy output, fever, weight loss, and stomal bleeding. The diagnosis is made by history and response to metronidazole.

Pouchitis usually responds to a course of antibiotics and continuous pouch drainage. Other complications include an incidence of obstruction after continent ileostomy of about 5%. Surgical intervention is mandatory when nonoperative therapy has been unsuccessful. The incidence of fistulas after creation of a continent ileostomy is approximately 10%. Fistulas most commonly originate in the pouch itself or at the base of the nipple valve. Pouch fistulas result from dehiscence of suture lines or, rarely, ileostomy tube erosion. These tracts may close with bowel rest, parenteral nutrition, and continuous pouch drainage. Fistulas from the base of the valve lead to incontinence, since ileal contents bypass the high-pressure zone of the nipple valve. These fistulas commonly arise with tearing of the sutures anchoring the pouch to the anterior abdominal wall. Valve fistulas rarely heal without operation. At laparotomy, the valve is excised, the pouch rotated, and a new valve constructed from the afferent tract.

Patient satisfaction with a continent ileostomy is excellent. Most patients note a marked improvement in their lifestyle, and almost all patients work and participate in social and recreational activities without restriction. These observations are understandable in that 90% of patients eventually have total continence after one or more procedures.[8] On the other hand, their enthusiasm is surprising considering that complications are quite frequent and often require major surgical intervention.

ILEOANAL POUCH

The most attractive of the continence-preserving alternatives is the ileoanal procedure, which consists of total abdominal colectomy, mucosal proctectomy, and endorectal ileoanal anastomosis. It removes the rectal disease without creating a perianal wound; preserves innervation to the anus, bladder, and genitals; and retains the usual pathway for defecation. Preoperatively, the rectum should be evaluated sigmoidoscopically. Active rectal disease requires topical 5-aminosalicylic acid or steroid enemas to minimize rectal inflammation and facilitate mucosectomy. The anorectal sphincter mechanism must be intact to prevent leakage of watery ileal contents. Use of this procedure in patients with poor sphincter function or fecal incontinence must be carefully individualized. Preoperative evaluation also allows the surgeon to be certain that patients undergoing this operation are highly motivated and willing to cope with potential postoperative complications.

After appropriate bowel preparation, the patient is brought to the operating room and placed in the modified lithotomy position. A midline incision is made and the abdomen explored to rule out evidence of CD. The colon is mobilized in the usual fashion. A few technical points should be stressed. Omentectomy may be inappropriate, since one study demonstrated a lower incidence of postoperative sepsis when the omentum was preserved.[1] Stapling of the distal ileum flush with the cecum is most important, as in preservation of the ileal branches of the ileocolic artery and vein. These vessels provide perfusion of the pouch after mesenteric division.[3] The pelvic peritoneum is incised and rectal mobilization begun. Dissection is carried ventrally to the level of the prostate in men and the midportion of the vagina in women. Posteriorly, the dissection is carried past the end of the coccyx. Mobilization of the rectum should be flush with the fascia propria to minimize damage to nearby nerves traveling to the urinary bladder and sexual organs. The sigmoid is transected and the colon is removed. The pathologist verifies the diagnosis of UC. When CD is suspected, the procedure should be abandoned and an ileorectal anastomosis or Brooke ileostomy constructed. Mucosal stripping is performed from a perineal approach. A solution of dilute epinephrine is injected into the submucosal plane to facilitate mucosectomy and minimize bleeding. The use of a Lone Star retractor facilitates exposure and minimizes damage to the sphincter mechanism (Fig. 16–5). The ex-

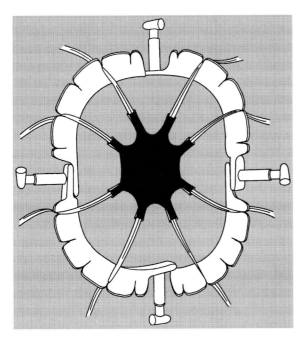

FIGURE 16-5. Lone Star retractor.

cised mucosa and remaining proximal rectum are removed, leaving a short cuff of denuded rectal muscle distally for about 4 cm above the dentate line. Attention is then directed towards creation of the ileal reservoir (Fig. 16–6). The terminal ileum is aligned to form a J and the pouch constructed with either a continuous absorbable suture or a stapling device. Both limbs of the J are approximately 15 to 20 cm in length, the exact length guided by where the pouch reaches deepest into the pelvis. The prospective apex of the pouch must reach beyond the symphysis pubis in order to accomplish a tension-free ileoanal anastomosis. Selective division of mesenteric vessels will allow for more length. Superficial incision on the anterior and posterior aspects of the small

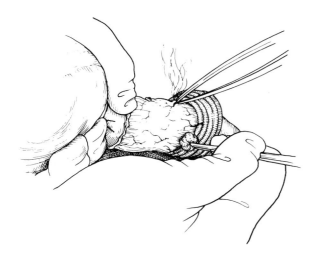

FIGURE 16-6. Rectal mucosal stripping by eversion of the rectal muscular layer and hemostasis. (From Utsunomiya, J., Iwama, T., and Inojo, M.: Total colectomy, mucosal proctectomy, and ileoanal anastomosis. Dis. Colon Rectum, *23*:459, 1980, with permission.)

bowel mesentery along the course of the superior mesenteric artery, and dissection of the ileal mesentery up to and anterior to the duodenum, are two additional important lengthening maneuvers.[3] The pouch is then pulled into the pelvis and the anastomosis carried out between the apex of the pouch and the dentate line (or by using the double-staple technique), approximating full-thickness bites of the pouch wall to the internal sphincter and anal mucosa. A proximal defunctioning loop ileostomy is created as already described (Fig. 16–2). Two suction drains are placed in the presacral space and brought out through the left lower quadrant. The abdomen is then closed.

Postoperative management is similar to that in patients who have had a low anterior resection. Ileostomy output can be quite high, since the stoma is more proximal than a Brooke ileostomy. Patients should be encouraged to keep themselves well hydrated. In some instances, antidiarrheal medication is prescribed.

Patients are usually discharged after 7 to 10 days in the hospital and return 2 to 3 months later to have the temporary ileostomy closed. Before closure, however, the pouch is thoroughly investigated. Digital rectal examination is used to assess anal sphincter tone and detect anastomotic strictures or defects. The pouch is examined endoscopically to ensure that the suture lines are healed, and a contrast study is performed to detect fistulas and sinus tracts. Only after confirmation that no pouch abnormalities are present is the ileostomy closed. Sphincter strengthening exercises should be encouraged in the period leading up to ileostomy closure, since they appear to improve functional results.[14] In 80% of patients, the ileostomy can be closed through a peristomal incision. However, in 20% of patients, the abdomen must be reopened.

Performing an ileoanal anastomosis is safe, with reported mortality rates ranging from 0 to 1%. In distinct contrast to mortality, however, morbidity after ileoanal procedures remains considerable.[16] Small bowel obstruction occurs in 20% of patients and results from adhesion formation to the large number of raw surfaces after colectomy, and from kinking at the ileostomy site. Most of the obstructive episodes occur in the immediate period after either procedure. Factors predictive of small bowel obstruction are a previous operation, twisting the ileostomy 180 degrees (as some authors promote to reduce fecal spillage into the defunctionalized pouch) and using a Brooke ileostomy in lieu of a loop ileostomy during the initial procedure.[10] Although an initial trial of nonoperative therapy is appropriate, surgical intervention is ultimately required in about 50% of patients who develop small bowel obstruction.

Although the incidence has steadily decreased with increasing surgical experience, pelvic sepsis still occurs in 5% of patients after an ileoanal procedure. The symptoms suggestive of pelvic sepsis are fever, leukocytosis, left lower quadrant fullness, and tenderness. Diagnosis is confirmed using computed tomography (CT), which demonstrates the presence of an abscess or of edematous tissues. Although most patients respond to antibiotics within 24 to 36 hours, patients with ongoing sepsis and a CT-diagnosed organized abscess should undergo early drainage, which is associated with less pelvic scarring and fibrosis and may allow for better long-term pouch compliance.

Stricture at the ileoanal anastomosis requiring surgery affects about 10% of patients. The culprit is usually anastomotic tension that also predisposes to infection from leakage. Most strictures can be fragmented digitally but occasionally the insertion of graded dilators is necessary. Rarely, a pouch advancement flap to relieve the stricture is needed.

Anastomotic separation is seen in approximately 10% of patients. If this combination is recognized during preileostomy closure contrast studies, or as a defect on digital examination, ileostomy closure should be delayed until complete clinical and radiographic evidence of healing. Local drainage procedures for an associated abscess or a direct repair of the separation are sometimes necessary. This aggressive approach will almost always be successful.[11]

Development of a pouch fistula to either the perineum or vagina is a particularly morbid event. Most patients require reinstitution of the diverting ileostomy and then repair of the fistula. Patients who develop a pouch fistula should be suspected of having Crohn's disease until proven otherwise, and an appropriate diagnostic work-up should be initiated. Salvage of the pouch can be expected in approximately one half of cases when the diagnosis is not CD.

The most common complication of the ileoanal procedure is pouchitis, occurring in up to one half of patients. Pouchitis occurs more commonly in patients who have extraintestinal manifestations of UC and is more common in patients with pancolitis than in those with left-sided or distal disease. Backwash ileitis does not predict the ultimate development of pouchitis. The etiology of this nonspecific inflammation is unclear but, as with the continent ileostomy, may be due to an overgrowth of anaerobic bacteria. Presenting symptoms are abdominal cramps, fever, pelvic pain, and a sudden increase in stool frequency. Treatment of pelvic reservoir pouchitis relies on the use of antibiotics such as metronidazole and ciprofloxacin. Although this regimen is almost always successful, occasionally steroid enemas or 5-aminosalicylates will be necessary. Patients with persistent pouchitis should be suspected of having CD. Uncommonly, an ileostomy with or without pouch excision is required for severe refractory pouchitis.

The number of bowel movements after successful ileoanal pouch procedures averages six per 24 hours. It should be pointed out that most patients are not particularly concerned with how often they defecate, since most can postpone defecation to accommodate social and recreational activities. Major incontinence is very unusual, although minor incontinence to mucus or stool, particularly at night, is seen in approximately 30% of patients. These patients are managed effectively with good perianal hygiene and the occasional use of a perineal pad. To obtain these results, however, approximately one half of patients regularly take a bulking agent or antidiarrheal medication to help regulate their bowels. Many patients also tend to eat less in the evening than at midday in order to minimize bowel movements

when they are going out or while sleeping. Total failure, defined as removal of the pouch, occurs in only 5% of cases and is usually caused by pelvic sepsis, undiagnosed CD, or an unacceptable stool frequency. Quality-of-life studies have also disclosed that more than 95% of patients are happy with their pouch and would not go back to an ileostomy.[24]

CONTROVERSIES

Several controversies currently exist about the ileoanal procedure. Some have questioned whether an ileoanal procedure can be used in CD or indeterminate colitis. One study has shown that only one of nine patients in whom an ileoanal pouch was done with a preoperative clinical diagnosis of CD retained a functioning pouch. Complications uniformly occur within months of ileostomy closure.[13] Others have also confirmed that patients with CD perform poorly after ileoanal pouch procedures.[4] Thus, we consider this disease a contraindication to an ileoanal pouch. However, in approximately 10% of patients, the ability to distinguish CD from UC is not possible. Patients with this condition, now called indeterminate colitis, manifest macroscopic and microscopic signs of both types of idiopathic inflammatory disease of the colon. Although some groups have documented good results of the ileoanal procedure in patients with indeterminate colitis,[13] other papers document a higher incidence of perineal complications and pouch failure.[18-21] Until the reasons underlying these discrepant data are uncovered, patients with indeterminate colitis should be counseled that undergoing an ileoanal procedure may predispose them to a higher incidence of pouch-related complications.

Another debated issue is whether ileoanal pouch procedures should be offered to elderly patients. Two reasons to avoid these procedures in older patients relate to the higher incidence of anal sphincter dysfunction with increasing age and the morbidity of reoperations in these medically at-risk patients. On the other hand, operations for rectal cancer with anastomosis to the anal sphincter are regularly carried out in patients in their seventh and eighth decades, and thus many surgeons contend that ileoanal pouches should also be made available. We believe that pouch procedures are feasible in suitably motivated elderly individuals who understand the risks and problems of this procedure. Perhaps the use of a double-stapled technique with preservation of the distal anal transition zone might improve function. Further studies are needed to fully resolve this issue.

Another controversy relates to the use of the ileoanal pouch in FP or UC patients who have established colorectal cancer. The presence of distant metastatic disease is generally a contraindication to an ileoanal pouch procedure. These unfortunate patients should be managed with segmental colectomy or abdominal colectomy with ileorectal anastomosis to facilitate early discharge and allow them to spend the rest of their lives relatively free of complications. Patients with middle and low rectal tumors, in accordance with basic principles of cancer surgery, are not eligible for this procedure. Ulcerative colitis patients with cecal cancers represent another unique subgroup of patients. The sacrifice of a long segment of adjacent distal ileum with its mesenteric vessels may limit positioning of the reservoir into the pelvis. If a tension-free anastomosis cannot be ensured, a Brooke ileostomy may be necessary. Studies examining the use of the ileoanal pouch in patients with locally invasive cancers of the colon and upper rectum have been conflicting. In a series from the Mayo Clinic, 13 UC patients with a carcinoma had postoperative complications and functional results identical to UC patients without cancer. Metastatic disease developed in only one patient.[30] In contrast, another study revealed that 2 of 12 UC patients with cancer who had an ileoanal pouch died of metastatic disease. Since both of these patients had Dukes stage C cancer, it is unclear that their course was adversely influenced by performing an ileoanal procedure.[28] This management approach is also encouraged by surgeons at the Lahey Clinic, where UC patients with cancer initially undergo an abdominal colectomy with ileostomy to accurately stage the disease. Patients with Dukes stage A cancer undergo an ileoanal pouch procedure within 3 to 6 months. For patients with Dukes stage B_1, B_2, or C, an observation period of 12 months is recommended to ensure that no recurrent disease develops.[33] Another reason to postpone the ileoanal pouch in these patients is to allow adjuvant chemoradiation treatment to proceed unhindered without any added morbidity from a pouch-anal anastomosis. Clearly, further work is needed to fully define the role of the ileoanal pouch in patients with an established carcinoma.

Many technical issues remain to be resolved. Some authors feel that the entire rectal mucosa does not need to be removed. They favor leaving 1 to 2 cm of distal mucosa behind, transecting the rectum just above the puborectalis, and stapling the pouch to the rectal remnant. The potential advantages of this approach include technical ease, since it avoids a mucosectomy and the perineal phase of the operation, less tension on the anastomotic line, and improved functional results because both sphincter injury is minimized and the anal transition zone with its abundant supply of sensory nerve endings is preserved. On the other hand, surgeons who oppose this operative approach contend that residual diseased mucosa is at risk for malignancy. Cancer within the rectal cuff has been reported.[29] In addition, the potential for continuing colitis in this residual mucosa is another concern. Rauh and co-workers have described a "short-strip pouchitis" that manifests as inflammation at the pouch anal anastomosis thought secondary to residual colitic mucosa.[26] In an effort to resolve these issues, two recent prospective randomized trials have demonstrated no significant differences in perioperative complications or functional results in those patients where a mucosectomy was done versus those patients where the distal rectal mucosa was preserved.[20,27]

Another controversial issue is the shape and size of the reservoir. It is clear based on physiologic studies that the addition of a reservoir decreases the pulse of activity of the terminal ileum and increases the storage capacity. These two features seem to enhance the results, particularly in the early postoperative period. A larger pouch may not necessarily be a better pouch, since its evacuation may be more difficult. It is unclear whether a J, S, H, or W pouch is to be preferred. Although one study suggests that a W pouch may be associated with decreased stool frequency,[23] a controlled study revealed no significant differences in operative complications or functional results in patients receiving a J or W pouch.[15] Since the number of patients in this study is relatively small, and because there have been no other randomized studies, we have not been inclined to change our practice of using a J pouch. Certainly, creation of a W pouch is more complicated, and if the procedure is to become universally applicable, it should be kept as simple as possible.

A final controversy that merits discussion relates to the routine use of a diverting loop ileostomy. Proponents of routine fecal diversion contend that postoperative complications are kept to a minimum. Loop ileostomy also obviates the problem of immediate severe diarrhea through a sphincter that has been damaged surgically by mucosectomy. On the other hand, many surgeons believe that the loop ileostomy is counterproductive. Notwithstanding the additional operation and increased hospitalization associated with its closure, morbidity of ileostomy closure is significant, as small bowel obstruction and anastomotic leaks are not uncommon. In addition, these ileostomies may be proximal in the small bowel and thus represent high-output stomas that can cause clinical dehydration. A recently published controlled trial of ileostomy versus no ileostomy in ileoanal pouch procedures concluded that a protective ileostomy did not reduce the incidence of pelvic sepsis. In fact, the ileostomy was associated with a higher incidence of pouch-specific complications. Functional results were similar in the two groups.[12] It appears that ileostomy can be safely avoided in those patients where there is no tension on the ileoanal anastomosis, the pouch has a good blood supply, the patient is in good general health, and no steroids are being used. It should be stressed that problems associated with the ileostomy or its closure such as dehydration, anastomotic leak, or bowel obstruction are easily managed with medical or surgical means. However, the development of a pouch-specific complication in those patients without an ileostomy is a particularly morbid event. Clearly, more work is needed to further resolve the issue of whether an ileostomy should be routinely used in this procedure.

CONCLUSIONS

The approach to the UC or FP patient requiring surgical intervention must begin with an open discussion concerning the pros and cons of each procedure. Surgeons should individualize treatment based on the patient's desires, fears, and expectations. In general, those patients desiring a minimum of complications without regard for continence should undergo total proctocolorectomy with Brooke ileostomy. Those patients wanting to preserve fecal continence but also willing to accept a number of potential postoperative complications that in some cases may necessitate a stoma should consider an ileoanal pouch. The risk of complications and the unknown long-term effects of continence-preserving surgery requires that patients be willing to undergo careful and regular follow-up. Patients not expected to comply with or take care of their continent ileostomy or ileoanal pouch should not be offered these procedures.

REFERENCES

1. Ambroze, W.L., Jr., Wolff, B.G., Kelly, K.A., et al.: Let sleeping dogs lie: Role of the omentum in the ileal pouch-anal anastomosis procedure. Dis. Colon Rectum, 34:563, 1991.
2. Barnett, W.O.: Current experiences with the continent intestinal reservoir. Surg. Gynecol. Obstet., 168:1, 1989.
3. Burnstein, M.J., Schoetz, D.R., Jr., Coller, J.A., et al.: Technique of mesenteric lengthening in ileal reservoir-anal anastomosis. Dis. Colon Rectum, 30:863, 1987.
4. Deutsch, A.A., McLeod, R.S., Cullen, J., et al.: Results of the pelvic-pouch procedure in patients with Crohn's disease. Dis. Colon Rectum, 34:475, 1991.
5. Dozois, R.R., Berk, T., Bulow, S., et al.: Surgical aspects of familial adenomatous polyposis. Int. J. Colorectal Dis., 3:1, 1988.
6. Dozois, R.R., Kelly, K.A., Ilstrup, D., et al.: Factors affecting revision rate after continent ileostomy. Arch. Surg., 116:610, 1981.
7. Farnell, M.B., van Heerden, J.A., Beart, R.W., Jr., et al.: Rectal preservation in nonspecific inflammatory disease of the colon. Ann. Surg., 192:249, 1980.
8. Fazio, V.W., and Church, J.M.: Complications and function of the continent ileostomy at the Cleveland Clinic. World J. Surg., 12:148, 1988.
9. Fonkalsrud, E.W.: Endorectal pull-through with ileal reservoir for ulcerative colitis and polyposis. Am. J. Surg., 144:81, 1982.
10. Francois, Y., Dozois, R.R., Kelly, K.A., et al.: Small intestinal obstruction complicating ileal pouch-anal anastomosis. Ann. Surg., 209:46, 1980.
11. Goloudeuk, S., Scott, N., Dozois, R., et al.: Ileol pouch-anal anastomosis: Reoperation for both related complications. Ann. Surg., 212:446, 1990.
12. Grobler, S.P., Hosie, K.B., and Keighley, M.R.B.: Randomized trial of loop ileostomy in restorative proctocolectomy. Br. J. Surg., 79:903, 1992.
13. Hyman, N.H., Fazio, V.W., Tuckson, W.B., et al.: Consequences of ileal pouch-anal anastomosis for Crohn's colitis. Dis. Colon Rectum, 34:653, 1991.
14. Jorge, J.N.N., Wexner, S.D., Morgado, P.J., et al.: Optimalization of sphincter function after restorative protocolectomy: A prospective randomized trial (Abstract). Dis. Colon Rectum, 36:P43, 1993.
15. Keighley, M.R.B., Yoshioka, K., and Kmiot, W.: Prospective randomized trial to compare the stapled double lumen pouch and the sutured quadruple pouch for restorative proctocolectomy. Br. J. Surg., 75:1008, 1988.
16. Kelly, K.A., Pemberton, J.H., Wolff, B.G., and Dozois, R.R.: Ileal pouch-anal anastomosis. Curr. Probl. Surg., 29:65, 1992.
17. Kock, N.G.: Intra-abdominal reservoir in patient with permanent ileostomy: Preliminary observation on a procedure resulting in fecal continence in 5 ileostomy patients. Arch. Surg., 99:223, 1969.
18. Koltun, W.A., Schoetz, D.J., Jr., Roberts, P.L., et al.: Indeterminate colitis predisposes to perineal complications after ileal pouch-anal anastomosis. Dis. Colon Rectum, 34:857, 1991.
19. Lichtiger, S.: Cyclosporine therapy in inflammatory bowel disease: Open label experience. Mt. Sinai J. Med., 57:315, 1990.
20. Luukkonen, P., and Jarvinen, H.: Stapled vs hand-sutured ileoanal anastomosis in restorative proctocolectomy. Arch. Surg., 128:437, 1993.
21. McIntyre, P.B., Pemerton, B.G., Wolff, R.R., et al.: Indeterminate colitis: Long-term outcome in patients after ileal pouch-anal anastomosis (Abstract). Dis. Colon Rectum, 36:P48, 1993.
22. Morowitz, D.A., and Kirsner, J.B.: Ileostomy in ulcerative colitis. Am. J. Surg., 141:370, 1981.
23. Nicholls, R.J., and Pezim, M.E.: Restorative proctocolectomy with ileal reservoir for ulcerative colitis and familial adenomatous polyposis: A comparison of three reservoir designs. Br. J. Surg., 72:470, 1985.
24. Pemberton, J.H., Phillips, S.F., Ready, R.R., et al.: Quality of life after Brooke ileostomy and ileal pouch-anal anastomosis: Comparison of performance status. Ann. Surg., 209:620, 1989.
25. Penna, C., Daude, F., Parc, R., et al.: Previous subtotal colectomy with ileostomy and sigmoidostomy improves the morbidity and early functional results after ileal pouch-anal anastomosis in ulcerative colitis. Dis. Colon Rectum, 36:343, 1993.
26. Rauh, S.M., Schoetz, D.J., Jr., Roberts, P.L., et al.: Pouchitis: Is it a wastebasket diagnosis? Dis. Colon Rectum, 34:685,
27. Seow-Choen, Tsunoda, A., and Nicholls, R.J.: Prospective randomized trial comparing anal function after hand sewn ileoanal anastomosis with mucosectomy versus stapled ileoanal anastomosis without mucosectomy in restorative proctocolectomy. Br. J. Surg., 78:430, 1991.
28. Stelzner, M., and Fonkalsrud, E.W.: The endorectal ileal pull-through procedure in patients with ulcerative colitis and familial polyposis with carcinoma. Surg. Gynecol. Obstet., 169:187, 1989.
29. Stern, H., Walfisch, S., Mullen, B., et al.: Cancer in an ileoanal reservoir: A new late complication. Gut, 31:473, 1990.
30. Taylor, B.A., Wolff, B.G., Dozois, R.R., et al.: Ileal pouch-anal anastomosis for chronic ulcerative colitis and familial polyposis coli complicated by adenocarcinoma. Dis. Colon Rectum, 31:358, 1988.
31. Turnbull, R.B., Hawk, W.A., and Weakley, F.L.: Surgical treatment of toxic megacolon: Ileostomy and colostomy to prepare patients for colectomy. Am. J. Surg., 122:325, 1971.
32. Turnbull, R.B., and Weakley, F.L.: Atlas of Intestinal Stomas. St. Louis, C.V. Mosby, 1967.
33. Wiltz, O., Hashmi, H.F., Schoetz, D.J., Jr., et al.: Carcinoma and the ileal pouch-anal anastomosis. Dis. Colon Rectum, 34:805, 1991.

Chapter 17

RESECTION OF THE COLON

ROBERT E. CONDON

This chapter concerns operations on the intraperitoneal large bowel. Resection of the colon is usually conducted for the removal of neoplasms, especially adenocarcinoma, and in the management of inflammatory bowel disease. Less frequently, colon resection is necessitated by ischemia caused by embolus or thrombosis. On occasion, resection may be indicated in the management of infectious diseases such as actinomycosis or for the complications of bacterial (typhoid) or parasitic (amebiasis) afflictions.

A number of operations, illustrated in previous versions of this text, are no longer performed with sufficient frequency to warrant inclusion today. Such procedures, which are of primarily historic interest, include the Mikulicz obstructive resections, staged resection using a preliminary colostomy, side-to-side bypasses for inflammatory bowel disease, "aseptic" anastomotic techniques, and colostomy constructed through the umbilicus.

The outcome following colon resection is better than is often assumed. A recent study of the end results in over 5,000 elderly patients having a colectomy for cancer indicated that the overall perioperative mortality was 5% and that survival in all comers was 63% at 2 years.[8]

An effective mechanical bowel preparation is an essential preliminary step in elective resections of the colon. Although occasional iconoclastic objections are recorded in the literature by surgeons who prefer to operate on a feces-filled colon,[4-6] nearly all surgeons evacuate the colon prior to operation. The most widely used and effective form of mechanical colon preparation is oral or nasogastric tube instillation of a relatively large volume of polyethelene glycol–electrolyte solution (Golytely, Colyte).[1,3]

Oral administration of poorly absorbed antibiotics is, in my view, also an essential step in elective preparation of the colon for resection.[2] Oral antibiotic administration reduces the residual bacteria in the colon at the time of operation to a concentration that is not infective. When properly done, oral antibiotic preparation is associated with a gratifying decrease in the incidence of postoperative infectious complications related to the resection, as well as with a decreased risk of postoperative anastomotic disruption (see Chapter 13).

Parenteral administration of antibiotics is also a popular current surgical practice and seems to have its major impact through a reduction in the overall incidence of nonrelated postoperative infections such as pneumonia and urinary tract infection. Many reports also indicate a small additional impact on the incidence of colon-related infectious complications with use of parenteral antibiotics.

SURGICAL ANATOMY

The colon is a mucosa-lined tube, which is surrounded by a thin but strong layer of connective tissue, the submucosa, and is covered by two layers of muscle, an internal circular layer and an external longitudinal layer, all of which are encased in serosa. The longitudinal muscle layer is complete around the circumference of the colon but is prominently gathered into three bundles, the taeniae coli. The taeniae are spaced more or less equidistantly around the circumference of the colon, one at the mesenteric border and the other two on the free borders of the colon. More or less prominent collections of serosa-encased fat, the appendices epiploicae, are found along the colon, especially on the left side, and are attached adjacent to the free taeniae. Each epiploic appendix contains a small arterial blood vessel. The greater omentum is attached along the anterior aspect of the transverse colon, but it can be dissected free from the bowel without compromising the omental blood supply.

Two vascular systems supply the colon. The superior mesenteric system supplies the ascending and transverse colon through the middle colic, ileocolic, and multiple right colic arteries (Fig. 17–1). The inferior mesenteric system supplies the descending and sigmoid colon through the left colic, multiple sigmoid, and superior hemorrhoidal arteries. The superior hemorrhoidal ar-

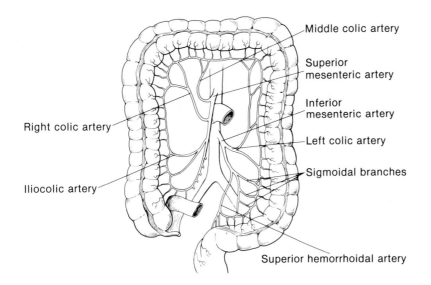

FIGURE 17-1. The arterial blood supply to the colon. The colon proximal to the splenic flexure is supplied via the superior mesenteric artery. Distal to the splenic flexure, the inferior mesenteric artery is the source.

tery is the terminal continuation of the inferior mesenteric artery after it has first given off its major proximal branch, the left colic artery, and the two or three branches that supply the sigmoid colon.

The marginal artery (Drummond's, Riolan's) forms a prominent collateral channel near the margin of the entire length of the colon from the region of the ileocecal valve to the proximal portion of the sigmoid colon. It is best seen in the territory between the middle colic and left colic arteries at which point it usually forms a well-defined vessel running parallel to and within 1 to 2 cm of the bowel. In the ascending and proximal transverse colon, the anastomotic channel is formed by the major terminal branches of the arterial supply, and its course is more irregular, often being a zigzag pattern. The same arrangement of anastomotic channels characterizes the terminal branches of the sigmoidal arteries supplying the sigmoid colon. Preservation of the marginal anastomotic blood supply is important in ensuring viability of the bowel ends used for anastomosis.

In general, the veins follow the arteries, except for the inferior mesenteric vein (Fig. 17–2), which swings away from the inferior mesenteric artery as it nears the aorta and travels superiorly, anterior to the renal pelvis, and

then behind the pancreas to join the splenic vein. The lymphatic drainage follows the arterial blood supply.

FUNDAMENTAL PRINCIPLES AND GENERAL TECHNIQUES OF RESECTION

Mobilization from the Gutters

The ascending and descending colon are each fixed to the retroperitoneum in the late stages of embryonic bowel development by a reflection of peritoneum from the bowel to the body wall. This peritoneal reflection can be cut and the bowel mobilized medially on its mesentery by blunt dissection (Figs. 17–3 and 17–4). The dissection is nearly bloodless, except at the hepatic and splenic flexures at which point there is regularly a small vessel. The dissection does not jeopardize the viability of the bowel, thus allowing the intraperitoneal colon to be mobilized quite freely. In portal hypertension, and often also in inflammatory bowel disease, secondary collateral vessels form in the normally avascular gutters and can lead to troublesome bleeding during mobilization of either the ascending or descending colon.

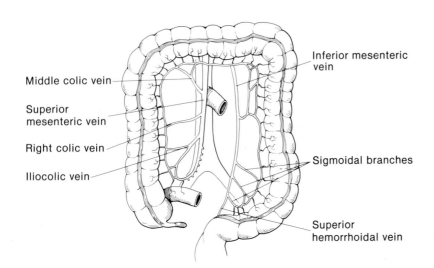

FIGURE 17-2. The venous drainage of the colon. For the most part, the veins parallel the arteries. The inferior mesenteric vein, however, is displaced to the left of its artery and courses beneath the pancreas to join the splenic vein.

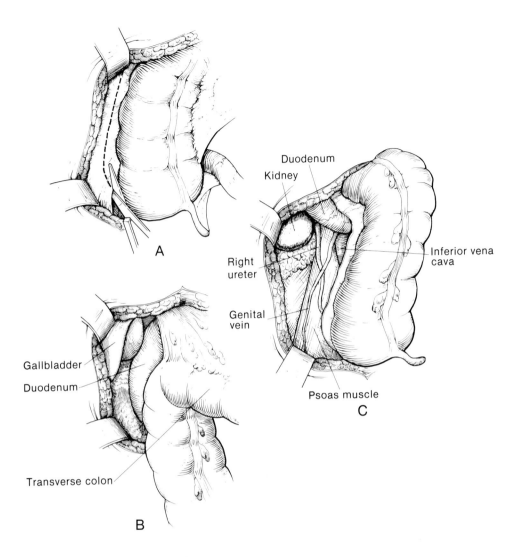

FIGURE 17-3. The right colon is mobilized from its gutter by cutting the peritoneal reflection beginning at the cecum and proceeding upward to the hepatic flexure (A). Medial traction and blunt dissection mobilize the ascending (B) and proximal transverse colon (C), exposing the psoas muscle, kidney, and duodenum. Care needs to be exercised in dissecting the base of the transverse mesocolon adjacent to the duodenum. No retroperitoneal structures should be sharply transected until the ureter has been definitely identified and protected.

The ureter, lying in the retroperitoneal tissues, will be visualized as the colon is mobilized medially. The ureter can be positively identified as it crosses anterior to the iliac artery on either side and can then be followed proximally and distally. If previous infection or dissection of the retroperitoneum has occurred, and identification of the ureters can be anticipated to present some difficulty, the ureters should be stented preoperatively. Unfortunately, the illuminated fiberoptic stents that formerly made ureteral identification very simple are no longer widely available.

Mobilization of the Splenic Flexure

Mobilization of the splenic flexure is fraught with the possibilities of hemorrhage from regional vessels or avulsion of the tip of the spleen or its capsule. Such events can be avoided by not retracting the splenic flexure inferiorly until after its attachments have been cut. The descending colon should first be mobilized from its gutter up to the region of the splenic flexure (Fig. 17-4). The omentum is next detached from the left transverse colon, and the omental dissection is carried to the region of the splenic flexure (Fig. 17-5).

Inferior traction on the splenic flexure should be avoided so that the attachments of the splenic flexure to the lower pole of the spleen will not be placed on tension sufficient to cause avulsion of a portion of the splenic capsule. Following mobilization of the omentum and the descending colon, blunt finger dissection along the superior plane of the left transverse mesocolon and immediately deep to the plane of the omentum can usually be made across the superior aspect of the splenic flexure. The flat and lienocolic ligament overlying the dissecting finger are bluntly crushed between thumb and finger. A large Kelly clamp is then passed from left to right with the deep blade following the path of the dissecting finger and the superficial blade placed between the spleen and the colon. The clamp is adjusted so that it will be a centimeter or more away from the colon when closed (Fig. 17-6). The tissues of the lienocolic ligament are sharply transected between the clamp and the flexure of the colon. There is always a prominent arterial branch located within the ligament. Once freed, the splenic flexure is mobilized inferiorly and medially by traction and blunt dissection, and any bleeding from the colic side of the pedicle is then controlled.

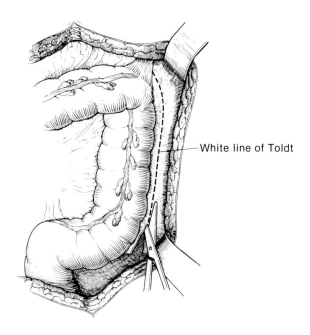

FIGURE 17–4. The descending colon is extracted from its gutter by first retracting the sigmoid colon medially and identifying the white line of Toldt in the flank. The peritoneum is incised from below upward following this line. Medial traction and blunt dissection complete the mobilization of the descending colon.

White line of Toldt

Mobilization of the Greater Omentum

The greater omentum is secondarily attached all along the transverse colon, usually beginning just distal to the hepatic flexure in the area overlying the duodenum, and continuing across to the region of the splenic flexure. The plane of attachment of the omentum to the transverse colon is ordinarily bloodless, except in cases of portal hypertension or inflammatory bowel disease. The fat content is thicker in the region of the hepatic flexure and some small blood vessels may cross the plane between the omentum and the bowel (see Fig. 17–5). In dealing with carcinoma involving the left transverse colon, the splenic flexure, or the proxi-

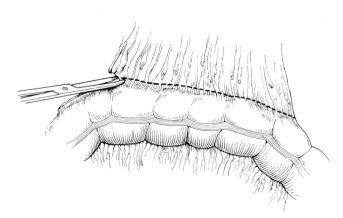

FIGURE 17–5. The greater omentum is mobilized by dividing its avascular attachment to the anterior aspect of the transverse colon. The line of incision begins just at or slightly above the taenia.

mal descending colon, the omentum or at least a portion of it should be resected in continuity with the colonic specimen. With carcinomas lying more distally in the descending or sigmoid colon, which require mobilization of the splenic flexure but not necessarily its resection, the omentum may be dissected away from the left transverse colon as a convenience in approaching the splenic flexure and to facilitate mobilization of the colon for anastomosis.

Instruments

Occlusion of the colon lumen proximal and distal to the proposed lines of resection is a useful precautionary step, although it may not be absolutely necessary if mechanical preparation of the bowel has been adequate. The most convenient clamps for providing such temporary occlusion are made with springy, flat blades; the blades are covered with cloth to provide traction (a laparotomy pad also can serve this purpose). The use of latex rubber tubing to cover the blades is less satisfactory, since it increases the bulk of the blade sufficiently that crush injury to the marginal arterial blood supply may occur.

A number of crushing clamps are available for application directly to the line of resection and are illustrated in Figure 17–7. The Rankin clamp was designed for "aseptic" bowel anastomosis but can serve equally well if an open technique is elected. A variety of stapling instruments have been used in various techniques of colon resection, the most useful of which is the EEA type of instrument.

Extent of Resection

Only the bowel tube need be resected when dealing with diverticulitis, inflammatory bowel disease, or a benign neoplasm. In such cases, the dissection of the mesentery can be at any convenient level, even immediately adjacent to the bowel. Usually the mesentery is transected about 7 to 10 cm from the bowel in order to reduce the number of blood vessels that need to be controlled (Fig. 17–8).

In resections for carcinoma, it is the lymphatic drainage that dictates the extent of resection.[7] Adequate extirpation of a carcinoma requires the sacrifice of a much larger block of tissue and its blood supply than is required for resection of the tumor per se. Margins of 5 cm on either side of a carcinoma are adequate regarding the bowel tube, but removal of the primary and secondary lymphatic drainage requires removal of the main arterial supply proximal and distal to the tumor as well as proximal dissection to the origin of the main blood supply to the tumor-bearing segment. The resection fields recommended for tumors in various locations are illustrated in Figure 17–9.

In all colon resections, the proximal and distal bowel should be mobilized so that the proposed anastomosis can be conducted without any tension. For lesions in the sigmoid and descending colon, this will require mobilization of the splenic flexure in nearly every case.

FIGURE 17-6. Mobilization of the splenic flexure. The descending colon should be mobilized first (see Fig. 17-4), then the omentum is mobilized from the left transverse colon (see Fig. 17-5). A forefinger is insinuated along the superior plane of the left transverse mesocolon beneath the lower pole of the spleen to emerge in the superior aspect of the left gutter (*A*). Much of the fat in the lienocolic ligament can be bluntly crushed between the thumb and forefinger. A large clamp is then passed from left to right, with the deep blade following the path of the dissecting finger and the superficial blade placed between the spleen and colon (*B*). The tissues of the lienocolic ligament are sharply transected between the clamp and the colon. The splenic flexure is then mobilized into the wound by medial and inferior traction, and any bleeding vessels on the colon side of the lienocolic ligament stump are clamped and ligated.

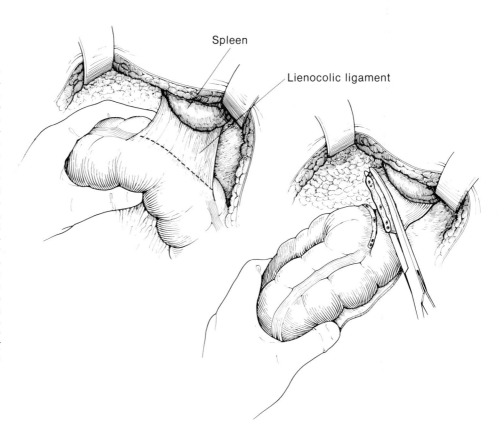

Obstructive Lesions

When cancer or another lesion brings about colonic obstruction, the most expeditious management is to resect the obstructing lesion and exteriorize the bowel ends. Alternatively, but less desirably, a proximal ileostomy or colostomy can be constructed for decompression, followed in a week or two by definitive resection. Anastomosis of the bowel is preferably avoided in emergency operations for obstruction for two reasons. First, the bowel wall proximal to the obstruction is likely to be edematous, and any anastomosis constructed in such bowel is tenuous. Second, antibiotic preparation of the bowel will not have been possible, and this increases the risk of anastomotic breakdown and its consequences. The preferable course is to exteriorize the bowel ends and to restore gastrointestinal continuity at a second operation conducted 6 to 8 weeks later.

When the distal bowel end cannot be brought to the abdominal wall as a mucous fistula, it may be closed with sutures or staples and left in situ. When this is done, the anus always should be manually dilated while the patient is still anesthetized. When such a closed end of bowel is left intraperitoneally, redissection and mobilization at a subsequent operation do not present undue problems. However, when the closed bowel end is located extraperitoneally in the pelvis (Hartmann procedure), remobilization and dissection of the bowel may be difficult. An abscess in the cuff is discovered with some frequency, and the intense inflammatory reaction in the extraperitoneal space often requires further sacrifice of bowel length before tissues suitable for anastomosis can be obtained. It is preferable to avoid a Hartmann procedure whenever possible.

Preparation of the Bowel for Anastomosis

Preservation of the adjacent marginal blood supply is important. A long length of devascularized and denuded bowel is not necessary for anastomosis. In fact, the ideal anastomosis involves denuding only a centimeter or less of the bowel end, a space just sufficient for the anastomosis to be completed without turning in any fat. Attached bits of serosal fat will need to be cleaned off around the circumference of the bowel being prepared for anastomosis. Sometimes a diverticulum is encountered in this process. If the diverticulum is close to the proposed line of resection, this line can be modified on an ad hoc basis to include removal of the diverticulum. If the diverticulum is sufficiently far away that it will not be included directly in the proposed line of anastomosis, it is most expeditiously handled by inverting it into the bowel and holding it there with a simple seromuscular suture. Remember that there is a small blood vessel in the wall of most diverticula.

Anastomosis preferably should not be conducted if the bowel wall is edematous because of obstruction or inflammation or if there is well-established peritonitis. Simple peritoneal contamination occurring immediately before or during operation should not deter construction of an anastomosis. However, established peritonitis with inflammation of the serosa in the region of the proposed anastomosis indicates that it should be deferred. The proximal end of the colon or ileum should be turned out as a temporary stoma. The distal end is preferably turned out as a mucous fistula, even if the distal segment contains diverticula or a sutured perforation that will later need to be resected. If a mucous fistula cannot be arranged, as is occasionally true in re-

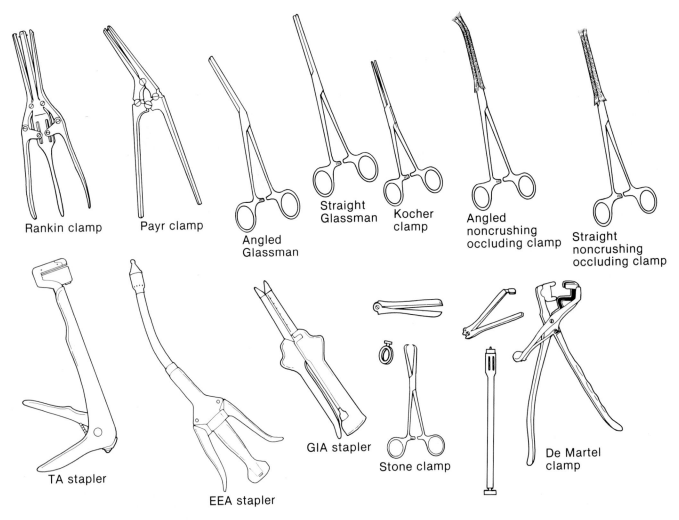

FIGURE 17-7. Useful instruments for colon resection.

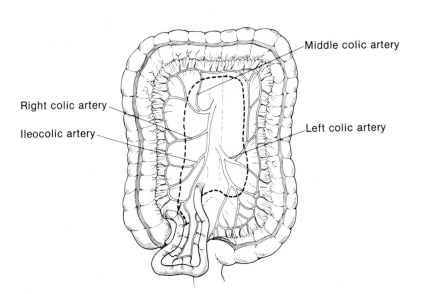

FIGURE 17-8. Division of the mesentery in colon resection for benign diseases, such as ulcerative colitis. Only the principal vessels are ligated. The extent of resection is dictated by the length of bowel that needs to be removed. The level of dissection in the mesentery is chosen at the surgeon's convenience.

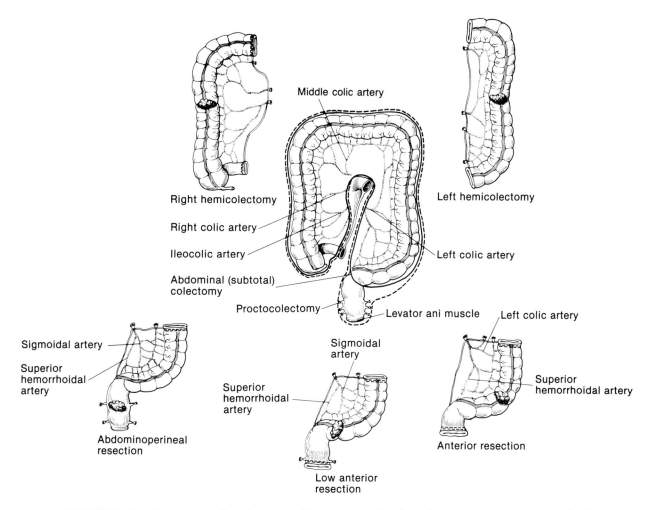

FIGURE 17-9. The extent of dissection and excision recommended for malignant tumors at various sites in the colon. The extent of resection is dictated by the need to remove the primary and secondary lymph node drainage of the tumor.

sections extending into the lower rectosigmoid, the distal bowel may be oversewn (Hartmann procedure).

Techniques of Anastomosis

Basically, an anastomosis is conducted between ileum or proximal colon and distal colon using end-to-end, end-to-side, or side-to-side techniques. Anastomoses may be sewn, either in one or two layers, or stapled, either alone or reinforced with sutures. In all anastomoses, the basic principle is that sutures or staples must engage the submucosa if the anastomosis is to be secure. Single-layer interrupted, sutured anastomoses and unreinforced stapled anastomoses best preserve blood supply to the bowel tissues within the anastomosis. Basic anastomotic techniques are illustrated in Figures 17–10 through 17–14.

Dilation of the Anus

Whenever a colon anastomosis or closure has been done and a proximal colostomy has not been placed, dilation of the anus under anesthesia is a wise precaution. The technique is that of the Lord stretch, although

very wide dilation is not needed. Fingers are serially inserted into the anal canal, gently but firmly distracting the sphincter until four fingers rest in the canal without constriction. The dilation must be done slowly to allow the mucosa of the anal canal, as well as the muscles of the sphincter, to stretch. Otherwise, a superficial mucosal rent may ensue. Four-finger dilation of the anus effectively prevents tight anal sphincter contraction for about 48 hours and thus obviates development of a functional closed loop leading to high pressure in the colon lumen, which then might cause local suture line seepage.

SPECIFIC OPERATIONS

Colotomy

Colotomy is useful for excision of a pedunculated benign polyp that is too large to be removed through a colonoscope. Large sessile polyps are better managed by segmental resection (see later discussion). The operation also is occasionally used to extract a foreign body from the rectosigmoid colon. After opening the abdo-

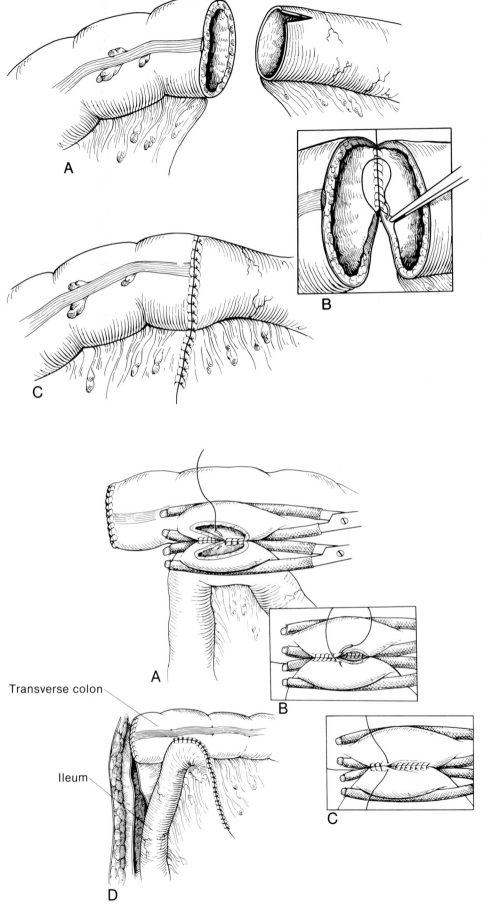

FIGURE 17-10. One-layer sutured end-to-end ileocolostomy. Interrupted nonabsorbable suture, such as braided 3-0 nylon, is employed. If needed, the antimesenteric border of the smaller diameter bowel segment can be incised (Cheatle back-cut) to make the diameter of the segments being anastomosed approximately equal (*A*). The sutures may be placed using running (*B*) or interrupted (*C*) technique. The same principles apply to one-layer colocolostomy.

FIGURE 17-11. *A* through *D*, Two-layer sutured side-to-side ileocolostomy. Similar principles apply to ileorectostomy and colorectostomy. The outer row is of interrupted nonabsorbable suture, such as 3-0 braided nylon; the inner row is of running absorbable material.

Transverse colon

Ileum

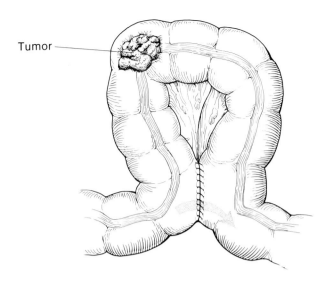

Tumor

FIGURE 17-12. Sutured side-to-side anastomosis. This technique is still used occasionally to bypass an obstructing tumor in cases of disseminated peritoneal carcinomatosis, but it has few other indications today.

men, the polyp or foreign body is located by palpation. Sometimes a polyp is elusive because of its soft consistency; it may be necessary to mobilize the colon to permit adequate palpation. Careful stripping of the bowel between the fingers usually will identify the polyp mass, and traction on the polyp will then identify the point of attachment of the stalk to the bowel wall. The colonic segment to be opened is isolated by cloth-shod occluding clamps.

The incision into the colon is made longitudinally in the anterior taenia (Fig. 17-15), overlying the point of attachment of the polyp stalk or the foreign body. For foreign bodies in the rectosigmoid, the colotomy is made in a slightly proximal position in the intraperitoneal distal sigmoid colon. The margins of the colotomy are grasped with Allis forceps and retracted, the polyp is identified and extracted, and the base of the stalk is suture ligated and then transected to remove the polyp. Foreign bodies, of course, are extracted manually or with instruments, often assisted by transmural manipulation.

The colotomy incision is closed longitudinally in one or two layers. For two-layer closure, a running stitch of absorbable suture is used to invert and close the mucosa; the seromuscular margins of the colotomy are then closed with interrupted or running nonabsorbable suture. For one-layer closure, interrupted nonabsorbable sutures or a stapler is employed. A longitudinal colotomy also can be closed transversely, and this formerly was the usual recommendation. Transverse closure, however, is unnecessary to preserve lumen diameter when the colotomy has been made through a taenia.

Segmental Sleeve Resection

Limited resection of the colon is primarily indicated for the removal of benign neoplasms. Segmental resection also will be applied occasionally in the management

of strictures or other focal lesions, and in resection of giant diverticula and similar benign entities. Even though the length of bowel to be resected is limited, wide mobilization of the colon with preservation of the marginal arterial blood supply needs to be undertaken. The only exception to the need for mobilization will involve selected lesions in the mid-sigmoid colon.

The mesenteric border of the colon is cleaned of fat and mesentery at convenient distances proximally and distally from the lesion to be excised. These two windows are connected by dissection through the mesentery, preferably preserving the marginal arterial arcade. A symmetric V excision into the mesentery can be done if convenient, but it is not necessary in every case. The objectives to be accomplished are (1) removal of the lesion with minimal borders, (2) preservation of the blood supply to the ends of bowel to be anastomosed in restoration of gastrointestinal continuity, and (3) end-to-end anastomosis, using either a single-layer or a double-layer technique.

A single-layer anastomosis technique is preferred because it better preserves blood supply (Fig. 17-16). A double-layer anastomosis adds an additional running, usually locking, stitch of absorbable suture, which coapts mucosa and submucosa but excludes the muscularis propria and serosa. An anastomosis also can be constructed using stapling techniques (see Figs. 17-13 and 17-14), although stapling rarely saves time compared with interrupted sutures in constructing a simple anastomosis.

Right Hemicolectomy and Ascending Colectomy

The difference in these two operations is that the hepatic flexure is resected in a right hemicolectomy. Ascending colectomy is most frequently indicated for removal of arteriovenous malformations in the region of the ileocecal valve and is also used to remove polyps and other benign lesions in the area of the cecum. Right hemicolectomy is most frequently done to remove a carcinoma of the right colon.

The cecum and ascending colon are mobilized, beginning by retracting the cecum medially and sharply transecting the lateral peritoneal fold at the inferior end of the right gutter. A finger is inserted into the gutter extraperitoneally, the cecum is retracted slightly medially, and then the peritoneal reflection from the body wall to the colon is sharply transected over the finger. These maneuvers are repeated sequentially as the dissection is carried superiorly to the hepatic flexure (see Fig. 17-3). The dissecting finger is advanced extraperitoneally around the hepatic flexure, which is then retracted inferiorly, and the peritoneal incision is carried across the superior aspect of the hepatic flexure and into the retroperitoneum near the lower pole of the kidney. Medial traction on the entire ascending colon now easily defines a dissection plane in the retroperitoneum, which is opened bluntly.

The distal ileum is similarly mobilized medially by traction and incision of the peritoneum overlying the psoas muscle until the right ureter is identified crossing the common iliac artery. The blunt retroperitoneal dis-

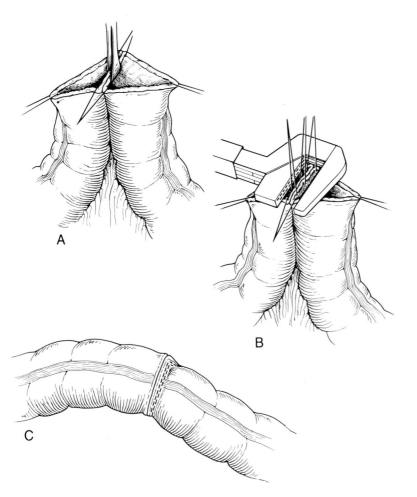

A

B

C

FIGURE 17-13. *A* through *C*, Everted triangulated single layer stapled end-to-end anastomosis. Each leg of the triangle is separately stapled.

section is continued superiorly along the lateral margin of the vena cava, preserving and pushing the gonadal vessels posteriorly until the level of the third portion of the duodenum is reached. The peritoneum between the lower pole of the right kidney and the anterior wall of the duodenum is finally transected. In all of this dissection, care is taken not to exert traction, which would disrupt the venous drainage of the colon. And, of course, the arterial blood supply also is carefully preserved. Most of this dissection will be without significant bleeding, although a small blood vessel is sometimes encountered in the region of the hepatic flexure. The appendiceal mesentery is mobilized from the distal ileum, transecting it if necessary.

In *ascending colectomy*, which is usually done for benign disease, the next step is to identify the major branch of the right colic artery, which supplies the colon immediately proximal to the hepatic flexure. A window is made through the mobilized mesentery immediately adjacent to the medial border of the ascending colon and just below this nutrient vessel. The mesenteric dissection is then carried inferiorly through the middle of the mesentery, outside the marginal vascular arcade, to the ileocolic artery. Careful inspection of the region of the ileocecal valve will determine if the ileocolic artery can be preserved. If so, the dissection is carried back to the bowel along the superior aspect of this artery, approaching the bowel immediately adjacent to the ileocecal valve. If not convenient, the ileocecal artery may be tran-

sected and the line of mesenteric dissection carried to the distal ileum approximately 5 cm proximal to the ileocecal valve (Fig. 17–17). Noncrushing occluding clamps are applied to the ileum and the right transverse colon. Paired crushing bowel clamps are applied at the proposed lines of bowel transection, and the specimen is removed. An ileoascending colostomy is constructed, usually employing an end-to-end anastomosis as illustrated in Figure 17–10.

Right hemicolectomy involves a similar mobilization of bowel. In addition, it is important to mobilize and remove the mesenteric lymph nodes adjacent to the origin of the right colic and middle colic arteries. Therefore, wide mobilization is carried out, following which a noncrushing occluding clamp is applied to the left transverse colon and a window is created in the mobilized transverse mesocolon just to the right side of the terminal branches of the middle colic artery (Fig. 17–18). The marginal vascular arcade is transected and the line of dissection is carried in the transverse mesocolon to the anterior aspect of the duodenum. The lymph nodes on the right side of the superior mesenteric and middle colic vessels should be resected; this dissection needs to proceed carefully, since these lymph nodes receive small blood vessels directly from the superior mesenteric artery and vein; careful dissection with precise hemostasis is required to avoid hemorrhage in this potentially difficult area. The base of the mesentery is transected, taking the ileocolic artery near its origins, and the dis-

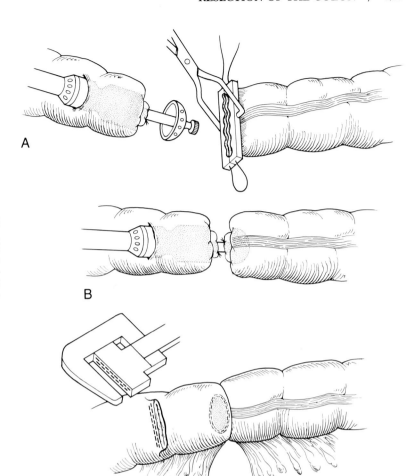

FIGURE 17-14. *A* through *C,* Principles of a stapled end-to-end anastomosis using the EEA stapler device. Pursestring sutures are used to pull the ends of bowel around the opened anvil of the device. The stapler cuts two circles of tissue (which should be checked for completeness) as the stapler is closed. The colotomy used to insert the stapler is closed with a TA-90 stapler or can be sutured.

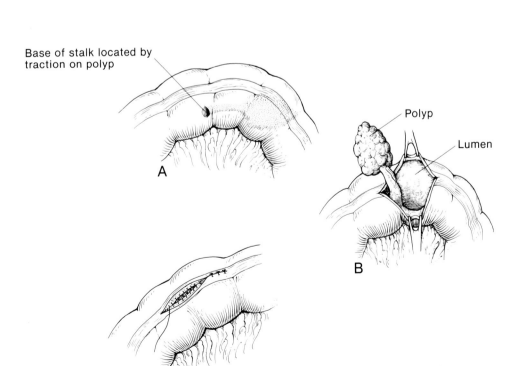

FIGURE 17-15. *A* through *C,* Colotomy for excision of a large benign polyp. A longitudinal incision in a taenia is employed and is closed longitudinally in one or two (illustrated) layers.

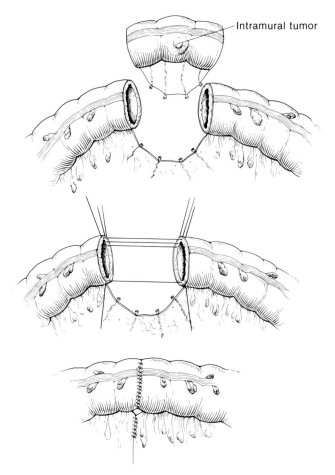

Intramural tumor

FIGURE 17-16. One-layer end-to-end colon anastomosis. Sutures are inserted from outside to inside on one end of the bowel, then are carried across and extracted inside to outside on the other bowel end. All sutures encompass only the seromuscular and submucosal layers of the bowel wall; the mucosa is excluded, although it is inverted as the sutures are tied. Initially, sutures are placed at the mesenteric and antimesenteric borders. The remainder of the sutures are then placed serially, as illustrated. Alternatively, if the bowel ends have some size disproportion, the third suture is placed halfway between the initial pair, then each of these segments is again divided by sutures placed at their midpoints and the process is continued, progressively dividing the bowel circumference into proportionately equal and smaller segments.

section is then continued to the distal ileum. A noncrushing occluding clamp is applied across the ileum, and paired crushing clamps are placed at the line of ileal transection. The technique is illustrated in Figure 17–3. Gastrointestinal continuity may be restored by either end-to-end (see Fig. 17–10) or end-to-side (see Fig. 17–11) ileotransverse colostomy.

Transverse Colectomy

Tumors in the mid–transverse colon are usually removed by transverse colectomy. Very occasionally, transverse colectomy may need to be employed in the management of a gastrocolic or gastrojejunocolic fistula or to remove necrotic bowel secondary to pancreatitis. In this operation, both the hepatic (see Fig. 17–3) and the splenic (see Fig. 17–6) flexures are mobilized. Cancers arising in the right transverse colon are sometimes most

conveniently managed by an extended operation that includes a right hemicolectomy together with excision of the transverse colon. Cancers arising in the distal transverse colon, clearly beyond the middle colic vessels but proximal to the splenic flexure, usually are resected by mobilizing the entire right colon, transecting the right transverse colon but preserving the hepatic flexure, and mobilizing the splenic flexure and the entire descending colon, resecting that portion proximal to the left colic artery. Gastrointestinal continuity is restored by end-to-end anastomosis (see Fig. 17–16).

Left (Descending) Colectomy

The usual indication for a left colectomy is a carcinoma arising in or just distal to the splenic flexure and proximal to the sigmoid flexure. The left colon is mobilized from its gutter by retracting the sigmoid colon medially and identifying the line of Toldt, which is sharply incised. Blunt extraperitoneal finger dissection with medial retraction of the descending colon permits progressive transection of the peritoneum in the gutter, proceeding superiorly to the region of the splenic flexure (Fig. 17–19). The splenic flexure is then mobilized, the dissection proceeding from right to left along the superior aspect of the transverse colon and the flexure (see Fig. 17–6). In some cases of cancer of the splenic flexure, the spleen must be resected in continuity with the colon in order not to compromise the dissection border around the primary tumor. In most cases, even though it violates the principle of including both the proximal and distal main arterial supply in the resected specimen, resection of cancers arising in the proximal descending colon can be conducted by transecting the left transverse colon just to the left of the middle colic vessels and preserving these vessels. The distal line of transection, depending on the location of the primary tumor, may allow preservation of the most proximal sigmoid arterial branches. However, if the tumor is lower in the descending colon, near the sigmoid flexure, one or more of the proximal sigmoidal arteries may need to be resected with the specimen. The left colic artery, and the sigmoidal arteries if necessary, are transected as they branch from the inferior mesenteric artery (see Fig. 17–9).

Noncrushing, lumen-occluding clamps are placed on the right transverse colon and sigmoid colon. A window is made in the mesentery immediately to the left of the main branches of the middle colic artery. The transverse mesocolon is incised, dissecting just lateral to the ligament of Treitz. With medial traction, the descending colon is bluntly mobilized medially to expose the aorta. In the last few centimeters of this dissection, the genital venous vessels and the ureter will be encountered and they need to be pushed posteriorly, the plane of dissection being carried just anterior to these structures.

Next, a window is made in the region of the sigmoid flexure, either proximal or distal to the upper sigmoidal arteries as dictated by the necessary margins of resection. The line of transection of the sigmoid mesocolon is carried medially, transecting arterial branches as they arise from the inferior mesenteric artery. The inferior

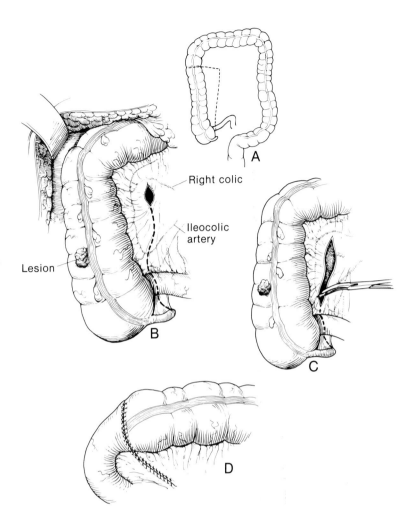

FIGURE 17–17. *A through D,* Ascending colectomy is usually done for benign disease affecting the region of the cecum or proximal ascending colon.

Right colic

Ileocolic artery

Lesion

mesenteric–superior hemorrhoidal arterial arcade is preserved. The line of dissection is carried close to the aorta, but it is not necessary to resect periaortic nodes. If such nodes are involved, the patient has disseminated disease, which will not be cured by resection of the primary colon tumor. The two lines of dissection are now connected in the retroperitoneum following the lateral border of the aorta and staying anterior to the left renal vein and the left kidney pedicle (see Fig. 17–18). The freely mobilized right colon and the sigmoid colon are approximated by an end-to-end anastomosis.

Anterior Sigmoid Resection

The common indications for anterior sigmoid resection are complicated diverticular disease and carcinoma arising in the mid–sigmoid colon. Anterior sigmoid resection differs from a low anterior resection in that the distal transection and anastomosis of the bowel are done intraperitoneally at the promontory of the sacrum. The entire descending colon (see Fig. 17–4) and splenic flexure (see Fig. 17–6) are mobilized. The left ureter is identified as it crosses the left common iliac artery and is preserved, as are the genital vessels (Fig. 17–20). After wide mobilization of the entire left colon and the sigmoid colon, the plane of resection in the mesentery is determined.

Resection of the sigmoid to remove carcinoma always involves more extensive resection than is necessary for benign disease, such as diverticulitis. For benign disease in the sigmoid colon, the left colic artery is preserved and the sigmoidal branches are transected as they arise from the superior hemorrhoidal arcade. The superior hemorrhoidal vessels also are preserved; only the involved segment of sigmoid colon is resected. The extent of resection for cancer is dictated by the need to remove the supplying arteries proximal and distal to the tumor and their associated draining lymph nodes. For cancer involving the proximal to mid–sigmoid colon, the inferior mesenteric artery is transected at or near its origin, sacrificing the left colic and all of the sigmoidal as well as the superior hemorrhoidal arteries. The bowel from the mid–descending colon distally to the sacral promontory will be excised. For cancer involving the mid- to distal sigmoid, in which the tumor is at least 10 cm proximal to the sacral promontory, the inferior mesenteric arcade is transected just after the origin of the left colic artery. Dissection is continued through the retroperitoneum medial to the superior hemorrhoidal arcade, which is to be excised. The bowel from the distal descending colon proximally to the junction of sigmoid and rectosigmoid distally will be resected.

Noncrushing occluding clamps are applied to the proximal descending colon, paired crushing bowel

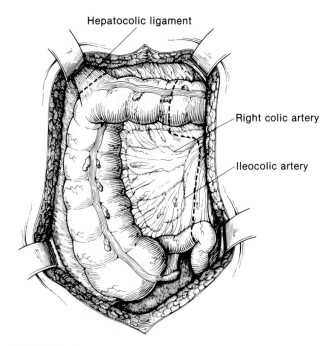

FIGURE 17-18. Right hemicolectomy. The hepatic flexure is mobilized in addition to the ascending colon (see Figs. 17–3 and 17–17). The right colic and ileocolic vessels are transected at or near their origin to permit excision of the lymph nodes at the root of the right colon mesentery.

most proximal portion of the rectosigmoid may be mobilized for a short distance from the anterior aspect of the sacrum by blunt retroperitoneal dissection. Crushing clamps in a pair are now placed across the distal sigmoid or upper rectosigmoid, the bowel is transected, and the specimen is removed. The proximal colon is mobilized sufficiently to permit end-to-end anastomosis to restore gastrointestinal continuity without tension.

Left Hemicolectomy

Left hemicolectomy simply combines descending colectomy, including resection of the splenic flexure, with anterior sigmoid resection. The operation may be necessitated by extensive tumors of the proximal sigmoid or the descending colon, which require resection of a wider field in order to remove all of the primary and secondary lymph node drainage of the primary tumor (Fig. 17–21). Following resection, the entire right colon and hepatic flexure are mobilized (see Figs. 17–3 and 17–17) and are rotated so that the right transverse colon proximally and the rectosigmoid distally can be anastomosed in end-to-end fashion. Alternatively, if restricted mesenteric length demands it, the proximal transverse colon can be closed by sutures or staples, and intestinal continuity can be restored by a side-to-end anastomosis.

Total Abdominal (Subtotal) Colectomy

In total abdominal colectomy, the entire intraperitoneal colon is removed. Total colectomy is indicated for the management of extensive inflammatory bowel disease or multiple polyposis prior to the appearance of carcinoma. Excision of lymphatics is unnecessary, excision of the bowel tube being the objective of the operation. Therefore, following mobilization of the colon from both gutters (see Figs. 17–3, 17–17, and 17–18) and mobilization of the hepatic and splenic (Fig. 17–6)

clamps are placed across the proposed line of colon transection, and the bowel is cut. The major portion of the specimen can now be lifted out of the wound and placed on traction. The proximal rectosigmoid is elevated by blunt dissection of its posterior attachments to the proximal sacrum, carrying the level of dissection about 1 to 2 cm below the point of entry of the superior hemorrhoidal vessels into the bowel. The pelvic peritoneum on the anterior and lateral aspects of the rectosigmoid is not opened in this operation, although the

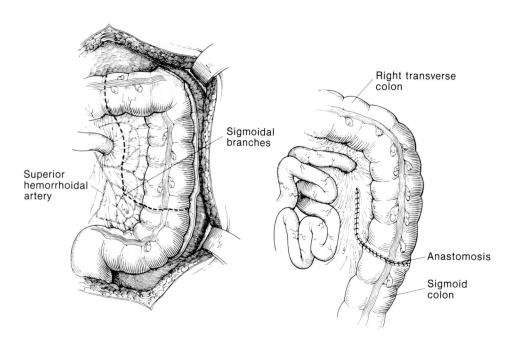

FIGURE 17-19. Left (descending) colectomy. The left colon is mobilized from its gutter (see Fig. 17–4) and the splenic flexure is mobilized (see Fig. 17–5). The mesentery and peritoneum are transected, preserving the middle colic, superior hemorrhoidal, and distal sigmoidal vessels. End-to-end anastomosis is done after mobilizing the hepatic flexure and right colon as necessary to relieve any tension.

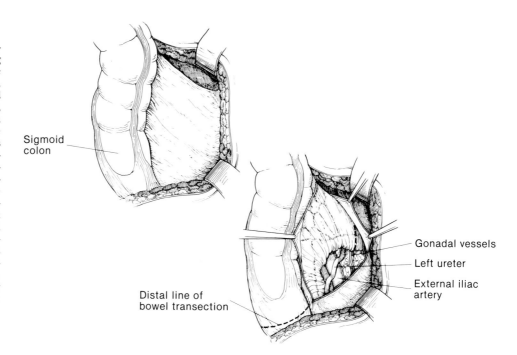

FIGURE 17-20. Anterior sigmoid resection. The descending colon and sigmoid flexure have been mobilized (see Figs. 17–4, 17–5, and 17–18). The sigmoid mesentery is mobilized medially, preserving the gonadal vessels and left ureter. For benign disease, the sigmoidal arteries are taken as they branch, preserving the inferior mesenteric–superior hemorrhoidal arcade. In resecting a mid-sigmoid cancer, however, the inferior mesenteric artery is transected just after giving off the left colic branch. For a more proximal sigmoid cancer, the inferior mesenteric artery is transected near its origin, including the left colic artery in the resected specimen. Bowel continuity is restored by end-to-end anastomosis (see Fig. 17–23).

flexures, the mesentery is transected at any convenient level that permits expeditious removal of the bowel with a minimum number of blood vessels needing to be ligated (Fig. 17–22).

Unless the distal ileum is involved, consideration may be given to preserving the ileocolic artery. The left colic artery is taken near its origin from the inferior mesenteric artery. The inferior mesenteric–superior hemor-

rhoidal arcade should be preserved unless all of the rectosigmoid colon is to be resected; in this case, the inferior mesenteric artery can be ligated near its origin.

The omentum may be separated from the transverse colon and left as an appendage of the greater curvature of the stomach. However, particularly in cases of inflammatory bowel disease, it is more efficient to transect the gastrocolic ligament and remove the omentum with the colon specimen. In cases of advanced inflammatory bowel disease, total proctocolectomy may be desirable.

In most cases, gastrointestinal continuity is re-established by end-to-end or end-to-side ileorectosigmoidostomy (Fig. 17–23). Sometimes the distal stump is over-

FIGURE 17-21. Left hemicolectomy involves resection of the bowel from the left transverse colon to the proximal rectosigmoid. It combines the technical maneuvers involved in descending (see Fig. 17–19) and sigmoid colectomy (see Fig. 17–20).

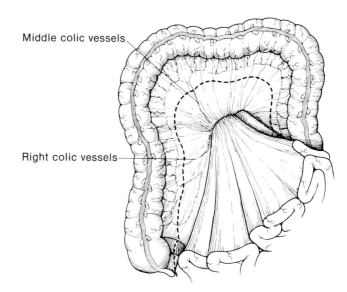

FIGURE 17-22. Total colectomy is performed for benign disease involving the entire colon. All of the intra-abdominal colon is mobilized. The blood vessels are taken at a convenient point in the middle of the mesentery.

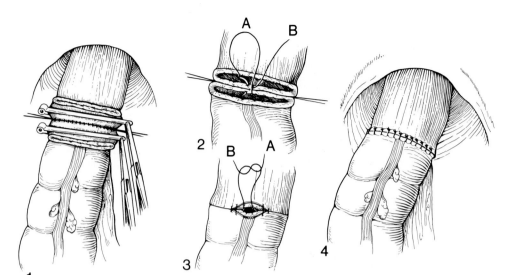

FIGURE 17-23. Anastomosis to the proximal rectosigmoid. A two-layer anastomosis of interrupted seromuscular nonabsorbable sutures and a running (alternatively, running locking) mucosal-submucosal absorbable suture is illustrated. A single layer anastomosis, omitting the inner mucosal suture, is also effective. In both techniques, the back row of seromuscular sutures is placed before the occluding clamps are removed.

sewn (Hartmann procedure), and an ileostomy is constructed. If an ileostomy is to be performed (see Chapter 16), the distal transected end of the rectosigmoid may be closed with staples or a running basting stitch under a Glassman clamp. This initial suture line is then buried by interrupted nonabsorbable seromuscular inverting sutures.

Loop Colostomy and Ileostomy

A loop colostomy or ileostomy is used for temporary diversion or decompression of the colon. For lesions in the rectum, a mid- or distal sigmoid colostomy is usually used. For lesions involving the sigmoid or descending colon, the colostomy usually is placed in the left transverse colon. For more proximal lesions, an ileostomy is used. The principles of these operations—sigmoid colostomy, left transverse colostomy, and ileostomy—are identical. The selected loop of bowel must have a mesentery of sufficient length to allow it to be brought above the level of the skin without tension. If the mesentery is not sufficiently long, additional mesenteric length must be secured. In a sigmoid colostomy or an ileostomy, a transverse incision of an avascular portion of the mesentery midway between the bowel and the retroperitoneum, with the line of dissection paralleling the bowel and preserving the arterial supply to the bowel, usually will provide sufficient additional mobilization. A second small window in the mesentery at the immediate bowel margin is made to provide passage for the device used to support the loop.

In the left transverse colon, a similar maneuver is often successful. However, in some patients, particularly obese ones, even wide incision of the transverse mesocolon will be insufficient to permit the bowel loop to be brought above the skin without tension. The splenic flexure would need to be mobilized to permit construction of the left transverse colostomy. In this special circumstance, it is better to abandon left transverse colos-

tomy and to mobilize the hepatic flexure and construct the colostomy in the right transverse colon. The functional results of a right transverse colostomy are the same as those of a left transverse colostomy. The technique of loop colostomy is illustrated in Figure 17-24. The same principles apply to loop ileostomy, the stoma usually being constructed about 20 to 30 cm proximal to the ileocecal valve. The stoma may be opened immediately if the bowel has been effectively prepared preoperatively. However, when constructed in unprepared bowel, opening a loop colostomy should be deferred for 12 to 24 hours to allow the bowel to seal to the subcutaneous tissues. If immediate decompression is required, as in cases of obstruction, a tube secured by a purse-string suture should be inserted into the proximal limb for the initial 12 to 24 hours, after which the stoma may be fully opened.

Divided Colostomy

In a divided colostomy, the ends of the bowel are separated, the proximal end being brought out as the colostomy. The distal end is brought out, through a separate stab wound, as a mucous fistula, although it may also be handled as a Hartmann procedure. The stoma should always be brought through the sheath of the rectus abdominis muscle in order to avoid later development of a peristomal hernia. If it is known that a colostomy will be required for only a short period, it is less imperative that it be constructed within the rectus sheath. However, if there is any question about the potential duration that the colostomy will need, the stoma should be constructed through the rectus sheath.

A divided colostomy may be opened in delayed fashion but usually is matured to skin immediately by suture. The technique is illustrated in Figure 17-25. An end colostomy or ileostomy is much easier to manage postoperatively, since a well-fitted collecting device can be

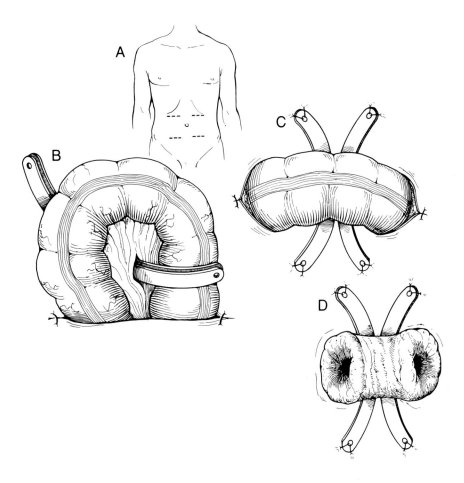

FIGURE 17-24. *A* through *D*, Loop colostomy. The loop of bowel is extracted through a conveniently placed transverse incision and is supported by a plastic bridge or a heavy rubber tube stent. If necessary, the ends of the incision are sutured so that the bowel is apposed to subcutaneous fat around its entire circumference. The bowel is not sutured to the peritoneum or fascia in adults, but the peritoneum should be sutured around the exiting bowel in infants to prevent herniation. Opening of the stoma is usually delayed for 24 hours.

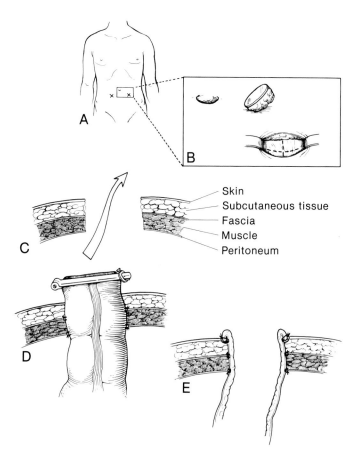

FIGURE 17-25. *A*, The preferred sites for a permanent stoma are within the rectus sheath and just below the waist (*X*); the site for the mucous fistula can be anywhere in the lower abdomen. *B*, A circular 2-cm button of skin and subcutaneous tissue is excised; a cruciate incision is made into the anterior rectus fascia; the rectus muscle is spread apart; and a circular 2-cm button of posterior sheath and peritoneum is excised. *C*, The stoma is manually dilated, and the closed end of the proximal bowel is drawn through. The bowel end should lie without tension 2 cm or more above the skin. *D*, Four-quadrant absorbable sutures anchor the colon to the peritoneum at the exit site. Similar nonabsorbable sutures anchor the colon to the anterior fascia; these sutures must not penetrate the mucosa of the bowel. The distal bowel end is extracted without tension as a mucous fistula through a stab wound at any convenient site and is held in position with a clamp or suture. After the main wound has been closed and protected, the end of the colostomy is opened and immediately sutured to skin (*E*) with interrupted absorbable sutures. These sutures successively include bowel submucosa at the end of the bowel segment, bowel wall 1 to 2 cm from the bowel end (to evert the stoma), and skin dermis at the edge of the stoma wound. Mucosa of bowel should abut the edge of skin without overlap. A collecting device is fitted. Postoperative ileus generally delays passage of stool for 1 to 3 days.

applied, something that is difficult to arrange with a loop stoma.

Colostomy Closure

Colostomy closure is not a minor procedure and should be conducted as an intra-abdominal operation after full bowel preparation. Attempts at local mobilization and closure without opening the abdomen are associated with an excess incidence of complications, whereas treating colostomy closure as a major open abdominal procedure results in no more complications than does any other elective colon operation.

The proximal and distal bowel segments are mobilized intraperitoneally, and the bowel is mobilized from its internal aspect to the level of the anterior fascia. Stone clamps are applied in pairs to each limb of bowel, the two segments of bowel are transected, the ends are withdrawn into the abdomen, and noncrushing occluding clamps are applied proximally and distally. A formal end-to-end anastomosis is then constructed. The short segment of bowel remaining in the body wall at the colostomy site is excised by sharply incising the mucosa-skin interface and bluntly mobilizing the bowel from the subcutaneous tissues. Sharp and blunt dissection frees the bowel from the fascia, and it is extracted. The mucous fistula site is similarly managed. The former stoma sites are closed only at the level of the peritoneum and posterior fascia; the remainder of the old stoma sites are packed open initially and are then allowed to close secondarily.

REFERENCES

1. Ambrose, N.S., Alexander-Williams, J., Johnson, M., et al.: The influence of polyethylene glycol (PEG) with a balanced electrolyte solution for bowel preparation on colonic microflora and colonic gas. Br. J. Surg., *69*:680, 1982.
2. Condon, R.E.: Intestinal antisepsis: Rationale and results. World J. Surg., *6*:182, 1982.
3. Davis, G.R., SantaAna, C.A., Morawski, S.G., and Fordtran, J.S.: Development of a lavage solution associated with minimum water and electrolyte absorption or secretion. Gastroenterology, *78*:991, 1980.
4. Hughes, E.S.R.: Asepsis in large-bowel surgery. Ann. R. Coll. Surg. Engl., *51*:347, 1972.
5. Irving, A.D., and Scrimgeour, D.: Mechanical bowel preparation for colonic resection and anastomosis. Br. J. Surg., *74*:580, 1987.
6. Johnston, D.: Bowel preparation for colorectal surgery (Editorial). Br. J. Surg., *74*:553, 1987.
7. Malassagne, B., Valleur, P., Serra, J., et al.: Relationship of apical lymph node involvement to survival in resected colon carcinoma. Dis. Colon Rectum, *36*:645, 1993.
8. Whittle, J., Steinberg, E.P., Anderson, G.F., and Herbert, R.: Results of colectomy in elderly patients with colon cancer, based on Medicare claims data. Am. J. Surg., *163*:572, 1992.

Chapter 18

LOW ANTERIOR RESECTION

ANTHONY M. VERNAVA, III / STANLEY M. GOLDBERG

Surgical resection of the primary tumor is the standard of care, and low anterior resection remains the procedure of choice, for most rectal cancers located in the high, mid, and even low rectum. Curative operative management remains divided between low anterior resection, abdominoperineal resection, and local excision. The decision between each of these options is based on the location and stage of the tumor, preoperative fecal continence of the patient, and the overall medical condition of the patient.

The treatment of rectal carcinoma has evolved over the past century but most rapidly over the past 20 years. Prior to the introduction of the circular intraluminal stapler, the abdominoperineal resection described by Miles[55] was the standard in operative management of rectal cancer. The advent of the circular intraluminal stapler in the 1970s obviated many of the technical prohibitions that formerly required the performance of an abdominoperineal resection. Since the introduction of the circular intraluminal stapler, additional technical refinements have been made and other surgical staplers have been introduced, effectively extending the limits of restorative resection down to the dentate line. The impact of the circular intraluminal stapler on the surgical management of rectal cancer was reviewed by Hackford[33] and is illustrated in Figure 18–1. This dramatic change in therapy has not been associated with any increase in treatment failure. Indeed, numerous comparisons between low anterior resection and abdominoperineal resection for rectal cancer demonstrate no significant therapeutic difference between the two procedures. It is not surprising, therefore, that "curative" anterior resection has overtaken abdominoperineal resection as the treatment of choice for most rectal cancers.

With the shift in therapeutic philosophy have come a number of controversies as the tension between the requirement to cure the patient is balanced against the desire to preserve sphincter function. For instance, as we extend the limits of restorative resection to the dentate line, the ideal distal margin for curative anterior resection becomes critically important. It appears that a distal margin of 5 or even 2 cm is not necessary for adequate distal clearance, but that a distal margin of 1 cm is adequate for most rectal cancers.[75] The lateral margins of resection remain important to potential cure and are a common cause of locoregional recurrence.[64] The extent of resection remains an area of debate among surgeons; radical pelvic lymphadenectomy[35] and complete mesorectal excision[38] continue to be recommended by some as useful in diminishing the rate of locoregional failure and improving survival. Endorectal ultrasound has become established as a precise tool to preoperatively stage rectal cancers (both to determine muscle wall invasion and to determine the presence of metastatic regional lymph nodes) as well as to follow patients after operation.[5–7,34,40,56] The technique can therefore help to distinguish between patients most likely to benefit from preoperative adjuvant radiation and chemoradiation therapy (i.e., TNM stage II and III disease) and those unlikely to derive any benefit from preoperative adjuvant therapy (i.e., TNM stage I). The controversy regarding adjuvant therapy for rectal cancer continues, most significantly with regard to whether preoperative therapy is preferred to postoperative therapy. This controversy has only somewhat abated since the National Institutes of Health (NIH) recommended, in 1990, routine postoperative adjuvant therapy for patients with TNM stage II and III rectal cancers.[11] Therapy recommended consists of intravenous 5-fluorouracil (5-FU) and high-dose pelvic irradiation (4,500 to 5,040 cGy). Certain prognostic indicators, such as DNA flow cytometric analysis,[14] continue to hold promise of being able to further stratify patients into recurrence risk groups that go beyond classic clinicopathologic staging, but are not yet sufficiently validated to recommend their routine application. Finally, several investigators have employed minimally invasive laparoscopic techniques in the performance of low anterior resection.[20,79] These results are preliminary and require additional evaluation.

These controversies notwithstanding, low anterior resection is an operation which, when well performed, of-

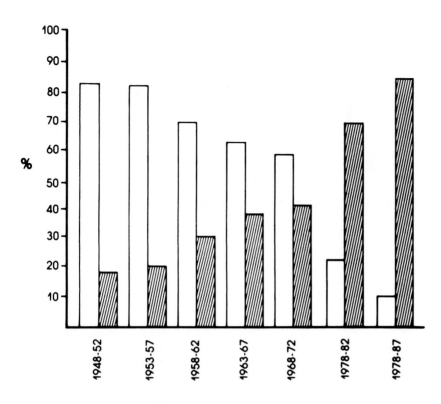

FIGURE 18-1. Trends in operation for rectal cancer: 1948–1988 (From Hackford, A.W.: The extent of major resections for rectal cancer. *In* Veidenheimer, M.C. [ed.]: Semin. Colon Rectal Surg., *1:*16, 1990, with permission.)

fers the patient with rectal cancer as high a probability of cure as that associated with any other operation, while maintaining the normal defecatory pathway. What follows is an attempt to provide a clinically useful review of the current status of low anterior resection in the management of rectal cancer, including operative technique, as well as some perspective on the evolving therapy of rectal cancer.

DEFINITION

A low anterior resection is any rectal resection that requires extraperitoneal rectal mobilization with an extraperitoneal colorectal or ileorectal anastomosis (Fig. 18–2). The anastomosis may be located in the middle or lower rectum (down to the dentate line) and may be either stapled or sutured. An operation resulting in an anastomosis to the intraperitoneal rectum (i.e., above the peritoneal reflection) is commonly referred to as a high anterior resection. A complete understanding of the anatomy of the lower abdomen and pelvis is essential to the successful and safe performance of low anterior resection and is illustrated in Figures 18–3 and 18–4.

HISTORY

Attempts to provide a restorative option following resection of a rectal cancer date back to Verneuil in 1873 and Kraske in 1885.[49] Kraske's method of transsacral ex-

tirpation of the tumor allowed the restoration of bowel continuity via an end-to-end anastomosis. Hochenegg provided an alternative technique of restorative resection by developing the first pull-through operation for rectal cancer in 1888.[41] Maunsell,[51] Weir,[78] Babcock,[3] Bacon,[1] Black,[8] Cutait,[13] and Turnbull[72] each subsequently described their own particular version of the pull-through operation. The difficulty in obtaining satisfactory results is illustrated by the plethora of approaches and anastomotic techniques described in these reports. Needless to say, none of these varied procedures gained

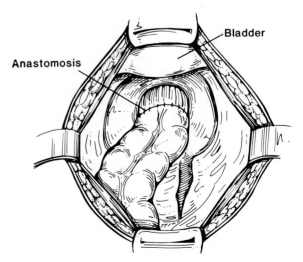

FIGURE 18-2. Extraperitoneal colorectal (or ileorectal) anastomosis.

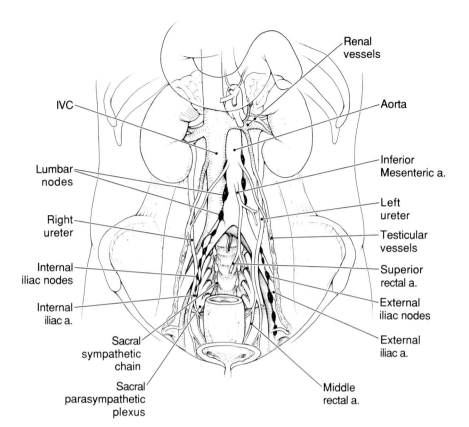

FIGURE 18-3. Anterior view of normal pelvic anatomy. (From Harnsberger, J.R., Vernava, A.M., and Longo, W.E.: Radical abdominopelvic lymphadenectomy in the treatment of rectal cancer [RAPL]: A historical perspective and its current role in the surgical management of rectal cancer. Dis. Colon Rectum, *37*:73, 1994, with permission.)

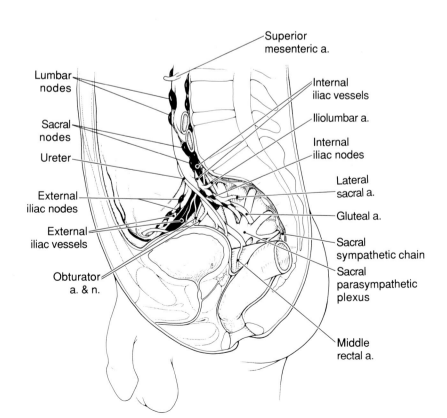

FIGURE 18-4. Lateral view of normal pelvic anatomy. (From Harnsberger, J.R., Vernava, A.M., and Longo, W.E.: Radical abdominopelvic lymphadenectomy in the treatment of rectal cancer [RAPL]: A historical perspective and its current role in the surgical management of rectal cancer. Dis. Colon Rectum, *37*:73, 1994, with permission.)

widespread acceptance among practicing surgeons because of the associated difficult complications, including sepsis and necrosis of the transposed colon, and because of the frequency of fecal incontinence after each of these operations.

In 1908, Miles described the technique of abdominoperineal resection.[55] The operation became the treatment of choice for all rectal cancers because Dukes, a prominent pathologist who practiced at St. Mark's Hospital in London with Miles, argued that the operation provided each patient with the best chance for cure by excision of most of the potentially involved lymphatics. Until the late 1970s, abdominoperineal resection with its permanent stoma was the procedure of choice for most patients with carcinoma of the rectum.

The modern anterior resection was initially described by Dixon and colleagues at the Mayo Clinic.[15] Anterior resection provided a restorative option compared to abdominoperineal resection, as well as to abdominosacral resection and the pull-through operations. However, the operation was not widely practiced, partly owing to surgeons' technical inability to perform a low anastomosis. Additionally, the widespread belief that more aggressive resection (i.e., abdominoperineal resection) was required to cure the patient limited the acceptance of anterior resection.

The advent of the circular intraluminal stapler obviated many of the technical difficulties involved with performing a low anastomosis. Additional technical refinements in the stapler, including the addition of a trochar on the body of the instrument, the introduction of the roticulating TA-55 stapler, and the use of the "double-staple" technique[22,30] have extended the limit of restorative resection to the dentate line. As familiarity with these instruments and their use has increased, the operation has become more widely practiced, and low anterior resection has now replaced abdominoperineal resection as the standard of therapy for most rectal cancers. This dramatic change in therapeutic philosophy has occurred with the clinical demonstration that low anterior resection is therapeutically equivalent to abdominoperineal resection.[37,45,53,80,82,84] Unfortunately, this alteration in management of low anterior resection reported in the medical literature has not translated into uniform practice in the community. In a pilot evaluation (unpublished) of management of rectal cancer in a community hospital over a recent 5-year period, fully 50% of patients with rectal cancers underwent abdominoperineal resection. These data are at odds with those present in the literature and demonstrate that the precise management of individuals with rectal cancer varies among clinicians. This variation seems to be based on the respective clinician's familiarity and proficiency with specific operative techniques and on their pre-existing clinical prejudices.

EXTENT OF RESECTION FOR RECTAL CANCER
Distal Margins

Since 1951, when Goligher, Dukes, and Bussey suggested that a 2-cm margin of normal rectum below the tumor was likely to result in treatment failure, a 5-cm distal margin has been the accepted therapeutic goal.[28] This 5-cm rule was based on the notion that distal tumor spread is common and that unless aggressive distal clearance is obtained, a higher rate of local recurrence will likely result. This notion is incorrect. Over the past 30 years, many patients have undergone complete rectal excision to satisfy this 5-cm distal clearance when a sphincter-saving procedure might otherwise have been employed. Currently, the increased experience with the intraluminal stapler, along with a trend toward sphincter preservation, has resulted in the acceptance of progressively shorter distal margins. This less aggressive therapeutic approach has not resulted in an increased incidence of treatment failures. Indeed, over the past 15 years, a number of investigators have published data suggesting that a 5-cm distal margin is too stringent a requirement.[5,22,28,30,37,45,53,54,63,75,80–82,84]

The literature contains abundant histologic justification for the acceptance of a distal margin that is less than 5 cm.[54,81] Most rectal cancers demonstrate no intramural, extrarectal, or lymphatic spread beyond the distal extent of the tumor. Whenever distal intramural or extrarectal spread is present, it is limited to within 2 cm in 95% of all cases.[63,80] Even patients with poorly differentiated tumors have been demonstrated to derive no significant benefit from a longer distal clearance.[18] It is not surprising, therefore, that sphincter-saving resection produces long-term clinical results equivalent to abdominoperineal resection in the treatment of most rectal carcinomas.[37,45,53,80,82,84] However, the acceptance of a distal margin less than 5 cm must be based on clinical data that clearly demonstrate that cure is not compromised. Pollet and Nicholls[63] could demonstrate no significant difference in either local recurrence or survival when distal margins greater than 2 cm were compared with distal margins less than 2 cm. Vernava and colleagues[75] demonstrated that a distal margin of 1 cm in a fresh, unpinned specimen was an adequate clearance for most rectal cancers.

Lateral Margins

A report by Quirke and colleagues[64] suggests that clearance of the lateral margins is essential for curative resection. In this report, 52 patients were treated for rectal carcinoma: 23 by abdominoperineal resection and 29 by sphincter-saving resection. Fourteen of the 52 patients (27%) had tumor-involved lateral margins. As one would expect, 11 of these 14 patients (85%) suffered a local recurrence. Contrarily, of the 38 patients with no evidence of tumor at their lateral margins, only 1 patient (3%) suffered a local recurrence. Since these data were published, we have altered our surgical technique so that the lateral excision of the mesorectum and the lateral ligaments is flush with the pelvic side wall. We routinely cauterize across the lateral ligaments, instead of ligating them as we previously did, in order to obtain a wider margin of excision. We recommend that the pathologist routinely ink and examine the lateral margins of excision. Those patients who have positive lateral margins should be considered candidates for postoperative radiation therapy.

Mesorectal Excision

According to Heald,[36,38,52] the source of most local recurrence after "curative" resection of rectal carcinoma is the microscopic spread of tumor into the mesorectum. In a standard low anterior resection, all of this tissue may not be resected, leaving residual micrometastatic disease present in the pelvis and dooming the patient to a local recurrence. Therefore, Heald advocates complete excision of the mesorectum along with the tumor. This excision actually extends below the distal margin of the resected bowel. His technique has resulted in the lowest published rate of local recurrence in the literature: 2.6 to 5%. This aggressive resection of the mesorectum is associated with a significantly higher anastomotic leak rate and Heald recommends consideration of temporary fecal diversion in those patients who have undergone total mesorectal excision and have an "ultralow" anastomosis (i.e., below 5 cm from the anal verge).

Radical Abdominopelvic Lymphadenectomy

Radical abdominopelvic lymphadenectomy for rectal cancer is based on the tenet that a primary cause of operative treatment failure is the presence of micrometastases in the residual, unresected, pararectal lymphatics and that the surgical removal of all this potentially involved lymphatic tissue will yield a lower rate of locoregional failure and improve survival. Figure 18–5 illustrates the lymphatic spread of rectal cancer based on the location of the tumor. This hypothesis has been present in the surgical literature since the 1950s. The data that claim to support or refute the concept are all poor and difficult to interpret.[2,19,26,42,57,70] A prospective, randomized, controlled study comparing conventional resection to radical abdominopelvic lymphadenectomy has not been done. The technique is more extensive than conventional resection, although at centers with experience with the procedure the operating time is only modestly prolonged and blood loss and postoperative hospitalization are not significantly increased. The extent of the operation is depicted in Figure 18–6.

The high incidence of postoperative urinary dysfunction and impotence have been major deterrents to the operation. There is evidence that selective preservation of the pelvic autonomic nerves is possible in this operation and that it ameliorates urinary and sexual dysfunction.[43] In a recent, comprehensive review of radical abdominopelvic lymphadenectomy for rectal cancer, Harnsberger and associates[35] found that despite increased morbidity with the operation there was sufficient evidence in the literature to warrant a prospective, randomized clinical trial evaluating the effect of surgical technique (i.e., conventional resection versus radical abdominopelvic lymphadenectomy) on patient outcome. At this time, however, there is not sufficient evidence to warrant the application of this radical technique on a routine basis.

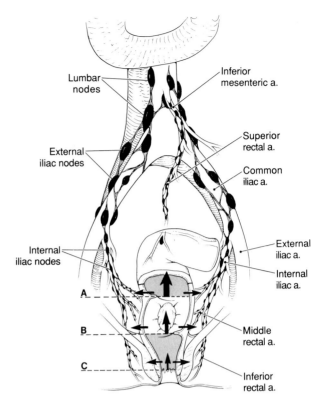

FIGURE 18-5. Normal lymphatic drainage of the rectum. *A,* Upper third of the rectum. Lymphatic drainage mainly occurs along the superior rectal artery (SRA) and inferior mesenteric artery (IMA) to the para-aortic nodes. Lymphatic drainage can also occur along the inferior mesenteric vein (IMV) to the paraportal lymphatics. *B,* Middle third of the rectum. Cephalad lymphatic drainage occurs along the SRA and IMA. Lateral lymphatic drainage occurs along the middle rectal vessels to the internal common iliac nodes. *C,* Lower third of the rectum. Lymphatic drainage is predominantly lateral and occurs along the middle and inferior rectal vessels to the internal iliac nodes. Cephalad drainage can also occur along the SRA and IMA. (From Harnsberger, J.R., Vernava, A.M., and Longo, W.E.: Radical abdominopelvic lymphadenectomy in the treatment of rectal cancer [RAPL]: A historical perspective and its current role in the surgical management of rectal cancer. Dis. Colon Rectum, *37*:73, 1994. Copyright Williams & Wilkins, 1994, with permission.)

Ligation of the Inferior Mesenteric Artery: High Versus Low

In 1952, Grinnell and Hiatt[32] discovered metastatic rectal cancer in lymph nodes located along the inferior mesenteric artery proximal to its bifurcation in 17% of patients undergoing abdominoperineal resection or low anterior resection. This fact stimulated them, and others, to suggest that a high ligation of the inferior mesenteric artery (i.e., at its origin at the aorta) would allow resection of these nodes and thereby improve survival. Unfortunately, there is no evidence that substantiates this notion; a prospective, randomized, controlled study evaluating the impact of the level of inferior mesenteric artery ligation on patient outcome has never been done. Rosi,[66] Grinnell,[31] and Pezim and colleagues[62] have each reported in retrospective, uncontrolled studies that the level of inferior mesenteric artery ligation has no impact on survival. It is impossible to coherently interpret these data. At the present time, the indication for high ligation of the inferior mesenteric artery is to improve mo-

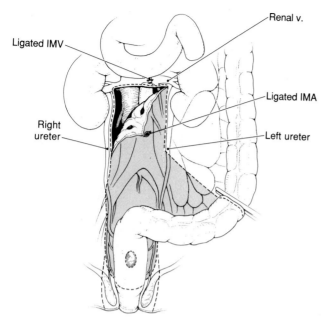

FIGURE 18-6. Operative boundaries of radical abdominopelvic lymphadenectomy. (From Harnsberger, J.R., Vernava, A.M., and Longo, W.E.: Radical abdominopelvic lymphadenectomy in the treatment of rectal cancer [RAPL]: A historical perspective and its current role in the surgical management of rectal cancer. Dis. Colon Rectum, *37*:73, 1994. Copyright Williams & Wilkins, 1994, with permission.)

bilization of the left colon to facilitate a tension-free anastomosis with the extraperitoneal rectum.

PATIENT SELECTION
General Considerations

The major factors that influence the selection of patients for low anterior resection include the location and size of the tumor; tumor mobility; tumor histologic grade and ploidy; the presence or absence of metastatic disease; the presence of obstruction; the adequacy of bowel preparation; and the body habitus, sex, and general medical condition of the patient. Most of these factors can be successfully assessed preoperatively and a preliminary determination made regarding the advisability of restorative resection. However, it is impossible to guarantee restoration of bowel continuity until after the rectum has been fully mobilized during the operation, particularly for very low lesions. Also, it is wise to counsel female patients that a hysterectomy or even a total abdominal hysterectomy may be required for adequate tumor resection.

It is important that the surgeon performing the operation be adept at several restorative techniques to ensure both the adequacy of resection and the highest probability of restoration of bowel continuity. The restorative techniques currently practiced include low anterior resection with a sutured or stapled anastomosis, the double-staple technique of low anterior resection, or a coloanal anastomosis. The abdominosacral approach can also be employed.

Location of the Tumor

The most important factor in patient selection for a low anterior resection is the site of the neoplasm. Lesions located in the upper one third of the rectum (i.e., 10 to 15 cm from the anal verge) are easily managed by anterior resection and the anastomosis can usually be either sutured or stapled, depending on the surgeon's preference. There is no difference in outcome based on the technique of anastomosis. Lesions located in the middle one third (i.e., 5 to 10 cm from the anal verge) and lower one third (i.e., 0 to 5 cm from the anal verge) of the rectum can be significantly more difficult to manage. The circular intraluminal stapler is ideally suited to the management of many of these lesions. The double-staple technique and the coloanal anastomosis are also suited to these low lesions. Any surgeon interested in the treatment of rectal carcinoma must be familiar with the various stapling and operative techniques available in order to provide a restorative option for these patients. A full description of each operative technique will be described further on.

In general, it is unwise to perform a low anterior resection for lesions located lower than 4 cm from the anal verge. A 1-cm distal margin is required as a minimum in all cases and a lesion located 4 cm from the anal verge would require an anastomosis at, or very near, the dentate line (i.e., a coloanal anastomosis). This represents the limit of restoration of bowel continuity after abdominal proctectomy. Also, anal canal length is approximately 2.5 to 4 cm. An infiltrating lesion located in this region may involve the sphincter complex and thereby require abdominoperineal resection for adequate removal. Favorable lesions (i.e., TNM stage I, <4 cm in size, involving <25% of the circumference of the bowel lumen) located below 10 cm from the anal verge can be managed by transanal excision.

Size and Mobility of the Tumor

Extremely large, bulky tumors are not candidates for primary restorative resection. They may, however, be candidates for a preoperative course of high-dose pelvic irradiation (4,500 to 5,000 cGy). This radiation therapy frequently shrinks a large tumor (i.e., downstages the tumor) and allows mobilization of a previously fixed tumor. In selected cases, a low anterior resection may then be feasible.

Tumor Fixation

Fixation of a rectal cancer to the pelvis is a relative contraindication to low anterior resection primarily because of the high risk of locally recurrent disease if the fixation is malignant and not inflammatory in nature. However, tumor fixation to contiguous pelvic structures should not necessarily contraindicate a restorative operation. En bloc resection of the uterus, posterior vaginal wall, seminal vesicles, prostate, bladder, or small intestine along with the rectum can be performed and should be done if necessary. Fixation of tumor to an adjacent organ or to the pelvis does not always indicate contiguous spread of the tumor. Indeed, tumor fixation may merely represent an inflammatory response by the adjacent tissue. When a tumor is resected, inflammatory fixation does not confer any increased risk of local recurrence or poorer survival. In a study of 625 patients who had undergone rectal excision, 169 (27%) patients had tumors that were fixed; 124 (20%) tumors were fixed by direct malignant spread and 45 (7%) by inflammatory tissue.[17] In those patients with lesions tethered by inflammatory tissue, there was no significant difference in either local recurrence or 5-year survival when compared with the patients with nonfixed tumors.

Histologic Grade, Degree of Differentiation, and Tumor Ploidy

Some authors consider poor tumor differentiation to be an absolute contraindication to restorative resection.[12] The evidence supporting that view is contradictory. It is clear that poorly differentiated tumors have a higher likelihood of local recurrence than do well-differentiated tumors. Five-year survival for patients with poorly differentiated tumors is also poorer. However, radical rectal extirpation (i.e., abdominoperineal resection) confers no survival advantage to patients with poorly differentiated tumors.[18] Moreover, poorly differentiated tumors are no more likely to recur after low anterior resection than after abdominoperineal resection.[18] Therefore, we do not consider poor tumor differentiation to be a contraindication to restorative resection. Rather, we consider histology and tumor differentiation along with other tumor characteristics when making a decision about operative management.

Tumor ploidy has recently emerged as a potential prognostic indicator in patients with colon and rectal cancer.[14,48,69] A recent review[14] of the subject suggests that nondiploid tumors are more likely to recur and have a poorer survival than diploid tumors. Despite the apparent association of nondiploid tumors with poorer outcome, there does not appear to be a relationship between nondiploid status and either advanced pathologic stage or poor histologic differentiation. Presently, there is not sufficient evidence to warrant using tumor ploidy in the operative decision between low anterior resection and abdominoperineal resection.

Sex and Body Habitus

Despite the clear advantage that modern operative stapling techniques have conferred on the performance of low anterior resection, there remain patients in whom it is impossible to perform the operation. These patients are usually obese men or women with a very narrow pelvis who have either a low or mid rectal lesion. In these patients, even the double-staple technique may be impossible because the TA stapler will not fit into the pelvis. In such cases, the rectum can be everted and a TA stapler applied, the rectum divided, and a double-staple anastomosis performed; or a coloanal anastomosis can be done.

CONTRAINDICATIONS TO LOW ANTERIOR RESECTION

Despite the therapeutic efficacy and psychologic and social advantage of restorative resection, there are patients who are not suited to the operation. Medically incapacitated patients unable to tolerate a prolonged anesthetic require palliative therapy. Local excision, fulguration, or intracavitary radiation should be considered in such cases.

Impaired Continence: The Effect of Low Anterior Resection on Continence and Sphincter Function

Preoperative gross fecal incontinence absolutely contraindicates the performance of a low anterior resection. Disastrous results can be anticipated whenever a low anterior resection is performed in an incontinent or marginally continent patient. Each patient should be questioned preoperatively about their bowel habits and a complete anorectal examination should be performed. If the patient is normally continent preoperatively, and the clinical evaluation of the anal sphincter complex is normal, then no additional evaluation is necessary and one may proceed with low anterior resection. On the other hand, equivocal cases should undergo anorectal manometry and any incontinent patient excluded from consideration for low anterior resection. Every patient undergoing operation should be informed that they will experience an increase in bowel frequency postoperatively. A temporary or permanent change in continence may also occur. Commonly, these changes in bowel frequency and continence gradually improve over the first postoperative year.

Anorectal physiologic evaluation reveals that rectal resection with a low anastomosis eliminates the reservoir capacity and decreases the compliance of the neorectum and uniformly results in an increase in the frequency of bowel movements.[10,44,61,74,83] This decrease in compliance, which seems to improve with time, appears to be the most important factor involved in the clinical changes in continence after anterior resection. There is also noted to be a drop in resting anal pressure that seems to be related to trauma to the internal anal sphincter that occurs during routine proper placement of the circular intraluminal stapler. This drop in resting pressure may or may not improve with time. Squeeze pressure also decreases after anterior resection, although it is unclear whether this is due to injury to the external anal sphincter or to the internal anal sphincter.

Advanced Age

Advanced age alone is not a contraindication to low anterior resection.[23] Good-risk, normally continent, elderly patients tolerate low anterior resection well and should not be denied the operation on the basis of age alone. Contrarily, advanced age can be associated with significant comorbid disease as well as deteriorating and even poor sphincter function. This fact can prove problematic for the surgeon because elderly patients frequently have significant difficulty adjusting to and caring for an intestinal stoma. Therapeutic considerations notwithstanding, the surgeon must determine whether or not the patient will tolerate the proposed procedure and the potential effect of the operation on the patient's lifestyle and decide in favor of the one with the least detrimental effect. A perineal colostomy is a devastating complication of low anterior resection and should be avoided.

Local Metastatic Disease

Any spread of tumor to the sphincter complex contraindicates any form of restorative resection; in such cases the sphincter complex must be removed to adequately resect the tumor. In patients with widespread pelvic metastases, the risk of malignant bowel obstruction also contraindicates low anterior resection, even as a palliative procedure. However, tumor fixation to the pelvis or to contiguous, resectable pelvic structures (e.g., posterior vaginal wall, prostate) is not an absolute contraindication to low anterior resection. Tumor fixation may represent merely an inflammatory response and en bloc resection may be possible.

Distant Metastasis

Distant metastatic disease is only a relative contraindication to low anterior resection. In the absence of extensive pelvic disease, low anterior resection can provide excellent palliation of the primary carcinoma. This is especially true in the patient who objects to having a stoma for the remaining time of his or her life. In such a case, low anterior resection eliminates the risk of complication from the local tumor and allows the patient to retain the normal defecatory pathway. The surgeon must weigh the risks of malignant obstruction or hemorrhage following low anterior resection versus the benefits of an unfettered lifestyle without an intestinal stoma. Finally, low anterior resection is an elective operation that requires full mechanical and antibiotic bowel preparation. The operation is relatively contraindicated as an emergency procedure. Those occasional individuals who present with an obstructing rectal carcinoma should undergo either a preliminary colostomy to decompress and prepare the bowel or a Hartmann procedure. Some authors have described safely performing an anastomosis in such cases by employing intraoperative, on-table colonic lavage[71] or the use of an intracolonic bypass device.[65]

OPERATIVE TECHNIQUE

General Considerations

In all cases of planned low anterior resection, an enterostomal therapist visits the patient preoperatively and the patient is counseled and marked for a permanent left-sided stoma should one prove necessary. The patient is also marked on the right for a possible temporary diverting loop ileostomy should the anastomosis require protection. After general anesthesia has been success-

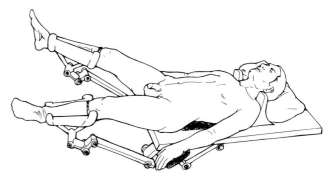

FIGURE 18-7. Modified lithotomy position. There must be no pressure on the peroneal nerve.

fully induced, a Foley catheter is inserted and the patient is placed in the modified lithotomy position (Fig. 18-7). This position allows easy access to the anorectum for a stapled anastomosis and also allows the performance of a combined synchronous abdominoperineal resection if sphincter preservation proves impossible. The patient's legs must be adequately padded and there should be no pressure on the peroneal nerve. Currently, we use boot-style stirrups (Allen stirrups), which are designed to have the foot bear the weight of the leg so that there is no pressure on the peroneal nerve. Sequential compression stockings are placed on both legs, where they remain functional throughout the procedure and postoperatively until the patient is sufficiently ambulatory. Perioperative low-dose subcutaneous heparin is also employed for prophylaxis of deep venous thrombosis. Care must also be taken that either arm is not hyperextended, which can cause a brachial plexus palsy.

A midline or infraumbilical abdominal incision is performed. An infraumbilical transverse abdominal incision provides excellent exposure to the sigmoid colon, rectum, and pelvis, and allows easy packing of the small bowel into the upper abdomen (Fig. 18-8). On the other hand, mobilization of the splenic flexure and visual assessment of the upper abdomen, including the liver, is difficult. A midline incision provides easy access to the entire abdomen and is routinely used for emergency operations and in patients who require multiple operations (e.g., patients with Crohn's disease). When the peritoneal cavity is entered, the entire abdomen is manually and visually explored. Any hepatic lesions suspicious for metastasis are biopsied now. The small bowel is packed away into the upper abdomen using several moist laparotomy pads. The patient is then placed in a modified Trendelenburg position to facilitate visualization in the pelvis. We routinely use headlights and fiberoptic-lighted abdominopelvic retractors during pelvic operations to ensure adequate illumination of the operative field. The rectal tumor is located and inspected. Aggressive manipulation of the tumor is avoided.

Mobilization of the Colon and Rectum

The sigmoid colon and left colon are mobilized by dividing the peritoneal attachments along the line of Toldt. The degree of mobilization performed depends

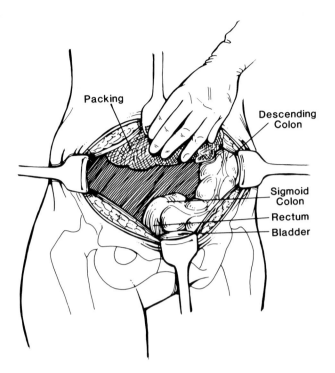

FIGURE 18-8. A transverse abdominal incision allows excellent exposure of the structures in the pelvis.

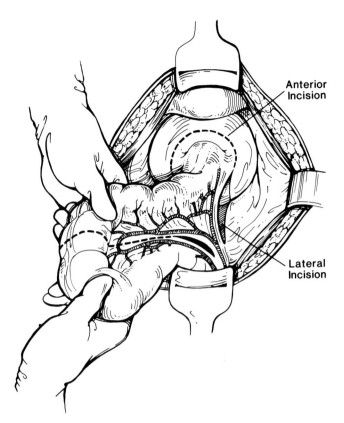

FIGURE 18-9. Following completion of colon mobilization, the pelvic peritoneum is incised laterally and then anteriorly.

on several factors, including the length of redundant colon present, the location of the rectal lesion, and the length of distal rectal resection required. It is always worthwhile to obtain sufficient mobilization of the colon at this point in the operation, since a tension-free anastomosis is essential. Under no circumstances should any tension on the anastomosis be accepted. One should not hesitate to fully mobilize the splenic flexure if necessary, even if this requires extension of the abdominal incision. It is also critical that the blood supply to the proximal colon be preserved and that the area of the proximal colon intended for the anastomosis be carefully inspected, making certain that it has adequate blood supply.

Following completion of colonic mobilization, the pelvic peritoneum is incised laterally (Fig. 18–9). Both ureters are identified and swept laterally, away from the area of dissection (Fig. 18–10). Ureteral stents are not routinely employed but are used in cases of large, bulky tumors; reoperative pelvic surgery; and in those patients who have undergone high-dose pelvic irradiation.

After both ureters have been identified and placed out of harm's way, the inferior mesenteric vessels are identified, doubly ligated, and divided (Fig. 18–11). As indicated earlier, high ligation of the inferior mesenteric vessels does not confer any survival or recurrence advantage, but may be necessary to improve mobilization of the left colon and allow the proximal colon to reach the rectal stump without tension.

The presacral space is now entered. We no longer employ blunt dissection in the presacral space; instead, we only use electrocautery and sharp dissection (Fig. 18–12). Significant difficulty can occur in the performance of the pelvic dissection, especially in patients with a very

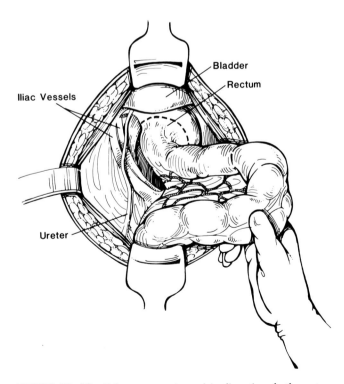

FIGURE 18-10. Prior to extensive pelvic dissection, both ureters must be identified and gently swept out of harm's way.

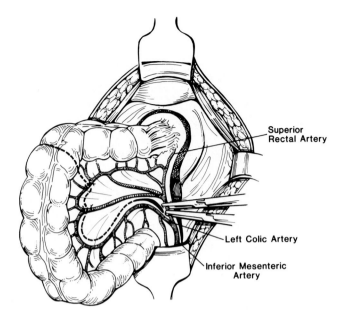

FIGURE 18-11. Ligation of the inferior mesenteric artery distal to the left colic artery.

Superior
Rectal Artery

Left Colic Artery

Inferior Mesenteric
Artery

deep and narrow pelvis. In such patients, we recommend dividing the sigmoid colon at the proximal line of resection prior to any further pelvic dissection. This maneuver allows increased mobility of the distal sigmoid colon and rectum and increases exposure in the pelvis. The rectum can be held completely to one side, allowing improved exposure of the lateral ligaments, as well as of the anterior and posterior dissection.

Mobilization of the Rectum and Resection of the Specimen

The initial step in rectal mobilization is entering the posterior space. This is done using electrocautery. Up-

ward tension is placed on the rectum and a tissue plane of loose areolar tissue becomes obvious, located between the sacrum and the thicker tissue of the mesorectum. This loose areolar tissue is divided with electrocautery along the concave shape of the sacral hollow down to the coccyx. Next, the retrosacral fascia, which is much thicker and tougher than this loose areolar tissue, will be encountered and should be divided using either electrocautery or scissors. Blunt dissection should not be used to divide the retrosacral fascia because of the risk of tearing into the rectum. The presacral space is an avascular plane and there should be no hemorrhage. The cause of any hemorrhage is usually an unligated vessel in the lateral ligaments or inadvertent entry into a presacral vein. Hemorrhage can also be caused during the anterior rectal mobilization if the prostate, seminal vesicles, or posterior vaginal wall have been entered. In such a case, the dissection should be redirected close to the rectal wall.

The lateral ligaments should be divided after the anterior and posterior dissection have been started (Fig. 18–13). We no longer routinely ligate the lateral ligaments. Instead, we divide the lateral ligaments with electrocautery in order to obtain wider lateral clearance. The middle rectal vessels located within the lateral ligaments are usually easily controlled with electrocautery. When necessary, they are ligated.

The entire mesorectum must be removed; therefore, the resection includes all of the soft tissue interposed between the bowel, the pelvic side walls, and the presacral fascia. Great care is taken to protect both ureters from injury.

In this manner, the rectum is circumferentially mobilized down beyond the lesion. Although a distal margin of 1 cm in the fresh unpinned specimen is adequate, in practice it is difficult to tell precisely how much distal margin is present with the rectum in situ and on stretch; therefore, as much rectum distal to the tumor as possi-

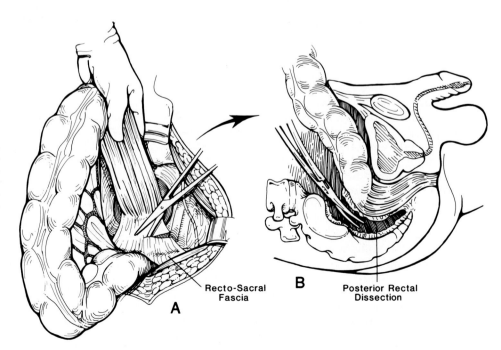

FIGURE 18-12. The presacral space is entered to perform the posterior rectal dissection. *A,* The rectosacral fascia is divided with scissors or electrocautery. *B,* The remaining posterior dissection is done using sharp or electrocautery dissection.

Recto-Sacral
Fascia

Posterior Rectal
Dissection

A

B

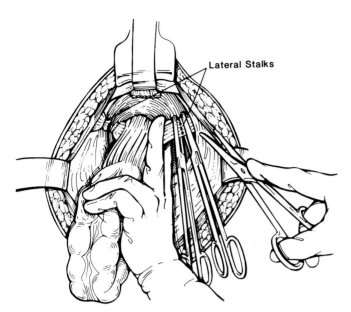

FIGURE 18-13. The lateral ligaments are divided sharply or with cautery. Ligation is not required and may limit the lateral excision.

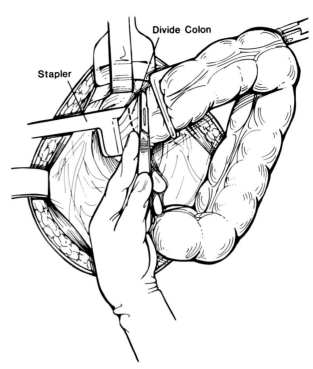

FIGURE 18-14. The bowel is divided between a TA stapler and a right-angled bowel clamp.

ble is resected. Prior to division of the rectum, a decision must be made concerning the method of anastomosis. If a stapled or sutured anastomosis is to be performed, the rectum can be divided at this point, distal to the lesion, between right-angled bowel clamps. If, however, the double-staple technique is to be employed, a roticulator TA-55 stapler should be placed around the rectum distal to the lesion and then fired (Fig. 18-14). The rectum can then be divided between the stapler and a right-angled bowel clamp. If the TA-55 stapler will not fit into the pelvis, the rectum can then be carefully everted through the anus and a TA-55 stapler applied to the everted rectum in the perineum and then fired. The rectum can then be divided and the specimen handed off.

Anastomotic Techniques

Suture Technique

The rectum is divided and handed off the operative field. Any mesentery around the cut edge of the bowel should be trimmed back a distance of 1 to 2 cm. It is both unnecessary and unwise to trim the mesentery any further from the edge of the bowel. The ends of the bowel must be viable after the mesentery has been trimmed.

A single-layer anastomosis is performed using interrupted 4-0 polyglycolic acid or 4-0 silk (Fig. 18-15). Traction sutures are placed in each corner of the anastomosis. The posterior row of sutures is placed first. Seromuscular sutures are placed and are spaced approximately 1 cm apart. After the entire row has been placed, these sutures are loosely but securely tied.

The bowel is then gently rotated, and in a similar fashion the anterior row of sutures is placed and then tied. This single, circumferential row of sutures is then reinforced with an additional full-thickness row of sutures

placed between each previously placed suture. This additional row of sutures acts to prevent any intraluminal anastomotic hemorrhage. Once again, there must be no tension on the anastomosis and the bowel must be viable. When the anastomosis is complete, the mesenteric defect is closed with a running absorbable suture.

End-to-Side Anastomosis

In some cases, an end-to-side anastomosis (i.e., end of rectum to side of colon) may be easier to perform than an end-to-end anastomosis. The distal end of the colon should be closed with sutures or a stapler. The side of the colon is brought down to the rectum and is then opened in a convenient location, making certain not to leave a long blind segment of colon (Fig. 18-16). As before, the anastomosis is performed using a single layer of interrupted 4-0 polyglycolic acid or silk sutures. The posterior row of sutures is placed first and the principles and technique of end-to-end anastomosis, previously outlined, are followed.

Stapling Techniques

Single-Staple Technique

After the distal rectum has been divided and the mesentery trimmed away from the proximal bowel edge, pursestring sutures of 2-0 polypropylene are placed in the proximal colon and in the distal rectal remnant. The sutures should be placed through the full thickness of bowel wall, including the very edge of the mucosa, not further than 5 mm from the bowel edge. Care must be taken so that an excessive amount of bowel is not in-

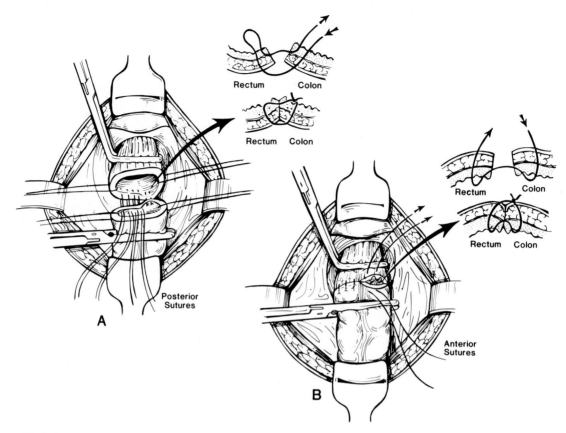

FIGURE 18-15. The single-layer suture technique. *A*, The posterior sutures are placed first. *B*, The anterior sutures are then placed.

cluded in the pursestring sutures, since this increases the difficulty of tying the suture securely around the post of the stapler.

The surgical assistant now performs the perineal portion of the operation. A stapler is chosen based on the size of the proximal colon and rectum. Generally, the size of the proximal colon is the limiting factor in choos-

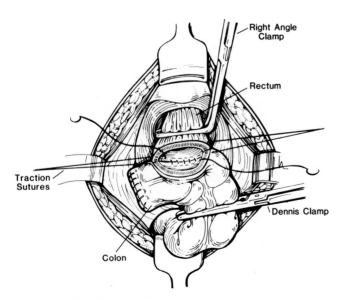

FIGURE 18-16. The Baker end-to-side anastomosis.

ing the size of the stapler. The assistant opens the stapler and verifies that a full staple cartridge has been loaded into the instrument. The anal canal is gently dilated with two fingers. The head of the stapler is lubricated with water-soluble jelly and is then gently passed through the anal canal into the distal rectum. The abdominal surgeon places a hand behind the rectum to feel the position of the tip of the stapler and then guides the advancement of the stapler until the head of the instrument protrudes through the open end of the rectum (Fig. 18–17). The stapler is opened and the distal pursestring suture is pulled taut around the post and securely tied. Any gaps in the pursestring suture should be reinforced with an additional suture. The proximal colon is now slid over the head of the stapler and its pursestring suture is tied securely around the post (Figs. 18–18 and 18–19).

Many times, the proximal colon is in spasm and is impossible to seat on the head of the stapler. There are several methods that can aid in relaxation of the bowel's smooth muscle. Glucagon, 1 mg intravenously, results in remarkable colonic relaxation. Bathing the colon in warm saline also will sometimes break spasm and allow gentle passage of the bowel onto the head of the stapler. Again, any gaps in the proximal pursestring suture should be closed by separate sutures.

The stapler is slowly closed (Fig. 18–20). No extracolonic tissue (i.e., fat or mesentery) should be included in the anastomosis. The stapler is fired only after making

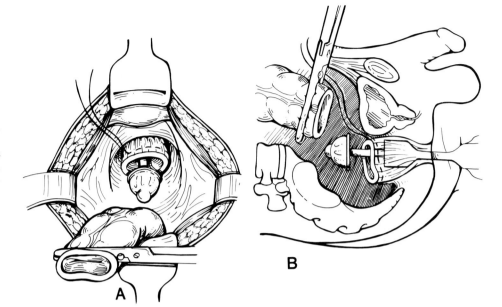

FIGURE 18-17. The head of the stapler is gently placed transanally (*A*) and is advanced until it protrudes through the cut edge of the rectum, (*B*) and the pursestring suture is tied.

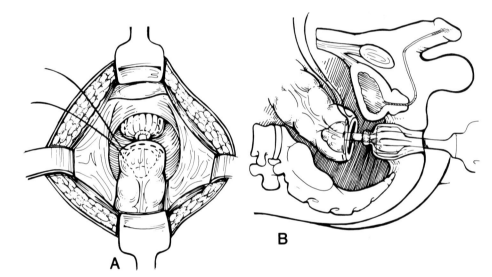

FIGURE 18-18. The proximal colon is gently advanced onto the stapler. *A*, Surgeon's view onto the stapler. *B*, Lateral view.

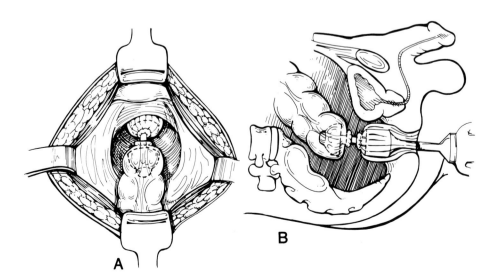

FIGURE 18-19. The proximal pursestring suture is then tied. *A*, Surgeon's view from the abdomen. *B*, Lateral view.

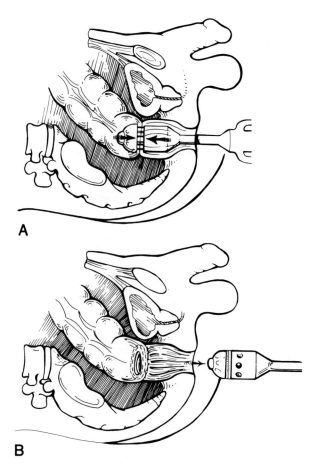

A

B

FIGURE 18-20. *A*, The stapler is closed slowly and is then fired. *B*, The anastomosis is completed and the stapler is gently withdrawn.

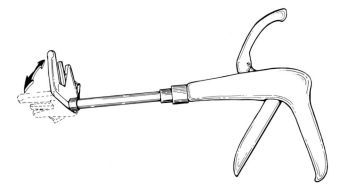

FIGURE 18-21. The roticulator TA-55 stapler. Note that the head is movable.

certain that it is securely closed. After being engaged, the stapler is opened and gently rotated back and forth. While the abdominal surgeon protects the anastomosis, the stapler is gently withdrawn. The assistant responsible for firing the stapler should now open the instrument and check the tissue donuts, making certain that the rings are complete. The surgeon must see these tissue rings, since incomplete rings indicate an incomplete anastomosis.

Checking the Anastomosis

After the completion of a stapled colorectal anastomosis, the staple line should be checked for integrity. A linen-shod clamp is placed on the colon proximal to the anastomosis. Rigid proctosigmoidoscopy is performed by the assistant, who should visualize the anastomosis. The patient is taken out of the Trendelenburg position, the pelvis is filled with sterile saline, and the bowel is insufflated with air distal to the anastomosis to check for any air leakage. In the presence of complete proximal and distal pursestring sutures in the tissue donuts, and when there is no air leakage, the anastomosis is complete.

Incomplete tissue donuts, or a persistent air leak when insufflation is performed, indicates an incomplete anastomosis, which requires reinforcement. The anas-

tomosis should not be taken down. If the anastomosis cannot be made airtight or if the surgeon is dissatisfied with the anastomosis for any reason, proximal fecal diversion should be employed.

Double-Staple Technique

As distal resection approaches the dentate line, the placement of the distal pursestring suture becomes progressively more difficult. A markedly obese patient and the narrow male pelvis can also hinder placement of the distal pursestring suture. These circumstances are ideally suited to the double-staple technique.[22,30]

Prior to division of the distal rectum, a TA-55 stapler is placed on the rectum below the lesion and is then engaged. A roticulator TA-55 can also be used for this task (Fig. 18–21) but can sometimes be difficult to fit into a narrow pelvis. The rectum is divided just proximal to the stapler after it has been fired and the specimen is removed. The security of the distal staple line is checked by having the operating assistant place a rigid proctosigmoidoscope through the anal canal into the rectal stump and insufflating with air while the rectal stump is under water. Any evidence of an air leak requires reinforcement of the staple line with sutures.

A circular intraluminal stapler with a trochar is used for the anastomosis. Such a device is produced by both Ethicon and U.S. Surgical (Fig. 18–22). The head is removed from the shaft of the instrument, making certain that the trochar attachment is in place in the instrument. The trochar is then retracted behind the body of the instrument (Fig. 18–23). Dilation of the anal canal is performed gently with two fingers and the stapler is carefully introduced into the rectum. Guided by the abdominal surgeon, whose hand is posterior to the rectum, the stapler is carefully advanced until its base is immediately adjacent to the staple line. Under direct vision, the stapler is opened, forcing the trochar through the rectal wall adjacent to the staple line (Fig. 18–24). (Care should be taken so that the trochar does not exit the rectum more than several centimeters from the staple line, since this could result in an ischemic area of rectum between the linear staple line and the circular staple line.) When completely opened, the trochar is removed. The head of the stapler is now placed into the

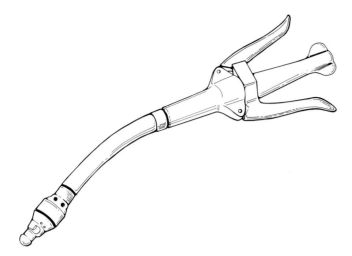

FIGURE 18-22. The C-EEA stapler. The head is detachable.

proximal colon and the pursestring suture is tied (Fig. 18–25). The head attachment is then snapped onto the stapler, which is then securely closed and fired (Figs. 18–26 and 18–27). The stapler is then opened, gently rotated, and withdrawn. The tissue donuts are inspected and the anastomosis is checked, as previously described, via rigid proctosigmoidoscopy and insufflation.

Drainage of the Presacral Space

After low anterior resection, we routinely drain the presacral space with soft, closed sump drains. These drains are left in place for approximately 24 to 48 hours unless there is pronounced drainage, in which case the drains are removed when the drainage significantly diminishes.

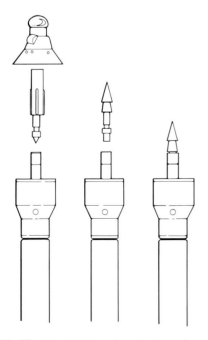

FIGURE 18-23. The C-EEA stapler with its trochar attachment.

POSTOPERATIVE CARE

Routine postoperative supportive care is employed with intravenous hydration, Foley catheter drainage, and sequential compression stockings. Nasogastric decompression is not routinely employed but is selectively used. Antibiotic prophylaxis is continued for 24 hours postoperatively and then discontinued. Oral intake is prohibited until evidence of the return of gastrointestinal function is manifest such as the passage of flatus or a bowel movement. Postoperative pain management is of paramount importance to ensure patient comfort, early and progressive patient ambulation, and to decrease morbidity. We liberally employ patient-controlled analgesic devices or epidural catheters for this purpose. The Foley catheter is left in place for at least 5 days and is then removed. Patients with an uncomplicated postoperative course are generally discharged between 6 and 9 days after operation.

RESULTS

Morbidity and Mortality

In the absence of significant comorbid disease, low anterior resection is associated with a 1 to 5% risk of death.[12,46,50] Urinary tract infection and urinary dysfunction remain the most common complications after low anterior resection. The incidence of urinary tract complications ranges, depending on the extent of pelvic dissection, from 7 to 70%.[42,46,47,50] This is not surprising when one considers the age of patients who typically present for management of rectal cancer, and the extensive pelvic dissection required. Permanent bladder paresis has been reported in as many as 15% of patients who have undergone a very low colorectal anastomosis.[47] The incidence of male sexual dysfunction after low anterior resection ranges from 40 to 100% and depends on the extent of pelvic dissection.[4,21,42,77] The risk of male sexual dysfunction after low anterior resection appears to increase with the age of the patient, with more aggressive pelvic lymphatic excision, and with lower resection. The incidence of wound infection is between 2 and 6%.[50]

Complications

Anastomotic Dehiscence

Early reports on low anterior anastomosis noted rates of anastomotic leak between 17 and 77%.[12] Goligher reported an overall anastomotic leakage rate of 49% following low anterior resection.[29] Technical advances and surgeon familiarity and proficiency with the technique have decreased the clinically significant anastomotic dehiscence rate to between 5 and 15%.[39,73] Factors that adversely influence the rate of anastomotic dehiscence include tension on the suture line, poor blood supply to the anastomosis, extracolonic tissue included within the anastomosis (i.e., fat), poor bowel preparation, and a postoperative pelvic collection of blood.[68]

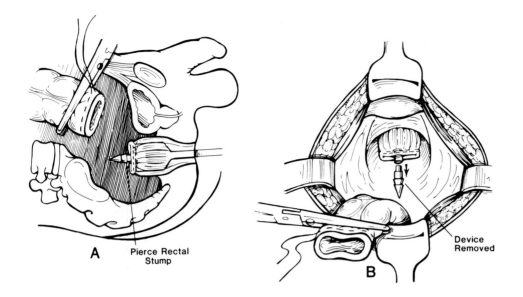

FIGURE 18-24. *A,* As the instrument is opened, the trochar slowly pierces the rectal wall. *B,* The trochar is then removed.

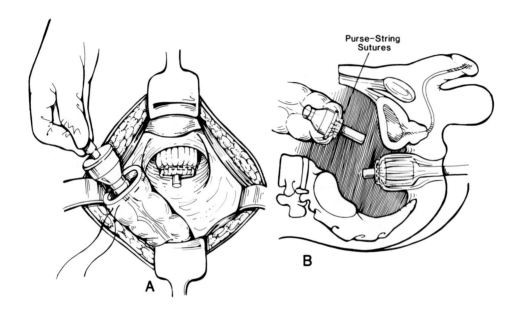

FIGURE 18-25. *A,* The proximal bowel is placed onto the head of the instrument. *B,* The purse-string suture is tied.

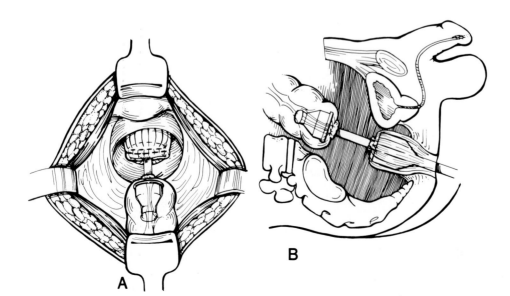

FIGURE 18-26. The head of the instrument is inserted into the stapling device. *A,* Surgeon's view from the abdomen. *B,* Lateral view.

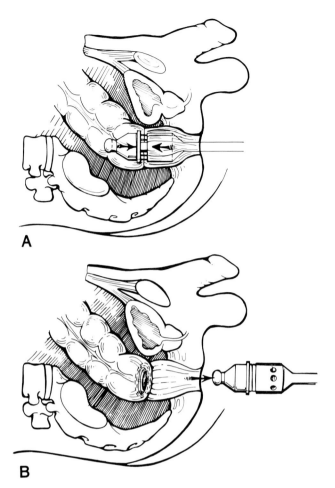

FIGURE 18-27. *A,* The stapler is closed and fired. *B,* The anastomosis is completed and the stapler is gently withdrawn.

Routine Proximal Colostomy

It is the opinion of the authors that proximal fecal diversion is not routinely indicated after an uncomplicated low anastomosis. Although fecal diversion does ameliorate the effects of any anastomotic dehiscence, it does not affect the rate of anastomotic dehiscence. Moreover, the creation of a diverting colostomy has its own consequent morbidity and mortality. Reported morbidity following colostomy closure approaches 50% in some series.[24,59] Nevertheless, proximal fecal diversion should be undertaken whenever the integrity of the anastomosis is suspect and it cannot be repaired to the surgeon's satisfaction.

Fecal Fistula

Fecal fistula following low anterior resection usually results from an anastomotic dehiscence. An uncomplicated fistula unassociated with sepsis will close spontaneously and requires no special therapy. Fistulas that include a septic focus require proximal fecal diversion and definitive therapy for resolution of the sepsis. In the presence of distal obstruction, malignancy, and recurrent inflammatory bowel disease, a fecal fistula will not heal and specific therapy with proximal fecal diversion may be required.

Anastomotic Stricture

There is usually some anastomotic narrowing during the immediate postoperative period. This may require up to 1 year to completely resolve. Indeed, swelling at the anastomotic site may become so severe in the immediate postoperative period as to produce a mechanical bowel obstruction. Management of these patients is expectant. The most severe cases can be treated by gently advancing a flexible sigmoidoscope to just beyond the anastomosis. This maneuver is risky, however, and may result in perforation of the anastomosis.

Local tissue edema, ischemia, and fibrosis are the causative factors. The anastomotic narrowing usually resolves over time until the lumen approaches the caliber of normal bowel. The entire healing process requires 3 months to 1 year and no specific therapy is usually required. Persistent tight anastomotic strictures do occur, however. They usually are a consequence of anastomotic dehiscence, with severe fibrosis and ischemia at the anastomosis. The incidence of this complication ranges between 1 and 31%.[9,37] Management of this type of stricture is by gentle dilation. A finger can be used for a low anastomosis, and Hegar dilators can be used for a higher anastomosis. One must remember that malignant recurrence can present as a tight anastomotic stricture that appears only several months after operation and does not respond to dilation. All chronic strictures should be biopsied and managed appropriately.

Anastomotic Hemorrhage

Significant anastomotic hemorrhage occurs in approximately 1% of patients undergoing low anterior resection and is usually due to inadequate hemostasis at the suture line.[50] Most patients are successfully treated by observation and transfusion of blood and coagulation factors as required. Rarely does a patient require reoperation for anastomotic hemorrhage.

Pelvic Abscess

Pelvic abscess is an unusual complication of low anterior resection, especially if the pelvic floor is left open. The presence of a pelvic abscess after low anterior resection usually indicates an anastomotic dehiscence. Gross fecal contamination during the operation and the accumulation of blood and exudate within the pelvis predispose the patient to abscess formation. The abscess can spontaneously drain through the colorectal anastomosis or via the vagina. If therapeutic intervention beyond administration of antibiotics is required, computed tomography–guided percutaneous drainage should be employed as the initial step. When open surgical drainage is necessary, it usually can be accomplished through the vagina or the rectum. The presence of peritonitis mandates an exploratory celiotomy.

Alterations in Bowel Function and Fecal Incontinence

Rectal resection with a low colorectal anastomosis is associated with loss of reservoir capacity and compliance that results in an increase in the frequency of bowel movements. Accommodation usually occurs over time, so that by the end of the first postoperative year, most patients have fully adjusted. The number of bowel movements usually decreases from seven to ten per day in the immediate postoperative period to between two and three per day at the end of 1 year. Those patients who continue to have unacceptably high bowel frequency can be managed with bulking agents, diphenoxylate hydrochloride and atropine, or codeine phosphate. Gross fecal incontinence is unusual following low anterior resection, provided that the patient was normally continent preoperatively. However, most patients do experience a minor change in continence after operation, especially following a very low anastomosis. Patients commonly complain of mild, intermittent incontinence to flatus and liquid stool. This change in continence is probably related to a transient stretch injury in the internal sphincter at the time the stapler was passed through the anal canal and should improve over time.

Local Recurrence

Local recurrence of cancer after low anterior resection is a troublesome and difficult complication to effectively treat. The risk of local recurrence largely depends on the pathologic stage. Currently, the incidence of local recurrence ranges between 2.6 and 30%.[36,38,67,75] Four potential mechanisms of local failure have been described.[27] They include the development of a new primary cancer, incomplete excision of the tumor in the pelvis, inadequate distal clearance of the bowel, and surgical implantation of exfoliated tumor cells on the anastomosis or other raw surfaces. The majority of local recurrences are probably due to incomplete excision of tumor in the pelvis either in the form of micrometastatic disease in the pararectal lymphatics or positive lateral margins, or gross tumor left on the pelvic sidewalls or sacrum.

Numerous factors influence the probability of local tumor recurrence and include TNM stage, tumor location, histology and degree of differentiation, tumor ploidy, distal margins, lateral margins, and the experience and technical ability of the operating surgeon. Tumors that are poorly differentiated, ulcerated, aneuploid, and advanced TNM stage all have a significantly higher risk of local recurrence than do their well-differentiated, nonulcerated, diploid counterparts. Low rectal tumors recur more frequently than do high rectal tumors. Patients that have tumors with these high-risk characteristics need not have the option of sphincter preservation foreclosed. Instead, they should be strongly considered for adjuvant chemoradiation therapy either before or after low anterior resection.

The cause of most local recurrence is probably residual pelvic disease and not shed tumor cells or a second primary carcinoma. Therefore, it is imperative to resect entirely the soft tissues surrounding the rectum. Additionally, wide pelvic dissection should be performed so that the lateral margins are free of disease. As mentioned earlier, the 1990 NIH consensus statement on rectal cancer recommends adjuvant chemoradiation

(i.e., intravenous 5-FU and high-dose [4,500 to 5,000 cGy] pelvic irradiation) for patients with TNM stage II and stage III rectal cancer.

Local pelvic tumor recurrence is very difficult to manage and curative re-resection is possible in fewer than 50% of patients. Salvage abdominoperineal resection is the treatment of choice. If necessary, pelvic exenteration can be performed. In a very few patients, a repeat low anterior resection may be possible. Intraoperative radiation therapy may be of benefit in some cases but it is not widely available.

REFERENCES

1. Bacon, H.E.: Evolution of sphincter muscle preservation and re-establishment of continuity in the operative treatment of rectal and sigmoidal cancer. Surg. Gynecol. Obstet., *81*:113, 1945.
2. Bacon, H., Dirbas, F., Myers, T., and Ponce de Leon, F.: Extensive lymphadenectomy and high ligation of the inferior mesenteric artery for carcinoma of the left colon and rectum. Dis. Colon Rectum, *1*:457, 1958.
3. Babcock, W.W.: Experiences with resection of the colon and the elimination of colostomy. Am. J. Surg., *46*:186, 1939.
4. Balslev, I. and Harling, H.: Sexual dysfunction following operation for carcinoma of the rectum. Dis. Colon Rectum, *26*:785, 1983.
5. Benyon, J., Foy, D.M.A., Roe, A.M., et al.: Endoluminal ultrasound in the assessment of local invasion in rectal cancer. Br. J. Surg., *73*:474, 1986.
6. Benyon, J., Mortensen, N.J.McC., Foy, D.M.A., et al.: Preoperative assessment of local invasion in rectal cancer: Digital examination, endoluminal sonography or computed tomography? Br. J. Surg., *73*:1015, 1986.
7. Benyon, J., Mortensoen, N.J.McC., Foy, D.M.A., et al.: Preoperative assessment of mesorectal lymph node involvement in rectal cancer. Br. J. Surg., *76*:276, 1989.
8. Black, B.M.: Combined abdomino-endo-rectal resection: Technical aspects and indications. Arch. Surg., *65*:406, 1952.
9. Blamey, S.L., and Lee, P.W.R.: A comparison of circular stapling devices in colorectal anastomoses. Br. J. Surg., *69*:19, 1982.
10. Carmona, J.A., Ortiz, H., and Perez-Cabanas, I.P.: Alterations in anorectal function after anterior resection for cancer of the rectum. Int. J. Colorectal Dis., *6*:108, 1991.
11. Consensus statement: NIH Consensus Development Conference, 1990 April 16–18;*8*:1.
12. Corman, M.L.: Low anterior resection. *In* Corman, M.L. (ed.): Colon and Rectal Surgery, 3rd ed. Philadelphia, J.B. Lippincott, 1993.
13. Cutait, D.E., and Figlioni, F.J.: A new method of colorectal anastomosis in abdominoperineal resection. Dis. Colon Rectum, *4*:335, 1961.
14. Dean, P., and Vernava, A.M.: Flow cytometric analysis of DNA content in colorectal carcinoma. Dis. Colon Rectum, *35*:95, 1992.
15. Dixon, C.F.: Surgical removal of lesions occurring in the sigmoid and rectosigmoid. Am. J. Surg., *46*:12, 1939.
16. Drake, D.B., Pemberton, J.H., Beart, R.W., Jr., et al.: Coloanal anastomosis in the management of benign and malignant rectal disease. Ann. Surg., *206*:600, 1987.
17. Durdey, P., and Williams, N.S.: The effect of malignant and inflammatory fixation of rectal carcinoma as prognosis after rectal excision. Br. J. Surg., *71*:787, 1984.
18. Elliot, M.S., Todd, I.P., and Nicholls, R.J.: Radical restorative surgery for poorly differentiated carcinoma of the mid rectum. Br. J. Surg., *69*:564, 1982.
19. Enker, W., Pilpshen, S., Heilweil, M., et al.: En bloc pelvic lymphadenectomy and sphincter preservation in the surgical management of rectal cancer. Ann. Surg., *203*:426, 1986.
20. Falk, P.M., Beart, R.W., Jr., Wexner, S.D., et al.: Laparoscopic colectomy: A critical appraisal. Dis. Colon Rectum, *36*:28, 1993.
21. Fazio, V.W., Fletcher, J., and Montague, D.: Prospective study of the effect of resection of the rectum on male sexual function. World J. Surg., *4*:149, 1980.
22. Feinberg, S.M., Parker, F., Cohen, Z., et al.: The double stapling

technique for low anterior resection of rectal carcinoma. Dis. Colon Rectum, 29:885, 1986.

23. Fitzgerald, S.D., Longo, W.E., Daniel, G.L., and Vernava, A.M.: Advanced colorectal neoplasia in the high-risk elderly patient: Is surgical resection justified? Dis. Colon Rectum, 36:161, 1993.

24. Freund, H.R., Raniel, J., and Juggia-Sulman, S.: Factors affecting the morbidity of colostomy closure: A retrospective study. Dis. Colon Rectum, 25:712, 1982.

25. Friis, J., Hjortrukp, A., and Nielson, O.V.: Sphincter-saving resection of the rectum using the EEA autostapler. Acta Chir. Scand., 148:379, 1982.

26. Glass, R., Ritchie, J., Thompson, H., and Mann, C.: The results of surgical treatment of cancer of the rectum by radical resection and extended abdominoiliac lymphadenectomy. Br. J. Surg., 72:599, 1985.

27. Goligher, J.C.: Treatment of carcinoma of the rectum. In Goligher, J.C. (ed.): Surgery of the Anus, Rectum and Colon, 5th ed. London, Bailliere Tindall, 1984, p. 590.

28. Goligher, J.C., Dukes, C.E., and Bussey, H.J.R.: Local recurrence after sphincter-saving excisions for carcinomas of the rectum and rectosigmoid. Br. J. Surg., 39:199, 1951.

29. Goligher, J.C., Graham, N.G., and DeDombal, F.T.: Anastomotic dehiscence after anterior resection of rectum and sigmoid. Br. J. Surg., 57:109, 1970.

30. Griffin, F.D., Knight, C.D., and Whitaker, J.M.: The double stapling technique for low anterior resection. Ann. Surg., 211:745, 1990.

31. Grinnell, R.: Results of ligation of the inferior mesenteric artery at the aorta in resections of carcinoma of the descending and sigmoid colon and rectum. Surg. Gynecol. Obstet., 120:1030, 1965.

32. Grinnell, R., and Hiatt, R.: Ligation of the inferior mesenteric artery at the aorta in resections for carcinoma of the sigmoid and rectum. Surg. Gynecol. Obstet., 94:526, 1952.

33. Hackford, A.W.: The extent of major resections for rectal cancer. In Veidenheimer, M.C. (ed.): Semin. Colon Rectal Surg., 1:16, 1990.

34. Harnsberger, J., Charvat, P., Longo, W.E., et al.: The role of intrarectal ultrasound (IRUS) in staging of rectal cancer and detection of extrarectal pathology. Am. Surg., (submitted).

35. Harnsberger, J.R., Vernava, A.M., and Longo, W.E.: Radical abdominopelvic lymphadenectomy in the treatment of rectal cancer (RAPL): A historical perspective and its current role in the surgical management of rectal cancer. Dis. Colon Rectum, 37:73, 1994.

36. Heald, R.J., Husband, E.M., and Ryall, R.D.H.: The mesorectum in rectal cancer surgery—the clue to pelvic recurrence. Br. J. Surg., 69:613, 1982.

37. Heald, R.J., and Leicester, R.J.: The low stapled anastomosis. Br. J. Surg., 68:198, 1981.

38. Heald, R.J., and Ryall, R.D.: Recurrence and survival after total mesorectal excision for rectal cancer. Lancet, 1:1479, 1986.

39. Heberer, G., Denecke, H., Pratshke, E., Teichmann, R.: Anterior and low anterior resection. World J. Surg., 6:517, 1982.

40. Hildebrandt, U., and Feifel, G.: Preoperative staging of rectal cancer by intrarectal ultrasound. Dis. Colon Rectum, 28:42, 1985.

41. Hochenegg, J.: Die sekrale Methode der Extirpation von MastdarmKrebsen nach Prof. Kraske. Wien. Klin. Wochenschr., 1:254, 272, 290, 309, 324, 348, 1888.

42. Hojo, K., Sawada, T., and Moriya, Y.: An analysis of survival and voiding, sexual function after wide ileopelvic lymphadenectomy in patients with carcinoma of the rectum, compared with conventional lymphadenectomy. Dis. Colon Rectum, 32:128, 1989.

43. Hojo, K., Vernava, A.M., Sugihara, K., and Katumata, K.: Preservation of urine voiding and sexual function after rectal cancer surgery. Dis. Colon Rectum, 34:532, 1991.

44. Horgan, P.G., O'Connell, P.R., Shinkwsin, C.A., et al.: Effect of anterior resection on anal sphincter function. Br. J. Surg., 76:783, 1989.

45. Jones, P.F., and Thomson, H.J.: Long term results of a consistent policy of sphincter preservation in the treatment of carcinoma of the rectum. Br. J. Surg., 69:564, 1982.

46. Kinn, A.-C., and Ohman, U.: Bladder and sexual function after surgery for rectal cancer. Dis. Colon Rectum, 29:43, 1986.

47. Kirkegaard, P., Hjortrup, A., and Sanders, S.: Bladder dysfunction after low anterior resection for mid-rectal cancer. Am. J. Surg., 141:266, 1981.

48. Kokal, W.A., Gardine, R.L., Sheibani, K., et al.: Tumor DNA content in resectable primary colorectal carcinoma. Ann. Surg., 209:188, 1989.

49. Kraske, P.: Zur Exstirpation hochsitzender Mastdarmkrebse. Verh. Dtsch. Ges. Chir., 14:464, 1885.

50. Manson, P.N., Corman, M.L., Coller, J.A., and Veidenheimer, M.C.: Anterior resection for adenocarcinoma: Lahey Clinic experience from 1963 through 1969. Am. J. Surg., 131:431, 1976.

51. Maunsell, H.W.: A new method of excising the two upper portions of the rectum and the lower segment of the sigmoid flexure of the colon. Lancet, 2:473, 1892.

52. McAnena, O., Heald, R.J., and Lockhart-Mummery, H.: Operative and functional results of total mesorectal excision with ultra-low anterior resection in the management of carcinoma of the lower one-third of the rectum. Surg. Gynecol. Obstet., 170:517, 1990.

53. McDermott, F., Hughes, E.S.R., Pihl, E., et al.: Long term results of restorative resection and total excision for carcinoma of the middle third of the rectum. Surg. Gynecol. Obstet., 154:833, 1982.

54. McDermott, F.T., Hugher, E.S.R., Phil, E., et al.: Local recurrence after potentially curative resections for rectal cancer in a series of 1008 patients. Br. J. Surg., 72:34, 1985.

55. Miles, W.E.: A method of performing abdominoperineal excision for carcinoma of the rectum and of the terminal portion of the pelvic colon. Lancet, 2:1812, 1908.

56. Milsom, J.W., and Fraffner, H.: Intrarectal ultrasonography in rectal cancer staging and in the evaluation of pelvic disease. Ann. Surg., 212:602, 1990.

57. Moriya, Y., Hojo, K., Sawada, T., and Koyama, Y.: Significance of lateral node dissection for advanced rectal carcinoma at or below the peritoneal reflection. Dis. Colon Rectum, 32:307, 1989.

58. Parks, A.G.: Transanal technique in low rectal anastomosis. Proc. R. Soc. Med., 65:975, 1972.

59. Parks, S.E., and Hastings, P.R.: Complications of colostomy closure. Am. J. Surg., 149:672, 1985.

60. Parks, A.F., and Percy, J.P.: Resections and sutured coloanal anastomosis for rectal carcinoma. Br. J. Surg., 69:301, 1982.

61. Pedersen, B.K., Huit, K., Olen, J., et al.: Anorectal function after low anterior resection for carcinoma. Ann. Surg., 294:133, 1986.

62. Pezim, M., and Nicholls, R.: Survival after high or low ligation of the inferior mesenteric artery during curative surgery for rectal cancer. Ann. Surg., 200:729, 1984.

63. Pollet, W.G., and Nicholls, R.J.: The relationship between the extent of distal clearance and survival and local recurrence rates after curative anterior resection for carcinoma of the rectum. Ann. Surg., 198:159, 1983.

64. Quirke, P., Durdey, P., Dixon, M.F., and Williams, N.S.: Local recurrence of rectal adenocarcinoma due to inadequate surgical resection: Histopathologic study of lateral tumour spread and surgical excision. Lancet, 2:996, 1986.

65. Ravo, B., Mishick, A., Addei, K., et al.: The treatment of perforated diverticulitis by one-stage intracolonic bypass procedure. Surgery, 102:771, 1987.

66. Rosi, P., Cahill, W., and Carey, J.: A ten year study of hemicolectomy in the treatment of carcinoma of the left half of the colon. Surg. Gynecol. Obstet., 114:14, 1962.

67. Rosen, C.B., Beart, R.W., Jr., and Ilstrukp, D.M.: Local recurrence of rectal carcinoma after hand sewn and stapled anastomosis. Dis. Colon Rectum, 28:305, 1985.

68. Schrock, T.R., Deveney, C.W., and Dunphy, J.E.: Factors contributing to leakage of colonic anastomoses. Ann. Surg., 177:513, 1973.

69. Scott, N.A., Rainwater, L.M., Wiegand, H.S., et al.: The relative prognostic value of flow cytometric DNA analysis and conventional clinicopathologic criteria in patients with operable rectal carcinoma. Dis. Colon Rectum, 30:523, 1987.

70. Stearns, M., and Deddish, M.: Five-year results of abdominopelvic lymph node dissection for carcinoma of the rectum. Dis. Colon Rectum, 2:169, 1959.

71. Thomson, W.H.F., and Carter, S.St.C.: On-table lavage to achieve safe restorative rectal and emergency colonic resection without covering colostomy. Br. J. Surg., 73:61, 1986.

72. Turnbull, R.B., Jr., and Cuthbertson, A.M.: Abdomino-rectal pullthrough resection for cancer and Hirschprung's disease. Cleve. Clin. Q., 28:109, 1961.

73. Vernava, A.M., Fitzgerald, S.D., Longo, W.E., and Kaminski, D.L.:

Sutured versus stapled colonic anasomosis: Does method affect outcome? Contemp. Surg., *43*:337, 1993.

74. Vernava, A.M., and Longo, W.E.: Other applications of colorectal physiology. *In* Wexner, S.D. (ed.): Colorectal Physiology: Investigation and Intervention. Semin. Colon Rectal Surg., *4*(4):144, 1992.

75. Vernava, A.M., Moran, M., Rothenberger, D.A., and Wong, W.D.: A prospective evaluation of distal margins in rectal cancer. Surg. Gynecol. Obstet., *175*:333, 1992.

76. Vernava, A.M., Robbins, P.L., and Brabbee, G.: Coloanal anastomosis for benign and malignant disease. Dis. Colon Rectum, *32*:690, 1989.

77. Walsh, P.C., and Schlegel, P.: Radical pelvic surgery with preservation of sexual function. Ann. Surg., *208*:391, 1988.

78. Weir, R.F.: An improved method of treating high-seated cancers of the rectum. JAMA, *37*:801, 1901.

79. Wexner, S.D., Johansen, O.B., Nogueras, J.J., and Jagelman, D.G.: Laparoscopic total abdominal colectomy: A prospective trial.

Dis. Colon Rectum, *35*:651, 1992.

80. Williams, N.S.: The rationale for preservation of the anal sphincter in patients with low rectal cancer. Br. J. Surg., *71*:575, 1984.

81. Williams, N.S., Dixon, M.F., and Hohnston, D.: Reappraisal of the 5-centimetre rule of distal excision for carcinomas of the rectum: A study of distal intramural spread and of patients' survival. Br. J. Surg., *70*:150, 1983.

82. Williams, N.S., Durdey, P., and Johnston, D.: The outcome following sphincter-saving resection and abdominoperineal resection for low rectal cancer. Br. J. Surg., *72*:595, 1985.

83. Williams, N.S., Price, R., and Johnston, D.: The long term effect of sphincter preserving operations for rectal carcinoma on function of the anal sphincter in man. Br. J. Surg., *67*:203, 1980.

84. Wolmark, N., and Fisher, B.: An analysis of survival and treatment failure following abdominoperineal resection and sphincter-saving resection in Dukes' B and C rectal carcinoma. Ann. Surg., *204*:480, 1986.

Chapter 19

ABDOMINOPERINEAL RESECTION

GEORGE E. BLOCK / ROGER D. HURST

The operative procedure for abdominoperineal resection of the rectum as practiced today is the lineal descendant of the operation described by Miles in 1908.[7] Miles adopted abdominoperineal resection as the alternative to perineal excision of the rectum. Following 57 perineal excisions by Miles, 54 patients experienced recurrence.

During the intervening 80 years since its introduction, the Miles operation has been modified by a number of surgeons. The recent modifications include the 1962 report of Rosi and co-workers,[8] who advocated excision of the entire mesentery of the inferior mesenteric artery rather than merely the mesentery of the rectosigmoid colon as described by Miles. In 1959, Child and Donovan[1] advised "stripping" of the aortoiliac regions to include these nodes, and Sterns and Deddish[9] described an extended pelvic lymphadenectomy as a logical expansion of the Miles operation. In 1979, we[2] reported enhanced survival by combining high ligation of the inferior mesenteric artery with a wide hypogastric node dissection. Improved survival and enhanced local control with wide pelvic lymph node dissection has also been reported by others.[4,6] This procedure, with some modification, remains our preferred operation and forms the basis of this chapter.

Although an adequate and curative operation can be performed without sacrifice of the anal sphincters for some tumors of the midrectum (6 to 10 cm from the anal verge) and a few small tumors of the lower rectum (<6 cm from the anal verge), abdominoperineal resection remains the standard operation against which the results of lesser procedures are measured. The operation is the procedure of choice for invasive carcinomas of the lower rectum, large tumors of the midrectum, epidermoid carcinomas of the anal canal that are refractory to radiation and chemotherapy, some uncommon lesions such as melanoma of the anus and rectum, large perianal tumors involving the anal canal, huge tumors of the rectosigmoid, certain rare tumors such as invasive chordoma and sarcoma, and recurrent rectal carcinoma following less extensive resection.

EXTENT OF OPERATION

The abdominoperineal resection is an operative translation of the anatomic knowledge of the pelvic viscera and the predictable sites of neoplastic extension from carcinoma of the rectum. It is a three-dimensional operation that takes into account the superior, inferior, lateral, and anteroposterior dimensions of spread. Omission of any one of these dimensions in the operative procedure is ill-founded because the rectum is still sacrificed and the patient is required to contend with a stoma, and male patients often with impotency, whereas one or more of the theoretical pathways of extension of the tumor are not removed. It appears logical, therefore, that in a functionally mutilating operation there is no place for pseudoconservatism in the performance of the procedure.

The extent of the operative procedure may be described by consideration of the predictable pathways of extension of carcinoma of the rectum or anus (Fig. 19–1). The superior axial lymphatic drainage of the rectum is via the mesorectum and the proximal lymph nodes along the branches of the inferior mesenteric artery. This pathway of extension is encompassed by ligation of the inferior mesenteric artery at its origin from the aorta and the total removal of the rectal mesentery including the entire mesorectum. Any inferior extension of the tumor within or adjacent to the wall of the rectum is excised by total removal of the rectum and anus, including the contents of the ischiorectal space. The lateral lymphatic drainage of the rectum is included by removal of the midrectal vessels, the hypogastric lymph nodes, and the levator sling, together with the lymph nodes along the common iliac artery. Of utmost importance is the clearance of the pararectal tissue for 360 degrees around the viscus. This dissection requires a vertical excision of pelvic contents to the walls of the internal obturator muscles laterally, to the sacrum posteriorly, and at least to the uterus and vagina or seminal vesicles anteriorly. All tissues between these structures must be included in the resection. Inferiorly, the perianal skin is removed in ac-

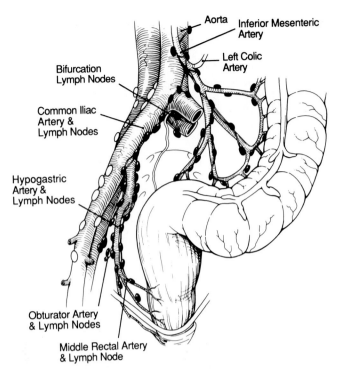

Aorta
Inferior Mesenteric Artery

Left Colic Artery

Bifurcation Lymph Nodes

Common Iliac Artery & Lymph Nodes

Hypogastric Artery & Lymph Nodes

Obturator Artery & Lymph Nodes

Middle Rectal Artery & Lymph Node

FIGURE 19-1. Lymphatic drainage of the rectum. The predictable sites of extension of the rectal carcinoma via the lymphatic system are excised in the procedure described in the text.

cordance with the lesion being treated—a wider excision is used for perianal and anal lesions than for rectal lesions.

At the termination of the procedure, there is a three-dimensional excision of the rectum that extends from the third portion of the duodenum superiorly to the aortoiliac vessels and sacrum posteriorly, the bladder anteriorly, and the muscular walls of the pelvis laterally. The ureters mark the lateral boundary of dissection at the pelvic peritoneum. The left ureter may be sacrificed if it is invaded by resectable tumor.

TECHNIQUE

Preparation of the Patient

Prior to operation, the location of the tumor measured from the anal verge is determined by proctoscopy, and histologic confirmation of the nature of the tumor is obtained. The surgeon should confer with the patient and family so that they understand the nature of the operation, the necessity for the operation, treatment options including alternative as well as adjuvant therapies, operative hazards, possible complications, and potential benefits. Most importantly, the patient should have a thorough understanding of the nature of a colostomy and possible impairment of sexual function. All appropriate candidates are given the opportunity for autologous blood donation. Additionally, male patients who may desire to father children in the future are advised to cryopreserve a sample of their sperm prior to the operation.

The bowel is cleansed mechanically by a combination of a liquid diet for 48 hours prior to operation and oral polyethylene glycol solution the evening prior to operation. Prophylactic antibiotics are appropriate; we prefer systemic prophylaxis given as cephazolin prior to operation and for one or two postoperative doses.

Specific medical problems such as anemia, cardiac arrhythmias, and hyperglycemia should be discovered and remedied prior to operation. Synchronous neoplasms of the colon are sought by endoscopy or air-contrast radiographs. If present, these lesions are included within the scope of the resection.

The patient is usually anesthetized with a general endotracheal anesthetic, but in certain instances conductive anesthesia may be appropriate.

Position of the Patient

After induction of anesthesia, an indwelling urinary catheter is inserted and the patient is placed in the lithotomy position with Lloyd-Davies stirrups. The position of the patient must ensure easy access to both the abdomen and the perineum. In most instances, the thighs are flexed approximately 30 degrees and abducted 30 to 40 degrees. Extreme abduction of the thighs is not necessary and may be harmful. The popliteal fossae and fibular heads are generously padded to avoid peroneal or tibial nerve palsies. The dependent legs are supported by elastic bandages to the knee or compression devices. A firm small pillow is placed beneath the sacrum so that the surgeon has easy access to the coccyx, and the anus is closed by a stout pursestring suture.

Incisions

The site of the descending colostomy is chosen preoperatively to avoid skin creases, scars, and bony prominences and is then checked for correctness by having the patient stand and sit. The appropriate sites are marked with an indelible pencil. We prefer to tattoo the colostomy site with absorbable ink prior to making the skin incision. An incision is chosen to afford adequate exposure but is placed so as not to interfere with the stoma.

Although a number of incisions may be used for the operation, most surgeons prefer either a midline incision, extending from above the umbilicus to the pubis, or a transverse incision. Our choice is a lower abdominal transverse incision extending across the abdomen at the level of the iliac crest. Depending on the abdominal configuration, this incision may be either midway or two thirds of the way from the umbilicus to the pubis. The stoma site is usually above the transverse incision and in the left lower quadrant with the vertical incision. The transverse incision affords superb exposure of the lower abdomen and pelvis and is cosmetically superior, is relatively painless, and resists disruption.

Upon opening the abdomen, a thorough exploration is made to ascertain the presence or absence of liver metastases, peritoneal implants, para-aortic lymph node involvement, the location and any fixation of the primary tumor, and the status of the peritoneal floor. In addition to direct observation and manual palpation, intraoperative ultrasound can be helpful in identifying liver metastases. If, upon initial exploration, the patient is deemed incurable or the tumor unresectable, the proposed abdominoperineal resection may be abandoned and a palliative procedure chosen instead.

Superior Dissection

The peritoneum is incised over the right common iliac artery and the incision is carried superiorly along the aorta to the level of the third portion of the duodenum (Fig. 19-2). On the left, the peritoneum is incised from the left common iliac artery lateral to the gonadal vessels and ureter, and this incision is carried superiorly to the left lumbar gutter. Between these two peritoneal incisions, the inferior mesenteric artery mesentery is swept toward the midline by sharp dissection, removing the underlying areolar, perivascular, and lymphatic tissue. During this dissection, both ureters are repeatedly identified and separated from inclusion in the dissection so that they form the lateral boundaries of the dissection at this level.

The periaortic areolar tissue and the lymph nodes situated adjacent to the inferior mesenteric artery are dissected free to expose the origin of the inferior mesenteric artery from the aorta. The inferior mesenteric artery is then divided between clamps and doubly suture ligated with nonabsorbable suture. Alternatively, the surgeon may elect to denude the inferior mesenteric artery of lymphatic tissue distal to the origin of the left colic artery and divide the arcade at this level. During this mesenteric dissection, tiny blood vessels and lymphatics adjacent to the iliac vessels and aorta are controlled by small metallic clips.

During the isolation of the inferior mesenteric artery, the superior pelvic ganglions of the pelvic autonomic nervous system and the nervi erigentes on each side will

come into view between the aortic adventitia and the developing mesenteric pedicle. This structure may be spared in the sexually active patient, and such a maneuver will help maintain male potency. If this is done, the lymphatic dissection is then carried out somewhat tediously behind the nervi erigentes so that, at the completion of the procedure, the aortoiliac node dissection is complete and the pelvic autonomic nerve pathways are free and traceable to the seminal vesicles or vagina and bladder.

The dissection continues inferiorly, removing the areolar tissue and lymphatics along the aorta and common iliac vessels to the bifurcation of the aorta superiorly and the iliac bifurcations laterally (Fig. 19-3). At the aortic bifurcation, the areolar tissue and lymph nodes at the aortocaval bifurcation are dissected free to expose the denuded aortic and vena caval bifurcations. Several large venous tributaries from the iliac veins to the adjacent lymph nodes and mesentery will be encountered and are controlled with clips. The lymphatic tissue so dissected will appear as an extension of the inferior mesenteric artery mesentery in the final specimen. Caudal dissection in the plane adjacent to the iliac veins brings the dissection into the presacral space at the promontory of the sacrum.

Posterior and Lateral Dissections

The posterior and lateral dissections are carried out together in complementary fashion. As the right and left lateral dissections proceed, the posterior dissection is facilitated, and together they ensure adequate pararectal clearance, total mobilization of the rectum, and extensive pelvic lymphadenectomy.

Posteriorly, the rectum is mobilized from the entrance to the presacral space at the bifurcation of the common iliac veins to well beyond the coccyx to expose the pubococcygeus portion of the levator sling. In order to avoid bleeding from vessels that traverse the presacral space, the posterior dissection is done under direct vision with the rectum retracted anteriorly by a Harrington retractor. This dissection is best accomplished with scissors; the blood vessels traversing the presacral space are controlled with small metallic clips prior to division.

The lateral dissection for adenocarcinoma of the rectum and epidermoid cancer of the anal canal differ in extent. For adenocarcinoma of the rectum, the lateral dissection proceeds from the denuded common iliac arteries along the hypogastric (internal iliac) arteries. For carcinoma of the anal canal, the external iliac vessels are also denuded to include their adjacent lymphatics. This dissection begins at the iliofemoral junction and proceeds superiorly to the bifurcation of the iliac vessels and is later supplemented by an obturator node dissection. For most rectal carcinomas, dissection of the external iliac nodes is superfluous. The lateral dissection for carcinoma of the rectum proceeds along the internal iliac vessels and their branches.

For this phase of dissection, the ureters (and, if appropriate, the nervi erigentes) are again identified and excluded from the dissection. The internal iliac arteries are stripped of all loose connective tissue and lymphat-

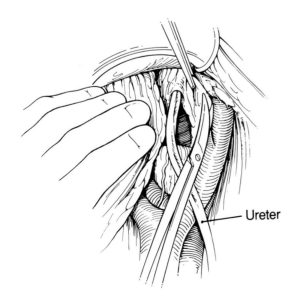

FIGURE 19-2. Abdominal phase. Right lateral peritoneal incision and ligation of the inferior mesenteric artery.

— Ureter

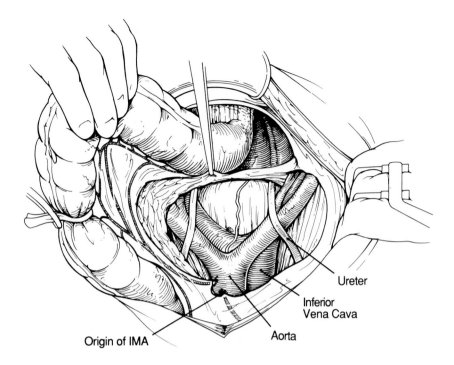

FIGURE 19-3. Abdominal phase. Dissection of the aortic, aortocaval, and common iliac nodes.

Ureter

Inferior Vena Cava

Aorta

Origin of IMA

ics, and the lymphatic tissue is dissected medially to be included in the final specimen. This dissection is carried inferiorly to the terminal branches of the internal iliac arteries. The midrectal vessels are identified at their origin from the internal iliac arteries and are ligated and divided at the pelvic walls. If sexual potency in the male is to be preserved, the dissection and transection of the midrectal arteries are accomplished medial to the course of the nervi erigentes within the lateral ligaments of the rectum. In the female patient, concomitant hysterectomy is often performed; at this time, the ovarian and uterine vessels are identified, ligated, and divided. Extensions of the tumor into the obturator fossa may be removed at this time or, alternatively, an obturator dis-

section may be accomplished after removal of the rectum (Fig. 19–4).

Upon completion of the posterior and lateral dissection, the rectum has been freed distal to the coccyx to the pubococcygeus muscle posteriorly and to the origins of the levators laterally so that the internal obturator muscles are cleared in their entirety and form the lateral margins of the dissection.

Anterior Dissection

After completion of the lateral and posterior dissections, the anterior dissection commences. Another equally satisfactory method is to incise the anterior peri-

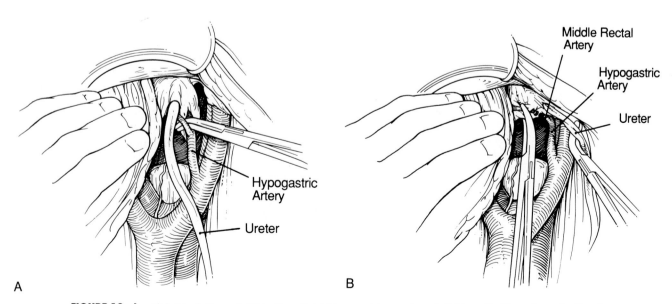

Hypogastric Artery

Ureter

Middle Rectal Artery

Hypogastric Artery

Ureter

A

B

FIGURE 19-4. Abdominal phase. A, Dissection of right hypogastric vessels and division of midrectal vessels. B and C, Removal of areolar tissue and lymphatics from the lateral pelvic walls and obturator fossa.

toneum at the time of the lateral dissection, carrying out the anterior dissection concomitantly with the lateral dissection so that the entire pelvis is dissected in a circular fashion. For descriptive purposes, we shall consider the anterior dissection separately.

In the female patient, the anterior dissection commences with a peritoneal incision in the sulcus between the anterior rectal wall and the posterior vaginal wall. If an en bloc hysterectomy is to be performed, the anterior peritoneal incision is made across the base of the bladder on the anterior vaginal wall. In males, the peritoneal incision is made posterior to the bladder. In both sexes, great care is taken to widely excise the pelvic peritoneum to include any neoplastic extensions in the cul-de-sac. Denonvilliers' fascia is incised beneath the peritoneum, and the connective tissue between the rectum and the seminal vesicles and prostate in men or the posterior wall of the vagina in women are dissected free onto the rectum (Fig. 19–5). If there is invasion or ad-

herence of the tumor to the prostate, seminal vesicles, or posterior vaginal wall, these structures are resected en bloc with the rectum.

The ureters are retracted laterally and are mobilized to their entrance into the bladder. If a single ureter is involved with tumor it may be sacrificed. If both ureters or the trigone of the bladder is invaded by tumor, a pelvic exenteration may then be required.

Transection of the Colon

After completion of the anterior dissection, the abdominal portion of the pelvic dissection is complete (Fig. 19–6). The pelvis is inspected for bleeding and a large pack is placed in the hollow of the sacrum while the colon is transected and the perineal excision proceeds.

The site for the division of the descending colon is now selected. Demarcation between viable and nonvia-

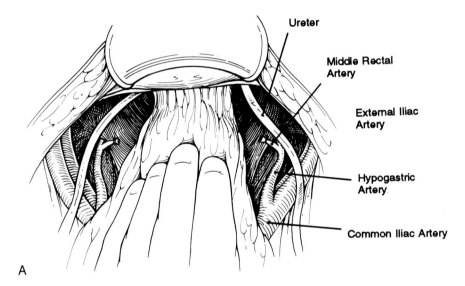

A

FIGURE 19-5. Abdominal phase. *A* and *B*, Anterior dissection. Separation of anterior rectum from bladder to expose seminal vesicles and prostate. *C*, View of pelvis upon completion of abdominal phase of the operation.

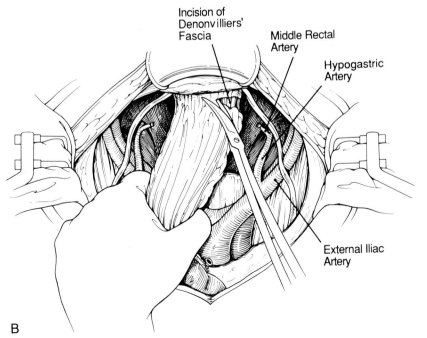

B

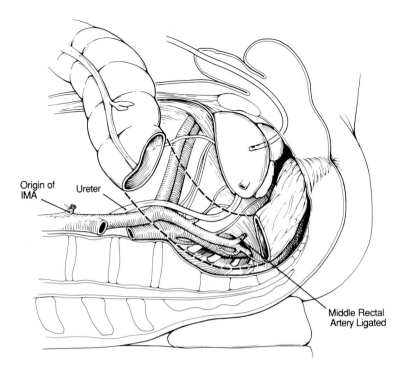

Origin of IMA

Ureter

Middle Rectal Artery Ligated

FIGURE 19-6. Abdominal phase. Midsagittal view of the pelvis upon completion of the abdominal phase.

ble bowel is usually obvious and most often is at the junction of the descending and sigmoid colon. A palpable pulse in the marginal artery must be confirmed to ensure adequate blood flow in the proximal segment. The peritoneum is incised and the mesentery is divided between hemostats on a line extending from the origin of the inferior mesenteric artery to the point of proposed division of the colon. The bowel is divided between noncrushing bowel clamps, or it may be conveniently divided by a GIA stapling device. The transected ends of the colon are covered with gauze sponges to minimize contamination. Although the abdominal colostomy may be constructed at this time, we prefer to defer this portion of the operation until the perineal dissection has been completed, the rectum has been removed, and the perineal wound has been closed.

Perineal Phase

The extent of the perineal incision varies with the lesion being treated. If the lesion is an anal canal carcinoma or a low rectal lesion that extends into the anal canal, an incision is chosen that extends from the coccyx and encompasses the ischial tuberosities laterally and the perineal body anteriorly. For higher or smaller lesions, a more conservative skin incision is indicated. In the female patient, the anterior extent of the perineal incision encompasses the posterior introitus if the posterior vaginal wall is to be resected.

The skin incision is deepened both to include the ischiorectal spaces and to expose the undersurface of the levator sling. We utilize the cutting phase of the electrocautery for the perineal dissection. The anococcygeal ligament is identified and transected immediately distal to the coccyx with a Mayo scissors. The left index finger of the operator is then inserted into the presacral space.

The entrance into the presacral space will be confirmed by a small gush of blood and fluid as the perineal wound is thus connected to the presacral space. The adequacy of the posterior dissection is then evaluated. If adequate, the exploring finger will be free in the presacral space. The levator sling is then prolapsed by the surgeon's index finger into the open perineal wound and is divided at its origin on the pelvic walls by the electrocautery. The division of the levator sling is begun at the coccyx (6-o'clock position) and is carried bilaterally anteriorly to the 10-o'clock and 2-o'clock positions (Fig. 19-7).

With this partial transection of the levator sling, the surgeon may then reach into the pelvis from the perineal wound and deliver the rectum and the rectosigmoid into the perineal wound so that the entire specimen is brought from the pelvis through the perineal wound and is exteriorized.

In the male patient, the only attachments of the rectum are a few remaining anterior fibers of the levator sling and Denonvilliers' fascia at the prostatic capsule. These are divided by electrocautery. If the rectal tumor extends into the prostatic capsule, a perineal prostatectomy can be accomplished at this time. In a female patient, the rectum and uterus are brought out through the posterior wound so that the remaining attachments are to the posterior vagina. The posterior vaginal wall may be excised when dealing with anterior rectal tumors; in smaller or posterior tumors, the rectovaginal septum may merely be divided if there is no hint of neoplastic extension into the vagina. If excised, the vaginal defect is easily reconstructed by interrupted, stout, absorbable sutures.

In most cases, the perineal wound may be closed primarily with interrupted subcutaneous and skin sutures. Closure is desirable, as it speeds convalescence and avoids the lengthy healing of a granulating perineal wound. The pelvis is drained with suction devices

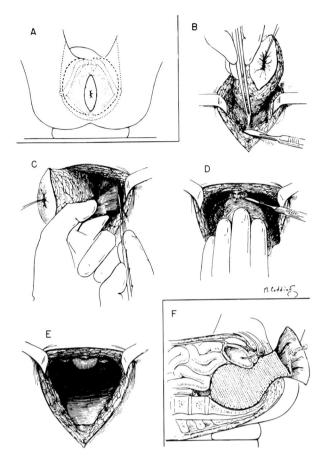

FIGURE 19-7. Perineal phase. *A*, Various skin incisions employed in the perineal phase. *B*, Transection of the anococcygeal ligament. *C*, Transection of the levator ani muscle. *D*, Separation of the anterior rectum from prostatic capsule. *E*, Perineal view upon completion of the perineal phase. *F*, Midsagittal section of the perineum and pelvis upon completion of the operation with tampon in place.

brought out through stab wounds in the buttocks. These pelvic drains should lie in the presacral space.

If the perineal excision is so extensive that perineal closure is difficult or impossible, the pelvis is packed with a large tampon of gauze enclosed in Owens surgical silk and the pelvic tampon is secured in place with stout sutures through the skin. This will allow early ambulation of the patient prior to removal of the pack approximately 5 to 6 days after operation.

Upon completion of the perineal phase, attention is again directed to the abdominal wound. Prior to further abdominal manipulation, the entire surgical team changes gloves and gowns.

Pelvic Closure and Colostomy Construction

Careful re-exploration of the abdomen and pelvis is made to search for bleeding. The pelvis now contains either suction drains or a pelvic pack. If adequate peritoneum has been preserved, the peritoneal floor may be closed. If there is not adequate peritoneum, or if closure is tenuous or under tension, the pelvic floor may be closed by an omental flap based on either the right or left gastroepiploic vessels. The omental flap is quite

useful both to protect against bowel herniation into the pelvic wound and to prevent small bowel injury if postoperative radiation is planned.

Prior to closing the pelvis, the surgeon may elect to clear obturator nodes from the obturator fossa. This is most easily accomplished after removal of the rectum, but this is not a dissection in continuity.

Following closure of the pelvis, an end colostomy is constructed. The stoma site should be over the body of the rectus abdominis muscle. The skin is incised, and the anterior fascia is excised as a thin ellipse 2 to 3 cm in length. The wound is carried through the posterior fascia and the colostomy is brought out via either an extraperitoneal or transperitoneal route. If transperitoneal, the defect created between the mesentery of the colon and the abdominal wall must be closed. The mesentery of the colon is fixed with a few stout sutures to the transversalis fascia at the stomal aperture to prevent future prolapse. Three to 4 cm of bowel should lie free without tension above the skin level. The abdominal wound is closed with wire sutures, and the subcutaneous tissue and skin are closed. Only after closure of the skin incision is the abdominal colostomy "matured." If a bowel clamp has been used at the time of transection of the colon, it is removed and absorbable interrupted sutures are placed to join the bowel wall and the dermis of the colostomy wound. If staples have been used to close the end of the descending colon, this closure is excised and the stoma is secured to the skin with interrupted sutures. A clear appliance is placed over the stoma, and the operative procedure is terminated.

POSTOPERATIVE CARE

Postoperatively, nasogastric decompression is maintained and the patient is kept fasting until bowel motility has returned. Presacral drains are left in place until the drainage is less than 25 ml/day (usually 3 to 4 days). If a pelvic pack has been used, it is removed in approximately 5 days; the wound is cleansed with saline irrigations and is allowed to heal by secondary intention. The bladder catheter is not removed until the patient is fully ambulatory and a cystometrogram has confirmed adequate bladder tone and contraction. Between 20 and 30% of patients will experience some degree of urinary retention that may require intermittent self-catheterization.[3] In almost all instances this is a temporary condition and normal bladder function returns within 3 months.[5]

REFERENCES

1. Child, G.C., and Donovan, A.J.: Abdominoperineal resection of the rectum. *In* Turell, R. (ed.): Diseases of the Colon and Anorectum. Philadelphia, W.B. Saunders, 1959, p. 459.
2. Enker, W.E., Laffer, U.T., and Block, G.E.: Enhanced survival of patients with colon and rectal cancer is based upon wide anatomic resection. Ann. Surg., *190*:350, 1979.
3. Kinn, A.C., and Ohman, U.: Bladder and sexual function after surgery for rectal cancer. Dis. Colon Rectum, *29*:43, 1986.
4. Koyama, Y., Moriya, Y., and Hojo, K.: Effects of extended systematic lymphadenectomy for adenocarcinoma of the rectum: Significant

improvement of survival rate and decrease of local recurrence. Jpn. J. Clin. Oncol., *14*:623, 1984.

5. Michelassi, F., and Block, G.E.: Morbidity and mortality of wide pelvic lymphadenectomy for rectal adenocarcinoma. Dis. Colon Rectum, *35*:1142, 1992.

6. Michelassi, F., Block, G.E., Vannucci, L., et al.: A 5 to 21 year follow-up and analysis of 250 patients with rectal adenocarcinoma. Ann. Surg., *208*:379, 1988.

7. Miles, W.E.; A method of performing abdomino-perineal resection for carcinoma of the rectum and the terminal portion of the pelvic colon. Lancet, *2*:1812, 1908.

8. Rosi, P.A., Cahill, W.J., and Carey, J.: A ten-year study of hemicolectomy in the treatment of carcinoma of the left half of the colon. Surg. Gynecol. Obstet., *114*:15, 1962.

9. Sterns, M.W., Jr., and Deddish, M.R.: Five year results of abdominopelvic lymph node dissection for carcinoma of the rectum. Dis. Colon Rectum, *2*:169, 1959.

Chapter 20

ABDOMINOSACRAL RESECTION

KENNETH ENG / S. ARTHUR LOCALIO

RATIONALE FOR ABDOMINOSACRAL RESECTION

Sphincter-saving operations have played an increasing role in the treatment of rectal cancer. Although technical aspects of low anastomoses have received most recent attention, there can be no complacency regarding the adequacy of radical resection. To minimize the risk of local recurrence, the resection should include not only an adequate distal margin, but also wide clearance of the lateral ligaments and the mesorectum beyond the tumor.

Sphincter function is dependent on preservation of the anal sphincters and their innervation. The uppermost component of the sphincter is the puborectalis sling. The lower limit of sphincter-saving resection in terms of pelvic clearance of tumor is also at the musculus puborectalis of the levator ani diaphragm. In order to carry out sphincter-saving resection in every case in which it is theoretically feasible, exposure must be adequate for complete mobilization to the levators and for precise measurement of the distal margin. Abdominosacral resection satisfies these requirements, but the operation should be assessed in the context of other currently available sphincter-saving operations.

Anterior Resection

Most surgeons perform anterior resection for lesions as low as they consider technically feasible and resort to abdominoperineal resection for the rest.[3,4] Anterior resection is suitable for most tumors in the upper third of the rectum. For many surgeons, the availability of staplers that allow end-to-end colorectal anastomosis has extended the range of anterior resection.[1,3,4] Although the stapler provides ease in performing low anastomoses, the problem of exposure for adequate radical resection remains. Even with the ingenious newer versions of these devices, which facilitate awkward anastomoses in the depths of the pelvis, the resection is limited to the area visible from the abdominal incision. Clearance of the tumor must not be jeopardized to save the sphincter.

Even in the hands of experienced surgeons, the abdominal approach alone cannot provide sufficient exposure for reliable resection of many midrectal cancers. In men, the abdominal exposure is limited to the level of the seminal vesicles. The anterior wall of the rectum below this level is obscured by the pubis. After thorough mobilization of the rectum, a midrectal tumor may be barely in view, and determination of an adequate distal margin will be in doubt. The wider pelvis in women may permit mobilization under direct vision to the levators, but obesity, an enlarged uterus, or previous inflammation and scarring may compromise this exposure.

Abdominoanal Resection

The coloanal anastomosis devised by Parks provides a means for anastomosis within the anal canal.[7] After abdominal mobilization and resection of the rectum, the anus is dilated and the mucosa is stripped from the remaining anorectal stump. The proximal colon is pulled through the muscular cuff and sutured perianally at the dentate line. The anastomosis may be performed using a stapler by inserting the distal pursestring suture from below.[3,4] Although the anastomosis is done as low as the dentate line, mobilization and resection of the cancer are carried out entirely by the abdominal route. Exposure is no different than for anterior resection. Unless one is willing to accept blind mobilization of the lower rectum, the method cannot allow radical resection to the levators in every case.

Abdominotranssphincteric Resection

One method for enhancing exposure for resection of midrectal tumors is the transsphincteric approach.[6] The levators and the anal sphincters are incised serially and are tagged with sutures for later reapproximation. This approach was used initially for local excision of benign tumors and early cancers, but Mason later described a combined abdominal and transsphincteric approach for radical resection of midrectal cancer. Although the method provides the necessary exposure for wide resection, it results in two intersecting suture lines when a radical resection and end-to-end anastomosis are performed. Anastomotic failure and pelvic sepsis might cause loss of the sphincter repair even when a protective colostomy is employed.

Abdominosacral Resection

Only abdominosacral resection provides the exposure for resection to the levators in every case without disturbing the sphincters of their innervation.[5] Excision of the coccyx allows direct visualization of the pelvis. The rectosigmoid stump is delivered through the posterior wound with an intact fascia propria, which contains rectal mesentery, perirectal fat, and lymphatics. The lowest portions of the lateral ligaments are divided by this posterior approach. The distal limit of the tumor is identified by palpation or sigmoidoscopy through the divided stump. The distal margin is measured with a ruler with no tension on the bowel. Only after this distal site is determined is the rectum cleared. Denonvilliers' fascia is incised, and the anterior wall of the rectum is cleared

to bare longitudinal muscle. The entire rectal mesentery is swept upward from the levators posteriorly and is included in the specimen. In this way, the widest possible clearance around the tumor is achieved (Fig. 20–1).

Resection to the puborectalis sling is possible in every case, regardless of individual variations in the patient's habitus. The proximal colon is delivered, and a sutured end-to-end anastomosis may be done. The anastomosis following the lowest resections may be facilitated by the circular end-to-end stapler.

SELECTION OF PATIENTS

The level of the cancer is determined by sigmoidoscopy with the patient in the knee-chest position. Patients with midrectal lesions 5 to 10 cm from the anal verge are candidates for abdominosacral resection. Lesions above these limits are treated by anterior resection. Lesions below the midrectal level are treated by abdominoperineal resection. This method of selection has been applied to all removable growths whether the operation is palliative or curative.

Selection of operation by sigmoidoscopy is limited by variations in mobility of the rectum and the length of the anal canal. The feasibility of abdominosacral resection may be accurately assessed by digital examination. The lower limit of the operation is at or just below the

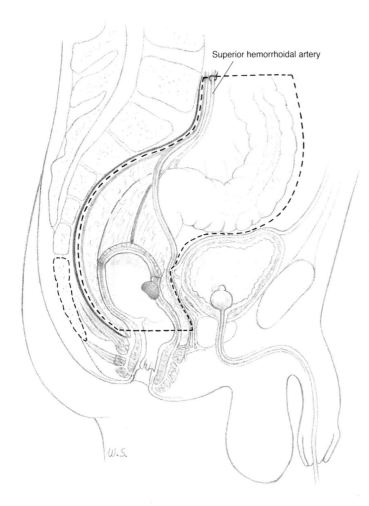

Superior hemorrhoidal artery

W.S.

FIGURE 20–1. Abdominosacral resection. Sagittal section showing extent of resection including the entire mesorectum and perirectal fat within the fascia propria to the level of the levator ani muscles.

puborectalis sling. The available distal margin is actually the distance from the puborectalis sling to the attachment of the tumor. This distance may be estimated by hooking the proximal interphalangeal joint of the examining finger on the puborectalis. The intraluminal extension of a tumor suitable for sphincter preservation may actually reach the top of the anal canal. The examining finger may slide beyond this point into the sulcus between the tumor and the rectal wall. If this attachment lies 2 to 3 cm above the puborectalis on digital examination, a margin of 3 cm or more will usually be attainable after mobilization.

Candidates for abdominosacral resection are examined in the lateral position. After mobilization of the rectum, the exposure in about 20% of midrectal cancers is adequate to complete the resection and anastomosis entirely through the abdominal approach. Only rarely has abdominosacral resection been abandoned in favor of abdominoperineal resection because an adequate distal margin could not be obtained. The preoperative measurements therefore predict quite accurately whether a sphincter-saving operation will be possible.

RESULTS

From 1966 to 1991, 954 consecutive patients with primary adenocarcinoma of the rectum were assigned to operation according to the level of the lesion as outlined in the section "Selection of Patients." The operation was an anterior resection in 468 patients, abdominosacral resection in 284 patients, and abdominoperineal resection in 199 patients. Three high-risk elderly patients had local excision only. Sphincter-saving resection was achieved in 79% of these patients.

Mortality and Morbidity

The risk of abdominosacral resection is comparable to that of anterior resection and abdominoperineal resection. The mortality rate was 2.4% after anterior resection, 1.4% after abdominosacral resection, and 1.5% after abdominoperineal resection in the study described. Morbidity following each of the three operations was also comparable, with the exception of anastomotic complications.

Anastomotic leaks were detected in 4% of the 752 patients undergoing anterior resection or abdominosacral resection. There were six leaks after 468 anterior resections (1.3%) and 23 leaks after 284 abdominosacral resections (8.1%).

The presence of the posterior wound in abdominosacral resection undoubtedly increases the detection rate for small leaks because of the easy egress of fecal matter by this route. In fact, most of the leaks (19 of 23) after abdominosacral resection resulted in a well-controlled posterior fistula. Nonetheless, the anastomosis after abdominosacral resection is lower than that after anterior resection and is, therefore, inherently more tenuous. Moreover, the posterior wound in close proximity to the anastomotic suture line may actually predispose to leakage. For this reason, the omentum is interposed between the anastomosis and the posterior wound whenever possible. All fistulas healed after temporary diversion of the fecal stream.

The anastomotic leakage rate after abdominosacral resection has improved from 9.7% in the first 15 years of the series to 5.5% in the last 10 years. This complication was seen in only 1 of 40 patients (2.5%) after abdominosacral resection with a stapled anastomosis in the most recent period. The stapled anastomosis after abdominosacral resection was associated with a leak rate comparable to anterior resection. Stapling is now the author's preferred method for anastomosis after abdominosacral resection.

Continence

Sphincter function following abdominosacral resection is normal in every case. As in all low rectal resections, loss of the rectosigmoid reservoir results in frequent small stools in the early postoperative period. However, the ultimate functional results following abdominosacral resection are indistinguishable from those following anterior resection.

Long-Term Survival

The crude 5-year survival rate for 553 patients after curative operations done from 1966 to 1981 was 63.8%. The 5-year survival rate was 67.8% for anterior resection, 67.9% for abdominosacral resection, and 51.4% for abdominoperineal resection (Table 20–1).

Pelvic recurrence affected 10.7% of our patients after anterior resection, 12.8% after abdominosacral resection and 12.5% after abdominoperineal resection (Table 20–2). Pelvic recurrence rates were 3.6% for Dukes A lesions, 9.4% for Dukes B lesions, and 22.3% for Dukes C lesions. There was no increase in the pelvic recurrence rate in patients undergoing sphincter-saving operations. Pelvic recurrence, like survival, was determined by the stage of disease and not by the operation performed.

Abdominosacral resection is the most reliable radical sphincter-saving operation for midrectal cancer that is too low for anterior resection. The posterior incision provides maximum exposure for wide resection of the tumor, a measured distal margin, and an accurate anastomosis. The procedure can be carried out consistently to the pelvic floor without disrupting the anal sphincters and their innervation. Sphincter function is consistently preserved. Mortality is no higher than for other radical rectal resections. Morbidity can be limited by the selective use of a protective colostomy. Addition of the posterior approach allows mobilization of the rectum to the levators in every case. Resection is limited only by the distance of the tumor from the sphincter and not by poor exposure due to obesity or a narrow pelvis. In our experience, abdominosacral resection extends the range of sphincter-saving resection beyond that possible with the abdominal approach alone, with no compromise in safety and no increased risk of local recurrence or death from cancer.

TABLE 20-1. CRUDE 5-YEAR SURVIVAL AFTER 553 CURATIVE RESECTIONS FOR RECTAL CANCER (1966-1981)

Operation	Dukes Classification	No. of Patients	5-Year Survivors	% 5-Year Survivors
Anterior resection (AR)	A	82	75	91.4*
	B	108	70	64.8
	C	71	32	45.0
	ALL	261	177	67.8†
Abdominosacral resection (ASR)	A	49	42	85.7
	B	56	42	75.0‡
	C	51	22	43.1
	ALL	156	106	67.9†
Abdominoperineal resection (APR)	A	35	27	77.1*
	B	48	25	52.1‡
	C	53	18	33.9
	ALL	136	70	51.4†

*Dukes A: APR versus AR, $P<.03$.
†Overall: APR versus AR, $P<.001$; APR versus ASR, $P<.004$.
‡Dukes B: APR versus ASR, $P<.015$.
Difference for other subsets not significant.

OPERATIVE TECHNIQUE

Position

The patient is placed in the right lateral decubitus position with the back and buttocks at the edge of the table (Fig. 20–2). An indwelling catheter is placed in the bladder and is taped to the thigh. The rectum is irrigated with normal saline until clear returns are obtained, followed by water irrigation to lyse exfoliated tumor cells. The incision sites are marked, the skin is prepared, and the patient is draped to provide simultaneous access to the abdominal and posterior wounds. Placement of a pillow between the knees allows access to the anus for digital evaluation of the anastomosis or insertion of a stapler.

The abdominal phase of the operation is identical to other radical operations for rectal cancer, but the surgeon must reorient his or her review of the anatomy from the horizontal to the vertical plane. This approach facilitates mobilization and delivery of the rectosigmoid stump and proximal colon through the posterior wound and obviates the need for turning and redraping the patient. The surgeon can return to the abdomen to further mobilize the proximal colon to avoid tension on the colorectal anastomosis or to perform a protective colostomy. The advantages of abdominosacral resection in the lateral position are analogous to the advantages of synchronous abdominoperineal resection in the Lloyd-Davies position.

Finally, in the event that resection and anastomosis can be achieved through the abdomen alone, or in the event that an adequate distal margin cannot be obtained, anterior resection or abdominoperineal resection may be performed without repositioning and redraping the patient.

Abdominal Incision

The abdomen is opened through an oblique incision starting between the left costal margin and the iliac crest, running parallel to the inguinal ligament and curving across the musculus rectus above the pubis (Fig. 20–2). The incision is carried through all layers of the abdominal wall.

TABLE 20-2. PELVIC RECURRENCE AFTER 553 CURATIVE RESECTIONS FOR RECTAL CANCER (1966-1981)

Operation	Dukes Classification	No. of Patients	Pelvic Recurrences	% Pelvic Recurrences
Anterior resection	A	82	2	2.4
	B	108	12	11.1
	C	71	14	19.7
	ALL	261	28	10.7
Abdominosacral resection	A	49	3	6.1
	B	56	4	7.1
	C	51	13	25.4
	ALL	156	20	12.8
Abdominoperineal resection	A	35	1	2.9
	B	48	4	8.3
	C	53	12	22.6
	ALL	136	17	12.5

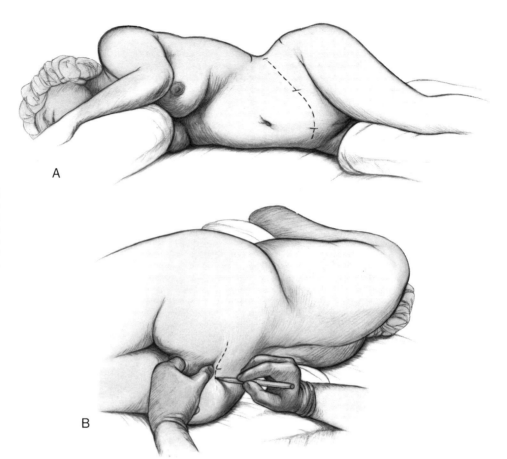

FIGURE 20-2. Abdominosacral resection. *A*, Patient is placed in the right lateral decubitus position with the right buttock and scapula at the edge of the table. Abdominal incision is marked. *B*, Posterior incision is marked at the sacrococcygeal joint.

The oblique incision affords excellent exposure of the splenic flexure and the pelvic organs. After thorough exploration of the abdomen, the small bowel is delivered from the abdomen and is protected by laparotomy pads. Little retraction is needed to keep the small bowel out of the way in the lateral position, since this maneuver is aided by gravity.

Mobilization of the Colon

The splenic flexure is mobilized (Fig. 20–3). The omentum is separated from the transverse colon by sharp dissection in the embryonic fusion plane. This dissection is carried far enough to the right to allow the transverse colon to rotate on the middle colic artery. The attachments of the omentum to the spleen may be divided at this time to allow the omentum to reach the pelvis. The left colon is drawn downward toward the patient's right side, and its lateral peritoneal attachments are divided. The peritoneal incision is carried down the lumbar gutter into the pelvis. The left gonadal vessels and the left ureter are identified and swept laterally (Fig. 20–4).

The colon is then drawn upward to the patient's left side, and the right leaf of the sigmoid mesentery is incised at its base. The right ureter is identified and swept laterally. The sigmoid mesentery containing the superior hemorrhoidal vessels and lymphatics is now easily swept upward from the aorta. This lymphovascular pedicle is isolated, clamped, divided, and suture ligated, usually at the level of the origin of the left colic artery (Fig. 20–5).

Mobilization of the proximal colon should be sufficient to allow it to lie loosely in the pelvis, conforming to the curve of the sacrum. The left colic artery may be divided at its origin when additional length is necessary, since the left colon is often tethered by this vessel. In that case, the marginal artery must be preserved, since the blood supply to the colon stump is now based on the middle colic artery. The mesosigmoid is divided to the site selected for the proximal margin. Cope-deMartel or other appropriate clamps are applied at this site and the colon is divided (Fig. 20–6). A stitch may be placed in the antimesenteric wall to aid in delivery of the proximal colon through the posterior wound without axial rotation.

Mobilization of the Rectum

The rectum is mobilized from the hollow of the sacrum by blunt dissection in the loose areolar plane anterior to the middle sacral artery and presacral venous plexus (Fig. 20–7). The peritoneal incisions at the base of the mesosigmoid are continued anteriorly to meet in the cul-de-sac, and the anterior wall of the rectum is freed to the level of the seminal vesicles or upper vagina.

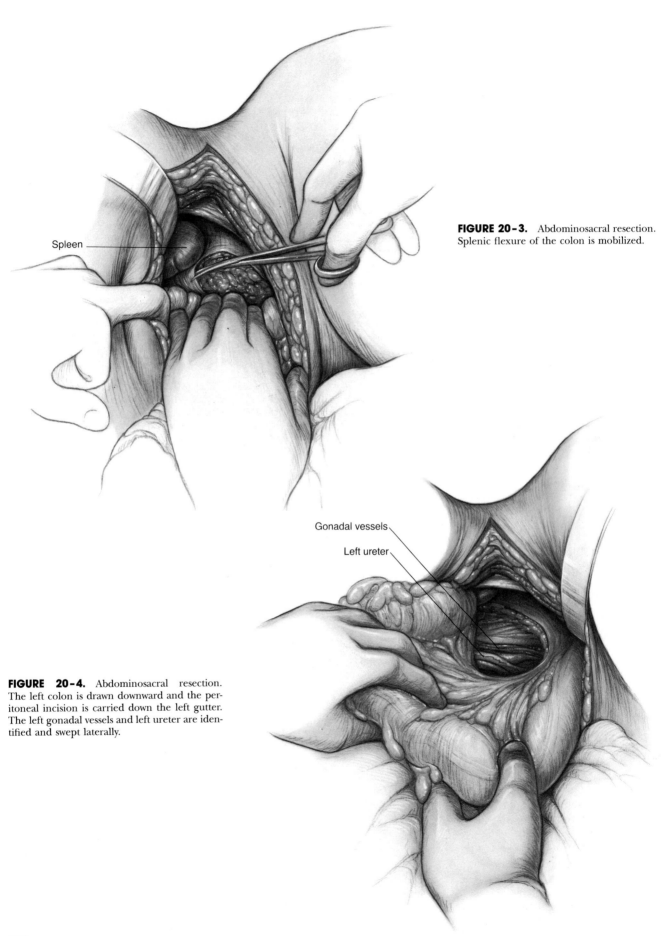

Spleen

FIGURE 20-3. Abdominosacral resection. Splenic flexure of the colon is mobilized.

Gonadal vessels

Left ureter

FIGURE 20-4. Abdominosacral resection. The left colon is drawn downward and the peritoneal incision is carried down the left gutter. The left gonadal vessels and left ureter are identified and swept laterally.

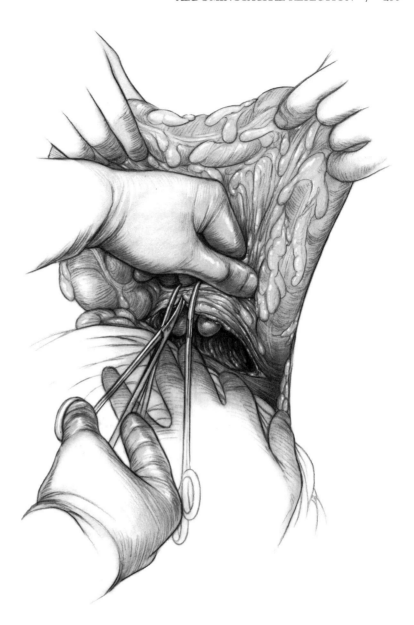

FIGURE 20-5. Abdominosacral resection. The colon is drawn upward, the right leaf of the sigmoid mesentery is incised, and the right ureter is identified. The superior hemorrhoidal vessels are then divided and ligated.

With the anterior and posterior dissections completed, the lateral ligaments of the rectum containing the middle hemorrhoidal vessels are identified. The left lateral ligament is divided first. The broad band of tissue that is the lateral ligament is dissected as far distally as possible, encircled with the finger, clamped near the pelvic side wall, divided, and ligated (Fig. 20-8). Upward displacement of the rectum now exposes the right lateral ligament, which is also encircled, divided, and ligated (Fig. 20-9).

The rectum has now been mobilized as completely as possible. The seminal vesicles or upper vagina are visible. The tip of the coccyx, the levator ani muscle diaphragm, and the puborectalis sling are palpable. If mobilization provides sufficient length to permit anterior resection, the operation is completed through the abdomen. For most midrectal cancers, posterior exposure will be necessary. Before proceeding to the posterior in-

cision, the pelvis is irrigated with saline, and meticulous hemostasis is achieved.

Posterior Dissection

A transverse incision is made over the sacrococcygeal joint (Fig. 20-10). Depression of the tip of the coccyx facilitates its disarticulation and excision (Fig. 20-11). Waldeyer's fascia is incised and the retrorectal space is entered. The opening is enlarged by blunt dissection, splitting the levators in the direction of their fibers. A transverse incision is suitable because it may be lengthened without limitation by the sacrum or the anus. If necessary, the gluteal muscles may be split for further exposure.

The rectosigmoid stump is now delivered through the posterior wound using the Cope-deMartel clamp as a handle. The lower rectum can now be mobilized further for wide lateral and distal clearance. The lowermost portions of the lateral ligaments that remain are divided at the pelvic side walls. The anterior surface of the rectum can be freed from the prostate or the lower vaginal wall. The posterior surface of the rectum is dissected to the puborectalis sling.

The extent of the tumor is determined, and the distal margin is measured with a ruler. With small tumors, the precise limits of the tumor may be determined by sigmoidoscopy through the rectosigmoid stump. The distal margin that is at least 3 cm from the lowest extension of the cancer is cleared of fat down to bare longitudinal muscle. A right-angle renal pedicle clamp is applied at this site (Fig. 20–12). The proximal colonic stump is then delivered, taking care to avoid axial rotation of the bowel. The latch of the Cope-deMartel clamp or the marking stitch is a convenient guide for maintaining proper orientation of the colon (Fig. 20–13). An extra 3 to 4 cm of proximal colon is pulled through posteriorly as illustrated in Fig. 20–13. This allows the suturing to be done without hindrance by the Cope-deMartel clamp.

Sutured Anastomosis

A series of interrupted Cushing stitches of 4-0 silk are placed (see Fig. 20–13). After all the sutures have been placed, they are tied and cut, retaining the first and the last to mark the corners of the anastomosis. The adjoining walls of the colon and rectum are incised. The cut edges should show brisk bleeding, indicating a good blood supply (Fig. 20–14).

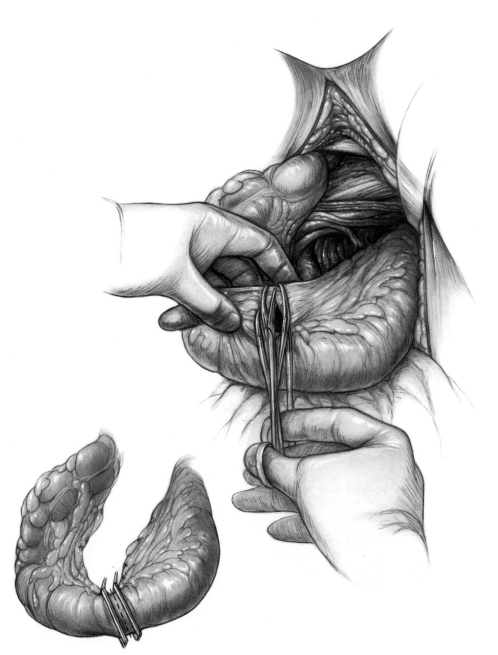

FIGURE 20-6. Abdominosacral resection. Division of mesocolon at proximal margin and division of colon between Cope-deMartel clamps.

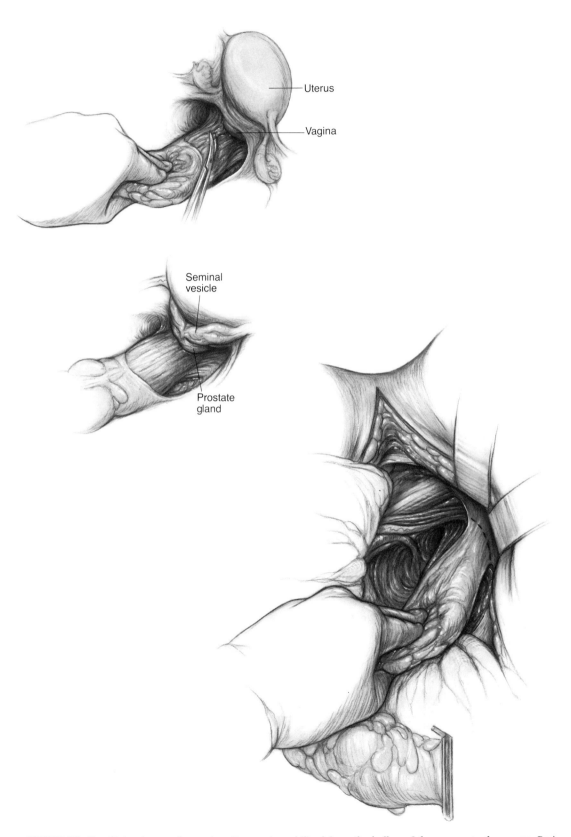

FIGURE 20-7. Abdominosacral resection. Rectum is mobilized from the hollow of the sacrum to the coccyx. Peritoneum in the cul-de-sac is incised and the rectum is dissected on Denonvilliers' fascia to the seminal vesicles or upper vagina.

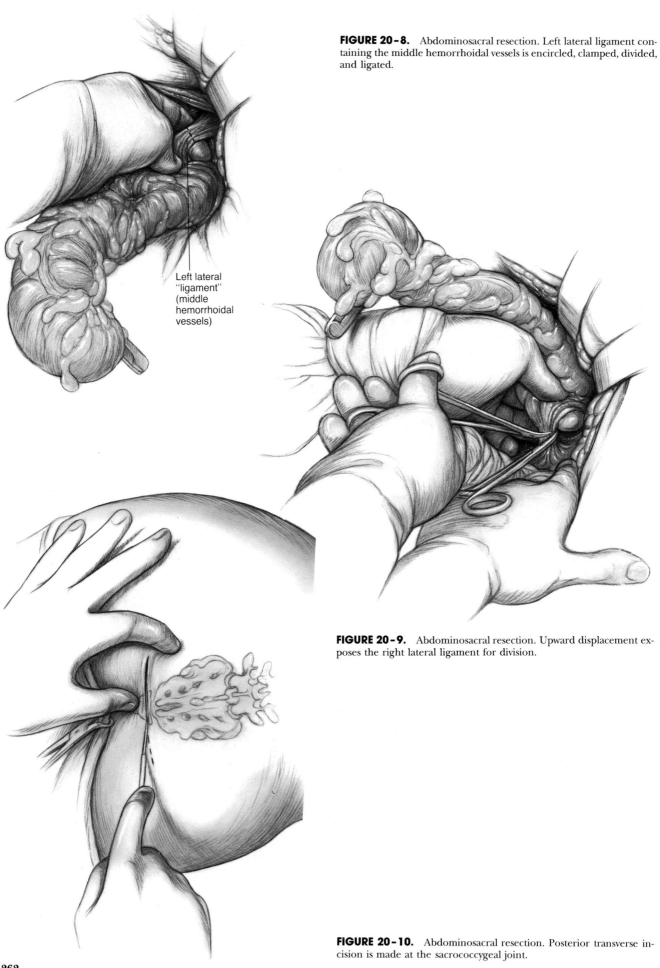

FIGURE 20-8. Abdominosacral resection. Left lateral ligament containing the middle hemorrhoidal vessels is encircled, clamped, divided, and ligated.

Left lateral "ligament" (middle hemorrhoidal vessels)

FIGURE 20-9. Abdominosacral resection. Upward displacement exposes the right lateral ligament for division.

FIGURE 20-10. Abdominosacral resection. Posterior transverse incision is made at the sacrococcygeal joint.

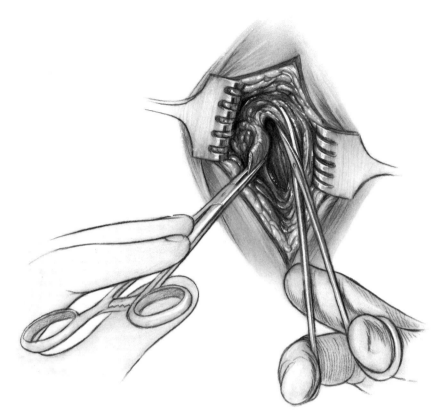

FIGURE 20-11. Abdominosacral resection. The coccyx is disarticulated with a knife and excised. Waldeyer's fascia is then incised and the retrorectal space is entered. This opening is enlarged by blunt dissection, splitting the levators in the direction of their fibers.

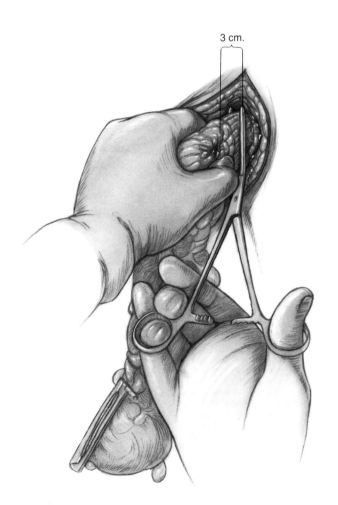

3 cm.

FIGURE 20-12. Abdominosacral resection. The specimen is delivered posteriorly with the fascia propria intact. Additional dissection is done to clear the pelvis completely to the levators. A distal margin of at least 3 cm is measured without tension. The rectum is cleared at this site and a right-angled renal pedicle clamp is applied.

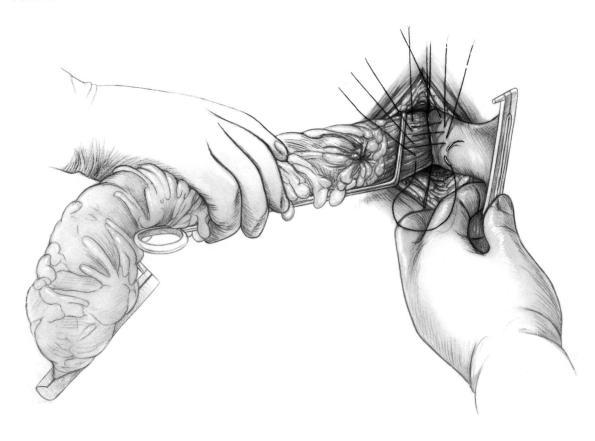

FIGURE 20-13. Abdominosacral resection. The proximal colon is delivered with care taken to avoid axial rotation. The first layer of interrupted nonabsorbable sutures is placed.

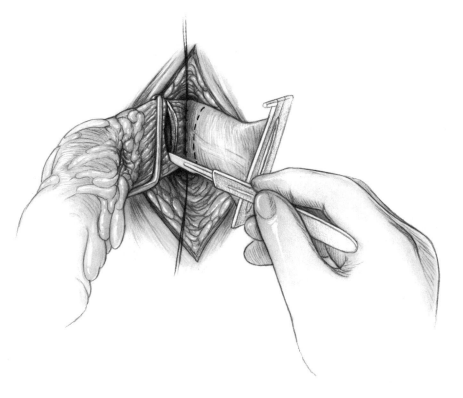

FIGURE 20-14. Abdominosacral resection. The adjoining walls of bowel are incised.

The second row of sutures is started at the center of the anastomosis, using a double-armed 4-0 chromic catgut or polyglycolic acid (Dexon) suture. This suture is tied and run in both directions as a full-thickness, loosely locked stitch (Fig. 20–15A). The remaining wall of the rectum is divided, and the specimen is removed. Excess proximal colon contained within the Cope-deMartel clamp is excised. The catgut suture is brought out at the corners of the anastomosis and the inner layer is completed using a continuous Connell suture (Fig. 20–15B). The outer layer is completed using interrupted Cushing sutures of 4-0 silk (Fig. 20–15C).

The pelvic and sacral wounds are now thoroughly irrigated with saline, and hemostasis is secured. The omentum is delivered through the posterior incision and is wrapped around the anastomosis. The position of the omentum may be maintained by tacking it to the levator ani with several sutures.

No attempt is made to close the defect in the pelvic peritoneum. Loops of small bowel will fill the pelvic

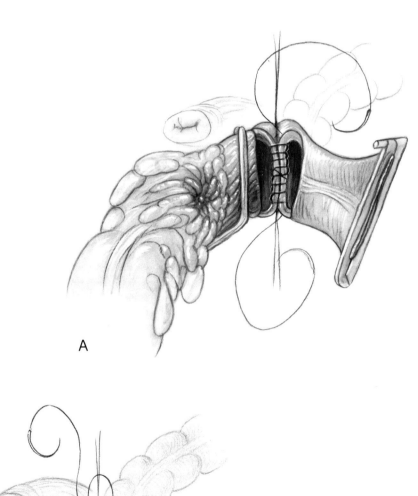

FIGURE 20-15. Abdominosacral resection. *A,* The inner layer is started as a running lock-stitch. *B,* The inner layer is completed as a continuous Connell suture. *C,* An outer layer of interrupted nonabsorbable sutures completes the anastomosis.

A

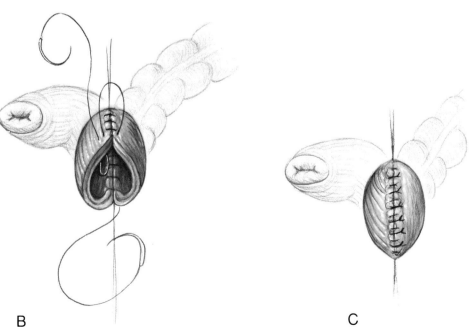

B

C

dead space and fluid accumulating in the pelvis can drain into the peritoneal cavity. As an added precaution, a soft closed suction drain of silicone rubber may be left in the pelvis. Drainage volumes of 100 to 250 ml are not unusual in the first 48 postoperative hours. The drain is removed as soon as possible.

Stapled Anastomosis

The end-to-end coloanal anastomosis may be facilitated by the use of a circular stapler (Fig. 20–16). After posterior delivery and full mobilization of the rectosigmoid stump, the rectum is cleared of fat at the level of the puborectalis. The rectum can be divided at or within the puborectalis sling. As the rectum is incised, a suture of O-polypropylene is inserted through the full thickness of the rectal wall from muscularis to mucosa. The incision is enlarged and the suturing continued circumferentially until the specimen is amputated and the pursestring suture is completed. With the patient in the lateral position, the stapler is easily inserted through the anus, allowing the surgeon to personally pass the instrument and to observe its appearance at the anorectal stump. The anorectal pursestring suture is tied around the shaft of the stapler. The distal suture may be inspected easily for inclusion of the entire circumference of rectum. A pursestring suture is placed in the proximal colon, and the bowel is guided down to the pelvis by the abdominal route. The proximal pursestring suture is tied over the anvil. The stapled anastomosis is completed under direct vision through the posterior wound.

Protective Colostomy

A protective colostomy should be employed when technical difficulties are encountered, when incomplete donuts are cut by the end-to-end stapler, and whenever any doubt exists as to the integrity of the anastomosis. We have employed completely diverting colostomy, loop colostomy, and cecostomy in this setting. Our current practice is to perform a lateral transverse colostomy brought through a wide defect in the abdominal wall and a small skin aperture (Fig. 20–17). This allows the colon to rise to the skin level, at which point a small lateral opening is sutured to the skin only. With adequate mechanical bowel preparation and a satisfactory anastomosis, complete diversion is unnecessary. In the first 5 to 9 postoperative days, intraluminal contents consist of only liquid and gas. A lateral opening, which bleeds off liquid and gas, prevents distention and offers sufficient protection. In fact, when bowel function returns, almost all stool is discharged through this lateral stoma. This colostomy may be closed in several weeks, often with local anesthesia.

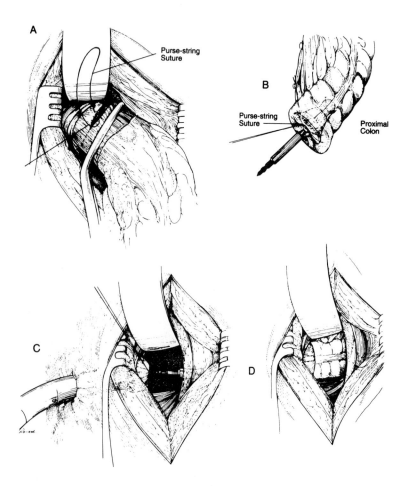

FIGURE 20–16. Abdominosacral resection. *A,* As the rectum is incised, a full-thickness suture of O-polypropylene is inserted. The incision is enlarged and the suturing continued circumferentially until the specimen is amputated and the pursestring suture is completed. *B,* A pursestring suture is placed in the proximal colon and tied over the anvil. *C,* With the patient in the lateral position, the stapler is easily inserted through the anus. The anorectal pursestring suture is tied around the shaft of the stapler. The proximal bowel is guided down to the pelvis by the abdominal route. *D,* The stapled anastomosis is completed under direct vision through the posterior wound. (From Eng, K.: Abdominosacral resection. *In* Daly, J.M., and Cady, B. [eds.]: Atlas of Surgical Oncology. St. Louis, Mosby-Year Book, 1993, p. 535, with permission.)

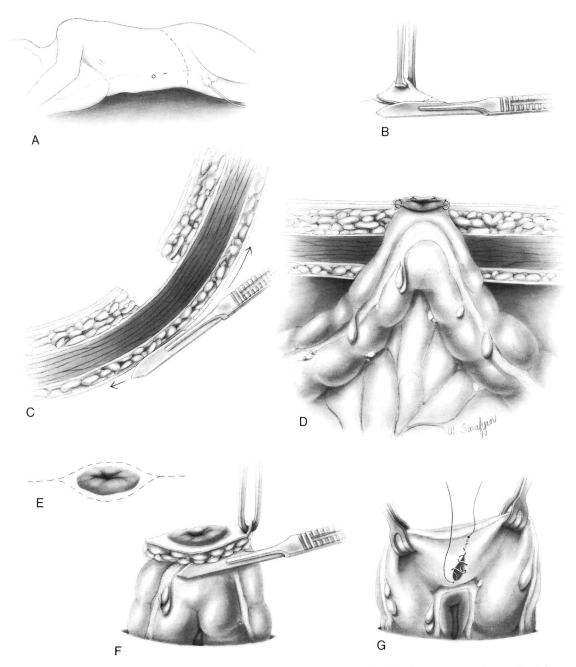

FIGURE 20-17. Abdominosacral resection. *A*, A protective colostomy is placed in the transverse colon to the right of the middle colic vessels. *B*, A 2-cm disk of skin is excised. *C*, The deep layers of the abdominal wall are incised to allow the colon to rise easily to skin level. *D*, A short, longitudinal incision is made in the antimesenteric wall of the colon, and the bowel is sutured to skin only. *E* through *G*, Colostomy closure without resection is usually possible.

REFERENCES

1. Beart, R.W., Jr., and Kelly, K.A.: Randomized prospective evaluation of the EEA stapler for colorectal anastomoses. Am. J. Surg., *141:* 143, 1981.
2. Eng, K., and Localio, S.A.: Simplified complementary transverse colostomy for low colorectal anastomosis. Surg. Gynecol. Obstet., *153:*734, 1981.
3. Goligher, J.C.: Recent trends in the practice of sphincter-saving excision for carcinoma of the rectum. *In* Jordan G.L., Jr. (ed.): Advances in Surgery. Chicago, Year Book Medical Publishers, 1979, p. 15.
4. Goligher, J.C.: Use of circular stapling gun with perianal insertion of anorectal purse-string suture for construction of very low colorectal or colo-anal anastomoses. Br. J. Surg., *66:*501, 1979.
5. Localio, S.A., Eng, K., and Coppa, G.F.: Abdominosacral resection for midrectal cancer: A fifteen year experience. Ann. Surg., *198:* 320, 1983.
6. Mason, A.Y.: Transsphincteric approach to rectal lesions. Surg. Ann., *9:*171, 1977.
7. Parks, A.G.: Transanal technique in low rectal anastomosis. Proc. R. Soc. Med., *65:*975, 1972.

Chapter 21

POSTERIOR AND PARASACRAL APPROACHES

DAVID A. ROTHENBERGER / STEVEN D. WEXNER

Posterior and parasacral approaches are methods of dissection designed to provide access to the presacral space and to the rectum itself. These approaches have played a varying role in the surgeon's armamentarium. They initially were a mainstay of the surgical extirpation of cancer of the rectum. Then they were used in a more limited role as a method to provide exposure for a low hand-sewn anastomosis after anterior resection of rectal cancer. Currently, posterior and parasacral approaches are almost never used as isolated approaches to malignant lesions of the rectum. They are used infrequently to expose and remove presacral lesions, to repair congenital anomalies, and to treat other benign conditions of the rectum.

HISTORICAL PERSPECTIVE

Kocher[15] in 1874 described a technique of excising the coccyx to allow excision of the rectum via a posterior approach. Kraske,[16] in a talk given to the Fourteenth Congress of the German Association of Surgeons in 1884, presented the procedure that still bears his name—that is, transsacral resection of cancer in the lower two thirds of the rectum with colostomy. He recognized that excising the coccyx alone was inadequate to expose the upper rectum and thus proposed a more radical posterior excision including a portion of the sacrum to gain appropriate exposure.[23] This became the preferred method of resection of rectal carcinoma in Europe during the latter portion of the nineteenth century. An alternative posterior approach, the transsphincteric dissection, was described by Bevan[3] in 1917, but it was not until 1970 when York-Mason[28] reintroduced this technique that it became more popular. These posterior approaches were supplanted by Miles'[20] abdominoperineal resection, which became the preferred method of treatment for rectal cancer in the early twentieth cen-

tury. In time, it became clear that not all rectal cancers had to be treated with an abdominoperineal resection. Equal survivorship often could be achieved by abdominal resection and low rectal anastomosis without the morbidity of a proctectomy and a permanent colostomy. The challenge was to find reliable methods of safely performing the low anastomosis. The posterior approach to the rectum became one of many techniques used for this purpose. In recent decades, low anterior anastomosis has become the normal method of restoring bowel continuity after rectal cancer resection and, for the most part, has replaced the posterior and parasacral approaches. Today, the most frequent indications for these approaches are the treatment of presacral cysts and tumors and the repair of imperforate anus. The modern surgeon often is so unfamiliar with these techniques (precisely because these approaches are used so rarely today) that he or she may avoid them even when they are indicated. This chapter is directed toward remedying this situation and to putting these approaches in their proper, limited perspective.

ANATOMY

A brief review of the relevant anatomy is important. The presacral space consists of the retrorectal space, the supralevator space, and the postanal space (see Fig. 34–5). It is really a potential space that normally contains mesenchymal tissue, the middle sacral artery, the superior rectal vessels, and branches of the sympathetic and parasympathetic nerves. The retrorectal space is the area between the upper two thirds of the rectum anteriorly and the sacral vertebrae posteriorly. The other anatomic boundaries are the lateral stalks of the rectum, ureters, and internal iliac vessels laterally; the pelvic peritoneal reflection superiorly; and the rectosacral fascia inferiorly (Fig. 21–1). The rectosacral fascia origi-

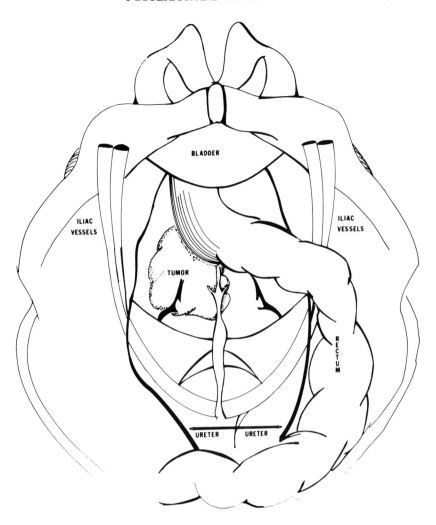

FIGURE 21-1. The anterior relationship of the rectum and a tumor to their pelvic structures.

nates at the periosteum of the fourth sacral vertebra and extends inferiorly and anteriorly to meet the rectum 3 to 5 cm cephalad to the anorectal ring.[14]

Caudad to the rectosacral fascia is the supralevator space, a U-shaped space situated on each side of the rectum. It is bordered superiorly by the peritoneum, laterally by the pelvic wall, medially by the rectum, and inferiorly by the levator ani muscles. Many lower presacral cysts and tumors occur in this space.

The postanal space is also a U-shaped space and connects the right and left ischiorectal fossae with each other posteriorly. The superficial postanal space is inferior to the anococcygeal ligament, and the deep postanal space is superior to the anococcygeal ligament but inferior to the levator ani muscle.

INDICATIONS

Rectal Carcinoma

The isolated posterior or parasacral approach should rarely, if ever, be used in the treatment of rectal carcinoma because there are now alternatives that provide excellent function and equivalent or better survival with less morbidity. Not surprisingly, there are very few re-

ports in the modern literature advocating the use of these approaches for rectal cancer. The transsacral approach is associated with a high rate of anastomotic breakdown (12%), fecal fistula (10%), and tumor recurrence (15%).[18,19] Christiansen[5] reports similar results in a small series. In a report published in 1977, York-Mason[28] reported satisfactory results in 89 patients treated with a posterior transsphincteric approach. Allgower and associates[1] reported similarly acceptable results in 1982.

A major objection to isolated posterior or parasacral approaches for rectal carcinoma is that complete proximal lymphadenectomy and pelvic clearance is impossible. To overcome this limitation, some surgeons advocate a combined abdominosacral approach, but this then negates the reputed advantages of minimal morbidity associated with local therapy.[18,19] The abdominosacral approach is discussed in detail in Chapter 20. Today, most rectal cancers are resected via an anterior approach with restoration of bowel continuity by a low colorectal anastomosis, often with the aid of stapling devices, or by a direct coloanal anastomosis.

Selected cases of lower or middle third rectal carcinoma may be treated by local means, thus avoiding the morbidity of a laparotomy and colostomy.[24] In general, transanal excision or endocavitary radiation are preferable to the posterior approaches for such tumors because they avoid the morbidity related to the incision; the risk of seeding the incision and postrectal tissues with tumor; and the problems of fecal fistula, anastomotic leak, and incontinence. Most cancers of the upper third of the rectum, which otherwise fit the criteria for curative local therapy, are best treated by anterior resection and low, stapled anastomosis or a coloanal anastomosis. In our experience, abdominoperineal resection is rarely, if ever, needed in a lesion of the upper third of the rectum and is needed in less than 10% of mid-rectal cancers.

An exception might be made in the high-risk patient in whom an early lesion is located proximally enough to make transanal excision or fulguration impossible and in whom endocavitary radiation is not technically feasible or is unavailable. Such a patient might benefit from a posterior approach to allow rectal excision with a primary anastomosis, thus avoiding much of the morbidity associated with an abdominal approach. In our experience, such patients are rare.

Palliative therapy of rectal cancer usually demands complete local clearance of the primary tumor if relief of local symptoms is to be achieved for longer than the short term. Usually, an anterior abdominal approach is best and is surprisingly well tolerated. Anastomosis is often possible and is safe. Local therapy often is not feasible because of the size and nature of the primary tumor, but it does work well in selected instances.[21] Posterior approaches offer little, if any, advantage and simply open up new tissue planes and incisions to problems of recurrence.

Benign Conditions of the Anorectum

The posterior approach is inappropriate for most villous tumors. Such benign lesions are usually amenable to either transanal excision or other forms of local therapy. In rare cases, an anterior resection is needed. Anterior resection is still, however, preferable to adding the morbidity of a posterior incision and the theoretical risk of violating tissue planes in the face of possible malignancy. In addition, the posterior transsacral method of resection is associated with significant risk of dehiscence and subsequent intractable colosacral fistula.[8] A "sacral anus" is one of the most dreaded complications of this procedure.

Rarely, the posterior approach may be of value in aiding transanal excision of a large villous lesion. If one finds that transanal excision is impossible at the most proximal portion of a tumor because of poor exposure, the posterior approach can be used to expose and mobilize, but not cut into, the rectum. An assistant can push the rectal wall inferiorly to allow the transanal operator to gain exposure and complete the excision of the tumor. This can be of great value but is rarely needed.

Other benign conditions of the rectum, such as a rectal stricture, a high rectovaginal fistula, or a rectoprostatic fistula, may be ideally suited for a posterior approach. Fortunately, such problems are rare. When present, however, a posterior approach with posterior proctotomy provides access to the anterior rectal wall to treat the fistula or to eliminate the rectal stricture by closing the proctotomy in a transverse manner.

Reconstruction of a major perineal laceration in small children can be difficult and often results in suboptimal continence. A recent report demonstrated the utility of a posterior sagittal approach to repair a fourth-degree perineal laceration sustained at 9 months of age resulting in a common rectovaginal orifice and complete fecal incontinence.[2] A $2^1/_2$-year-old girl underwent this repair involving precise identification of the striated muscle complex and allowing reconstruction with complete continence.

Presacral Cysts and Tumors

Posterior and parasacral approaches are still useful for presacral lesions, with either concomitant coccygectomy or sacrectomy. Prior to a decision regarding the method of approaching a presacral lesion, consideration must be given to its size and location. Finne[6] has established certain helpful criteria. He noted that the risk of malignancy in presacral lesions increases from 4% in neonates to 95% in older pediatric age group. In adults, only 10% of cystic presacral lesions are malignant, whereas solid lesions carry a 60% risk of malignancy.[6] For practical purposes, lesions with central nervous system or skeletal involvement will require posterior laminectomy, sacral resection, or both. A posterior approach is required for adequate visualization of the neuroanatomy and preservation of uninvolved structures. In most cases of malignancy and high-lying lesions, a combined abdominosacral approach is best (see Chapter 20). Midsacral soft tissue masses without osseous involvement are probably best approached transabdominally, because early control of the vascular pedicle is feasible. The middle sacral vessels generally feed the tumor and can be ligated prior to extensive mobilization (Fig. 21–1). Low presacral cysts are amenable to parasacral extirpation after coccygectomy.

In a Mayo Clinic series, 80% of 120 presacral lesions were successfully and completely excised through a posterior approach.[13] Some authors caution that only tumors less than 5 cm in diameter should be removed by the posterior approach, as lesions larger than this have a high incidence of metastases and recurrence after inadequate resection.[25]

Cloacal Malformations

Peña and deVries[22] introduced the posterior sagittal anorectoplasty for repair of imperforate anus in 1982. Since then, this posterior approach has been used widely for a variety of cloacal malformations.[4,10] Hedlund and associates[9] recently summarized an experience of 30 patients with imperforate anus treated by this technique. Anorectal manometry studies performed 5 to 10 years postoperatively showed that anal resting tone and anal squeeze pressures were subnormal in most patients. Rectal volume and sensation to balloon distention, however, were within normal range. A rectal-anal inhibitory reflex was demonstrated in 9 of 30 patients. Soiling was more common in patients with a very low anal resting tone, defined as less than 40 cm H_2O, and a low anal squeeze pressure, defined as less than 100 cm H_2O. Constipation was more common in patients with a large rectal volume, defined as greater than 150 ml. Correlation between anal manometry and clinical results was not perfect. They did find that rectal atresia patients showed near normal results and that there was no difference in results between bulbar and prostatic fistula patients.[9] The techniques used for this indication are discussed in detail in Chapter 35 and will not be discussed further here.

TECHNIQUE

Preliminaries

Full mechanical and antibiotic bowel preparation should be performed in every patient. Although the operation may proceed without contamination, bone and cartilage will be exposed and the bowel lumen might be inadvertently entered. For these reasons, a prophylactic broad-spectrum antibiotic should be routinely employed. A fiberoptic headlight provides good visualization in what can otherwise be a deep, dark hole. The patient is placed in the prone-jackknife position with hips elevated on a Kraske-type roll (see Fig. 34–1).

Incision and Dissection

The incision can be made parallel to the sacrococcygeal joint, perpendicular to the coccyx, or in a lazy S next to the coccyx (see Fig. 34–10). If a paracoccygeal approach is desired, it should be made on the side on which the tumor is predominantly based. The incision is carried through the skin, subcutaneous tissue, and fat until the sacrum, coccyx, and anococcygeal ligament have all been identified. Weitlaner, Gelpi, or other self-retaining retractors, such as the Lone Star (Lone Star Manufacturing, Houston, TX) that provide good lateral retraction and adequate visibility should be used for the duration of the procedure. The fibrous coccygeal insertions of the anococcygeal ligament and the pubococcygeus are divided along the midline to reveal the levator ani muscles. The presacral space is entered (Fig. 21–2; also see Figs. 34–5, 34–11, and 34–12). Blunt and sharp dissection is performed to gradually free the rectum, cyst, or presacral tumor from adjacent structures. If a cyst is present, it should be left adherent to the coccyx, since recurrence rates are higher without coccygectomy.[6,26] Gemsenjäger[7] strongly advocates a transverse incision and division of pelvic floor muscles to expose the anorectum. He believes this provides a better exposure of the supralevator space and the distal rectum than does a longitudinal incision. The authors have no experience with transverse dissection, but it is an attractive approach. Regardless of the dissection technique utilized, great care should be taken throughout the procedure to avoid inadvertent rectal wall injury.

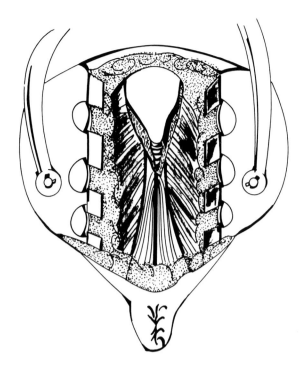

FIGURE 21-2. Entering the presacral space through a posterior incision.

Transsphincteric Approach

The posterior transsphincteric approach allows a wider and more distal exposure by using a left parasacral incision from the midsacrum to the anal verge. The incision can be widened by incising through the lower portion of the gluteus muscle. This technique calls for division of the external sphincter, puborectalis, and levator ani muscles along the lines of the incision. All divided muscles must be tagged step by step so that they can be later identified for appropriate reapproximation. The surgeon must remember that the nerve supply to these muscles lies lateral to the incision. The internal sphincter muscle is also divided, leaving only the mucosa and submucosa intact. This incision can easily be converted to a proctotomy if necessary. Today, such a distal posterior exposure is almost never needed, and the posterior transsphincteric approach, popularized by York-Mason,[28] is rarely necessary. Huber and von Flue[11] abandoned the transsphincteric approach of York-Mason and stated that "by cutting directly onto the rectum by diathermy, the operation is simpler and does not require reconstruction of the sphincter apparatus."

Coccygectomy

Additional proximal exposure can be achieved by performing a coccygectomy. For presacral lesions, it is useful to insert one or two fingers into the rectum to help accurately assess the thickness of the rectal wall.[26] In this manner, the presacral lesion can be delivered into the wound and carefully separated from the posterior rectal wall (Fig. 21–3). Disarticulation of the coccyx from the fifth sacral vertebra is achieved by grasping the coccyx between the surgeon's thumb and forefinger and flex-

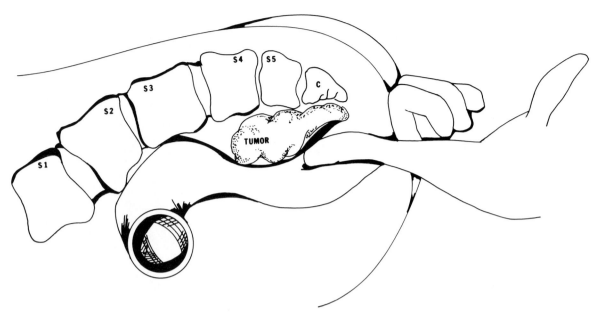

FIGURE 21-3. Transrectal palpation allows digital assessment of the thickness of the rectal wall and can aid in exposure and delivery of a presacral tumor.

ing it anteriorly (see Fig. 34–12). The intercoccygeal joint is then sought with the point of the scalpel or electrocautery, and the joint is divided. In elderly patients, the coccyx sometimes cannot be separated by a scalpel or cautery because of osteoarthritic changes. In such cases of fusion, an osteotome, a chisel and mallet, or a saw can be used.

Sacrectomy

The distal sacrum and its associated nerve roots can be resected through the posterior approach if even more proximal exposure is needed. This is especially useful for presacral tumors that have osseous involvement. The decision regarding the number of distal sacral vertebrae to excise is based on the size of the lesion and its relationship to the sacrum (Fig. 21–4). The lower two sacral vertebrae and their nerves can be sacrificed if necessary without fear of a significant neurologic deficit.[12,14,17,27] However, it is imperative that the third sacral nerve root, which runs in an inferoanterior direction, be preserved on at least one side to avoid incontinence.

The approach is similar to that already described for coccygectomy. A midposterior axial, curvilinear, or horizontal incision is used to expose the levator ani muscle and coccyx (see Fig. 34–10). The anococcygeal ligament is detached from the coccyx, and the coccyx is then excised. The middle sacral artery is tied or electrocoagulated. The central decussating fibers of the levator ani muscle are bluntly separated in the midline to better expose the cephalad aspect of the presacral space (i.e., the supralevator space and the posterior wall of the rectum). This may provide enough exposure to handle the problem.

If more exposure is needed, a distal sacrectomy is per-

formed (Fig. 21–4). To gain the requisite exposure, the gluteus maximus muscles can be detached bilaterally, and the sacroiliac ligaments can be divided. Sacral mobilization is continued by lateral division of the sacrospinous and sacrotuberous ligaments and anterior division of the piriform muscles. When dividing the piriform muscles, care must be taken to identify and preserve the sciatic nerves and inferior gluteal vessels. The final portion of the dissection is the division of the superiorly based sacroiliac ligaments and the anterior longitudinal ligament. The sacrum is excised using a saw. The presacral lesion, coccyx, and sacral segments can then be lifted en bloc from the field.

Proctotomy

As noted earlier, a proctotomy is occasionally useful to deal with a rectal stricture or a high rectovaginal or rectoprostatic fistula. Occasionally, this approach can also be useful for selected tumors of the rectum.

The posterior rectal wall is exposed by either a coccygectomy or sacrectomy depending on the precise location of the problem for which the operation is performed. A posterior proctotomy is performed in a linear manner with cautery exposing the anterior rectal wall. If dealing with a fistula, a layer closer is achieved and one tries to rotate the rectal wall such that it is no longer adjacent to the fistula into the vagina or prostate. It is helpful at times to interpose adjacent tissues between the organs involved in such a fistula. A stricture can be corrected by closing the defect transversely. A neoplasm can be excised submucosally and the resulting defect is approximated, generally using polyglycolic acid sutures. The posterior proctotomy wound is closed transversely to correct strictures but may be closed vertically if it does

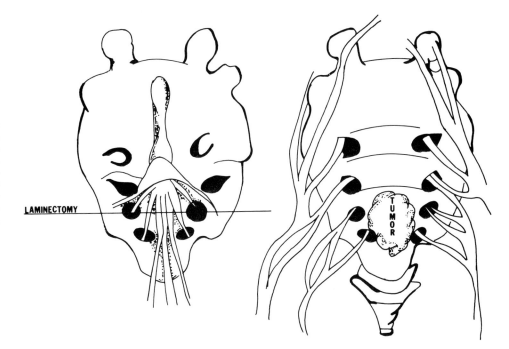

FIGURE 21-4. The relationship of a presacral tumor to nerve roots and the sacrum. The distal two sacral segments, and their associated nerves, may be resected without inducing significant neurologic deficit. In performing sacral laminectomy, care should be taken to preserve the third sacral nerve root, at least unilaterally.

LAMINECTOMY

not compromise the lumen, using either one- or two-layer technique.

Proctectomy

If a proctectomy is to be performed through a posterior approach, a coccygectomy, and usually a distal sacrectomy, are necessary for exposure. Mobilization of the rectum is done with special care to avoid injury anteriorly, at which point the rectum may be adherent to the vagina or prostate. The peritoneum may be opened anterior to the rectum and a Penrose drain placed around the rectum for traction. By pulling the bowel inferiorly, the superior rectal vessels are exposed and ligated. The rectum can then be divided between clamps at the desired level and an anastomosis performed.

Wound Closure

Meticulous hemostasis throughout the dissection is critical to ensure adequate exposure and minimize risks of postoperative hematoma and abscess. Performance of the dissection with electrocautery is helpful, as the small vessels often retract superiorly under the anterior lip of the sacrum after division. The middle and lateral sacral vessels are particularly prone to bleeding.

Inadvertent rectal injury can be recognized by insufflating air into the rectum via a proctoscope while the rectum is covered with saline. Any defects must be repaired with inversion of the mucosa. Since a large dead space results from these posterior approaches, a large, soft closed suction drain should be placed in the wound and delivered through a separate paraincisional stab wound. The wound should then be irrigated and closed in layers with reapproximation of the levator ani muscle and the anococcygeal ligament with 3-0 polyglycolic acid

sutures. The skin is approximated with a 4-0 subcuticular polyglycolic acid suture.

CONCLUSION

Posterior and parasacral approaches to rectal lesions have for the most part been replaced by other surgical techniques. Carcinomas and strictures can usually be treated through a standard laparotomy with a per anum low stapled anastomosis. Coloanal anastomosis, abdominoperineal resection, transanal excision, fulguration, endocavitary radiation, and other local techniques complete the modern colorectal surgeon's armamentarium.

The lesions that are most often potentially curable with a posterior or parasacral procedure are presacral cysts and tumors. Most low-lying benign presacral cystic lesions are curable by a posterior excision with an en bloc coccygectomy. High-lying presacral tumors, tumors larger than 5 cm, and those that require proximal sacrectomy are best approached by either an abdominal or a combined abdominal-transsacral approach. Resection of lesions such as anterior sacral meningocele and chordoma should be contemplated only with a multidisciplinary team. If one is careful to work within these constraints and guidelines, the posterior and parasacral approaches remain highly valuable techniques, although they are very limited in their application.

REFERENCES

1. Allgower, M., Durig, M., Hochstetter, A.V., and Huber, A.: The parasacral sphincter-splitting approach to the rectum. World J. Surg., 6:639, 1982.
2. Applebaum, H., and Atkinson, J.B.: The posterior sagittal ap-

proach for reconstruction of severe rectovaginal injuries. J. Pediatr. Surg., 26:856, 1991.

3. Bevan, A.D.: Carcinoma of the rectum—treatment by local excision. Surg. Clin. North Am., 1:1233, 1917.

4. Brain, A.J.L., and Keily, E.M.: Posterior sagittal anorectoplasty for reoperation in children with anorectal malformations. Br. J. Surg., 76:57, 1989.

5. Christiansen, J.: Excision of mid-rectal lesions by the Kraske sacral approach. Br. J. Surg., 67:651, 1980.

6. Finne, C.O., III: Presacral tumors and cysts. In Cameron, J.L. (ed.): Current Surgical Therapy—2. Toronto, B.C. Decker, 1986, p. 482.

7. Gemsenjäger, E.: Transverse pelvic floor division for the posterior approach to the rectum and anus. Int. J. Colorect. Dis., 4:67, 1989.

8. Goligher, J.: Treatment of carcinoma of the rectum. In Surgery of the Anus, Rectum, and Colon. London, Bailliere Tindall, 1984, p. 599.

9. Hedlund, H., Peña, A., Rodriguez, G., and Maza, J.: Long-term anorectal function in imperforate anus treated by a posterior sagittal anorectoplasty: Manometric investigation. J. Pediatr. Surg., 27:906, 1992.

10. Hendren, W.H.: Cloacal malformations: Experience with 105 cases. J. Pediatr. Surg., 27:890, 1992.

11. Huber, A.K., and von Flue, M.: Parasacral surgery for curative treatment of rectal cancer. Int. J. Colorect. Dis., 6:86, 1991.

12. Huth, J.F., Dawson, E.G., and Eilber, E.R.: Abdominosacral resection for malignant tumors of the sacrum. Am. J. Surg., 148:157, 1984.

13. Jao, S.-W., Beart, R.W., Jr., Spencer, R.J., et al.: Retrorectal tumors. Mayo Clinic experience, 1960–1979. Dis. Colon Rectum, 28:644, 1985.

14. Johnson, W.R.: Retrorectal tumors. In Goldberg, S.M., Gordon, P.H., and Nivatvongs, S. (eds.): Essentials of Anorectal Surgery. Philadelphia, J.B. Lippincott, 1980, p. 215.

15. Kocher, T.D.: Exstirpatic recti nach vorheriger excision des steissbeins. Cent. Chir., 10:145, 1874.

16. Kraske, P.: Quoted in Corman, M.L. (ed.): Colon and Rectal Surgery. Philadelphia, J.B. Lippincott, 1985, p. 393.

17. Localio, S.A., Eng, K., and Ranson, J.H.C.: Abdominosacral approach for retrorectal tumors. Ann. Surg., 191:555, 1980.

18. Localio, S.A., Eng, K., and Coppa, G.F.: Abdominal sacral resection for midrectal cancer. A fifteen year experience. Ann. Surg., 198:320, 1983.

19. Localio, S.A., and Eng, K.: Abdominal sacral resection. In Beahrs, O.H., Higgins, G.A., and Weinstein, J.J. (eds.): Colorectal Tumors. Philadelphia, J.B. Lippincott, 1985, p. 185.

20. Miles, W.E.: Pathology of spread of cancer of rectum and its bearing upon surgery of cancerous rectum. Surg. Gynecol. Obstet., 52:350, 1931.

21. Moran, M., Rothenberger, D.A., Lahr, C.J., et al.: Palliation for rectal cancer. Resection? Anastomosis? Arch. Surg., 122:640, 1987.

22. Peña, A., and deVries, P.: Posterior sagittal anorectoplasty: Important technical considerations and new applications. J. Pediatr. Surg., 17:796, 1982.

23. Perry, E.G., and Hinrichs, B.: A new translation of Professor Dr. P. Kraske's zur exstirpation hochsitzender mastdarmkrebse. Aust. N. Z. J. Surg., 59:421, 1989.

24. Rothenberger, D.A., and Finne, C.O., III: The case against routine radical surgery for early rectal cancer. In Simmons, R.L., and Udekwa, A.O. (eds.): Debates in Clinical Surgery. Chicago, Year Book Medical Publishers, 1990, p. 54.

25. Schittek, A., Clausen, K.P., and Minton, J.P.: Mesenchymona of the retrorectal space: A case report and review of the literature. J. Surg. Oncol., 25:85, 1984.

26. Spencer, R.J., and Jackman, R.J.: Surgical management of precoccygeal cysts. Surg. Gynecol. Obstet., 115:449, 1962.

27. Stener, B., and Gunterberg, B.: High amputation of the sacrum for extirpation of tumors: Principles and technique. Spine, 3:351, 1978.

28. York-Mason, A.: Trans-sphincter approach to rectal lesions. Surg. Ann., 6:171, 1977.

Chapter 22

ANATOMY AND PHYSIOLOGY OF THE ANUS AND RECTUM

JOHN H. PEMBERTON / ALAN P. MEAGHER

The anatomy and physiology of the anorectum—the terminal portion of the alimentary tract that maintains enteric continence and facilitates defecation—although intensely investigated, continues to be the subject of debate and speculation. Several dogmatic versions of anatomy, and more particularly of physiology, have been modified as a result of newer research using novel methodology that quantifies not only parameters of anorectal motility but also the function of the pelvic floor muscles. The goals of this chapter are to describe the functional anatomy of the anorectum and pelvic floor, particularly from the viewpoint of the surgeon performing pelvic and anal surgery, to detail recent changes in our understanding of anorectal and pelvic floor physiology, and to describe the role abnormal physiology may play in the etiology of several common anorectal disorders.

EMBRYOLOGY

The hindgut, cloaca, proctodeal pit, and anal tubercles are the precursors of the structures of the anorectum. The hindgut forms the portion of the rectum cranial to the pubococcygeal line, whereas the cloaca forms the portion below it. The urogenital and intestinal tracts terminate in the cloaca before week 5 of gestation (Fig. 22–1). At week 6, caudal migration of the urorectal septum separates the tracts (Fig. 22–2). The cloacal part of the anal canal is lined by both ectodermal (from the anal pit) and endodermal elements and, after breakdown of the anal membrane, is the origin of the anal transition zone.

The anal tubercles are ectodermal in origin and become joined posteriorly and anteriorly to encircle the proctodeal pit (Fig. 22–3). Anteriorly, the tubercle forms part of the perineal body, which completely separates the rectum from the urogenital tract.

Imperforate anus results from nonunion of the proctodeum and the rectum, whereas membranous imperforate anus is a result of failure of the anorectal membrane to disintegrate. Rectovaginourethral or bladder fistulas occur if the urorectal septum does not divide the cloaca completely. The external sphincter forms at the same time as the perineal body; the perineal body separates the early "cloacal sphincter" into urogenital and anal portions (Fig. 22–2B). The internal sphincter is formed later from enlarging fibers of the circular muscle of the rectum. During development, the external anal sphincter (EAS) migrates caudally, whereas the internal anal sphincter (IAS) migrates cephalad. Finally, it is generally agreed that the blood supply, venous return, and lymphatic drainage above the anal transition zone are portal in origin, whereas below this zone they are systemic.

ANATOMY

Rectum

Varying in length with age, sex, and body habitus, the rectum is described by anatomists as beginning at the S3 vertebral body, but surgeons describe it as beginning at the sacral promontory.[45] The rectum descends caudally, following the curve of the sacrum first downward and then forward for a distance of 13 to 15 cm to end at the anorectal ring, or the top of the anal canal (Fig. 22–4). This ring is formed by the pelvic floor muscles (the puborectalis muscle, in particular) and the EAS and IAS (Fig. 22–5). The anal canal continues below the anorectal ring by turning abruptly downward and backward to terminate at the anal verge.

The rectum has three lateral curves. The upper and lower curves are convex to the right, whereas the middle curve is convex to the left (Fig. 22–6). On the intraluminal aspect of these curves are the valves of Houston.

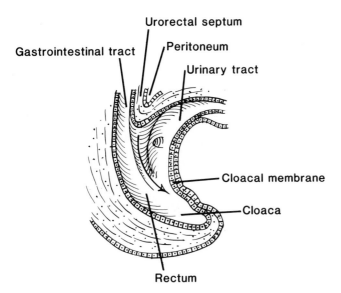

FIGURE 22-1. The embryo at week 5 of gestation. Note that the urinary and gastrointestinal tracts end in a common cloaca. The urorectal septum will migrate caudally.

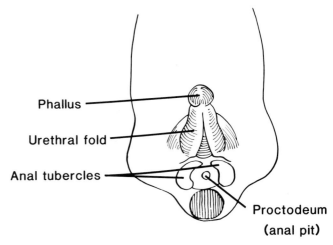

FIGURE 22-3. The proctodeum, or anal pit, is surrounded by the anal tubercles. The anterior tubercle forms part of the perineal body.

These infoldings incorporate all layers of the rectal wall except the longitudinal muscle layer. The middle valve is the most consistent and usually marks the level of the anterior peritoneal reflection.[44] When the curves are straightened by rectal mobilization, the rectum "lengthens" by about 5 cm.

Intraluminally at the rectosigmoidal junction, the transverse folds characteristic of the sigmoid colon give way to the smoother rectal mucosa (Fig. 22-7).[163] *Externally* at the rectosigmoidal junction, the three taeniae coli can be seen to disappear as they spread to encircle the rectum as the longitudinal muscle layer (see Fig. 22-4). This is sometimes difficult to appreciate, however. Additional clues are that the rectum has no epiploic tags, sacculations, or obvious mesentery.[45]

The wall of the rectum consists of four layers: mucosa, submucosa, and the circular and longitudinal muscle layers (Fig. 22-7). In the upper one third of the rectum, peritoneum covers its exterior on the anterior and lat-

eral sides (see Figs. 22-4 and 22-6; Fig. 22-8), wrapping around to nearly encircle the rectum except for the short mesorectum. In the middle third, only the anterior aspect of the rectum is covered, as the mesorectum is very short and thick. The lower portion of the rectum is devoid of peritoneum. The anterior peritoneal reflection shows considerable variation; in men, the level of the peritoneum above the anal verge is about 7 to 9 cm; in women, it is between 5 and 7.5 cm.[44] The peritoneum is reflected from the rectum to form the perirectal fossa laterally. In men, the anterior peritoneum reflects onto the seminal vesicles and bladder, and in women it reflects onto the vagina and uterus (Fig. 22-8). High in the rectum, the peritoneum is closely applied to the longitudinal muscle coat. In the middle third, however, a layer of fat is interposed between the peritoneum and the longitudinal muscle.

Rectal Relationships (Fig. 22-9)

Posteriorly, the rectum is related to the sacrum, coccyx, levator ani muscles, the medial sacral vessels, and

FIGURE 22-2. The embryo at weeks at 6 to 7. The urorectal septum has migrated caudally to separate the urinary and gastrointestinal tracts. The common cloacal membrane (*A*) has now been separated (*B*).

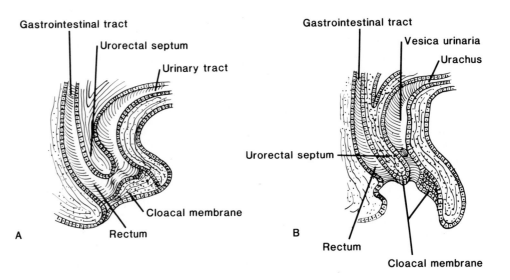

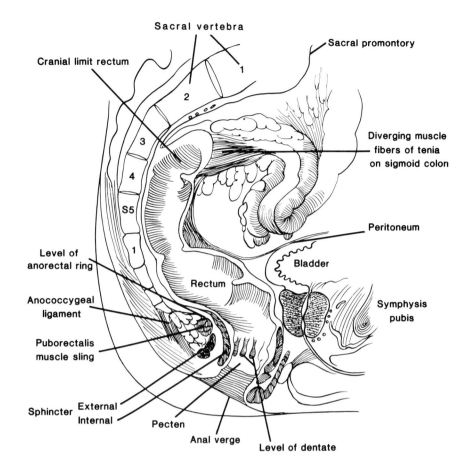

FIGURE 22-4. The course of the rectum through the pelvis. The rectum descends downward from S3 to the most proximal level of the coccyx and then downward and forward to end at the level of the anorectal ring. The fibers of the taeniae coli diverge at the level of S2–S3, providing an external visual landmark indicating the beginning of the rectum proper.

the roots of the sacral nerve plexus. Anteriorly, in men, the *extraperitoneal* rectum is related to the prostate, seminal vesicles, vas deferens, and urinary bladder. In women, the extraperitoneal rectum lies behind the posterior vaginal wall.

Fascial Relationships and Attachments (Fig. 22-10)

The *fascia propria* (fascial capsule) envelops the vessels and lymphatics in the posterior extraperitoneal portion of the rectum. This fascia is continuous with the visceral pelvic fascia. Below the anterior peritoneal reflection, condensations of this fascia on each side of the rectum are termed the lateral ligaments and attach the rectum to the lateral pelvic side walls. These ligaments support the rectum and must be divided to facilitate rectal mobilization. *Accessory branches* of the middle hemorrhoidal

artery sometimes traverse these attachments, but the main arteries (if present at all) do not. Autonomic nerves do pass through the lateral ligaments to the sacrum.[129]

The sacrum and coccyx are covered by *presacral fascia* (Figs. 22–10 and 22–11). This fascia also covers the median sacral vessels. From the S4 level, the *rectosacral* fascia (fascia of Waldeyer), a part of the parietal pelvic fascia, runs downward and forward to reflect onto the fascia propria above the anorectal ring (Fig. 22–11A). This is a variable layer that may be sharply incised to facilitate complete posterior rectal mobilization[27] (Fig. 22–11B).

Anteriorly, the extraperitoneal rectum is also covered by tough *visceral pelvic fascia* (Denonvilliers' fascia) that extends from the peritoneal reflection downward to the urogenital diaphragm, parallel to the rectum and dorsal to the urogenital structures, and attaches laterally to the lateral ligaments (Fig. 22–12). This fascia separates the

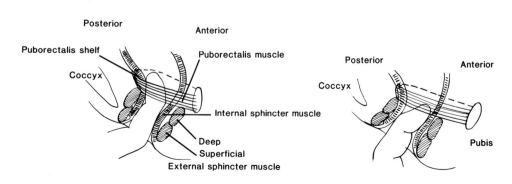

FIGURE 22-5. The anorectal ring is composed of the puborectalis muscle and the deepest portion of the external anal sphincter. The ring is most easily palpated *posteriorly* as the puborectalis "shelf."

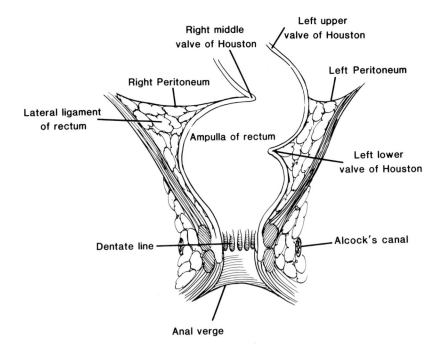

FIGURE 22-6. The curves of the rectum. The upper and lower curves are convex to the right, whereas the middle curve is convex to the left. The three valves of Houston are also seen. Note the peritoneum is reflected from the rectum at the level of the middle valve.

rectum from the prostate and seminal vesicles or vagina (see Fig. 22–10) and should be entered high near the peritoneal reflection and during anterior rectal mobilization for benign disease in order to separate these structures from the rectum.

Anal Canal

The anal canal extends from the anorectal ring above to the hairy skin of the anal verge below (Fig. 22–13). At rest, the anal canal is closed, its lateral walls opposed so that an anterior posterior slit is formed.[114] The anal verge is attached to the perineal raphe anteriorly and the anal raphe posteriorly.

Circumferentially, the anal canal is related to the IAS and EAS. Posteriorly, the anal canal is also related to the coccyx, laterally it is related to the ischiorectal fossa and its contents, and anteriorly it is related to the urethra in men and to the lower vagina and perineal body in women.

Epithelium of the Anal Canal

Approximately 2 cm cranial to the anal verge is a line of anal valves (Fig. 22–13). This landmark is the pectinate or dentate line and is located at the junction of the middle and distal thirds of the internal sphincter. Above each valve is a pit or anal crypt. Connected to the anal crypts are a variable number of glands (four to ten) that traverse the submucosa to terminate in the submucosa, IAS, or the intersphincteric plane (Fig. 22–14). If obstructed, these glands are the source of perianal abscesses and fistulas.

Cranial to the anal valves, but still in the anal canal, the mucosa is pleated into 12 to 14 columns (columns of Morgagni) (see Figs. 22–7 and 22–13). The mucosa above the valves in the area of the columns consists of several layers of cuboidal cells (Fig. 22–15). This mu-

cosa gives way, at variable distances around the anal canal (0.5 to 1 cm), to a single layer of columnar cells that is characteristic of rectal epithelium. The color of the mucosa also changes: from 0.5 to 1 cm above the dentate line, the mucosa is deep purple changing to the characteristic pink of the rectal mucosa.[45] This area above the dentate line is the *anal transition zone.*

Caudal to the dentate line, the anal canal is lined by modified squamous epithelium devoid of hair and

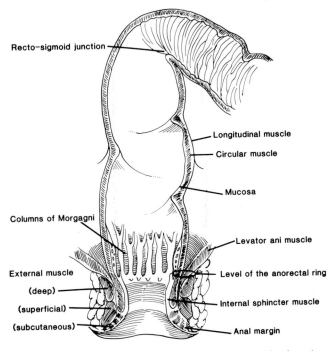

FIGURE 22-7. The corrugated mucosa of the sigmoid colon gives way to the smooth mucosa of the rectum. Compared with Figure 22–6, the rectum has been "stretched" and the curves straightened. The layers of the rectal wall are also depicted.

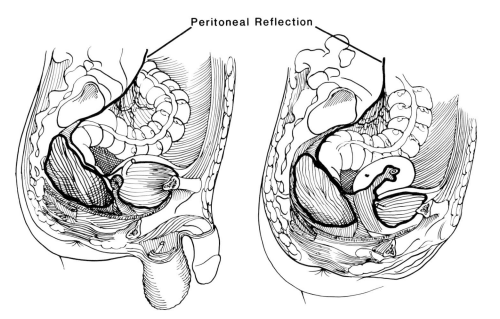

FIGURE 22-8. The reflections of the peritoneum in men and women.

glands, which appears smooth, thin, and stretched.[45] Further caudally, this modified squamous epithelium changes to squamous epithelium with hair and glands at the anal verge (Fig. 22–15). It is important to remember that none of the mucosal boundaries described here are at the same level at all places around the circumference of the anal canal.[157]

Anal Canal Musculature

SMOOTH MUSCLE. (Fig. 22–16). The IAS is a continuation of the circular muscle of the rectum and ends with a pronounced rounded edge about 1 to 1.5 cm caudal to the dentate line and slightly cranial to the terminus of the EAS.[45] The IAS is 2.5 to 4 cm in length and about 0.5 cm thick.

LONGITUDINAL ANAL MUSCLE. Anatomic descriptions of this muscle, which lies between the IAS and EAS, are particularly varied.[83] Superiorly, it is continuous with the longitudinal muscle of the rectal wall and pubococcygeus muscle,[163] whereas inferiorly, fibers course through the IAS and EAS, with some gaining attachment to the perianal skin. These dermal terminations are called the corrugator cutis ani.

STRIATED MUSCLE. The EAS is slightly longer than the IAS and occupies a position outside the IAS, enveloping it throughout its length (Fig. 22–16). The EAS is an elliptic cylinder of muscle that is continuous with the puborectalis muscle superiorly, whereas inferiorly it becomes subcutaneous and lies laterally and more caudally than the IAS. The EAS is divided into deep and superficial compartments. Posteriorly, the EAS is attached to the skin superficially and to the sacrococcygeal raphe and coccyx more deeply and is continuous with the puborectalis muscle at the level of the anorectal ring. Anteriorly, the EAS is attached to the skin superficially, to the transverse perineus muscle slightly more deeply, and proceeds most deeply with the puborectalis muscle toward the pubis at the level of the anorectal ring.

The *levator ani plate* consists of three muscles that

form the posterior pelvic diaphragm (Fig. 22–17). The *iliococcygeus* muscle originates from the ischial spine and obturator fascia and passes caudally, posteriorly, and medially to be inserted on the sacrum (at S4 and S5) and the anococcygeal raphe. The *pubococcygeus* muscle originates from the obturator fascia and pubis and passes posteriorly, caudally, and medially to decussate with fibers from the contralateral side. The posterior line of demarcation is the anococcygeal raphe. The fibers from the medial part of the pubococcygeus fuse with the perineal body, prostate, and vagina and form part of the longitudinal muscle bundle as it travels in the intersphincteric plane.

The *puborectalis* muscle (Figs. 22–17 and 22–18) arises with the pubococcygeus from the pubis and urogenital diaphragm and proceeds posteriorly alongside the anorectal junction. Fibers from one side join with fibers from the other to form a sling behind the rectum at the anorectal ring. This ring is an important landmark (see Fig. 22–5); incising it almost always results in fecal incontinence.

Whether the puborectalis muscle and EAS should be considered as one anatomic muscle group is the subject of continuing controversy. Perhaps the best evidence that the two are of the same striated muscle complex is provided by Wendell-Smith[158] and Wood.[163]

OTHER MUSCLES. The pelvic diaphragm fixes the pelvic viscera and provides a firm wall against which increased abdominal pressure is exerted during defecation, coughing, laughing, and lifting. The bilateral involuntary *rectococcygeus* muscles arise from the coccyx and pass forward and downward to blend with the longitudinal muscle fibers of the rectum and pelvic fascia; these muscles tether the rectum to the coccyx. The *coccygeus* muscles are also bilateral but are voluntary. They arise from the ischial spine and insert into the fifth sacral vertebra and coccyx. These muscles support the rectum and bring the coccyx forward during squeezing. The *superficial transverse perineus muscle* (see Fig. 22–16) arises from the pubis and inserts into the central perineal ra-

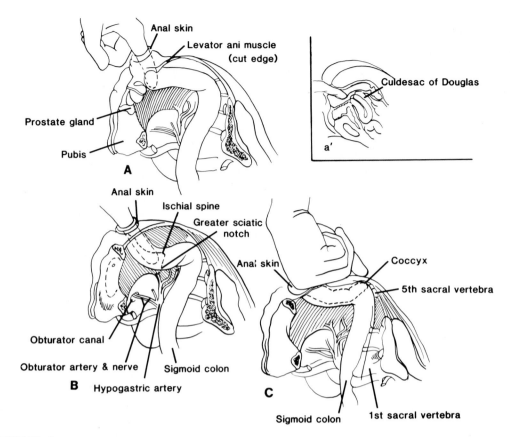

FIGURE 22-9. Relationships of the rectum palpable to the examining finger. Anteriorly, the prostate (*A*) and vagina and uterus (*a'*) are easily palpated. Laterally, the ischial spine, pelvic side wall, and levator plate are palpable (*B*). Posteriorly, the coccyx and presacral space can be palpated readily (*C*).

phe and perhaps also in the EAS. The function of this muscle is to fix the central tendon. The *deep transverse perineus muscle* (Fig. 22–16) arises from the ischium bilaterally. In men, these muscles merge with the external urinary sphincter and act to voluntarily cut off the urinary stream.

Para-anal and Pararectal Spaces

There are several important potential spaces in the anorectal region that have surgical relevance (Figs. 22–19 through 22–21).[44]

The apex of the *ischiorectal space* is at the origin of the levator ani muscles from the obturator fascia (Figs. 22–19 and 22–21). This space is bounded inferiorly by the perineal skin, anteriorly by the transverse muscles of the perineum, posteriorly by the sacrotuberous ligament and gluteus maximus muscle, medially by the EAS and levator ani, and laterally by the external obturator muscle. In the lateral wall of this space is Alcock's canal, through which the pudendal vessels and nerves course. There is a potential extension of this space anteriorly, which courses above the urogenital diaphragm. The contents of this space include fat, the inferior hemor-

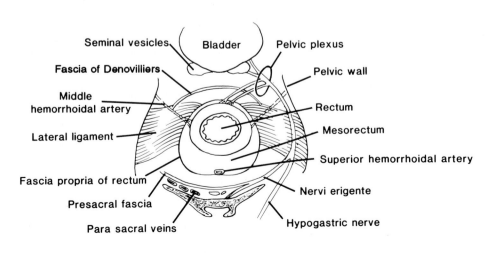

FIGURE 22-10. The pelvis viewed from above showing the major fascial, neural, and arterial structures.

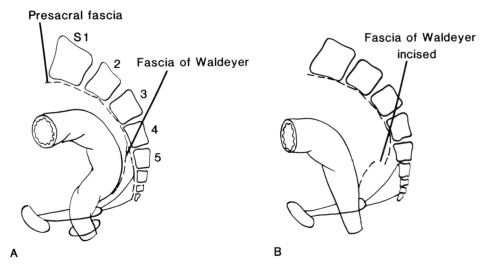

FIGURE 22-11. The presacral and Waldeyer's fasciae. *A,* Waldeyer's fascia reflects from the presacral fascia *above* the anorectal ring. Cutting the fascia (*B*) frees the rectum *posteriorly,* facilitating complete mobilization.

rhoidal vessels and nerves, and the scrotal or labial vessels.

The *perianal space* (Figs. 22–19 and 22–21) surrounds the anal verge, is continuous with the fat of the buttocks laterally, and extends into the intersphincteric space. Its contents are the most caudal part of the EAS, the external hemorrhoidal plexus, and the inferior hemorrhoidal vessels. This space is bound down tightly because the corrugator cutis runs through it. The *intersphincteric space* (see Fig. 22–19) is a potential space between the IAS and the EAS and is continuous with the perianal space. The bilateral *supralevator spaces* (Figs. 22–19 through 22–21) are bounded superiorly by the peritoneum, laterally by the obturator fascia, medially by the rectum, and inferiorly by the levator plate. These spaces can connect to each other posteriorly behind the rectum, deep to the anococcygeal raphe but superficial to the rectosacral fascia. The *submucous space* begins at the dentate line and extends cranially to join the submucosa of the rectum proper. The internal hemorrhoidal plexus is in this space.

The *superficial postanal space* (Fig. 22–20) is continuous with the superficial ischiorectal fossa posteriorly, deep to the skin but superficial to the anococcygeal ligament. The *deep postanal space* (see Fig. 22–20), in contrast, connects the deeper parts of the ischiorectal fossa together posteriorly behind the anal canal, deep to the anal coccygeal ligament but superficial to the anococcygeal raphe. Horseshoe abscesses usually occur through this space but also may occur in the superficial postanal space (Fig. 22–21).

The *retrorectal space* (see Fig. 22–20) begins cranial to the rectosacral ligament between the rectum and the sacrum and is continuous with the retroperitoneal space above. Its boundaries are the fascia propria of the rectum anteriorly, the presacral fascia posteriorly, and the lateral rectal ligaments laterally. This plane is avascular; the fascia propria protects the mesorectal vessels, and the presacral fascia invests the presacral vessels.

Vasculature

The major arterial blood supply to the rectum and anal canal is provided by the superior and inferior hem-

orrhoidal (superior and inferior rectal) arteries, whereas the middle hemorrhoidal (rectal) artery has a variable contribution depending on the size of the superior hemorrhoidal artery (Fig. 22–22).

The superior hemorrhoidal artery is a direct continuation of the inferior mesenteric artery once it crosses the left common iliac vessel. It descends in the sigmoid mesocolon to the level of S3, at which point it bifurcates into right and left branches and then further bifurcates into anterior and posterior branches.[40] These branches enter the rectal wall to gain access to the submucosa and then descend to the level of the columns of Morgagni in the anal canal. About five identifiable branches of these arteries reach the level of the anal canal, with predominance at the right posterior, right anterior, and left lateral positions (Fig. 22–23). There tends to be a paucity of extramural midline arterial anastomoses both anteriorly and posteriorly along the length of the rectum.

The *inferior hemorrhoidal arteries* are branches of the internal pudendal artery, which is itself a branch of the internal iliac artery. They pierce the EAS to reach the submucosa of the anal canal and then ascend in this plane.

A substantial *middle hemorrhoidal artery* tends to be present if the superior hemorrhoidal artery is small. This artery arises from the internal iliac artery or the internal pudendal artery[129] and reaches the rectal wall by traversing the supralevator space on top of the levator ani musculature but deep to the levator fascia. The artery *does not* traverse the lateral stalks but may send minor branches through them.

Although there are relatively few, if any, *extramural* anastomoses between these arteries, there is little doubt that a rich *intramural* anastomotic network is present.[163] These observations support the clinical fact that division of both the superior hemorrhoidal and middle hemorrhoidal arteries (if present) does not result in necrosis of the rectum.

Venous drainage of the rectum and anal canal runs with the arterial supply. Drainage through the superior hemorrhoidal vein is into the portal system, whereas drainage through the middle and inferior hemorrhoidal veins is into the systemic system. There are free anastomoses between all of these venous channels.[150]

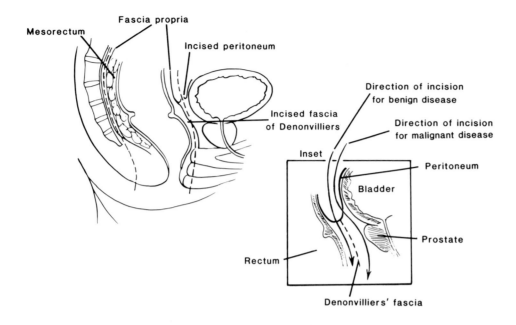

FIGURE 22-12. Fascial relationships anteriorly. In men, the peritoneum reflects from the bladder onto the rectum. Denonvilliers' fascia runs *parallel* to the rectum, separating the rectum from anterior structures. *Anterior* mobilization is accomplished by incising posteriorly through Denonvilliers' fascia; the "correct" plane can readily be bluntly developed.

Lymphatic drainage likewise follows the vascular supply (Fig. 22–24). Drainage from the upper two thirds of the rectum ascends with the superior hemorrhoidal artery to reach the inferior mesenteric nodes. The lower third of the rectum drains not only into the inferior mesenteric nodes but also into the internal iliac nodes. Lymphatic drainage from the anal canal above the dentate line courses to the inferior mesenteric nodes and internal iliac nodes. Drainage below the dentate line is usually to the inguinal lymph nodes but can be to the inferior mesenteric nodes and to nodes along the course of the inferior hemorrhoidal artery. Retrograde lymphatic spread below the level of a rectal cancer commonly occurs only if extensive involvement of proximally draining lymphatic and venous channels has occurred.[118]

Finally, dye injection studies by Block and Enquist[16] have shown that lymphatic drainage in women could spread to the posterior vaginal wall, uterus, broad ligament, ovaries, and cul-de-sac. Perhaps spread through

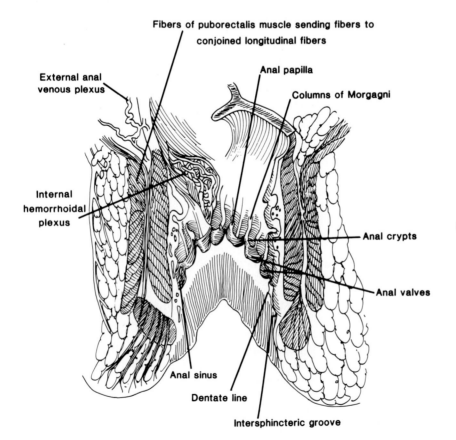

FIGURE 22-13. The anal canal.

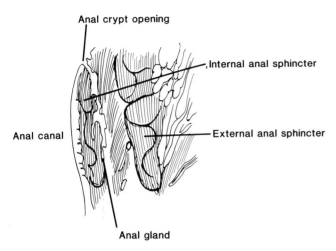

FIGURE 22-14. An anal gland connected to an anal pit.

these channels occurs only if proximal lymphatic and venous channels are blocked.

Innervation

The extrinsic innervation of the rectum and upper part of the anal canal includes both sympathetic and parasympathetic nerves. In general, the *sympathetic response* consists of inhibition of contraction of smooth muscle of the rectum with contraction of the IAS, and the *parasympathetic response* is the stimulation of contraction of the rectal wall, but relaxation of the IAS.

The *sympathetic* supply to the rectum arises from L1–L3, exiting as lumbar sympathetics to join the aortic plexus (superior hypogastric plexus, hypogastric plexus) (Fig. 22–25). Some fibers from this plexus join the inferior mesenteric plexus around the base of the inferior mesenteric artery, and continue along this artery to supply the rectum. Other fibers continue over the aortic bifurcation caudally into the presacral plexus. As they continue caudally, many fibers pass caudolaterally to-

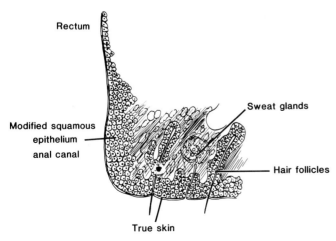

FIGURE 22-15. The epithelial lining of the anal canal.

wards the pelvic plexus (inferior hypogastric plexus). These fibers often coalesce into several identifiable bundles, the so-called right and left hypogastric nerves, which lie adjacent to the posterolateral aspect of the rectum. The pelvic plexus lies on the side wall of the pelvis deep to the peritoneum but superficial to the endopelvic fascia, at about the level of the lower third of the rectum lateral to the lateral stalks (Fig. 22–10). Branches from the pelvic plexus innervate the rectum, via the lateral stalks, and the anal canal, bladder, and sexual organs. Branches from the presacral plexus also pass directly to the posterior aspect of the rectum.[88]

Parasympathetic innervation of the rectum originates from the anterior roots of S2, S3, and S4—the nervi erigentes (Fig. 22–25). Branches of these nerves may pass cephalad into the presacral plexus, laterally and forward to join with the sympathetic nerves in the pelvic plexus, or directly to the posterior surface of the rectum. Parasympathetics pass upwards to the inferior mesenteric plexus to be distributed with the superior hemorrhoidal artery to the rectum, and through the mesocolon to the sigmoid and descending colon. Other parasympathetics are distributed from the pelvic plexus to the bladder, genitals, and IAS. An important subdivision of the pelvic plexus (inferior hypogastric plexus) is the *periprostatic* plexus, which is adjacent to the rectum and prostate and supplies parasympathetic and sympathetic input via *anterolateral* connections to the prostate, seminal vesicles, corpora cavernosum, vas deferens, urethra, ejaculatory ducts, and bulbourethral glands (Fig. 22–25). Fortunately, termination of these fibers occurs above Denonvilliers' fascia and thus can be protected by careful dissection below it (see Figs. 22–10 and 22–12).[75] Erection of the penis is controlled by parasympathetic input (sympathetic input does inhibit vasoconstriction, thereby increasing vascular engorgement), whereas sympathetic inflow causes emission and parasympathetic inflow causes ejaculation.[65]

The *somatic pelvic nerves* arise from S3, S4, and S5 and cross the pelvic floor under the levator ani fascia. The levator muscles are supplied by these nerves, as is the anal canal. The pudendal nerve arises from S2, S3, and S4 and enters the perineum from Alcock's canal. Branches of the pudendal nerves are the inferior hemorrhoidal, perianal, and dorsal penile or clitoral nerves (Fig. 22–25).

Anal Canal

INTERNAL ANAL SPHINCTER. The motor supply to the IAS is sympathetic (L5) and parasympathetic (S2, S3, and S4). The tone of the IAS is mediated by both sympathetic and parasympathetic fibers[163]; contraction of the IAS, however, is predominantly sympathetically mediated.[19] Relaxation of the IAS occurs as part of an intramural (intrinsic) reflex called the rectoanal sphincter inhibitory response. It has now been demonstrated that the nonadrenergic, noncholinergic neurotransmitter mediating IAS relaxation is very likely to be nitric oxide.[120,153] Distention of the rectal wall above the anorectal ring causes relaxation of the IAS.

LONGITUDINAL ANAL MUSCLE. Little is known about the

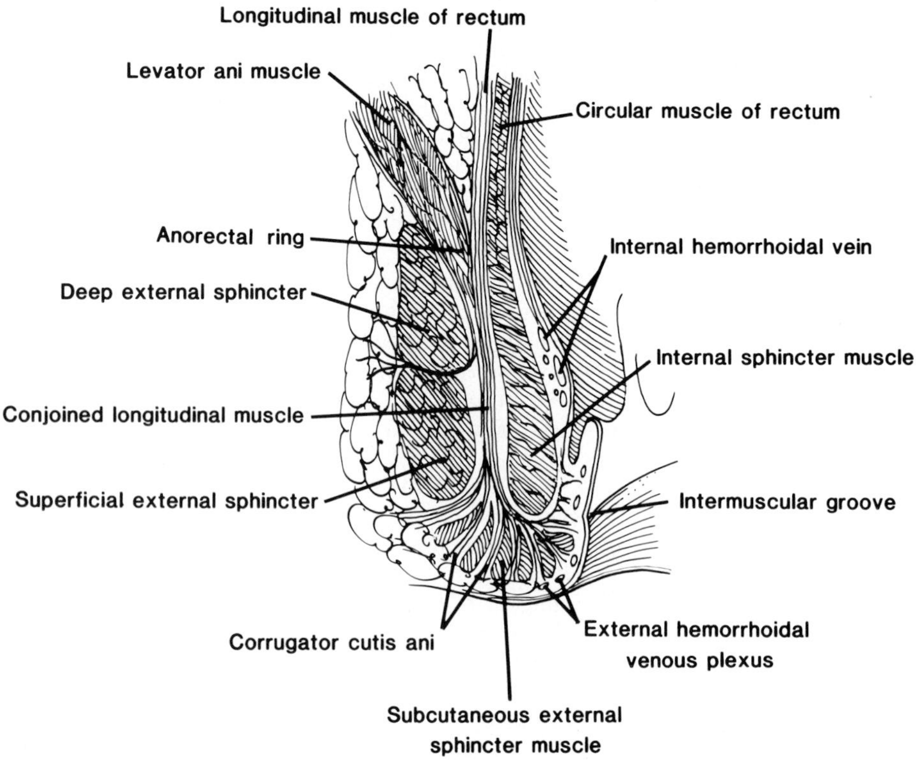

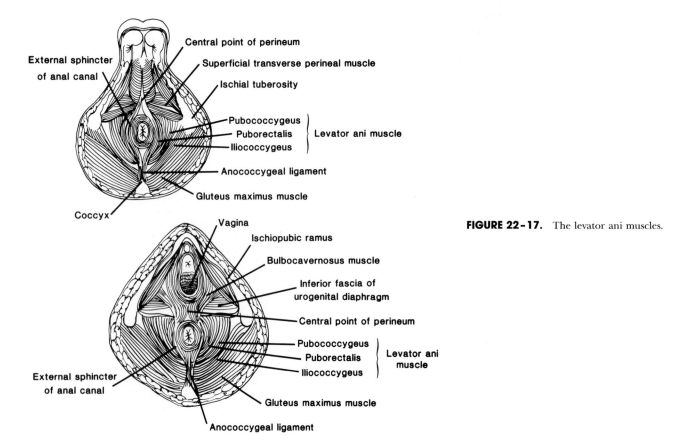

Longitudinal muscle of rectum

Levator ani muscle

Circular muscle of rectum

Anorectal ring

Internal hemorrhoidal vein

Deep external sphincter

Internal sphincter muscle

Conjoined longitudinal muscle

Superficial external sphincter

Intermuscular groove

Corrugator cutis ani

External hemorrhoidal
venous plexus

Subcutaneous external
sphincter muscle

FIGURE 22-16. The voluntary and involuntary muscles of the anal canal.

External sphincter
of anal canal

Central point of perineum

Superficial transverse perineal muscle

Ischial tuberosity

Pubococcygeus
Puborectalis   } Levator ani muscle
Iliococcygeus

Anococcygeal ligament

Gluteus maximus muscle

Coccyx

Vagina

Ischiopubic ramus

Bulbocavernosus muscle

Inferior fascia of
urogenital diaphragm

Central point of perineum

Pubococcygeus
Puborectalis   } Levator ani
Iliococcygeus   muscle

External sphincter
of anal canal

Gluteus maximus muscle

Anococcygeal ligament

FIGURE 22-17. The levator ani muscles.

nerve supply of this smooth muscle. It appears to show true sphincteric specialization by generating spontaneous tension.[102] It is distinct from the IAS, as stimulation of muscarinic receptors causes contraction rather than relaxation.

EXTERNAL ANAL SPHINCTER. (Figs. 22–25 and 22–26). Motor supply to the EAS travels in the pudendal nerve (S2 and S3) and the perineal branch of S4. There is crossover of the fibers at the cord level such that unilateral transection of a pudendal nerve does not abolish function of the EAS.[164]

LEVATOR ANI. (Fig. 22–26). The motor supply of the puborectalis muscle is controversial; the pudendal nerve alone, direct pelvic branches of S3 and S4 alone, or a combination of the two provides motor innervation. The pubococcygeus and iliococcygeus muscles are supplied on their superior aspects by S4 and on their inferior aspects by perineal branches of pudendal nerves.

Sensation

ANAL CANAL. (Fig. 22–27). From 1 to 1.5 cm above the anal valves to the anal verge, the anal canal epithelium contains free nerve endings, Meissner's corpuscles (touch), Krause's bulbs (cold), Golgi-Mazzoni bodies (pressure), and genital corpuscles (friction).[33,133] Sensation is carried in the inferior hemorrhoidal branch of the pudendal nerve.

RECTUM. Although many nonmyelinated nerve fibers exist, organized endings are generally lacking in the rectal mucosa. Receptors for rectal distention likely lie outside the rectal wall itself.[75,130,139] Sensation from the rectum is carried in parasympathetic nerves S2, S3, and S4.

Anatomic Rectal Mobilization

Rapid, complication-free mobilization of the rectum can be achieved by an "anatomic" dissection of the perirectal structures. Such an anatomic dissection achieves its goals rapidly and safely.

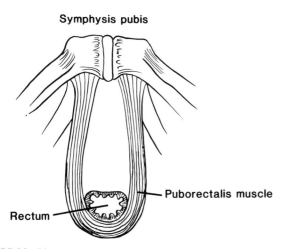

Symphysis pubis

Puborectalis muscle

Rectum

FIGURE 22–18. The puborectalis muscle from above. The puborectalis muscle lies adjacent to the anorectal junction laterally and swings around to encircle the sphincter posteriorly.

Elevation of the Sigmoid

After freeing the sigmoid colon from any developmental lateral abdominal wall attachments, the white line of Toldt is incised, and the gonadal vessels and underlying left ureter are swept laterally (Fig. 22–28A and B). By firm elevation of the sigmoid loop, the inferior mesenteric artery is then placed on stretch, making identification of the superior hemorrhoidal artery easier. With the forceps, the tissue clinging to the superior hemorrhoidal artery (superior rectal artery) is swept directly posteriorly, opening a window in the sigmoid mesentery immediately below the superior hemorrhoidal artery at the level of the aortic bifurcation. The tissue separated from the superior hemorrhoidal artery contains the aortic plexus and, caudally, the presacral plexus and right and left hypogastric nerves.

Pelvic Dissection

The arch of the superior hemorrhoidal artery is followed forward toward the rectum, which by strong upward traction is oriented in an anterior and posterior direction. Again, using the forceps or scissors, the tissue behind the superior hemorrhoidal artery is pushed downward, and, once across the promontory, the retrorectal space is easily entered (Fig. 22–28C). Using the scissors, this space is developed sharply downward to about S3 and then downward and forward to the rectosacral fascia at the level of S4. If easily seen, the rectosacral fascia is then sharply incised. If not, the posterior dissection is carried laterally by sweeping hand motions that loosen the perirectal areolar tissue. Sharply transecting the rectosacral fascia then allows safe blunt finger dissection to the level of the levator raphe (Fig. 22–28D). By using this technique to enter the pelvis behind the rectum, the hypogastric nerves and the hypogastric plexus are protected throughout their course. There is no anatomic or physiologic benefit to be gained by pursuing an *intramesenteric* dissection.[37]

Lateral Mobilization

The peritoneum on both sides of the rectum is incised so that the incisions meet in the midline over the rectum in the retrovesical or vaginal pouch (Fig. 22–28E). Sweeping hand motions, posteriorly and laterally, are then made on each side of the rectum, loosening and elevating the perirectal tissue. There are no nerves or vessels in this plane, as they lie on the sidewall near the ureters. By elevating the rectum out of the pelvis, the lateral ligaments can be better identified.

Anterior Dissection

After incising the peritoneum over the retrovesical or retrovaginal pouch, sharp dissection is carried posteriorly toward the rectum, thus incising Denonvilliers' fascia (Fig. 22–28F, G, and H). For malignant disease, Denonvilliers' fascia is not entered until well below the level of the seminal vesicles or at about the midvaginal level. The dissection proceeds sharply between the rec-

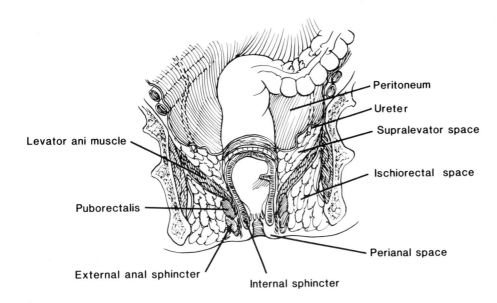

FIGURE 22-19. Coronal diagram of the para-anal and pararectal spaces.

tum and Denonvilliers' fascia to the level of the lower prostate or midvagina. The periprostatic plexus is adjacent to this dissection, but its fibers are sent to the genitals and prostate *above* Denonvilliers' fascia; they should therefore be protected by staying close to the rectum.

Division of the Lateral Stalks
(Fig. 22–28*I*)

Only after anterior and posterior dissections are complete can the lateral ligaments be adequately defined and accurately divided. This is because traction of the rectum will not tent the ligaments if the posterior and anterior rectal attachments are present. The ligaments are defined by finger dissection. The thumb is placed anteriorly between the rectum and Denonvilliers' fascia

and is swept around and down toward the index finger, which has been positioned posteriorly underneath the lateral structures. A pinching motion thus defines the ligaments bilaterally. The ligaments are then divided and ligated close to the rectum in benign disease and laterally in malignant disease. If the superior hemorrhoidal artery is small, there is a higher chance that significant bleeding will occur from branches of the middle hemorrhoidal artery in the lateral ligaments. The pelvic plexus of nerves is quite lateral, being adjacent to the pelvic side walls so that even relatively wide division of the lateral ligaments should not result in nerve damage. Problems do arise when the levators are excised radically, as fibers from the pelvic plexus run adjacent to the superior surface of the levator ani. Intersphincteric proctectomy in patients with benign disease, however,

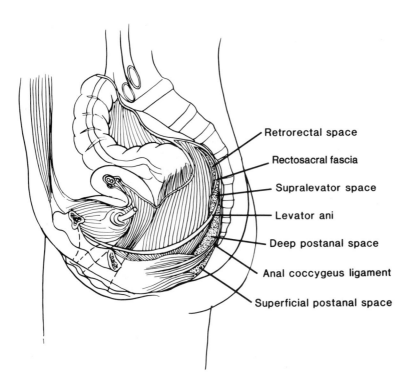

FIGURE 22-20. Lateral diagram of the posterior pararectal spaces.

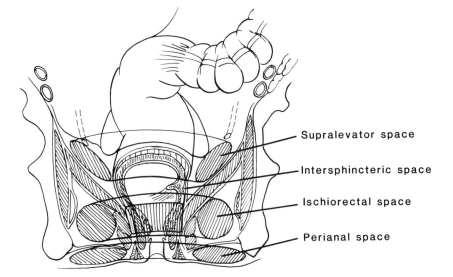

FIGURE 22-21. Coronal diagram of the para-rectal and para-anal spaces illustrating how an abscess can track posteriorly from one lateral space to gain access to the contralateral space.

Supralevator space

Intersphincteric space

Ischiorectal space

Perianal space

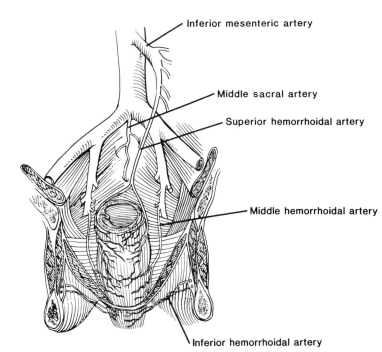

Inferior mesenteric artery

Middle sacral artery

Superior hemorrhoidal artery

Middle hemorrhoidal artery

Inferior hemorrhoidal artery

FIGURE 22-22. The vasculature of the rectum and anal canal. If present, the middle hemorrhoidal artery is small and lies immediately on top of the levator ani musculature and *not* in the lateral rectal stalks.

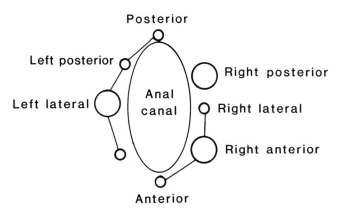

FIGURE 22-23. The positions of the three major (and five minor) arterial branches often identifiable at the level of the anorectal ring. This distribution is identical to the location of the major and minor internal hemorrhoidal groups.

preserves the pelvic plexus. After this dissection is completed, using a hand-sewn or stapled low anterior anastomosis, ileoanal or coloanal anastomosis, or intersphincteric proctectomy, bladder and sexual function should be normal.

Conclusion

A nerve-preserving relatively bloodless, nonperforating, rapid, and safe mobilization of the rectum can be accomplished if (1) the retrorectal space is sharply developed just behind the superior hemorrhoidal artery, (2) the rectosacral ligament is sharply incised, (3) the anterior dissection is carried out deep to Denovilliers' fascia, and (4) anterior and posterior dissections are completed before defining and ligating the lateral ligaments.

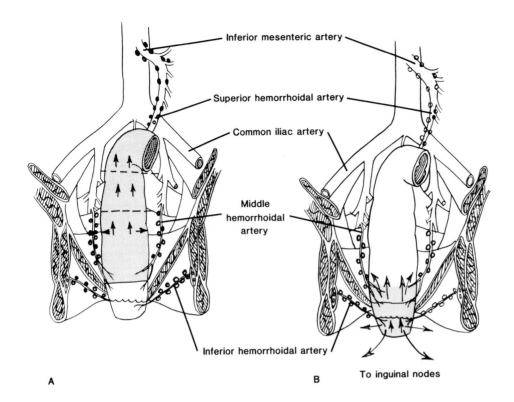

Inferior mesenteric artery

Superior hemorrhoidal artery

Common iliac artery

Middle hemorrhoidal artery

Inferior hemorrhoidal artery

To inguinal nodes

A

B

FIGURE 22-24. The lymphatic drainage of the rectum and anal canal. The ''watershed'' is the dentate line; tumors above this line may shed cells into the internal iliac and inferior mesenteric nodal chain (A), whereas tumors below this line may shed cells into the inguinal lymph node chain (B).

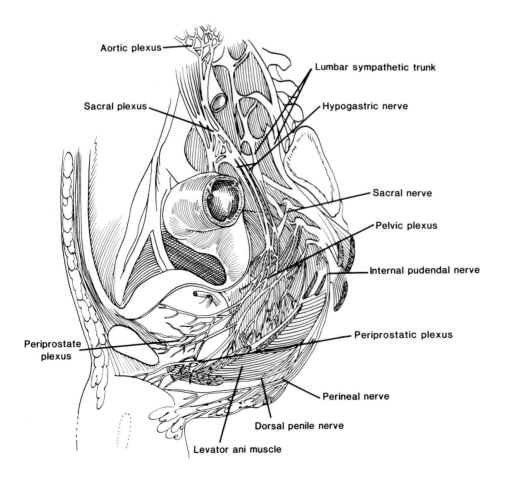

Aortic plexus

Sacral plexus

Lumbar sympathetic trunk

Hypogastric nerve

Sacral nerve

Pelvic plexus

Internal pudendal nerve

Periprostate plexus

Periprostatic plexus

Perineal nerve

Dorsal penile nerve

Levator ani muscle

FIGURE 22-25. The innervation of the rectum, anal canal, and anterior structures. The sympathetic hypogastric nerves, together with the parasympathetic nerves arising from S2–S4, join in the pelvic plexus.

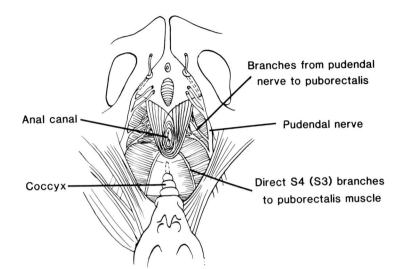

FIGURE 22-26. Innervation of the puborectalis muscle and other muscles of the levator plate.

Physiology

The mechanisms that maintain anorectal continence and facilitate defecation are related and complex. A clearer understanding of anorectal physiology has been made possible by the introduction of several newer methodologies designed to quantitate parameters of anorectal motility. Renewed appreciation of the clinical importance of anorectal physiology can be seen in the relatively recent explosion of interest in disordered anorectal function. The pathophysiologic bases of fecal incontinence, constipation, expulsion disorders, rectal intussusception, rectal prolapse, solitary rectal ulcer, rectocele, posterior rectal hernia, and obstructed defecation are undergoing intense investigation—causes are being hypothesized and treatments are being proposed.

Factors Maintaining Fecal Continence

Continence depends on the ability to defer the "call to stool" to a socially convenient time and place. The factors responsible for maintaining anorectal fecal continence are (1) the anal canal high-pressure zone (anal sphincter mechanism); (2) the anorectal angle and coordinated activity of the pelvic floor musculature; (3) anorectal sensory and reflex mechanisms; (4) distensibility, "tone," and capacity of the rectum; (5) rectal motility and evacuability; (6) colonic transit; (7) anal canal motility; and (8) stool volume and consistency.[109]

Anal Canal High-Pressure Zone

The mean length of the anal canal high-pressure zone is 4 cm. Women have a shorter anal canal than men (mean 3.7 versus 4.6 cm).[95] During anal sphincter squeeze, the anal canal lengthens, whereas during straining it shortens.[66]

RESTING PRESSURE. The EAS and IAS envelop the anal canal and are responsible for maintaining resting and generating squeeze pressures. Stepped pull-through manometric techniques, which measure intraluminal pressure, show a graduated increase in pressure proximally to distally in the anal canal (Fig. 22-29). The highest resting pressures are recorded 1 to 2 cm proximal to the anal verge. The mean anal canal resting pressure is approximately 90 cm H_2O ($\pm$SEM).[46] Resting pressure is lower in women than in men[121] and may be lower in older subjects.[4]

Resting pressure may be distributed unequally (Fig. 22-30) around the circumference of the anal canal because of the anatomic arrangement of the anal sphincter and pubococcygeus muscles (see Fig. 22-29). Posteriorly, resting pressure is highest proximally and lowest near the anal verge.[24,147] McHugh and Diamant,[86] in careful manometric studies, showed that anterior resting pressures in women were highest distally in the anal canal, but in men they were highest proximally. The IAS contributes about 85% of the resting tone of the anal canal.[42] Dividing the IAS in the presence of a normal EAS weakens tone but does not entirely abolish it.

EAS tone is maintained during the day and is present, though reduced, during sleep.[39] Coughing and the Valsalva maneuver increase EAS activity.[39,66] With the exception of the cricopharyngeus and paraspinus muscles, the EAS and the levator complex are the only striated muscles that maintain a constant tonus. This tone is mediated by a low sacral reflex. Straining to defecate, however, usually renders the EAS electrically silent.

SQUEEZE PRESSURE. Squeeze pressure is generated by contraction of the EAS and the puborectalis muscle; intra-anal canal pressures are increased more than two times greater than resting levels during maximum effort.[66]

Squeeze pressure may also be distributed unequally around the anal canal. Taylor and co-workers[147] found that squeeze pressures in the proximal anal canal were highest posteriorly and lowest anteriorly. In the midanal canal, squeeze pressure was distributed equally. In the distal anal canal, squeeze pressure was highest anteriorly and lowest posteriorly.

Maximum squeeze pressure elevation lasts less than 1 minute, as the sphincter fatigues rapidly after that time (Fig. 22-31).[66,114] Because squeeze efforts generate high pressure briefly, the squeeze mechanism likely acts effectively only to prevent leakage upon presentation of enteric content to the proximal canal at inopportune

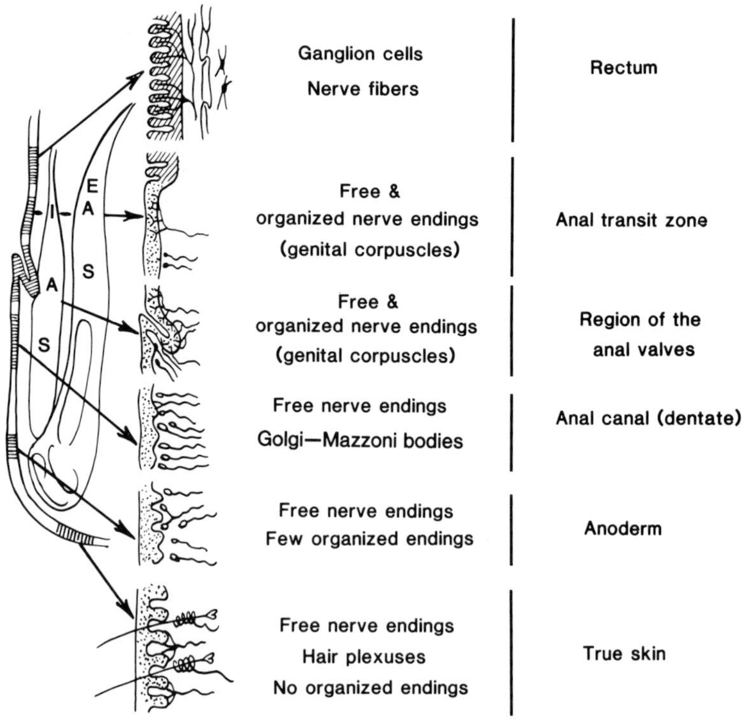

Ganglion cells
Nerve fibers
Rectum

Free &
organized nerve endings
(genital corpuscles)
Anal transit zone

Free &
organized nerve endings
(genital corpuscles)
Region of the
anal valves

Free nerve endings
Golgi—Mazzoni bodies
Anal canal (dentate)

Free nerve endings
Few organized endings
Anoderm

Free nerve endings
Hair plexuses
No organized endings
True skin

FIGURE 22-27. Distribution of sensory nerves in the anorectum.

times. Squeeze pressure, therefore, is probably not responsible for maintaining fecal continence from hour to hour. A mechanism that does provide continence is the pressure differential between the rectum (6 cm) and the anal canal (90 cm H_2O).

Anorectal Angle

Another mechanism that helps to maintain hour-to-hour fecal continence, particularly of solid content, is the configuration of the pelvic floor, formed predominantly by the anteriorly directed pull of the puborectal muscle as it envelops the anorectum at the level of the anorectal ring (Fig. 22–32). The result of these anatomic relationships is the *anorectal angle*. Barkel and colleagues found that the mean (±SD) angle was 102 ± 18 degrees at rest in the left lateral position. Standing changed the angle slightly, but sitting widened the angle significantly to 119 ± 17 degrees. Sphincter squeeze, a maneuver that augments anorectal continence, and the Valsalva maneuver, which stresses continence, sharpened the angle to 81 ± 19 degrees and 87 ± 23 degrees, respectively ($P < .05$, lying position) (Fig. 22–33). It has been found that if the angle is normal (puborectalis muscle is competent) but the sphincter is inadequate, continence of solid stool usually is maintained.[156]

The puborectalis muscle also has the property of continuous resting electrical activity, even during sleep. Parks[106] assigned anatomic importance to the anorectal angle in that it enables the anterior wall of the rectum to act as a "flap valve" at the level of the anorectal ring: when intra-abdominal pressures rose, the anterior wall of the rectum would be forced against the top of the anal canal, thus preventing leakage (Fig. 22–34).

The effectiveness of the anorectal angle in situations in which intrarectal pressure may surpass resting anal canal pressure, such as during the Valsalva maneuver or with lifting or coughing, may be augmented by a "flutter valve" effect.[114] The proximal anal canal is subjected to greater forces than is the surrounding gut; this situation could be created by flattening the walls of the anal canal as they pass through an anteroposterior slit in the pelvic diaphragm. This mechanism would have the effect of forcing the walls together during the periods of suddenly increased intra-abdominal pressure (Valsalva, lifting, coughing, and laughing), thus helping to maintain fecal continence (Fig. 22–35).

The angulation between the rectum and anal canal must be overcome in order to evacuate solid enteric content. This is accomplished by squatting; the angle is straightened to greater than 110 degrees by flexing the hips 90 degrees. Straightening of the anorectal angle is augmented by straining, which usually causes the puborectalis muscle and EAS to become electrically silent, although this does not always occur.[66] With the angle overcome, content passes into the anal canal.

In a novel experiment, Finlay and colleagues[38] investigated movements of the pelvic floor during expulsion of air and liquid. They found that expulsion of air was achieved by a sharpening of the anorectal angle and increased anal canal and intrarectal pressures. Conversely, expulsion of liquids was achieved by a widening of the anorectal angle, decreasing anal canal pressure, and increasing intrarectal pressure.

However, the importance of the anorectal angle is controversial. Bartolo and colleagues have demonstrated that during a Valsalva maneuver the anterior rectal wall does not contact the upper sphincter, suggesting that the flap-valve theory is incorrect.[10] Although continence may be improved following the operation of postanal repair, the outcome does not correlate with the change in angle, and in the operation of anterior

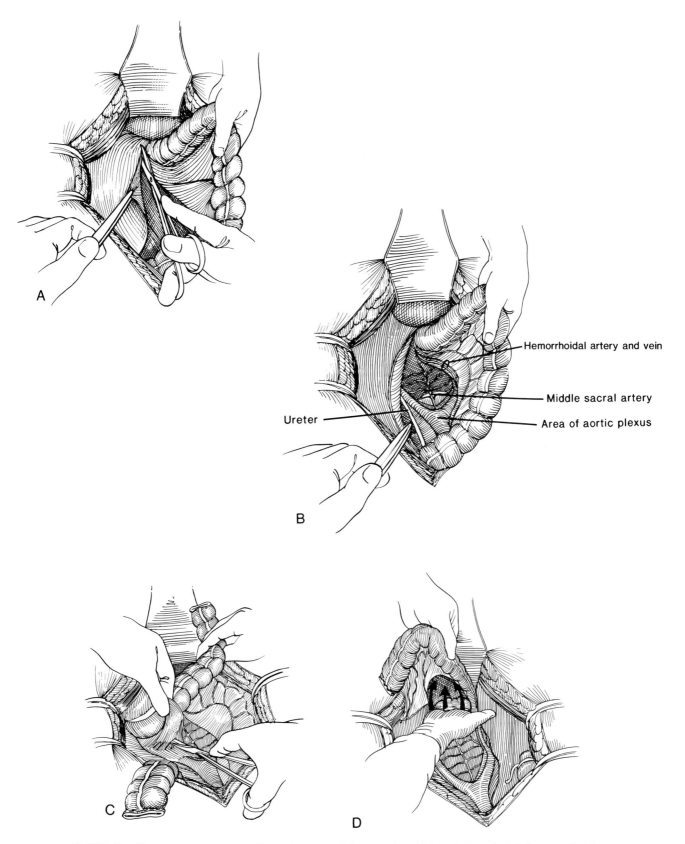

FIGURE 22-28. Pelvic dissection. *A,* The peritoneum of the mesosigmoid is incised on the left by retracting the sigmoid colon firmly out of the pelvis. *B,* The ureter is easily visualized at this point. The mesenteric "window" (underneath the tented superior hemorrhoidal artery and vein) is made carefully, in benign disease, so as not to disturb the aortic plexus. *C,* Access to the presacral (retrorectal) space is achieved by pulling the sigmoid colon up and forward using sharp dissection. *D,* Careful blunt dissection frees the rectum posteriorly to the level of Waldeyer's fascia. *Arrows* indicate the motion of the hand used to loosen the lateral peritoneum and perirectal tissue. *Illustration continued on following page*

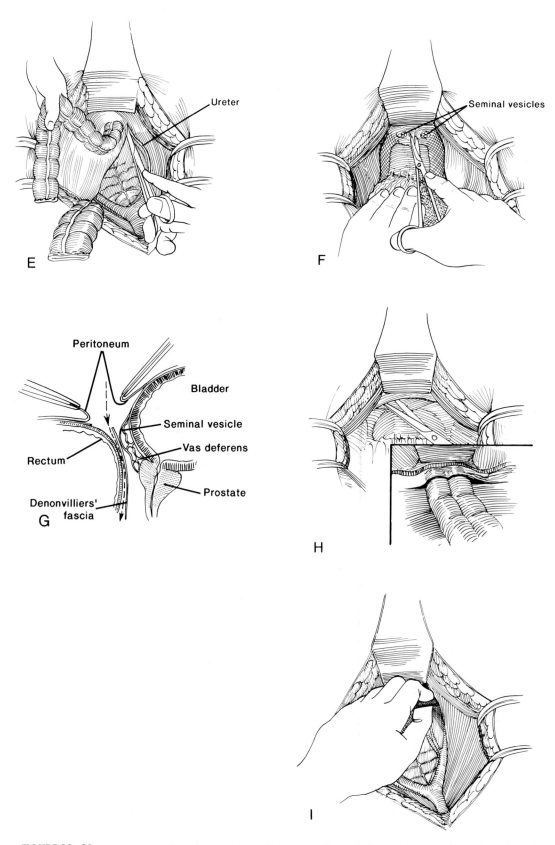

FIGURE 22-28. *Continued E,* The right ureter is usually now seen beneath the peritoneum. The peritoneal incisions meet in the depths of the pouch of Douglas. *F,* The peritoneum is incised. *G* and *H,* Denonvilliers' fascia is pierced with the scissor, allowing access to a bloodless plane posterior to the seminal vesicles (vagina) but anterior to the rectum. This plane is developed with the fingers to the level of the midprostate (or midvagina). *I,* After the lateral peritoneal fascia and lateral rectal tissue are loosened down to the level of the lateral stalks, the stalks themselves are loosened by lifting motions of the dissecting hand. Stalks are defined by pinching motions and, if feasible, they are ligated bilaterally.

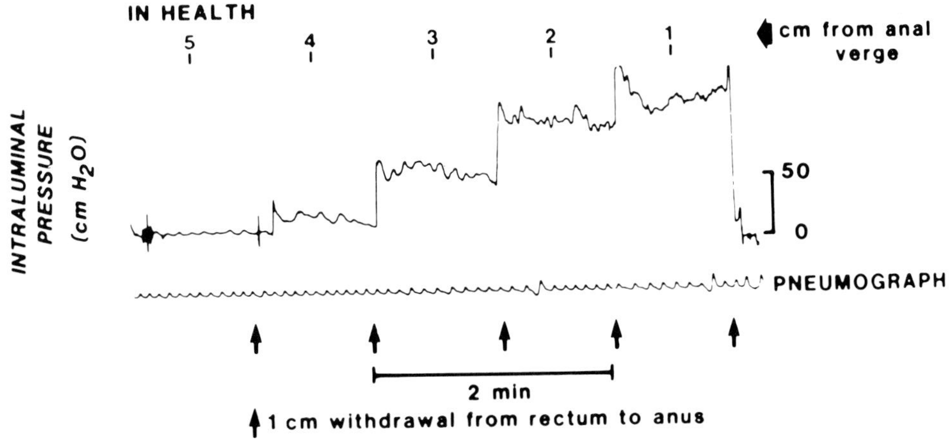

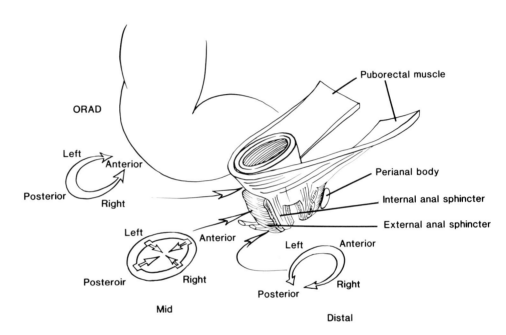

FIGURE 22-29. Perfused single-channel recording of resting anal canal pressure. At 5 cm from the anal verge, the intrarectal pressure is 5 mm Hg. Stepwise withdrawal of the probe shows the highest resting pressure to be 1 to 2 mm proximal to the anal verge.

FIGURE 22-30. The anatomy of the anorectum might explain radial variations in resting pressure. The puborectalis muscle swings around behind the anal canal at its most proximal limit; posterior resting pressures are thus higher than anterior resting pressures. In the midcanal, radial pressures are equally distributed. In the most distal part of the canal, resting pressures are lowest posteriorly and highest anteriorly. (From Taylor, B.M., Beart, R.W., Jr., and Philips, S.F.: Longitudinal and radial variations of pressure in the human anal sphincter. Gastroenterology, *86:*693, 1984, with permission.)

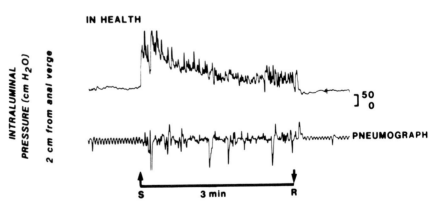

FIGURE 22-31. Anal canal squeeze pressure, in one quadrant, recorded by an indwelling perfused probe positioned 2 cm proximal to the anal verge. The overall duration of elevated pressure was 3 minutes, but the highest incremental pressure was recorded for less than 1 minute.

sphincteroplasty, continence also improves despite the anorectal angle becoming significantly more obtuse.[119,105]

Anorectal Sensation

Sensory mechanisms allow discrimination of the character of enteric content (gas, liquid or solid stool) and detection of the need to pass that content. The site of

these sensory receptors is either in the rectal muscularis or in the surrounding pelvic floor musculature.[160] Moreover, investigators studying patients after coloanal anastomosis, in whom all of the rectal mucosa and most of the rectal muscularis had been removed, found that discrimination persisted. The ability to detect intrarectal pressure differentials was hypothesized by Goligher and Hughes[46] to be important in discriminating content

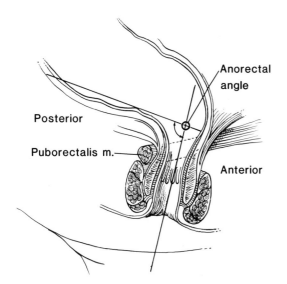

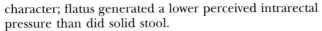

FIGURE 22-32. The angulation between the rectum and anal canal. This angle is formed by the anteriorly directed pull of the puborectalis muscle and is measured at the intersection of a line drawn through the center of the anal canal and a line drawn along the posterior wall of the rectum.

Posterior

Puborectalis m.

Anorectal angle

Anterior

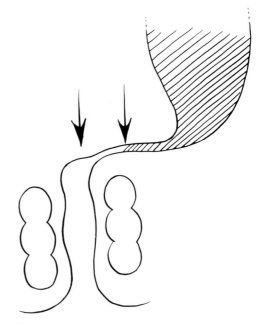

FIGURE 22-34. The "flap valve" effect of the anorectal angle.

character; flatus generated a lower perceived intrarectal pressure than did solid stool.

Duthie and Bennett[32] found that acute sensation resided only in the mucosa of the proximal anal canal. Bartolo and colleagues[10] have confirmed these observations by determining that sensation was most acute in the region of the anal valves. Enteric content, therefore, would have to gain access to the anal canal in order to be distinguished. This would occur if the internal sphincter relaxed in response to rectal distention.

Rectal Anal Sphincter Inhibitory Response

With acute rectal distention, the rectal wall contracts slightly, the proximal portion of the anal canal relaxes (presumably, the IAS), and the distal portion contracts (EAS). This is the rectal anal sphincter inhibitory re-

sponse (RASIR) (Fig. 22–36). Sensory receptors for this response are located in the rectum, and it is likely that the response is mediated by the inhibitory neurotransmitter nitric oxide.[19,101] Shepherd and Wright[134] originally observed that the response might be mediated at the level of the spinal canal. It is now clear that the reflex is due to intramural nerves.[81] The reflex can return, to some extent, following coloanal anastomosis,[78] probably due to nerves growing across the anastomosis. Rapid intermittent balloon distentions cause *prolonged* relaxation of the internal sphincter, whereas continuous distention initially causes the sphincter to relax, with a slow return to resting tone over time.[19] The mechanism mediating this return to baseline resting pressure is likely to be exponential adaptation of the rectum to distention.[3]

The role of the rectal anal sphincter inhibitory re-

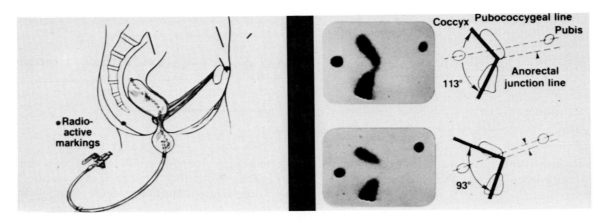

FIGURE 22-33. Scintigraphic imaging of the movements of the anorectal angle. *Left*, Balloon device in place filled with ^{99m}Tc-labeled water. Radioactive markers lie over the pubis and coccyx. *Right*, Scintigraphic image of the anorectal angle at rest (*top*) and during squeeze (*bottom*). To the right are diagrams of the same images. During squeeze, the angle narrows to 93 degrees and the anorectal junction (the level of the pelvic floor) ascends.

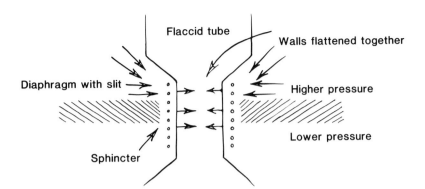

FIGURE 22-35. The "flutter valve" effect present at the pelvic floor.

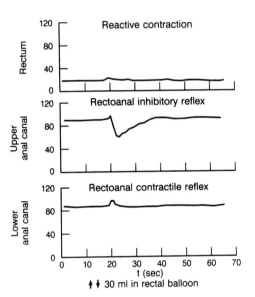

FIGURE 22-36. The rectal anal sphincter inhibitory response is composed of three parts: (1) reactive rectal muscular contraction, (2) relaxation of the internal anal sphincter with decreased resting anal canal pressure, and (3) contraction of the external sphincter. The decrease in resting pressure lasts approximately 20 seconds and always returns to baseline.

sponse is not fully understood. Duthie and Bennett[32] hypothesized that such transient relaxation of the IAS would allow the enteric content to come into contact with the sensitive mucosa of the proximal anal canal (the anal transition zone); its character could then be recognized. If rectal distention continued unabated, however, the external sphincter was inhibited and the perceived need to evacuate became urgent. In an inter-

esting study, Miller and colleagues[92] documented that this sampling response occurred in healthy ambulatory patients between four and ten times per hour. These observations confirm those of Ihre,[61] who found that each passage of enteric content into the rectum is accompanied by internal sphincter relaxation and EAS and puborectalis muscle contraction.

Although this is an attractive hypothesis, its ultimate importance is disputed by findings that after ileoanal anastomosis, the response often cannot be recorded, yet continence is not seemingly affected.[14] Moreover, Ihre[61] found that if enteric content came in contact *only* with the tissues of the anal canal, a distinction between gas and stool could not be made. Finally, Read and Read[123] found that continence to large volumes of saline infused into the rectum was unaffected when local anesthesia was applied to the mucosa of the anal canal.

Rectal Distensibility ("Compliance") and Capacity

The rectum accommodates passively to distention—intraluminal pressure remains low, whereas intraluminal volume increases (Fig. 22–37). The maximal tolerable volume in healthy individuals approximates 400 ml, yet intraluminal pressure remains less than 20 mmHg. By plotting the slope of $\Delta V/\Delta P$, the distensibility of the rectum can be calculated. Heppell and colleagues[55] found it to be 16.8 + 2 ml/cm H_2O (mean + SEM) in seven healthy volunteers. Whether the rectum possesses the gastric fundal property of receptive relaxation—that is, relaxation in *anticipation* of filling from above—is unknown. Rectal distensibility is altered by inflammatory bowel disease so that instead of a distensible "bag," the

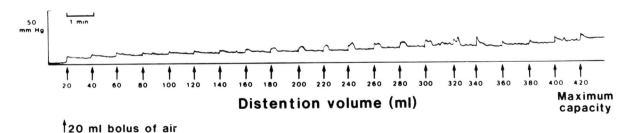

FIGURE 22-37. Effect of distention of an intrarectal balloon on rectal motility. Rectal accommodation ensures little rise in intraluminal pressure even at 420 ml of inflation.

rectum becomes a "lead pipe" conduit for stool between the sigmoid colon and the anal sphincters; patients with active chronic ulcerative colitis invariably have frequency, urgency, tenesmus, and episodes of incontinence that are caused by loss of rectal wall "compliance."

Motility of the Rectum and Anal Canal

Rectum

Resting intraluminal rectal pressure approximates 5 mmHg. Infrequent, small-amplitude contractions have been recorded in the rectum; these do not change in frequency or amplitude as intraluminal volume increases. The mean ($\pm$ SEM) amplitude of these waves is about 10 ± 3 cm H_2O, which is very low. There are three types of rectal contractile activity: (1) simple contractions at a frequency of 5 to 10 cycles/min; (2) contractions (about 3 cycles/min) but with amplitudes of up to 100 cm H_2O; and (3) slow contractions of high amplitude, which appeared to propagate.[130,159] More recently, rectal motor complexes have been described. These are bursts of strong, sustained contractions with an amplitude of up to 50 cm H_2O lasting 3 to 10 minutes and occurring every 80 to 90 minutes during the day and every 50 to 60 minutes during the night.[72,103] Connell[25] found that a gradient for intraluminal contractile activity existed that increased in frequency from the sigmoid colon to the rectum; the hypothesis would be that such a gradient would impede the aboral flow of content. Moreover, pressures within the rectum and anal canal equalize intermittently, either during "sampling"[92] or when content is emptied into the rectum.[61]

Anal Canal

The anal canal exhibits a unique motility pattern; small oscillations of pressure occur at frequencies of about 15 cycles/min with an amplitude of about 10 cm H_2O superimposed on the resting tone (Fig. 22–38). In addition, irregular anal waves with amplitudes of greater than 20 cm H_2O have been observed.[104] An ultraslow wave also can be recorded in 40% of normal subjects,[54] the mean duration of which is 33 seconds with an amplitude of 30 to 100 cm H_2O.[66] There is also a slow wave gradient in the anal canal, the frequency of the slow wave being highest distally.[48,66,112] This would tend to pro-

pel the content back into the rectum, keeping the canal itself clean and ensuring continence.

Characteristics of Rectal Filling and Emptying

Instilling large volumes of material into the rectum results in progressive accommodation to the increasing volume. Importantly, however, the infused material does not remain solely in the rectum; recent studies have shown that about half promptly refluxes into the sigmoid colon and remains there. When evacuation occurs, the sigmoid colon empties first into the rectum, and *then* the rectal volume is evacuated (Fig. 22–39).[98] These results suggest that the sigmoid colon in health plays an active role in maintaining overall continence; only when sufficiently filled would the sigmoid colon empty a portion of its contents into the rectum. Other relationships between the more proximal bowel and the rectum were investigated recently by Kellow and associates[65]; upon distention of the rectum with a balloon, duodenocecal transit during fasting and after feeding was slowed when compared with control values. Gastric emptying also was delayed by rectal distention in studies performed by Youle and Read.[165]

Contribution of Colonic Motility to Fecal Continence

Movements of the Colon Seen Radiographically[73]

RETROGRADE PROPULSION. These contractions originate in the transverse colon, migrate toward the cecum, and may retard the aboral progression of feces.

SEGMENTAL, NONPROPULSIVE MOTILITY. These movements are composed of retrograde *and* anterograde contractions in a single segment of colon and are *not* responsible for aboral progression. Transit through the distal colon is faster than through the right colon.

MASS MOVEMENTS. These movements are characterized by propulsion of large fecal boluses over long segments of the colon. They occur infrequently and have also been seen during defecation. The entire rectum, sigmoid colon, and descending colon empty together.

Electrical Events

Two types of activity are seen in the human colon—slow waves and spike bursts. Slow waves originate in the circular muscle of the colon, are infrequent, and may produce contractions. The longitudinal muscle exhibits a distinctly different slow wave frequency than does the

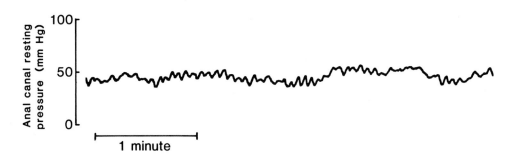

FIGURE 22–38. Single-channel recording of anal canal motility. Superimposed on the resting pressure are small oscillations of pressure that occur at a frequency of 15 cycles/min with an amplitude of about 10 mmHg.

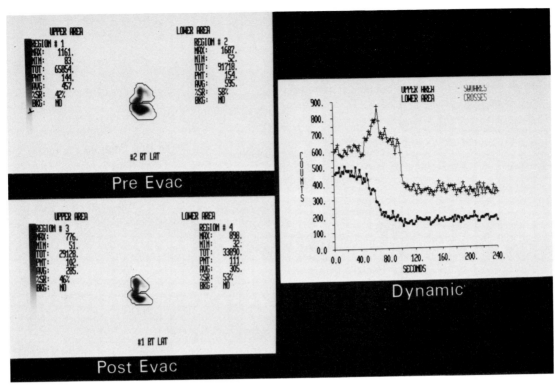

FIGURE 22-39. Patterns of normal rectal filling and emptying. Evacuation dynamics are obtained by gamma-camera imaging of ^{99m}Tc-labeled artificial stool. The infused artificial stool disperses into the sigmoid colon and rectum (*upper left*). A postevacuation scan is seen on the lower left of the figure. On the right side of the figure is a dynamic record of evacuation from the sigmoid colon (*squares*) and rectum (*crosses*). Note that the sigmoid colon empties into the rectum first (counts decrease in the sigmoid and rise in the rectum) and then both evacuate together. The mean evacuation among healthy volunteers is approximately 75% of the stool mass.

circular muscle, but activity of both is linked.[60] These properties of the colonic slow wave differ from the slow wave of the stomach and small bowel. In general, the slow wave frequency is 11 cycles/min proximally, decreasing to about 6 cycles/min in the sigmoid. The site of a possible colonic pacemaker in humans is unknown. In the cat, the pacemaker is in the transverse colon.[23] Torsoli and colleagues[152] found that the transverse and left colon generate pressure waves at greater frequencies than does the right colon; the higher the frequency of contraction, the more the impediment to aboral flow. The rectal slow wave frequency is about 20 cycles/min; a gradient is thus observed between colon and rectum.

Interestingly, recordings of intraluminal pressure from the "rectosigmoid" have shown an area of elevated pressure[51] and high frequency of phasic contraction.[25] Such specialized motility at this site could help prevent the uncontrolled aboral progression of stool from the sigmoid colon to the rectum. Although it is doubtful that a true sphincter (O'Beirne) exists at the rectosigmoid junction, storage at this level is probably facilitated by the firm nature of the stools.[110]

Spike bursts are associated with contractions. Two patterns of colonic spike burst activity have been recorded in humans: short bursts (few seconds) and long bursts (approximately 30 seconds). Reliable correlations between these electrical events and organized movements have not been made.

Stool Volume and Consistency

Colonic absorption of water reduces the 1,000 to 1,500 ml of small bowel content introduced into the cecum each day to about 150 ml/day.[115] This volume is passed with a frequency of three stools per day to three stools per week. The consistency of the stool is usually firm.

If the consistency or volume of the stool changes dramatically, the continence mechanism could be stressed: if small pellets of hard stool are introduced slowly into the rectum, rectal distention and, in turn, perception of the presence of enteric content likely does not occur. Indeed, Bannister and colleagues[5] showed that volunteers defecated large deformable stools more readily and with less strain than small hard pellets. Ambroze and colleagues[2] demonstrated that semisolid stool is more completely evacuated than either solid or liquid stool. Conversely, large volumes of liquid stool emptied rapidly into the rectum may quickly overcome the continence mechanism and incontinence would occur, even in healthy individuals.

The influence of stool volume and consistency in maintaining continence is likely greater than previously believed. By simply changing the character of the stool in some incontinent patients with low resting and squeeze pressures and an obtuse anorectal angle, *continence can be restored.*

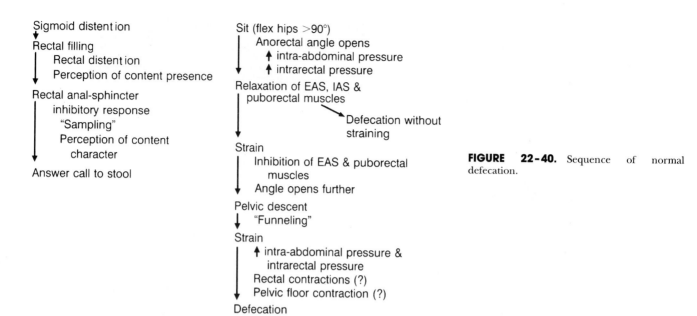

Sigmoid distention
↓
Rectal filling
  Rectal distention
  Perception of content presence
↓
Rectal anal-sphincter
  inhibitory response
    "Sampling"
  Perception of content
    character
↓
Answer call to stool

Sit (flex hips >90°)
↓ Anorectal angle opens
    ↑ intra-abdominal pressure
    ↑ intrarectal pressure
Relaxation of EAS, IAS &
  puborectal muscles
↓   → Defecation without
                      straining
Strain
↓ Inhibition of EAS & puborectal
     muscles
   Angle opens further
Pelvic descent
↓ "Funneling"
Strain
↓ ↑ intra-abdominal pressure &
      intrarectal pressure
   Rectal contractions (?)
   Pelvic floor contraction (?)
Defecation

FIGURE 22-40. Sequence of normal defecation.

Sequence of Defecation (Fig. 22–40)

The sequence of defecation in healthy subjects begins when the volume of enteric content in the sigmoid becomes sufficiently large to trigger contractions, which empty the content into the rectum. Rectal distention follows, and the sensations of the presence of content and its character are perceived. Intermittent but progressive rectal distention initiates the rectoanal sphincter inhibitory response, and the precise nature of the rectal content is determined.

If the choice is made to evacuate the rectum, the sitting position is assumed; sitting renders the anal rectal angle less acute than at rest. Intrarectal and intraabdominal pressure then rises. Such pressure increases result in reflex relaxation of the EAS, IAS, and puborectalis muscles. Some normal subjects then pass the content without straining. Others, however, must strain to initiate rectal emptying. With straining, the EAS, IAS, and puborectalis muscles relax further and the pelvic floor descends, forming a funnel, the outlet of the funnel being the top of the anal canal.

With the pelvic floor descended; a funnel formed; the anorectal angle obtuse; and the EAS, IAS, and puborectalis muscles relaxed, increased intra-abdominal pressure is transmitted directly to the fecal bolus, expelling it. Whether contraction of the rectal wall or the pelvic floor muscles occurs during evacuation is unknown. Furthermore, the contribution of colonic emptying to normal defecation is unknown presently, although it likely plays some role. When emptying is complete, a "closing reflex"[9] occurs, during which the EAS and the puborectalis muscles transiently contract. This reflex promotes recovery of tonic activity of the IAS and closes the anal canal.

Disordered Anorectal Physiology

With the caveat that *normal* anorectal physiology is incompletely understood, several physiologic observations have been made in patients with anorectal disorders.

Hemorrhoids

Hemorrhoids are generally considered to result from downward displacement of specialized cushions of mucosal and submucosal tissue.[150] This theory is supported by the finding of higher sensory thresholds in the upper anal canal mucosa in patients with hemorrhoids, due to the less sensitive rectal mucosa being displaced into the upper anal canal.[127] A high resting anal canal pressure is common in patients with hemorrhoids. In the past, increased IAS activity has been thought to be responsible for this, and the finding of ultraslow waves in 40% of patients with hemorrhoids compared to 8% of controls has been used to support this theory.[50] However, more detailed recent studies have included direct pressure measurement of the anal cushions during rest, coughing and straining, and anal ultrasonography.[141,143] It was found that the IAS is not significantly thicker in patients with hemorrhoids than controls, and it is likely that the high anal pressures are related to increased vascular pressure in the anal cushions, rather than increased IAS activity.

Fissure-in-Ano

Resting anal canal pressure is higher in patients with anal fissures than in controls,[22] the normal internal sphincter relaxation response is followed by an overshoot,[97] and ultraslow waves can be recorded in up to 80% of patients with fissure.[49,131] Whether the high resting pressure and the slow waves are the cause or result of the fissure is unclear. However, these high pressures have been demonstrated to correlate with decreased anodermal blood flow,[132] and this may contribute to the pain and chronicity of this disorder.[43] Topical glyceryl trinitrate, a nitric oxide donor, has been demonstrated to reduce anal pressure in normals.[79] However, the results of further investigations regarding its role in anal fissure, in which chronic fibrotic changes in the IAS are prominent,[18] are awaited.

Rectal Prolapse

The pathogenesis of complete and occult rectal prolapse is intussusception of the rectum. This has been clearly and convincingly documented by Broden and Snellman[17] and Theuerkauf and co-workers[148] (Fig. 22–41). It is not a hernia; herniation of the pouch of Douglas is a common *concomitant* feature of complete rectal prolapse, but it is not the cause. Why the rectum undergoes intussusception is unknown. Interestingly, prolapse may have a familial tendency, and those with progressively systemic sclerosis are predisposed to developing prolapse.[84,77]

Porter[116] performed electromyography in patients with rectal prolapse and found complete and *protracted* inhibition of the puborectalis muscle with straining, which might predispose to prolapse. Because some patients with rectal prolapse also had abnormal descent of the perineum and fecal incontinence, Parks and associates[108] proposed that with prolonged straining at defecation, the pudendal and pelvic nerves would be progressively stretched until injury occurred; the puborectalis and EAS muscles thus become denervated. The puborectalis muscle and the EAS would thus be lax and allow prolapse to progressively form. However, pelvic floor abnormalities cannot be directly responsible for the rectal intussusception itself, which begins 6 to 8 cm *above* the puborectalis muscle.

Disordered defecation with excessive straining is common in patients with prolapse, although this may be due to rather than be the cause of the prolapse.[84] What may occur is that patients have difficulty expelling the content, thus prompting them to strain at stool for prolonged periods of time. Straining sometimes occurs because the puborectalis muscle fails to relax appropriately.[128] In response to the prolonged increase in intra-abdominal pressure, the lax rectum begins to undergo intussusception into itself. With continued straining, the pelvic floor muscles and the EAS may become partially denervated because the pudendal and pelvic nerves are stretched repeatedly. Episodes of incontinence

are the result. As the rectum descends further, patients experience a feeling of continual fullness and strain even more at stool. Eventually, the intussusception is exteriorized. One problem with this hypothesis is that some patients with complete rectal prolapse have no abnormalities of puborectalis or EAS innervation and are not incontinent.

Fecal incontinence accompanies prolapse in 30 to 80% of cases.[161] This may be related to the chronic straining and subsequent pudendal neuropathy.[108] In addition, recurrent prolapse is likely to cause stretch injury to the IAS and EAS. Furthermore, the constant presence of a partly intussuscepted rectum may cause prolonged lowering of IAS tone due to the rectoanal inhibitory reflex,[36] and this may partly be responsible for the incontinence affecting patients with internal prolapse.[62]

Constipation of Childhood

In patients with suspected Hirschsprung's disease, the diagnosis is often made manometrically; the lack of intramural ganglion cells is reflected in a lack of the normal rectal anal sphincter inhibitory response. In other children with constipation but without Hirschsprung's disease, high resting anal canal pressures and loss of rectal sensitivity have been observed.[90]

Pruritus Ani

Eyers and Thomson[34] and Allan and co-workers[1] found that most patients with pruritus ani had normal rectal and anal canal resting pressures but an exaggerated rectal anal sphincter inhibitory response.

Proctalgia Fugax

"Spasm" of the puborectalis, levator ani, and external sphincter muscles is a likely source for the pain associated with proctalgia. It is reported by about 15% of the general population.[149] Recently, a hereditary form of proctalgia fugax associated with constipation and a

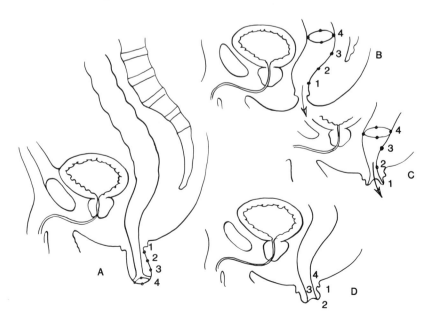

FIGURE 22–41. Cause of rectal prolapse is intussusception of the rectum. *A*, Radiopaque beads are clipped to the prolapse in positions 1 to 4. *B*, The prolapse is reduced. *C*, The patient strains. Bead at position 1 appears first. *D*, Continued straining. Bead at position 2 appears next, followed by bead at position 3, and then those at position 4. (From Theuerkauf, F.J., Beahrs, O.H., and Hill, J.R.: Rectal prolapse: Causation and surgical treatment. Ann. Surg., *171*:819, 1970, with permission.)

grossly thickened, myopathic internal sphincter has been reported.[64] However, proctalgia fugax may be a heterogeneous condition, and Harvey[53] performed motility studies in two patients with frequent episodes of proctalgia and found that episodes of pain were associated with contractions of the sigmoid colon.

Irritable Bowel Syndrome

Several authors have found that the rectum and sigmoid colon of patients with irritable bowel syndrome (IBS) are hypertonic and hypersensitive and exhibit increased contractile activity (frequency and amplitude).[8,159] Moreover, there is an enhanced colonic motor response to meals, stress, and luminal distention.

Pelvic Radiation

Varma and colleagues[155] showed that after pelvic radiation for prostatic cancer in men, maximum anal canal resting pressure and anal canal length were reduced when compared with controls. Moreover, they documented submucosal and intramural nerve plexus damage in these patients; however, the striated muscles were not affected.

Fecal Incontinence

Disorders of the anus and rectum are the most common causes of chronic fecal incontinence, although other etiologies such as cerebral or spinal lesions, multiple sclerosis, diabetes, or severe diarrhea may also cause incontinence.[21,121,142]

Biopsies of the EAS and puborectalis muscles in patients with chronic fecal incontinence often demonstrate histologic changes characteristic of denervation injury with partial reinnervation.[108] Electromyographic changes have confirmed these changes; single-fiber studies have demonstrated increased fiber density, and the terminal motor latency of the pudendal nerve (the time from stimulating the pudendal nerve at the ischial spine to recording an evoked response in the EAS) is prolonged, whereas the latency of the nerve more proximally is usually normal.[67,68,136,162]

It is now recognized that most cases of chronic major fecal incontinence, a disorder generally affecting women, are the result of childbirth.[144] During normal vaginal delivery, the pudendal nerve, which supplies the EAS and pelvic floor muscles, is damaged. The injury may be due to stretching or compression by the fetal head. It has been shown that the pudendal nerve terminal motor latencies are prolonged for up to 3 months following delivery, and the EAS shows electromyographic evidence of denervation followed later by reinnervation.[135] There is also a decrease in anal sensation following childbirth.[26] The neural damage is more likely when the fetal head is large, when the second stage of labor is prolonged, or when forceps are used.[135] The above-mentioned changes are not seen following cesarian section.

It has been recognized for some time that direct damage to the anal sphincters may occur during childbirth, because of perineal tears or midline episiotomies. However, recent studies using anal endosonography have demonstrated that sphincter defects following vaginal delivery can be demonstrated in as many as 87% of women.[29]

Fecal incontinence due to childbirth does not generally occur until many years later, and the changes in anorectal function in these intervening years are not well characterized. It is known that denervation of the pelvic floor is associated with perineal descent, a condition in which the lax perineum lies at a lower point than normal in relation to the bony pelvis and in which the perineum often descends further upon straining at stool (Fig. 22–42). In patients with perineal descent it has been demonstrated that 60 seconds of simulated straining at stool results in a temporary worsening of

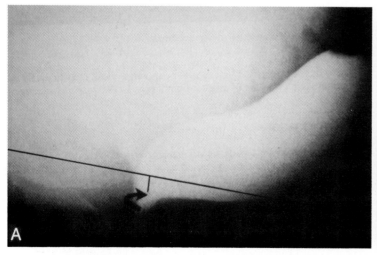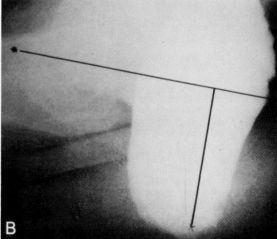

FIGURE 22–42. Defecating proctogram. A, Normal position of the rectum, anorectal angle, and anal canal. B, Gross perineal descent. (From Barthram, C.I., and Makieu, P.H.G.: Radiology and the pelvic floor. In Henry, M.M., and Swash, M. (eds.): Coloproctology and the Pelvic Floor. Pathophysiology and Management. London, Butterworth's, 1985, with permission.)

pudendal neuropathy, with an increase in the pudendal nerve terminal motor latency.[82] Repeated straining may eventually result in incontinence. Chronic straining at stool, with consequent pudendal neuropathy and perineal descent, may also be responsible for some cases of neurogenic fecal incontinence in nulliparous women and in men. However, pudendal neuropathy and perineal descent alone do not account for all the electrophysiologic findings in fecal incontinence.[9] Fecal incontinence, which occurs when rectal pressure exceeds anal pressure, is a complex condition often involving abnormalities of the EAS, IAS, and rectum.

In addition to low squeeze pressures, manometric studies of patients with incontinence usually demonstrate a low resting anal pressure, indicating IAS damage.[140] Abnormally frequent and abnormally prolonged relaxations of the IAS have been demonstrated manometrically and electromyographically, and the IAS electromyogram frequency is decreased in patients with fecal incontinence when compared to controls.[35,80,140] Ultrastructural changes in the IAS have been demonstrated in patients with neurogenic incontinence, with loss of smooth muscle cells, disruption of the relationship of remaining cells, stretching of the elastic tissue, and increased collagen fibril content.[80,145] In vitro studies have demonstrated abnormal adrenergic control and cholinergic sensitivity, suggesting possible autonomic denervation.[80,137,138]

Occasionally, patients with chronic fecal incontinence have normal resting and squeeze pressures, with impaired rectal sensation to balloon insufflation. They fail to contract their EAS in time to compensate for reflex relaxation of the IAS, and can leak small amounts of fluid before they perceive this leakage and voluntarily contract their EAS. Such cases accounted for 8% of cases of incontinence in one series.[140] Other patients have a "hypersensitive" rectum with abnormally high pressure contractions in response to infusion of saline,[122] although these cases are only associated with incontinence when there is also some sphincter weakness.[140] In other patients, decreased rectal compliance appears to be important.[162]

Constipation

The known and suspected causes of constipation are legion. Although it is imperative that relatively obvious causes for constipation (such as endocrine or metabolic disorders, effects of drugs, psychological imbalance, faulty diet, congenital problems such as megacolon or megarectum, rectal tumors, or sigmoid volvulus) be sought, the causes in most patients with severe *chronic* constipation seen by surgeons are colonic dysmotility, disordered defecation, or a combination of both.

Colonic Dysmotility

One form of colonic dysmotility is slow-transit constipation. This term describes an idiopathic disorder of colonic motility characterized by a radiologically normal colon but prolonged transit time. It is primarily a disorder of young women. Intervals between stools gradually become longer until they occur a week or more apart. Fiber supplements, such as psyllium, paradoxically worsen the symptoms. Most patients take laxatives in increasingly large amounts until they are unable to pass a stool spontaneously. The cause of slow-transit constipation has variously been ascribed to an abnormality of the myenteric plexus,[71] abnormal colonic neuronal neuropeptides,[30] impaired motor response to cholinergic stimulation,[12] deficient rectal sensation (no call to stool), laxative abuse, psychological problems, and reduced stool volume. Rectal physiology is abnormal in some patients with slow-transit constipation, with a decreased frequency of rectal motor complexes[11] and an absence of the normal increase in rectal myoelectric activity following eating.[13] Along with the colonic inertia of this condition, gastric and small bowel transit is often slow.[154]

The other major disorder of colonic motility is the constipation-predominant variant of IBS. The likely pathophysiology of IBS is an enhanced motor response of the colon to meals, stress, and luminal distention. Patients with constipation-predominant IBS, unlike those with slow-transit constipation, have episodes of diarrhea and a normal colonic transit time, and they respond appropriately to stool bulking agents.

Abnormal Defecation

Abnormal defecation results from failure of the striated muscles of the pelvic floor to relax upon straining (anismus), failure of the internal sphincter to relax upon rectal distention (Hirschsprung's disease), laxity of the pelvic floor (descending perineum syndrome), rectal intussusception (occult rectal prolapse), complete rectal prolapse (procidentia), anterior rectal herniation (rectocele), posterior rectal herniation, and deficient or ignored rectal sensation. Of these, only Hirschsprung's disease is well characterized pathophysiologically and the role of surgery clearly defined; the aganglionic segment of rectum is removed (or bypassed) and a normal pattern of defecation is restored by a pull-through operation. Hirschsprung's disease, descending perineum syndrome, and rectal prolapse have already been discussed.

Anismus

The clinical findings in patients with anismus include an inability to initiate defecation, incomplete evacuation, a history of manual disimpaction, assuming contorted postures for defecation, laxative and enema abuse, leakage, and rectal "pain."

It has been proposed that the cause of symptoms in patients with anismus is failure of the puborectalis and EAS to relax during defecation straining.[117] This results in a failure of the anorectal angle to straighten during defecation (Fig. 22–43). In some patients with anismus, these muscles not only do not relax during defecation, but paradoxically contract, and many patients are unable to defecate a fluid-filled balloon.[117] However, studies of defecation using plugs, catheters, balloons, or radiology are artificial and findings of paradoxic

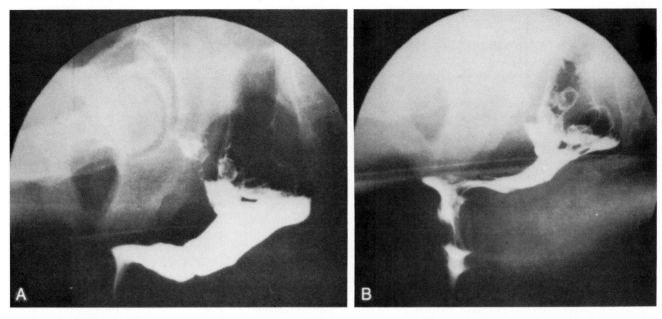

FIGURE 22–43. Series of defecating proctograms illustrating failure of the anorectal angle to widen in response to straining (anismus). (From Bartolo, D.C.C.: Pelvic floor disorders. *In* Schrock, T.R. (ed.): Perspectives in Colon and Rectal Surgery, Vol. 1. St. Louis, Quality Medical Publishing, 1988, with permission.)

contraction may be due to conscious or unconscious restraint by the patient. Findings consistent with paradoxic contraction have been noted in healthy controls and patients who are not constipated.[63,66] In one study, there was no correlation between electromyographic evidence of anismus and the ability of the patient to evacuate the rectum or symptoms of obstructed defecation.[93] Others have demonstrated that patients who evacuate poorly on proctography often do not strain sufficiently to raise their intrarectal pressure enough to defecate.[126] However, of the patients with standard manometric and electrophysiologic evidence of anismus, there may be a core of patients who do suffer paradoxic contraction outside the anorectal laboratory. Twenty per cent of patients with standard electrophysiologic evidence of anismus also demonstrated paradoxic contraction when studied with ambulatory electrophysiologic equipment.[31]

Rectal Herniation

Ihre and Seligson[62] documented by scintiradiography that stool can preferentially fill a rectocele instead of being evacuated (Fig. 22–44). In order to defecate, some women place a finger in the vagina and push backward while straining. Other patients extract the stool digitally from the rectocele, whereas others push up on the perineum.

It is clear that a rectocele can cause difficult defecation and that surgical repair facilitates defecation. However, when is a rectocele functionally significant? The mere presence of a rectocele is meaningless because many women with a rectocele have no problem with defecation.

Posterior hernias have also been described. Upon straining, the posterior rectal wall *appears* to herniate backward and downward through the levator plate (Fig. 22–45). The cause of this defect is unclear. One explanation may be that if the pubococcygeus muscle remains relaxed upon straining, the rectum would progressively protrude into it. The result of such a defect may be that increases in intraabdominal pressure, rather than expelling the stool, merely balloon the rectum posteriorly and caudally, thus making defecation difficult to initiate and complete.

Disturbed Sensation

If the presence of content within the rectum cannot be perceived, stool accumulates and is not expelled. Some investigators have found that in constipated patients, the rectal anal sphincter inhibitory response is blunted. Often the rectum is concomitantly enlarged, but it is not known if this is a primary (congenital) or secondary (acquired) phenomenon. Sometimes patients will ignore the sensation that stool is in the rectum. If this becomes a habit, large volumes of stool accumulate and subsequently become difficult and painful to pass. This may be caused by behavioral problems. Read and colleagues[124] found that 30% of women who were constipated did not experience a desire to defecate. Although the rectal anal sphincter inhibitory response was normal, very large volumes of rectal distention were required to induced sensation.

Evaluation and Management

A flow diagram of the physiologic evaluation of a chronically constipated patient is shown in Figure 22–46. Individual studies are described further on. If there is a *primary colonic cause* for constipation and the pelvic floor functions normally, ileorectostomy may be indicated if symptoms warrant. If the pelvic floor functions abnormally, pelvic floor retraining through operant con-

assessment.[89] Subjects ingest one capsule (in which 20 markers have been placed) each morning for 3 days: abdominal x-ray films are taken on days 4 and 7. Transit through the right, left, and rectosigmoid segments of the colon can be calculated. By this method, transit time through each segment is about 11.5 hours, and total transit time is approximately 36 hours. Men have significant shorter whole colon transit times than do women (33 ± 4 hours versus 47 ± 4 hours; $P < .05$), but age has no effect on colonic transit. More recently, the use of oral radionuclide in the assessment of colonic transit has become established,[87,20] although at present it is not clear that this more expensive technique offers practical advantages.

Although measuring colonic transit is very helpful in assessing patients presenting with constipation,[111] delayed colonic transit does not necessarily mean the colon is abnormal. In one study, normal volunteers were asked to suppress the urge to defecate as much as possible for 1 week, and this resulted in prolonged right colonic, rectosigmoid, and total colonic transit times, consistent with "slow transit constipation."[69] Indeed, such voluntary suppression of defecation also delays a gastric emptying.[151]

Tests of Colonic and Anorectal Function

Anorectal Manometry

Anorectal manometry (ARM) quantifies resting and squeeze pressures of the anal canal high-pressure zone, defines the maximum capacity and distensibility of the rectal ampulla, and measures the presence and appearance of the rectal anal sphincter inhibitory response.

No one technique of manometry is superior to others. What is important is that a range of normal values ob-

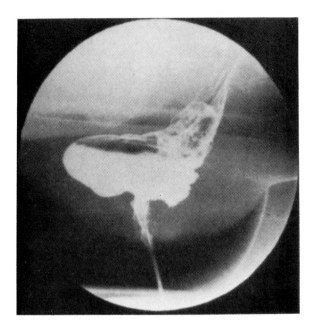

FIGURE 22-44. Defecating proctogram showing filling of a large anterior rectocele. (From Bartolo, D.C.C.: Pelvic floor disorders. *In* Schrock, T.R. (ed.): Perspectives in Colon and Rectal Surgery, Vol. 1. St. Louis, Quality Medical Publishing, 1988, with permission.)

ditioning[15] may be helpful. Anatomic problems causing evacuation difficulties, such as rectocele, rectal prolapse, or aganglionosis, are managed surgically.

Colonic Transit Study

The colonic transit test quantifies the transit time of small radiopaque markers through the colon. A recent modification of an earlier technique has simplified the

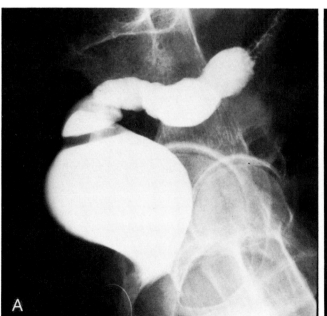
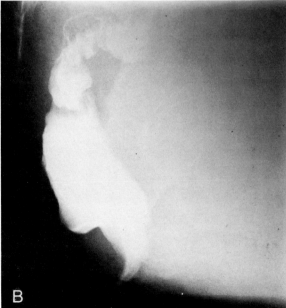

FIGURE 22-45. Defecating proctograms showing "herniation" of the rectum into the pelvic floor posteriorly at rest (*A*) and with straining (*B*).

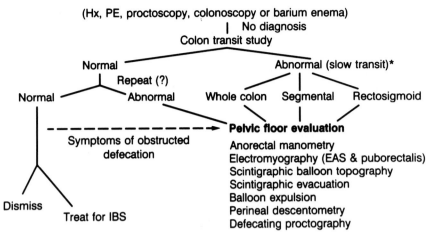

(Hx, PE, proctoscopy, colonoscopy or barium enema)

| No diagnosis

Colon transit study

Normal · · · Abnormal (slow transit)*

Repeat (?)

Normal · · · Abnormal

Whole colon · Segmental · Rectosigmoid

Pelvic floor evaluation

Symptoms of obstructed defecation

Anorectal manometry
Electromyography (EAS & puborectalis)
Scintigraphic balloon topography
Scintigraphic evacuation
Balloon expulsion
Perineal descentometry
Defecating proctography

Dismiss

Treat for IBS

*If symptoms of nausea, vomiting, "heartburn", bloating and/or rapid postprandial distention are present, motility studies of the proximal gut are indicated to exclude a generalized intestinal pseudeo-obstruction

FIGURE 22–46. Flow diagram of evaluation of the severely constipated patient. Patients who have difficulty defecating should undergo pelvic floor examination even if results of colon transit studies are normal.

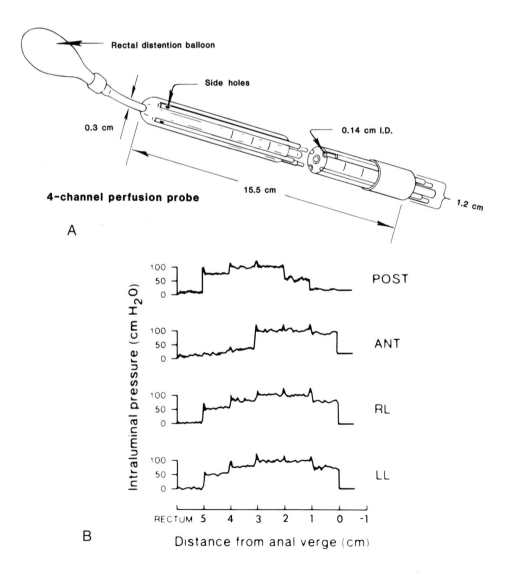

Rectal distention balloon

Side holes

0.3 cm

0.14 cm I.D.

15.5 cm

4-channel perfusion probe

1.2 cm

A

Intraluminal pressure (cm H$_2$O)

100
50
0
POST

100
50
0
ANT

100
50
0
RL

100
50
0
LL

RECTUM 5 4 3 2 1 0 -1

B

Distance from anal verge (cm)

FIGURE 22–47. *A,* Schematic diagram of a 4-channel Plexiglas probe used to perform anorectal manometry. The channels are perfused via a pneumohydraulic perfusion system. The balloon is used to elicit the rectal anal sphincter inhibitory response. (From Taylor, B.M., Phillips, S.F., and Spencer, R.J.: The ileoanal anastomosis. Assessment of continence. *In* Dozois, R.R. (ed.): Alternatives to Conventional Ileostomy. Chicago, Year Book Medical Publishers, 1985, with permission.) *B,* Four-quadrant pull-through resting anal canal pressure recording. Posteriorly, relative pressures are greatest high in the anal canal and least low in the anal canal. Anteriorly, these relationships are reversed. Resting pressures show little variation in the lateral quadrants (see Fig. 22–30).

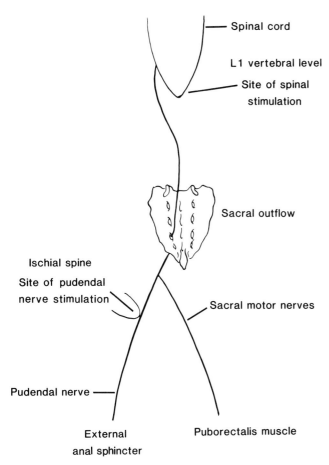

FIGURE 22-48. Sites at which nerve stimulation is performed.

ception (occult rectal prolapse). In addition, defecating proctograms are used to calculate resting and straining anorectal angles. The problem is that positive findings are often misinterpreted, since rectal intussusception sometimes occurs in healthy individuals.

Electromyography

The EAS and puborectalis muscles are studied. Measurements are carried out during rest, during sphincter squeeze, during a Valsalva maneuver in which defecation is actively prevented, and during a straining maneuver simulating attempted defecation. Sphincter defects may also be mapped, although it appears that endoanal ultrasonography maps defects equally well, while causing less pain.[28]

A standard concentric needle is used for initial electromyograhic assessment. Single-fiber techniques are useful for calculation of fiber density of the EAS and puborectalis muscle (see "Fecal Incontinence").

Nerve Stimulation

Spinal and terminal motor latencies are determined by stimulating either transcutaneously over L1 and L4 (spinal motor latency of EAS and puborectalis muscles) or at the exit of the pudendal nerve from the pudendal canal (pudendal nerve terminal motor latency), and recording the arrival of the stimulus at the puborectalis muscle and EAS (Fig. 22-48).

Scintigraphic Balloon Topography (see Fig. 22-33)

This study demonstrates movements of the anorectal angle and pelvic floor with low radiation exposure using scintigraphic techniques. In health, maneuvers such as sphincter squeeze and a Valsalva maneuver narrow the angle and lower the junction.[7] In patients with disorders of continence, these normal movements of the anorectal angle and junction may be disturbed.[113]

Scintigraphic Evacuation (see Fig. 22-29)

In order to quantitate the efficiency of evacuation and determine patterns of evacuation, a test has been developed that radiolabels artificial stool.[98] This scintigraphic imaging material is infused into the rectum to a preestablished maximal rectal capacity. Subjects evacuate and a gamma camera records the pattern and calculates the efficiency of evacuation. Patients with disorders of continence may demonstrate abnormal emptying efficiency and patterns of evacuation.[113]

Mucosal Sensation

Measuring electrosensitivity and temperature sensation in the anal canal are novel techniques designed to quantify the usually subjective parameter of anal canal sensation. Roe and co-workers[127] found that sensory thresholds were elevated in patients with incontinence and hemorrhoids but were reduced (sensation was heightened) in patients with fissure. The more complex

tained from healthy volunteers is available, to which results of ARM from patients with anorectal disorders can be compared.

The results of ARM using a perfused four-channel methylmethacrylate (Plexiglas) probe with four 0.14-cm channels oriented 90 degrees apart are shown in Figure 22-47. The channels are perfused with normal saline (37°C) at the rate of 0.3 ml/min via a low-compliance, pneumohydraulic perfusion system. A balloon attached to a catheter that transverses the middle of the probe allows assessment of the inhibitory reflex and rectal capacity.

This technique provides a sequential pull-through resting pressure profile of the anal canal in four quadrants. The test is repeated, and the subject is asked to squeeze as long as possible with the probe positioned sequentially in the proximal, middle, and distal anal canal. The probe is then repositioned in the proximal anal canal, and the rectal balloon is inflated and immediately deflated in 5-ml increments in order to elicit proximal anal canal relaxation (the rectal anal sphincter inhibitory response).

Defecating Proctography

The defecating proctography examination has gained increasing popularity (see Fig. 22-42 through 22-45).[8,74,85] The primary usefulness of defecating proctography is in determining the presence of rectal intussus-

technique of measuring temperature sensation likewise showed impairment of sensation in patients with incontinence.[91]

REFERENCES

1. Allan, A., Ambrose, N.S., Silverman, S., and Keighley, M.R.B.: Physiological study of pruritus ani. Br. J. Surg., 75:576, 1987.
2. Ambroze, W.L., Pemberton, J.H., Bell, A.M., et al.: The effect of stool consistency on rectal and neorectal emptying. Dis. Colon Rectum, 34:1, 1991.
3. Arhan, P., Devroede, G., Persoz, B., et al.: Response of the anal canal to repeated distension of the rectum. Clin. Invest. Med., 2:83, 1979.
4. Ayoub, S.E.: Arterial supply to the human rectum. Acta Anat. (Basel), 100:317, 1978.
5. Bannister, J.J., Davison, P., Timms, J.M., et al.: Effect of stool size and consistency on defecation. Gut, 28:1246, 1987.
6. Bannister, J.J., Gibbons, C., and Read, N.W.: Preservation of faecal continence during rises in intra-abdominal pressure: Is there a role for the flap valve? Gut, 28:1242, 1987.
7. Barkel, D.C., Pemberton, J.H., Pezim, M.E., et al.: Scintigraphic assessment of the anorectal angle in health and after ileal pouch-anal anastomosis. Ann. Surg., 208:42, 1988.
8. Bartolo, D.C.C.: Pelvic floor disorders. In Schrock, T.R. (ed.): Perspectives in Colon and Rectal Surgery, Vol. 1. St. Louis, Quality Medical Publishing, 1988, p. 1.
9. Bartolo, D.C.C., Read, N.W., Jarratt, J.A., et al.: Differences in anal sphincter function and clinical presentation in patients with pelvic floor descent. Gastroenterology, 85:68, 1983.
10. Bartolo, D.C.C., Roe, A.M., Locke-Edmunds, J.C., et al.: Flap-valve theory of anorectal continence. Br. J. Surg., 73:1012, 1986.
11. Bassotti, G., Betti, C., Antonietta, M., and Morelli, A.: Prolonged (24-hour) manometric of rectal contractile activity in patients with slow transit constipation. Digestion, 49:72, 1991.
12. Bassotti, G., Chiarioni, G., Imbimbo, B.P., et al.: Impaired colonic motor response to cholinergic stimulation in patients with severe chronic idiopathic (slow transit type) constipation. Dig. Dis. Sci., 38:1040, 1993.
13. Bassotti, G., Morelli, A., and Whitehead, W.E.: Abnormal rectosigmoid myoelectric response to eating in patients with severe idiopathic constipation (slow-transit type). Dis. Colon Rectum, 35:753, 1992.
14. Beart, R.W., J.R., Dozois, R.R., Wolff, B.G., and Pemberton, J.H.: Mechanisms of rectal continence: Lessons from the ileoanal procedure. Am. J. Surg., 149:31, 1985.
15. Bleijenberg, G., and Kuijpers, J.H.C.: Treatment of spastic pelvic floor syndrome with biofeedback. Dis. Colon Rectum, 30(2):108, 1987.
16. Block, I.R., and Enquist, I.F.: Studies pertaining to local spread of carcinoma of the rectum in females. Surg. Gynecol. Obstet., 112:41, 1961.
17. Brodén, B., and Snellman, B.: Procidentia of the rectum studied with cineradiography. A contribution to the discussion of conservative mechanisms. Dis. Colon Rectum, 11:330, 1968.
18. Brown, A.C., Sumfest, J.M., and Rozwadowski, J.V.: Histopathology of the internal and sphincter in chronic anal fissure. Dis. Colon Rectum, 32:680, 1989.
19. Burleigh, D.E., and D'Mello, A.: Neural and pharmacologic factors affecting motility of the internal anal sphincter. Gastroenterology, 84:409, 1983.
20. Camilleri, M., and Zinsmeister, A.R.: Towards a relatively inexpensive, noninvasive, accurate test for colonic motor disorders. Gasteoenterology, 103:36, 1992.
21. Caruana, B.J., Wald, A., Hinds, J.P., and Eidelman, H.: Anorectal sensory and motor function in neurogenic fecal incontinence. Comparison between multiple sclerosis and diabetes mellitus. Gastroenterology, 100:465, 1991.
22. Cerdan, F.J., de Leon, A.R., Azpiroz, F., et al.: Anal sphincter measures in fissure-in-ano before and after lateral internal sphincterotomy. Dis. Colon Rectum, 25:198, 1982.
23. Christensen, J.: Motility of the colon. In Johnson, L.R. (ed.): Physiology of the Gastrointestinal Tract. New York, Raven Press, 1987, p. 665.
24. Coller, J.A.: Clinical application of anorectal manometry. Gastroenterol. Clin. North Am., 16:17, 1987.
25. Connell, A.M.: The motility of the pelvic colon: Motility in normals and in patients with asymptomatic duodenal ulcers. Gut, 2:175, 1961.
26. Cornes, H., Bartolo, D.C.C., and Stirrat, G.M.: Changes in anal canal sensation after childbirth. Br. J. Surg., 78:74, 1991.
27. Crapp, A.R., and Cuthbertson, A.M.: William Waldeyer and the rectosacral fascia. Surg. Gynecol. Obstet., 138:252, 1974.
28. Deen, K.I., Kumar, D., Williams, J.G., et al.: Anal sphincter defects. Correlation between endoanal ultrasound and surgery. Ann. Surg., 218:201, 1993.
29. Deen, K.I., Kumar, D., Williams, J.G., et al.: The prevalence of anal sphincter defects in fecal incontinence: A prospective endoscopic study. Gut, 34:685, 1993.
30. Dolk, A., Broden, G., Holmstrom, B., et al.: Slow transit chronic constipation (Arbuthnot Lane's disease). An immunohistochemical study of neuropeptide-containing nerves in resected specimens from the large bowl. Int. J. Colorect. Dis., 5:181, 1990.
31. Duthie, G.S., and Bartolo, D.C.C.: Anismus: The cause of constipation? Results of investigation and treatment. World J. Surg., 16:831, 1992.
32. Duthie, H.L., and Bennett, R.C.: The relation of sensation in the anal canal to the functional anal sphincter. A possible factor in anal continence. Gut, 4:179, 1963.
33. Duthie, H.L., and Gairns, F.N.: Sensory nerve-endings and sensation in the anal region of man. Br. J. Surg., 47:585, 1960.
34. Eyers, A.A., and Thomson, J.P.S.: Pruritus ani: Is anal sphincter dysfunction important in aetiology? BMJ, 2:1549, 1979.
35. Farouk, R., Duthie, G.S., Pryde, A., et al.: Internal and sphincter dysfunction in neurogenic fecal incontinence. Br. J. Surg., 80:259, 1993.
36. Farouk, R., Duthie, G.S., Bartolo, D.C.C., and MacGregor, A.B.: Restoration of continence following rectopexy for rectal prolapse and recovery of the internal anal sphincter electromyogram. Br. J. Surg., 79:439, 1992.
37. Fazio, V.W., Fletcher, J., and Montague, D.: Prospective study of the effect of resection of the rectum on male sexual function. World J. Surg., 4:149, 1980.
38. Finlay, J.G., Carter, K., and McLeod, I.: A comparison of intrarectal infusion of gas and mass on anorectal angle and anal canal pressure (Abstract). Br. J. Surg., 73:1025, 1986.
39. Floyd, W.F., and Walls, E.W.: Electromyography of the sphincter ani externus in man. J. Physiol., 122:599, 1953.
40. Foster, M.E., Lancaster, J.B., and Leaper, D.J.: Leakage of low rectal anastomosis: An anatomic explanation? Dis. Colon Rectum, 27:157, 1984.
41. Frenckner, B.: Function of the anal sphincters in spinal man. Gut, 16:638, 1975.
42. Frenckner, B., and Euler, C.V.: Influence of pudendal block on the function of the anal sphincters. Gut, 16:482, 1975.
43. Gibbons, C.P., and Read, N.W.: Anal hypertonia in fissures: Cause or effect. Br. J. Surg., 73:443, 1986.
44. Goldberg, S.M., Gordon, P.H., and Nivatvongs, S.: Essentials of Anorectal Surgery. Philadelphia, J.B. Lippincott, 1980.
45. Goligher, J.C.: Surgery of the Anus, Rectum and Colon, 5th ed. London, Bailliere Tindall, 1984.
46. Goligher, J.C., and Hughes, E.S.R.: Sensibility of the rectum and colon: Its role in the mechanism of anal continence. Lancet, 1:543, 1951.
47. Gowers, W.: The anatomic action of the sphincter ani. Proc. R. Soc. Med., 26:77, 1877.
48. Hancock, B.D.: Measurement of anal pressure and motility. Gut, 17:645, 1976.
49. Hancock, B.D.: The internal sphincter and anal fissure. Br. J. Surg., 64:92, 1977.
50. Hancock, B.D., and Smith, K.: The internal sphincter and Lord's procedure for haemorrhoids. Br. J. Surg., 62:833, 1975.
51. Hardcastle, J.D., and Mann, C.V.: Study of large bowel peristalsis. Gut, 9:512, 1968.
52. Hardcastle, J.D., and Parks, A.G.: A study of anal incontinence and some principles of surgical treatment. Proc. Soc. Med. 63(Suppl):116, 1970.
53. Harvey, R.F.: Colonic motility in proctalgia fugax. Lancet, 2:713, 1979.

54. Haynes, W.G., and Read, N.W.: Ano-rectal activity in man during rectal infusion of saline: A dynamic assessment of the anal continence mechanism. J. Physiol., 330:45, 1982.
55. Heppell, J., Kelly, K.A., Phillips, S.E., et al.: Physiologic aspects of continence after colectomy, mucosal proctectomy, and endorectal ileo-anal anastomosis. Ann. Surg., 195:435, 1982.
56. Heppell, J., Pemberton, J. Kelly, K.A., and Phillips, S.F.: Ileal motility after endorectal ileoanal anastomosis. Surg. Gastroenterol., 1:123, 1982.
57. Heppell, J., Taylor, B.M., Beart, R.W., Jr., et al.: Predicting outcome after endorectal ileoanal anastomosis. Can. J. Surg., 26:132, 1983.
58. Hinton, J.M., and Lennard-Jones, J.E.: Constipation: Definition and classification. Postgrad. Med. J., 44:720, 1968.
59. Hoffman, M.J., Kodner, I.J., and Fry, R.D.: Internal intussusception of the rectum: Diagnosis and surgical management. Dis. Colon Rectum, 27:435, 1984.
60. Huizinga, J.D., Chow, E., Diamant, N.W., and El-Sharkawy, T.Y.: Coordination of electrical activities in muscle layers of the pig colon. Am. J. Physiol., 252:G136, 1987.
61. Ihre, T.: Studies on anal function in continent and incontinent patients. Scand. J. Gastroenterol., 25(Suppl.):1, 1974.
62. Ihre, T., and Seligson, U.: Intussusception of the rectum—internal procidentia: Treatment and results in 90 patients. Dis. Colon Rectum, 18:391, 1975.
63. Jones, P.N., Lubowski, D.Z., Swash, M., and Henry, M.M.: Is paradoxical contraction of puborectalis muscle of functional importance? Dis. Colon Rectum, 30:667, 1987.
64. Kamm, M.A., Hoyle, C.H.V., Burleigh, D.E., et al.: Hereditary internal anal sphincter myopathy causing proctalgia fugax and constipation. A newly identified condition. Gastroenterology, 100:805, 1991.
65. Kellow, J.E., Gill, R.C., and Wingate, D.L.: Modulation of human upper gastrointestinal motility by rectal distension. Gut, 28:864, 1987.
66. Kerremans, R.: Morphological and Physiological Aspects of Anal Continence and Defaecation. Arscia, Ultgavin, Brussel, 1969.
67. Kiff, E.S., and Swash, M.: Normal proximal and delayed distal conduction in the pudendal nerves of patients with idiopathic (neurogenic) faecal incontinence. J. Neurol. Neurosurg. Psychiatr., 47:820, 1984.
68. Kiff, E.S., and Swash, M.: Slowed conduction in the pudendal nerves in idiopathic (neurogenic) faecal incontinence. Br. J. Surg., 71:614, 1984.
69. Klauser, A.G., Voderholzer, W.A., Heinrich, C.A., et al.: Behavioral modification of colonic function. Can constipation be learned? Dig. Dis. Sci., 35:1271, 1990.
70. Krevsky, B., Malmud, L.S., D'Ercole, F., et al.: Colonic transit scintigraphy: A physiologic approach to the quantitative measurement of colonic transit in humans. Gastroenterology, 91:1102, 1986.
71. Krishnamurthy, S., Schuffler, M.D., Rohrmann, C.A., and Pope, C.E., II: Severe idiopathic constipation is associated with a distinctive abnormality of the colonic myoenteric plexus. Gastroenterology, 88:26, 1985.
72. Kumar, D., Williams, N.S., Waldron, D., and Wingate, D.L.: Prolonged manometric recording of anorectal motor activity in ambulant human subjects: Evidence of periodic activity. Gut, 30:1007, 1989.
73. Kumar, D., and Wingate, D.L.: Fecal continence, defecation and colorectal motility. B. Colorectal motility. In Henry, M.M., and Swash, M. (eds.): Coloproctology and the Pelvic Floor: Pathophysiology and Management. London, Butterworths, 1985, p. 47.
74. Kuijpers, H.C., and Strijk, S.P.: Diagnosis of disturbances of continence and defecation. Dis. Colon Rectum, 27:685, 1984.
75. Lane, R.H.S., and Parks, A.G.: Function of the anal sphincters following colo-anal anastomosis. Br. J. Surg., 64:596, 1977.
76. Lee, J.F., Mauer, V.M., and Block, G.E.: Anatomic relations of pelvic autonomic nerves to pelvic operations. Arch. Surg., 107:324, 1973.
77. Leighton, J.A., Valdovinos, M.A., Pemberton, J.H., et al.: Anorectal dysfunction and rectal prolapse in progressive systemic sclerosis. Dis. Colon Rectum, 36:182, 1993.
78. Lewis, W.G., Holdsworth, P.J., Stephenson, B.M., et al.: Role of the rectum in the physiological and clinical results of coloanal and colorectal anastomosis after anterior resection for rectal carcinoma. Br. J. Surg., 79:1082, 1992.
79. Loder, P.B., Kamm, M.A., Nicholls, R.J., and Phillips, R.K.S.: Topical glyceryl trinitrate: Reversible chemical sphincterotomy. Dis. Colon Rectum., 36:P22, 1993.
80. Lubowski, D.Z., Nicholls, R.J., Burleigh, D.E., and Swash, M.: Internal anal sphincter in neurogenic fecal incontinence. Gastroenterology, 95:997, 1988.
81. Lubowski, D.Z., Nicholls, R.J., Swash, M., and Jordan, M.J.: Neural control of internal anal sphincter function. Br. J. Surg., 74:668, 1987.
82. Lubowski, D.Z., Swash, M., Nicholls, R.J., and Henry, M.M.: Increase in pudendal nerve terminal motor latency with defecation straining. Br. J. Surg., 75:1095, 1988.
83. Lunniss, P.J., and Phillips, R.K.S.: Anatomy and function of the anal longitudinal muscle. Br. J. Surg., 79:882, 1992.
84. Madden, M.V., Kamm, M.A., Nicholls, R.J., et al.: Abdominal rectopexy for complete prolapse: Prospective study evaluating changes in symptoms and anorectal function. Dis. Colon Rectum, 35:48, 1992.
85. Mahieu, P., Pringot, J., and Bodart, P.: Defecography. I. Description of a new procedure and results in normal patients. II. Contribution to the diagnosis of defecation disorders. Gastrointest. Radiol., 9:247, 253, 1984.
86. McHugh, S.M., and Diamant, N.E.: Anal canal pressure profile: A reappraisal as determined by rapid pullthrough technique. Gut, 28:1234, 1987.
87. McLean, R.G., Smart, R.C., Gaston-Parry, D., et al.: Colon transit scintigraphy in health and constipation using oral iodine-131-cellulose. J. Nucl. Med., 31:985, 1990.
88. Meagher, A.P., Adams, W.J., and Lubowski, D.Z.: Autonomic nerves cross the plane of posterior rectal dissection. Dis. Colon Rectum, 36:P25, 1993.
89. Metcalf, A.M., Phillips, S.F., Zinsmeister, A.R., et al.: Simplified assessment of segmental colonic transit. Gastroenterology, 92:40, 1987.
90. Meunier, P., Marechal, J.M., and DeBeaujeu, M.J.: Rectoanal pressures and rectal sensitivity studies in chronic childhood constipation. Gastroenterology, 77:330, 1979.
91. Miller, R., Bartolo, D.C.C., Cervero, F., and Mortensen, N.J.: Anorectal sampling: A comparison of normal and incontinent patients. Br. J. Surg., 75:44, 1988.
92. Miller, R., Bartolo, D.C.C., Cervero, F., and Mortensen, N.J.: Anorectal temperature sensation: A comparison of normal and incontinent patients. Br. J. Surg., 74:511, 1987.
93. Miller, R., Duthie, G.S., Bartolo, D.C.C., et al.: Anismus in patients with normal and slow transit constipation. Br. J. Surg., 78:690, 1991.
94. Mundy, A.R.: An anatomical explanation for bladder dysfunction following rectal and uterine surgery. Br. J. Urol., 54:501, 1982.
95. Nivatvongs, S., Stern, H.S., and Fryd, D.S.: The length of the anal canal. Dis. Colon Rectum, 24:600, 1981.
96. Northover, J.M.A.: Hereditary internal anal sphincter myopathy causing proctalgia fugax and constipation. A newly identified condition. Gastroenterology, 100:805, 1991.
97. Nothmann, B.J., and Schuster, M.M.: Internal anal sphincter derangement with anal fissures. Gastroenterology, 67:216, 1974.
98. O'Connell, P.R., Kelly, K.A., and Brown, M.L.: Scintigraphic assessment of neorectal motor function. J. Nucl. Med., 27:460, 1986.
99. O'Connell, P.R., Pemberton, J.H., and Kelly, K.A.: Motor correlates of defecation after ileal pouch-anal anastomosis (Abstract). Dig. Dis. Sci., 30:785, 1985.
100. O'Connell, P.R., Stryker, S.J., Metcalf, A.M., et al.: Anal canal pressure and motility after ileoanal anastomosis. Surg. Gynecol. Obstet., 166:47, 1988.
101. O'Kelly, T.J., Brading, A., Mortensen, N.J.McC.: Nerve mediated relaxation of the human internal anal sphincter: The role of nitric oxide. Gut, 34:689, 1993.
102. O'Kelly, T.J., Brading, A., and Mortensen, N.J.McC.: In vitro response of the anal canal longitudinal muscle layer to cholinergic and adrenergic stimulation: Evidence of sphincter specialization. Br. J. Surg., 80:1337, 1993.
103. Orkin, B.A., Hansan, R.B., and Kelly, K.A.: The rectal motor complex. J. Gastrointest. Motil., 1:5, 1989.
104. Orkin, B.A., Hanson, R.B., Kelly, K.A., et al.: Human anal motility

while fasting and during sleep. Gastroenterology, *100*:1016, 1991.

105. Orrom, W.J., Miller, R., Cornes, H., et al.: Comparison of anterior sphincteroplasty and postanal repair in the treatment of idiopathic fecal incontinence. Dis. Colon Rectum, *34*:305, 1991.

106. Parks, A.G.: Anorectal incontinence. Proc. Soc. Med., *68*:681, 1975.

107. Parks, A.G., Porter, N.H., and Hardcastle, J.: The syndrome of the descending perineum. Proc. Soc. Med., *59*:477, 1966.

108. Parks, A.G., Swash, M., and Urich, H.: Sphincter denervation in anorectal incontinence and rectal prolapse. Gut, *18*:656, 1977.

109. Pemberton, J.H., and Kelly, K.A.: Achieving enteric continence: Principles and applications. Mayo Clin. Proc., *61*:586, 1986.

110. Pemberton, J.H., and Phillips, S.F.: Colonic absorption. *In* Schrock, T.R. (ed.): Perspectives in Colon and Rectal Surgery. St. Louis, Quality Medical Publishing, 1988, p. 89.

111. Pemberton, J.H., Rath, D.M., and Ilstrup, D.M.: Evaluation and surgical treatment of severe chronic constipation. Ann. Surg., *214*:403, 1991.

112. Penninckx, F., Kerremans, R., and Beckers, J.: Pharamacological characteristics of the nonstriated anorectal musculature in cats. Gut, *14*:393, 1973.

113. Pezion, M., Pemberton, J.H., Philips, S.F., et al.: The immobile perineum: Pathophysiologic implications in severe constipation (Abstract). Dig. Dis. Sci., *32*:924, 1984.

114. Phillips, S.F., and Edwards, D.A.W.: Some aspects of anal continence and defaecation. Gut, *6*:396, 1965.

115. Phillips, S.F., and Giller, J.: The contribution of the colon to electrolyte and water conservation in man. J. Lab. Clin. Med., *81*:733, 1973.

116. Porter, N.H.: A physiological study of the pelvic floor in rectal prolapse. Ann. Coll. Surg. Engl., *31*:379, 1962.

117. Preston, D.M., and Lennard-Jones, J.E.: Anismus in chronic constipation. Dig. Dis. Sci., *30*:413, 1985.

118. Quer, E.A., Daklin, D.C., and Mayo, C.W.: Retrograde intramural spread of carcinoma of the rectum and rectosigmoid: A microscopic study. Surg. Gynecol. Obstet., *96*:24, 1953.

119. Rainey, J.B., Donaldson, D.R., and Thomson, J.P.S.: Postanal repair: Which patients derive most benefit? J. R. Coll. Surg. Edinb., *35*:101, 1990.

120. Rattan, S., and Chakder, S.: Role of nitric oxide as a mediator of internal anal sphincter relaxation. Am. J. Physiol., *262*:G107, 1992.

121. Read, N.W., Harford, W.V., Schmulen, A.C., et al.: A clinical study of patients with fecal incontinence and diarrhea. Gastroenterology, *76*:747, 1979.

122. Read, N.W., haynes, W.G., Bartolo, D.C.C., et al.: Use of anorectal manometry during rectal infusion of saline to investigate sphincter function in incontinent patients. Gastroenterology, *85*:105, 1983.

123. Read, M.G., and Read, N.W.: The role of anorectal sensation in preserving continence. Gut, *23*:345, 1982.

124. Read, N.W., Timms, J.M., Barfield, L.J., et al.: Impairment of defecation in young women with severe constipation. Gastroenterology, *90*:53, 1986.

125. Ritchie, J.: Pain from distention of the pelvic colon by inflating a balloon in the irritable colon syndrome. Gut, *14*:125, 1973.

126. Roberts, J.P., Womack, N.R., Hallan, R.I., et al.: Evidence for dynamic integrated proctography to redefine anismus. Br. J. Surg., *79*:1213, 1992.

127. Roe, A.M., Bartolo, D.C.C., and Mortensen, N.J.: New method for assessment of anal sensation in various anorectal disorders. Br. J. Surg., *73*:310, 1986.

128. Rutter, K.R.P.: Electromyographic changes in certain pelvic floor abnormalities. Proc. Soc. Med., *67*:53, 1974.

129. Sato, K., and Sato, T.: The vascular and neuronal composition of the lateral ligament of the rectum and the rectosacral fascia. Surg. Radiol. Anat., *13*:17, 1991.

130. Scharli, A.F., and Kiesewetter, W.B.: Defecation and continence: Some new concepts. Dis. Colon Rectum, *13*:81, 1970.

131. Schouten, W.R., and Blankensteijn, J.D.: Ultra slow wave pressure variations in the anal canal before and after lateral internal sphincterotomy. Int. J. Colorect. Dis., *7*:115, 1992.

132. Schouten, W.R., Briel, J.W., and Auwerda, J.J.A.: Relationship between anal pressure and anodermal bloodflow: The vascular pathogenesis of anal fissure. Dis. Colon Rectum., *36*:P11, 1993.

133. Schuster, M.M.: Motor action of rectum and anal sphincters in continence and defecation. *In* Cade, C.F., and Heidel, W. (eds.): Handbook of Physiology, Section 6: Alimentary Canal, Vol. 4, Washington, D.C., American Physiological Society, 1968, p. 2121.

134. Shepherd, J.J., and Wright, P.G.: The response of the internal anal sphincter in man to stimulation of the presacral nerve. Am. J. Dig. Dis., *13*:421, 1968.

135. Snooks, S.J., Setchell, M., Swash, M., and Henry, M.M.: Injury to the innervation of pelvic floor sphincter musculature in childbirth. Lancet, *2*:546, 1984.

136. Snooks, S.J., and Swash, M.: Nerve stimulation techniques. *In* Henry, M.M., and Swash, M. (eds.): Coloproctology and the Pelvic Floor: Pathophysiology and Management. London, Butterworths, 1985, p. 112.

137. Speakman, C.T.M., Hoyle, C.H.V., Kamm, M.A., et al.: Adrenergic control of the internal anal sphincter is abnormal in patients with idiopathic fecal incontinence. Br. J. Surg., *77*:1342, 1990.

138. Speakman, C.T.M., Hoyle, C.H.V., Kamm, M.A., et al.: Decreased sensitivity of muscarinic but not 5-hydroxytryptamine receptors of the internal anal sphincter in neurogenic fecal incontinence. Br. J. Surg., *79*:829, 1992.

139. Stephens, E.D., and Smith, E.D.: Ano-rectal Malformation in Children. Chicago, Year Book Medical Publishers, 1971.

140. Sun, W.M., Donnelly, T.C., and Read, N.W.: Utility of a combined test of anorectal manometry, electromyography, and sensation in determining the mechanism of "idiopathic" fecal incontinence. Gut, *33*:807, 1992.

141. Sun, M.W., Peck, R.J., Shorthouse, A.J., and Read, N.W.: Hemorrhoids are associated not with hypertrophy of the internal anal sphincter, but with hypertension in the anal cushions. Br. J. Surg., *79*:592, 1992.

142. Sun, M.W., Read, N.W., and Donnelly, T.C.: Anorectal function in incontinent patients with cerebrospinal disease. Gastroenterology, *99*:1372, 1990.

143. Sun, M.W., Read, N.W., and Shorthouse, A.J.: Hypertensive anal cushions as a cause of the high anal canal pressures in patients with hemorrhoids. Br. J. Surg., *77*:458, 1990.

144. Swash, M.: Fecal incontinence. Childbirth is responsible in most cases. BMJ, *307*:636, 1993.

145. Swash, M., Gray, A., Lubowski, D.Z., and Nicholls, R.J.: Ultrastructural changes in internal anal sphincter in neurogenic fecal incontinence. Gut, *29*:1692, 1988.

146. Swash, M., and Snooks, S.J.: Electromyography in pelvic floor disorders. *In* Henry, M.M., and Swash, M. (eds.): Coloproctology and the Pelvic Floor: Pathophysiology and Management. London, Butterworth's, 1985, p. 88.

147. Taylor, B.M., Beart, R.W., Jr., and Phillips, S.F.: Longitudinal and radial variations of pressure in the human anal sphincter. Gastroenterology, *86*:693, 1984.

148. Theuerkauf, E.J., Jr., Beahrs, O.H., and Hill, J.R.: Rectal prolapse: Causation and surgical treatment. Ann. Surg., *171*:819, 1970.

149. Thompson, W.G., and Heaton, K.W.: Proctalgia fugax. J. R. Coll. Phys. Lond., *14*:247, 1980.

150. Thomson, W.H.F.: The nature of haemorrhoids. Br. J. Surg., *62*:542, 1975.

151. Tjeerdsma, H.C., Smout, A.J., and Akkermans, L.M.: Voluntary suppression of defecation delays gastric emptying. Dig. Dis. Sci., *38*:832, 1993.

152. Torsoli, A., Ramorino, M.L., and Crucioli, V.: The relationships between anatomy and motor activity of the colon. Am. J. Dig. Dis., *13*:462, 1968.

153. Tottrup, A., Glavind, E.B., and Svane, D.: Involvement of the L-arginine-nitric oxide pathway in internal anal sphincter relaxation. Gastroenterology, *102*:409, 1992.

154. Van Der Sijp, J.R., Kamm, M.A., Nightingale, J.M., et al.: Disturbed gastric and small bowel transit in severe idiopathic constipation. Dig. Dis. Sci., *38*:837, 1993.

155. Varma, J.S., Smith, A.N., and Busuttil, A.: Function of the anal sphincters after chronic radiation injury. Gut, *27*:528, 1986.

156. Varma, K.K., and Stephens, D.: Neuromuscular reflexes of rectal continence. Aust. N.Z. J. Surg., *41*:263, 1972.

157. Walls, E.W.: Observations of the microscopic anatomy of the human anal canal. Br. J. Surg., *45*:504, 1958.

158. Wendell-Smith, C.P.: Quoted in Wood, B.A.: Anatomy of the anal sphincters and pelvic floor. *In* Henry, M.M., and Swash, M.

(eds.): Coloproctology and the Pelvic Floor: Pathophysiology and Management. London, Butterworth's, 1985.

159. Whitehead, W.E., Engel, B.T., and Schuster, M.M.: Irritable bowel syndrome: Physiological and psychological differences between diarrhea-predominant and constipation-predominant patients. Dig. Dis. Sci., *25:*404, 1980.

160. Winckler, G.: Remarques sur la morphologie et l'innervation du muscle releveur de l'anus. Arch. Anat. Histol. Embryol. (Strasb.), *41:*77, 1958.

161. Williams, J.G., Wong, W.D., and Jensen, L., et al.: Incontinence and rectal prolapse: A prospective manometric study. Dis. Colon Rectum, *34:*209, 1991.

162. Womack, N.R., Morrison, J.F.B., and Williams, N.S.: The role of pelvic floor denervation in the etiology of idiopathic faecal incontinence. Br. J. Surg., *73:*404, 1986.

163. Wood, B.: Anatomy of the anal sphincters and pelvic floor. *In* Henry, M.M., and Swash, M. (eds.): Coloproctology and the Pelvic Floor: Pathophysiology and Management. London, Butterworth's, 1985, p. 3.

164. Wunderlich, M., and Swash, M.: The overlapping innervation of the two sides of the external anal sphincter by the pudendal nerves. J. Neurol. Sci., *59:*97, 1983.

165. Youle, M.S., and Read, N.W.: Effect of painless rectal distension on gastrointestinal transit of solid meal. Dig. Dis. Sci., *29:*902, 1984.

Chapter 23

DIAGNOSIS OF ANORECTAL DISEASE

TERRY C. HICKS / FRANK G. OPELKA

More is missed by not looking than by not knowing.
                                    Thomas McCrae 1870–1935

The diagnosis of anorectal disease can be made in the majority of cases if the examiner listens to the patient, asks the right questions, and performs a complete proctologic examination.

TAKING THE HISTORY

Patients with anorectal complaints are often reluctant to seek help because of fear that the examination will be painful or because of anxiety that they may have cancer. The examiner should put the patient at ease and impart a concerned, attentive, and confident attitude. The chief complaint may be specific and dramatic, such as rectal bleeding or severe pain, but often it is vague or nonspecific, and the patient may have difficulty describing symptoms. Having little knowledge of the anorectal region, many patients assume erroneously that any complaint is caused by hemorrhoids. After the chief complaint is elicited, the provider should allow the patient to briefly elaborate on the present illness, with interruption as necessary to establish the time of onset, duration and frequency of symptoms, previous attacks, and treatment given.

The examiner should ask other detailed and specific questions relative to the chief complaint and other anorectal symptoms.

Bleeding

If there is any bleeding, what is the color of the blood—is it bright, dark, maroon, or black? Where is the blood noted—is it on the toilet tissue, the surface of the stool in the toilet bowl, mixed in the stool, or in mucus? Does the blood drip or is it on the underclothing? What is the quantity of blood? How long has the patient had this problem?

Bright red blood usually implies an origin in the anus, rectum, or lower colon. Blood on the stool surface sug-

gests an anal origin, whereas blood mixed in the stool usually comes from a site above the anus. In clinical settings where blood is found mixed in the stool, a total colonic examination is required to rule out proximal lesions. Blood that drips into the commode during or after a bowel movement usually is from prolapsing internal hemorrhoids. The passage of blood and mucus may be seen with inflammatory bowel disease or cancer and also warrants a thorough examination. Patients tend to overestimate the quantity of blood ("It filled the commode"). Intermittent bleeding over a number of years is usually from internal hemorrhoids or an anal fissure. Regardless of the amount of blood, the duration of bleeding, or an apparent hemorrhoidal source, a complete proctologic examination is necessary to accurately determine the cause.

Pain

Patients with acute anal pain seek treatment early, whereas those with chronic discomfort usually delay. Where is the pain? Is it related to bowel movements? Acute pain with a tender perianal lump suggests a thrombosed hemorrhoid or abscess. Abscesses are often associated with a continuous throbbing pain. Burning pain during or after a bowel movement is usually due to an anal fissure, particularly if it is associated with constipation and bright blood. Deep rectal pain may be caused by an abscess in the deep posterior or anterior anal spaces or supralevator areas; it may be accompanied by chills, fever, and urinary retention. Sporadically occurring nocturnal attacks of deep rectal pain lasting a few minutes are characteristic of proctalgia fugax, fleeting rectal pain of unknown origin. Some authorities believe it is due to rectal or levator muscle spasm.[8,9] Chronic, vague, deep rectal pain and associated perineal or genital pain require careful evaluation, although often no organic cause can be found. The pain is often attributed to atypical coccygodynia, levator muscle syndrome, or mental depression. Coccygeal pain is often challenging for the physician because rarely is an ano-

310

rectal source identified. Although patients often give a history of trauma to this area, this rarely correlates with a demonstrable pain nidus.

External Lump or Swelling

If a lump or swelling is acute and painful, the examiner should think of an acutely thrombosed hemorrhoid or abscess. Nonacute conditions include external hemorrhoids, skin tags, anal papillae, warts, perineal cysts, comedones, and rarely, anal or perianal neoplasms (squamous cell carcinoma, Bowen's disease, or extramammary Paget's disease).

Prolapse

Is prolapse related to bowel movements? Does it recede spontaneously or require digital pressure? Prolapse occurring with defecation or straining that requires digital reduction is most likely caused by third-degree internal hemorrhoids. Prolapse with progressive pain and swelling that does not reduce with digital pressure is probably due to circumferential hemorrhoidal prolapse with thrombosis and strangulation. Complete rectal prolapse is chronic, gets progressively larger, is fairly easy to reduce, and is associated with loss of sphincter tone and incontinence. On examination, complete rectal prolapse is characterized by circumferential sulci, whereas hemorrhoidal prolapse presents with a radial orientation of sulci.

Change in Bowel Habits

What is the patient's bowel habit? Has there been a change? Patients have great variations in their bowel consistency and frequency, and any significant deviation deserves an appropriate clinical evaluation. It is important for the clinician to document any changes in the patient's medication history, dietary history, or operations (i.e., gallbladder, vagotomy, or small bowel) that may be contributory to the bowel habit complaints. Is there constipation or diarrhea? What is the caliber and shape of the stool? Any persistent change in bowel habits raises the possibility of colon or rectal cancer. Any change from normal sized stools to small-caliber or ribbon stools suggests possible anal carcinoma or stricture. Frequent small stools with tenesmus, blood, and mucus strongly suggest rectal carcinoma.

Anal or Perianal Drainage

Is there fecal drainage or mucus seepage? Does it contain pus or blood? Is there associated perineal swelling? Intermittent perineal drainage associated with recurrent swelling is characteristic of a chronic abscess or fistula. Perianal hidradenitis, infected inclusion cysts, warts, comedones, pruritus ani, and neoplasms may also cause drainage.

Perianal Itching

Although pruritus is normally seen in healing anorectal wounds, itching is also associated with anorectal disease, particularly if there is drainage or large external hemorrhoids or tags, which cause difficulty in cleansing. Itching as the primary symptom, without obvious anorectal disease, is classified as idiopathic and may be related to neurodermatitis, dietary habits (caffeine, chocolate, and dairy products), sensitivity to local creams or ointments, or extensive cleansing (see Chapter 24). Bowen's and Paget's disease may also present with pruritus ani.

Fecal Incontinence

Patients with fecal incontinence should be questioned concerning previous anorectal surgery and anorectal trauma. Women should be asked about the possibility of obstetric tears or injuries. A determination should be made whether incontinence is for flatus only, for diarrhea, or for formed stools. Minor incontinence is usually transitory and associated with diarrhea. Major incontinence is extremely distressing to the patient. Concomitant conditions (neuromuscular diseases, diabetes mellitus), medications, pelvic radiation, and gastroenteritis may play a role. Patients with chronic rectal prolapse also may have incontinence (see Chapter 29).

Additional History

The physician also should inquire about the patient's general health, specifically about any loss of strength or vitality, or loss of appetite or weight. A history of previous illnesses, including current medications, should be documented. In taking the family history, determine whether the grandparents, parents, siblings, or other close relatives of the patient have had colon or rectal cancer or polyps. Also, ask about the possibility of familial polyposis, cancer-prone family history syndrome, breast cancer, endometrial carcinoma, ovarian carcinoma, or inflammatory bowel disease. In today's social climate, a sexual history may reveal behavior patterns that increase the risk of anorectal trauma or infections. This history is elicited by asking whether the patient is heterosexual, homosexual, or bisexual. Further questions will follow as appropriate to the clinical presentation. It is also important to document if the patient is receiving anticoagulants or has been treated with radiation or chemotherapy. The physician must also document conditions that may require the patient to receive prophylaxis for subacute bacterial endocarditis prior to invasive procedures.

ANORECTAL EXAMINATION

The examiner may have formed an opinion of the probable diagnosis after taking a history. If not, he or she should have in mind a differential diagnosis of several conditions to be sought during the examination. The differential diagnosis will determine the focus of the anorectal exam. Most patients require anal inspection, digital palpation, anoscopic exam, and proctosigmoidoscopy. Certain conditions require drainage, biopsy, excision, or specimen collection. Although a specifically designed examination room is desirable, a regular examining room is suitable, provided that it has proctologic instruments and equipment listed in Table 23–1.

Inspection

After the patient has been appropriately positioned (Fig. 23–1),[5] the buttocks are gently retracted for inspection. The areas to be observed include the buttocks (look for lumps, scars, or skin abnormalities) and the sacrococcygeal area (look for pilonidal pits, sinuses, cysts, or old scars). The anus is observed for discharge, rashes, external hemorrhoids (skin-covered), skin tags, thrombosed hemorrhoids (purple, tender lumps), protruding internal hemorrhoids (mucosa-covered), prolapsed anal papillae (white and firm), anal scarring, or deformity. The anus is inspected further by gentle perineal eversion and traction. A search is made for fissures, sentinel piles, enlarged papillae, erosion, or traumatic tears. The perianal area is also inspected for signs of inflammation, thickening, maceration, moistness, excoriations, lumps, swelling, drainage areas, or tumor. If one or more drainage areas are found, anorectal fistula is suspected; a differential diagnosis includes infected inclusion cysts, furuncle, and hidradenitis.

Digital Palpation

External palpation of the perianal area is performed to evaluate any lumps, swelling, or drainage. Fistula tracks often can be palpated and their direction traced toward the anus. Using a well-lubricated glove or finger cot, the examiner inserts the index finger gradually into the

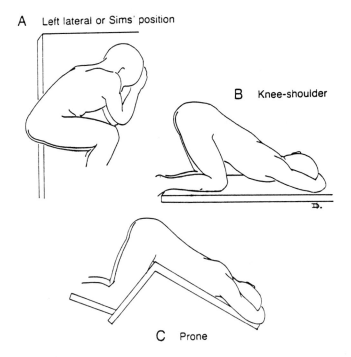

FIGURE 23–1. Positions of patient for anorectal examination. *A,* Left lateral (Sims') position. *B,* Knee-shoulder position. *C,* Prone (jackknife) position using proctoscopy table. (From Hill, G.J., II: Outpatient Surgery, 2nd ed. Philadelphia, W.B. Saunders, 1980, with permission.)

anus. For patient comfort, the physician should align the examining finger with its narrowest diameter parallel to the normal anterior-posterior configuration of the anus. The intersphincteric groove is identified just inside the anal verge. Increased thickness or spasm of the internal sphincter muscle should be noted. As the finger is inserted further, the examiner assesses for presence of pain, tightness, scarring, or stricture. The anal canal and dentate line are palpated for ulcers or fissures, irregularity, scarring, enlarged anal papillae, or tumor. Sphincter tone is assessed, and if it is excessively relaxed or atonic, external sphincter "squeeze" is tested by asking the patient to tighten those muscles. If contraction is poor, the examiner should search for a possible sphincter defect. The finger is inserted further through the anus, and the anorectal ring is identified by noting the thick puborectalis muscle that forms a sling around the anus posteriorly and produces a sharp posterior anorectal angle. The ability of the patient to contract the puborectalis muscle and the strength of its contraction should be noted.

The lower rectum is then examined, beginning anteriorly by palpating the prostate or cervix. The rectum is circumferentially examined for muscosal, intermuscular, or extrarectal pathologic conditions. A search is made for a polyp, mass, tenderness, or induration. A sessile, villous tumor is especially difficult to palpate if the examiner is not acutely aware of subtle changes in the consistency of the rectal mucosa. The examiner should note tumor location, size, ulceration, and mobility. The pelvic side walls and posterolateral sacrococcygeal area should be examined for any adenopathy. Internal hemorrhoids usually are not palpable unless they are enlarged from

TABLE 23–1. EXAMINING ROOM PROCTOLOGIC INSTRUMENTS AND EQUIPMENT

DISPOSABLE ITEMS
  Gloves or finger cots
  Lubricants
  Tissue paper
  Swabs
  Disinfectants
  Disposable enemas

LIGHTING
  Good room lighting
  Gooseneck-type light for perineal inspection
  Light source for scopes

DIAGNOSTIC EQUIPMENT
  Anoscopes
  Proctosigmoidoscopes

DIAGNOSTIC-ASSISTANCE MACHINES
  Electrocoagulation machine
  Water suction device or equivalent suction machine

ACCESSORIES
  Probes
  Crypt hooks
  Biopsy forceps
  Suction tubes
  Specimen containers
  Slides and stool culture materials
  Fecal occult blood testing kits

chronic prolapse, in which case longitudinal folds may be felt. The cul-de-sac is examined for the presence of a shelf or pelvic mass. The depth of the digital exam varies with the experience and the finesse of the examiner and is not necessarily related to finger length. After digital examination, the finger should be checked for gross blood.

Anoscopic Examination

An anoscope is essential for examining the anal canal. Either a beveled or slotted type may be used. Short anoscopes are not satisfactory because they do not allow full visualization of the anal canal. The slotted type has the disadvantage of having to be withdrawn, rotated, and reinserted several times to examine the entire anal circumference. Beveled scopes allow for rotation without complete withdrawal. An adequate anoscope is the modified Hirschman's type (Fig. 23–2), which is available in large, medium, and small diameters. These scopes are equipped with a proximal fiberoptic light attached to the handle. It is preferable to use a large size, but if the anus is tight or narrow, it is necessary to use a smaller size.

As the lubricated anoscope is introduced slowly, the patient should be asked to strain in order to produce anal relaxation. After full-length insertion, the obturator is withdrawn, and the handle of the scope is controlled with the left hand. The right hand is used for suctioning or swabbing and for manipulating probes, crypt hooks, and biopsy instruments for obtaining specimens. During anoscopy, the entire anal circumference is inspected. If the beveled scope is not fully withdrawn as each segment is visualized, it can be inserted and rotated successively without replacing the obturator or pinching the sensitive anoderm, and the 360-degree circumference can be observed.

Internal hemorrhoids are evaluated and graded (Table 23–2) by asking the patient to strain with the anoscope at the dentate line and noting the degree of bulging and amount of descent below the line (see Chapter 26).

Anal fissures are located most commonly in the posterior or anterior midline and are typically associated with a sentinel pile and an enlarged anal papilla. Fissures found in the lateral positions demand further clinical investigation. Indolent fissures with edema and purplish discoloration of the anal skin suggest the possibility of inflammatory bowel disease, primary syphilis, tuberculosis, or leukemia[4] (see Chapter 25). Abscesses and fistulas begin with infection in anal crypts at the dentate line. When a fistula is suspected because of an external secondary drainage site on the anoderm,[7] a search should be made for the primary opening. Suspicious anal crypts may be probed or observed for drainage of pus. Attempts to probe external fistula tracks should be made cautiously because doing so can be painful, and there is danger of causing a false passage (see Chapter 27). During anoscopy, a search is made for tumors, polyps, papillae, and atypical ulcerations. Biopsies, cultures, and smears are taken as indicated.

Proctosigmoidoscopy

Proctosigmoidoscopy is indicated for most patients with anorectal or colonic symptoms as part of the initial visit. Exceptions include those patients with painful thrombosed hemorrhoids, acute fissures, abscesses, or severe stricture, or when there is suspicion of acute inflammatory bowel disease or diverticulitis. Rigid proctosigmoidoscopy (RS) has been replaced by flexible fiberoptic sigmoidoscopy (FFS) in the evaluation of rectal bleeding, changes in bowel habits, diarrhea, constipation, weight loss, anemia, and abdominal pain. Flexible sigmoidoscopy is better tolerated, easier to perform, reaches further into the colon, and uses improved optics compared to rigid proctosigmoidoscopy.[6] Rigid scopes are usually 25 cm long and are made in diameters of 12, 15, and 19 mm (Fig. 23–3). The average length of insertion of the rigid scope by experienced endoscopists is only 17 to 19 cm, whereas the average depth of insertion of a flexible scope is 55 cm. The flexible scopes are available in varying lengths, but the most popular length is 65 cm (Fig. 23–4). Flexible fiberoptic sigmoidoscopy is also used for cancer screening in asymptomatic patients older than 45 years of age. Rigid scopes are best used today to remove stool, foreign bodies, and blood from the rectum to facilitate an examination. The rigid scope most accurately measures the distance of tumors or masses from the anal verge.

PREPARATION. Preparation for rigid proctosigmoidos-

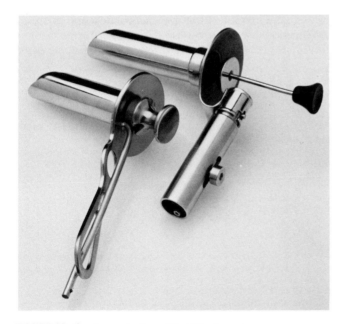

FIGURE 23–2. Large-sized modified Hirschman's anoscopes.

TABLE 23–2. CLASSIFICATION OF INTERNAL HEMORRHOIDS

First-degree	Enlarged, nonprolapsing vascular cushions
Second-degree	Prolapsing cushions, reduce spontaneously
Third-degree	Prolapsing cushions, reduce manually
Fourth-degree	Prolapsing cushions, nonreducible

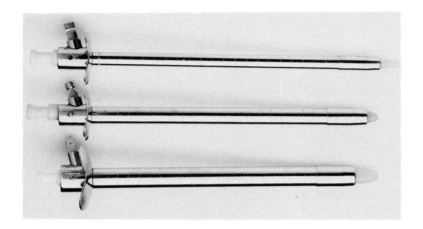

FIGURE 23-3. Large-, medium-, and small-diameter Welch Allyn rigid sigmoidoscopes.

copy consists of a single disposable enema given 30 minutes before the examination. For flexible fiberoptic sigmoidoscopy, two enemas are given, one about 1 hour before and another 30 minutes before the examination. However, recent studies have indicated that in some patients one enema is sufficient.

INSERTION. Proctosigmoidoscopy is usually performed immediately after anoscopy. The scope is carefully inserted through the anus, and the adequacy of the preparation is immediately determined. The lumen of the bowel must be clean and empty; mucus and liquid stool can be removed by suction. With insufflation and suction as needed, the scope is passed cephalad, and the vascular pattern is noted. Inflammation, granularity, friability, and ulceration obscure the vascular pattern and may indicate inflammatory bowel disease. The primary objective of insertion is to advance the tip of the scope by keeping the lumen in view. The endoscopist should avoid overinsufflation with air, as this leads to increased patient discomfort and can increase the difficulty of the examination because the angles in the normal colon become more pronounced. Experienced endoscopists may use several torquing maneuvers and techniques to limit discomfort and maximally advance the instrument. The scope is advanced to the fullest extent possible, but the examination should be terminated if the patient experiences severe discomfort. When the view is blind, it is

helpful to withdraw the scope and find the fold or turn that indicates lumen direction. Length of insertion does not necessarily correlate with actual location of the scope tip, since the sigmoid loop may be stretched and may not extend as far proximally as indicated by the distance the scope has been inserted. Note is made of any pathologic condition encountered on insertion, but the primary examination is performed upon withdrawal of the scope. After maximal insertion, the scope is withdrawn, with visualization of the entire lumen circumferentially and inspection for potential blind spots behind folds and turns. Note is made of mucosal inflammation, ulceration, diverticular disease, polyps, submucosal tumors, carcinoma, or vascular lesions. Abnormal areas and neoplasms may be biopsied, but it seems more prudent to perform this at the time of a subsequent colonoscopy. The advantages of delaying these biopsies are twofold. First, during a colonoscopy, synchronous lesions may be identified that will require biopsies; second, any complication that occurs from biopsy in the unprepared setting may magnify the complications. Polyps may be biopsied, but need not be removed, since subsequent colonoscopy and polypectomy are indicated.

COMPLICATIONS. Complications of rigid proctosigmoidoscopy and flexible fiberoptic sigmoidoscopy are rare. Perforation has been reported but should not occur if the lumen is kept in view and the tip of the scope is not

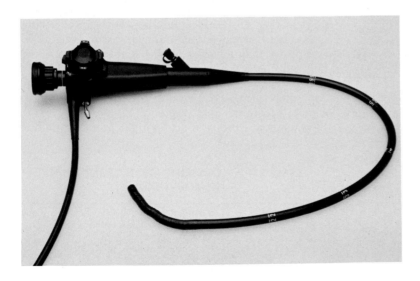

FIGURE 23-4. Pentax 65-cm flexible fiberoptic sigmoidoscope.

forcefully advanced. Since sedation is not used, the patient's response of pain should alert the examiner to stop and pull back. If perforation should occur, as evidenced by free intra-abdominal air or signs of peritonitis, immediate hospitalization, intravenous resuscitation, and antibiotics are indicated. The need for laparotomy should be decided on a case-by-case basis.

Significant bleeding seldom occurs after biopsy during flexible fiberoptic sigmoidoscopy because the forcep jaws are small. However, serious bleeding can result after biopsy when larger forceps are used during rigid proctosigmoidoscopy. Bleeding after biopsy usually stops spontaneously, but if bleeding from a small artery is noted, it should be controlled by pressure and coagulation.

Explosion has occurred during electrocoagulation, although it is a rare event. It is possible because methane and hydrogen are normally present in colon gas. When rigid proctosigmoidoscopy is performed, explosion can be prevented by replacing colon gas with room air by repeated insufflation and suction. Diathermy machines should not be used during flexible fiberoptic sigmoidoscopy unless the entire colon has been prepared. In the event of an explosion, the proximal colon may be severely lacerated and perforated. An emergency operation is needed to repair or resect damaged areas.

SPECIAL DIAGNOSTIC EXAMINATIONS

Diagnosis of most anorectal disease can be made after completion of routine examinations, but some conditions require additional special procedures.

BARIUM CONTRAST STUDIES. The rectum and rectosigmoid are best visualized by direct rigid proctosigmoidoscopy or flexible fiberoptic sigmoidoscopy. However, if there is a severe rectal stricture or an obstruction in the rectum that prevents passage of a sigmoidoscope, colonic contrast studies using barium or water-soluble agents may provide needed information. Soluble contrast studies may also image the colon in acute inflammatory conditions like diverticulitis or ischemia. Small bowel studies may also be necessary if the history or anorectal findings suggest Crohn's disease.

COLLECTION OF STOOL SPECIMENS. Specimens for smear, culture, warm stage examination, or toxin assays should be obtained from patients with atypical anal ulcers, diarrhea, or colitis. These tests will help to identify infectious diarrhea, amebiasis, anal syphilis, herpes, gonorrheal proctitis, AIDS-related infections, *Clostridium difficile* toxin, or lymphogranuloma.

DEFECOGRAPHY. This special radiographic procedure is indicated in rectal prolapse and in some cases of incontinence and constipation. Defecography allows for fluoroscopic evaluation of rectal evacuation. It may help identify pelvic floor anomalies. It requires skilled radiologists with special equipment.

ANAL FISTULOGRAMS. These studies are often confusing but may be helpful in complicated fistulas. Recently, computerized tomography (CT) –directed fistulograms have been found to be helpful in tracing complex fis-

tulas, and CT scans may also be helpful in localizing deep ischioanal and supralevator space abscesses.

ANAL MANOMETRY. Instruments that measure anorectal pressure increase our knowledge of the physiology of fecal incontinence and pelvic floor dysfunction. Manometry can establish resting sphincter function, voluntary sphincter squeeze, rectoanal inhibitory reflexes, and the minimal and maximal sensory volumes.

ANAL ELECTROMYOGRAPHY. This examination can be helpful in evaluating incontinence when a neurogenic cause is suspected. Such conditions include difficult childbirth, which may injure pudendal nerves, mengingomyelocele, and cauda equina lesions. Incontinent patients may have sphincter defects from trauma mapped out using electromyography to isolate the cut ends of the sphincter for repair.

ENDORECTAL ULTRASOUND (ERUS). Recently, endorectal ultrasound has gained favor in staging the depth or penetration of rectal carcinomas. Increasing experience may also identify perirectal adenopathy. Endorectal ultrasound can map external sphincter defects in patients with traumatic incontinence.

COMPUTERIZED AXIAL TOMOGRAPHY (CAT) AND MAGNETIC IMAGING RESONANCE (MRI). The role of these two diagnostic modalities for staging and postoperative follow-up of colon and rectal cancer patients is still being defined. Both modalities provide an overall preoperative staging accuracy of 74%. MRI has proven to be more accurate than CT in detecting perirectal extension of tumor; however, the detection of lymph node metastases has a higher degree of accuracy with CT than with MRI.[1-3,11] The emerging role of endorectal ultrasound may displace both of these examinations for staging of rectal cancer.

CORRELATION OF HISTORY AND PHYSICAL FINDINGS

In arriving at a diagnosis of anorectal disease, the examiner must correlate information learned from the history with objective findings noted on the physical examination. The correct diagnosis should be apparent if the history and examination have been conducted in a thorough and methodical manner. Next, the examiner must determine if the physical findings are the cause of the patient's complaint.[10] Are the symptoms out of proportion or incongruent with the objective proctologic diagnosis? For example, are uncomplicated hemorrhoids the cause of the patient's severe anal pain? Finally, the examiner must decide if the proctologic condition requires surgery or a trial of conservative medical management.

REFERENCES

1. Butch, R.J., Stark, D.D., Wittenbert, J., et al.: Staging rectal cancer by MR and CT. Am. J. Roentgenol., *146:*1155, 1986.
2. Freeny, P.C., Marks, W.M., Ryan, J.A., and Bolen, J.W.: Colorectal carcinoma evaluation with CT: Preoperative staging and detection of postoperative recurrence. Radiology, *158:*347, 1986.

3. Guinet, C., Buy, J.-N., Ghossain, M.A., et al.: Comparison of magnetic resonance imaging and computed tomography in the preoperative staging of rectal cancer. Arch. Surg., *125*:385, 1990.
4. Hicks, T.C., and Ray, J.E.: Rectal and perineal complaints. *In* Polk, H.C., Jr., Stone H.H., and Gardner, B. (eds.): Basic Surgery, 3rd ed. East Norwalk, CT, Appleton-Century-Crofts, 1987, p. 455.
5. Hill, G.J., II: Outpatient Surgery, 2nd ed. Philadelphia, W.B. Saunders, 1980.
6. Marks, G., Boggs, H.W., Castro, A.F., et al.: Sigmoidoscopic examination with rigid and flexible fiberoptic sigmoidoscopes in the surgeon's office. A comparative prospective study of effectiveness in 1,012 cases. Dis. Colon Rectum, *22*:162, 1979.
7. Ray, J.E.: Hemorrhoids, anal fissure and anal fistula. *In* Conn. H.F. (ed.): Current Therapy. Philadelphia, W.B. Saunders, 1975, p. 331.
8. Rubin, R.J.: Proctalgia fugax. *In* Fazio, V. (ed.): Current Therapy in Colon and Rectal Surgery. Philadelphia, B.C. Decker, 1990, p. 68.
9. Salvati, E.P.: The levator syndrome and its variant. Gastroenterol. Clin. North Am., *16*:71, 1987.
10. Shackelford, R.T., and Zuidema, G.D. (eds.): Surgery of the Alimentary Tract, 2nd ed., Vol. III. Philadelphia, W.B. Saunders, 1982, p. 381.
11. Thompson, W.M., Halvorsen, R.A., Foster, W.L., Jr., et al.: Preoperative and postoperative CT staging of rectosigmoid carcinoma. Am. J. Roentgenol., *146*:703, 1986.

Chapter 24

PRURITUS ANI

THOMAS H. DAILEY

Pruritus ani is a symptom complex consisting of an intense itch and burning discomfort of the perianal skin. It has a multiplicity of causes, several of which may coexist. It is frequently nocturnal and recurrent and is associated with varying degres of skin breakdown, weeping, maceration, lichenification, and superinfection. Pruritus ani is often refractory to treatment until the cause is identified and appropriate therapy is instituted. Many patients' symptoms can be treated successfully, even without a specific etiology being determined. The following is a useful clinical guide for surgeons treating this often vexing condition.

HISTORY

Taking a detailed medical, surgical, and dermatologic history leads to a rational, efficient, and successful work-up, diagnosis, and treatment. It is crucial to establish the exact nature and periodicity of all perianal symptoms and their relationship to defecation and anal hygiene habits, dietary intake, allergies, medications, and exercise. Systemic illnesses that are associated with pruritus ani include diabetes mellitus, hyperbilirubinemia, and blood dyscrasias (leukemias and aplastic anemia). Chronic diarrhea or constipation, when associated with pruritus ani, should be investigated because inflammatory bowel disease, infectious diarrhea, or intestinal parasites may be involved.

Previous anorectal surgery that may lead to anatomic deformities, physiologic alterations of continence, or both, must be carefully noted, as must specifics regarding a history of sexually transmitted diseases, the patient's sexual orientation, chronic vaginitis, and immune status. Allergies, especially to topical medications, are commonly associated with pruritus ani. An exhaustive list of medications (oral and topical) must be made, as well as proprietary agents (e.g., soaps, deodorants, perfumes) and suppositories; note those containing antibiotics, estrogens, steroidal compounds, and the "caine" preparations. Dermatologic conditions often related to pruritus ani include psoriasis, seborrhea, intertrigo, and nonspecific neurodermatitis. A brief review of the patient's domestic and occupational stresses is often enlightening.

PHYSICAL EXAMINATION

Patients with pruritus ani are generally healthy, vigorous males (male:female ratio, 4:1), aged 20 to 50 years.[24] Examination often may not yield any etiologic clues.[13] Remote skin lesions may indicate the cause of pruritus ani: for example, psoriatic lesions of the nails, elbows, or knees; seborrheic dermatitis of the scalp; scratchy marks secondary to neurodermatitis of dermatophytic infections of the fingers or toes; or scabies and pediculosis in the groin.

Examination of the perineum should be done with the patient in the prone–jackknife position. Bright light and a magnifying glass are essential. The patient is examined initially without an enema or perianal cleansing. Digital rectal examination should include evaluation of sphincteric competence by measuring the strength of resting and maximum contractions. The consistency of the stool should be noted (especially if it is pasty and adherent), as should any anal or vaginal soiling by stool, blood, or pus seen on the patient's perineal skin or undergarments.[4] Scrapings for microscopic study must be done on skin that is free of greasy medications. The skin is then gently cleansed to allow careful inspection, culture, and biopsy when indicated. A disposable enema is administered prior to anoscopy and sigmoidoscopy.

Anoscopy and endoscopic examination of the rectum may reveal a variety of common disorders, such as inflammatory bowel disease, infectious proctitides, or growths that should be appropriately cultured or biopsied. Purged stools can be studied later for ova and parasites if indicated. Colonoscopy and barium enemas are rarely of diagnostic value and should be reserved for special indications.

DIAGNOSIS AND TREATMENT

After a thorough history and careful examination, the surgeon usually will be able to assign the cause of the patient's symptoms to one or more of the four following categories: leakage, sensitivities, dermatoses, and infections. It is important to recognize, however, that many patients will ultimately defy clear diagnostic categorization and by exclusion will be placed in a primary "idiopathic'' group. Such patients can still be successfully treated by a variety of simple measures outlined in the following discussion.

Leakage

Seepage of moisture from the anal canal onto the perineal skin causes inflammation and gross and microscopic fissuring, which may progress to ulceration with attendant exudation and suppuration. This leads to debilitating pain and disability. Invariably the patient experiences difficulty establishing anal hygiene and, predictably, initiates a variety of local measures that may prove of little benefit. In fact, such self-treatment often exacerbates the condition; medical consultation is then sought.

A common anorectal cause of leakage is hemorrhoids, especially the prolapsing variety. They are best demonstrated by the Valsalva maneuver during anoscopy. Anal mucosal prolapse is seen in women, mostly anteriorly, and often as a result of a difficult vaginal delivery; care must be taken not to overlook an associated vaginitis or urinary tract infection. Anal fissures are often heralded by a ''sentinel'' tag with surrounding dermatitis, especially posteriorly (Fig. 24–1). Anorectal fistulas cause pruritus during periods of drainage of pus from the external opening(s). Prolapsing anal papillae (fibromas),

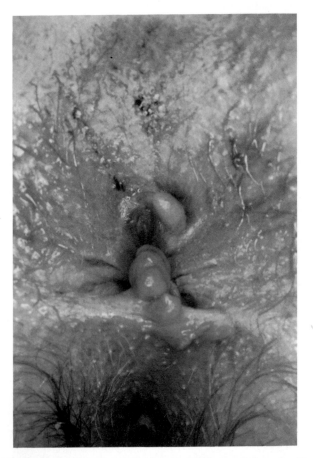

FIGURE 24-1. Anterior and posterior midline anal fissures with ''sentinel'' tags and associated pruritus. The patient is in the prone position.

low-lying anorectal polyps, and villous tumors may cause an irritating mucoid anal discharge. Anoscopy affords easy differential diagnosis of these lesions.

Surgical correction of these anorectal disorders is indicated only in those patients in whom the disorders are clearly causing the pruritus. No more than 15% of patients with pruritus ani will be helped by surgery.[6] Surgical candidates must be carefully selected only after an aggressive course of conservative therapy fails over a 6-week period. Excellent results in controlling pruritus ani have been reported with the use of rubber band ligation, operative hemorrhoidectomy,[18] and other appropriate anorectal procedures.

The introduction of anorectal manometry and cinedefecography has led to the identification of internal rectal prolapse (sigmoidorectal intussusception) as a cause of anal leakage that can be surgically cured in many cases. Manometric studies showed that patients with pruritus ani have anal leakage at lower volumes of water instilled into the rectum.[3,11] They also showed that the internal anal sphincter may have an exaggerated rectoanal inhibitory response to rectal dilation; thus, an inappropriate sphincteric relaxation leads to leakage and pruritus ani. Another study indicated that coffee may play a role in reducing internal sphincter pressure.[24]

Chronic constipation, particularly if it progresses to fecal impaction, may lead to chronic leakage of mucus, stool, and irritative alkaline secretions. Efforts should be directed toward establishing complete rectal emptying, emphasizing a high-fiber diet, psyllium bulk-formers, and increased hydration. If this regimen fails, daily rectal washouts using a bulb syringe with warm tap water may be necessary to ensure complete evacuation of the rectum.

Diarrhea, either episodic or chronic, can cause pruritus ani. It usually is self-limited; a cause need not be sought initially. However, if symptoms persist despite treatment of the diarrhea, appropriate culture and mucosal biopsies are indicated to diagnose specific enteric infections or inflammatory bowel disease. Pruritus ani may result from leakage of alkaline stool and mucus in susceptible individuals. In such cases, an acid skin preparation containing steroids or oral lactobacillus therapy may prove beneficial during acute episodes.

Sensitivities

The perianal skin is abundantly supplied with a dense network of sensory nerve endings for pain and itch. Irritation of the exposed skin on the perineum can be caused by alkaline intestinal secretions, ingested chemicals, and a wide variety of medications and foods.

Foods that commonly cause pruritus ani include tomatoes, coffee, tea, caffeinated colas, beer, chocolate, citrus, and similar products.[12] Excluding all these items from the diet and then introducing them, one by one in increasing amounts, allows one to identify the offending item(s) as symptoms reappear. A ''threshold'' amount that can be tolerated without causing recurrent pruritus can then be determined and should be reproducible. Coffee and tomatoes are the most common offenders and should be reintroduced first. "Hot" condiments (e.g., spices, peppers, chili) should be discontinued in susceptible patients. Milk products may cause an irritating, pasty, adherent stool; this can be eliminated in most patients by the addition of psyllium or methylcellulose bulk-forming agents.

Medications taken orally, such as colchicine and quinidine, occasionally cause pruritus ani. Antibiotics are also offenders through their action in altering colonic flora. A direct systemic effect in producing pruritus ani has been demonstrated by the intravenous injection of hydrocortisone sodium phosphate.[19] Various topical preparations containing antibiotics or anesthetic "caines" produce a violaceous, intensely itchy rim of inflammation that corresponds to the area of contact with the medication (Fig. 24–2). Topical allergy is simply confirmed by patch testing with the presumed allergen. Such a chemical found in toilet tissue has recently been identified.[5] Successful withdrawal of the suspected agent is diagnostic.

Chemicals contained in various scented soaps, toilet tissues, deodorants, and lotions can cause severe perianal itching. Patients often "polish" the perianal skin with harsh paper or bath towels in an effort to thoroughly "sterilize" the area that itches. This causes further painful fissuring and excoriation. Alcohol-based anal wipes cause painful burning which, perversely, temporarily relieves ("extincts") the itching; however, the effect is short-lived. It is preferable to use a soothing, water-soluble emolient cream (Balneol) applied with cotton balls several times a day, after defecation, and at bedtime. Further relief can be afforded by simultaneously placing a thin pledget of unsterile cotton against the anus. This protects the excoriated areas from further abrasion by the opposite buttock and absorbs sweat, reactive seepage, and anal discharge. Thus, epithelialization necessary for complete cure is promoted.

Dermatoses

Dermatoses can be divided into benign and malignant conditions. Among the benign lesions, psoriasis (Fig. 24–3) commonly extends from the perianal skin into the intergluteal fold; it is scaly, erythematous, and usually associated with distant skin or fingernail lesions. Similarly, seborrheic dermatitis can be seen in multiple sites distant from the anus. Comedones are easily diagnosed as multiple, yellow, cutaneous, perianal cysts that are rarely pruritic but may be related to the chronic use of commonly used fluorinated steroids.[20] Telltale scratch marks elsewhere on the skin will aid in the diagnosis of perianal neurodermatitis. Lichen sclerosis of the vulva and perineum is pruritic and responds to high concentrations of topical corticosteroids.[14] A magnifying glass and strong suspicion will uncover pediculosis pubis and scabies. Appropriate medications are promptly curative, but reinfection must be watched for.

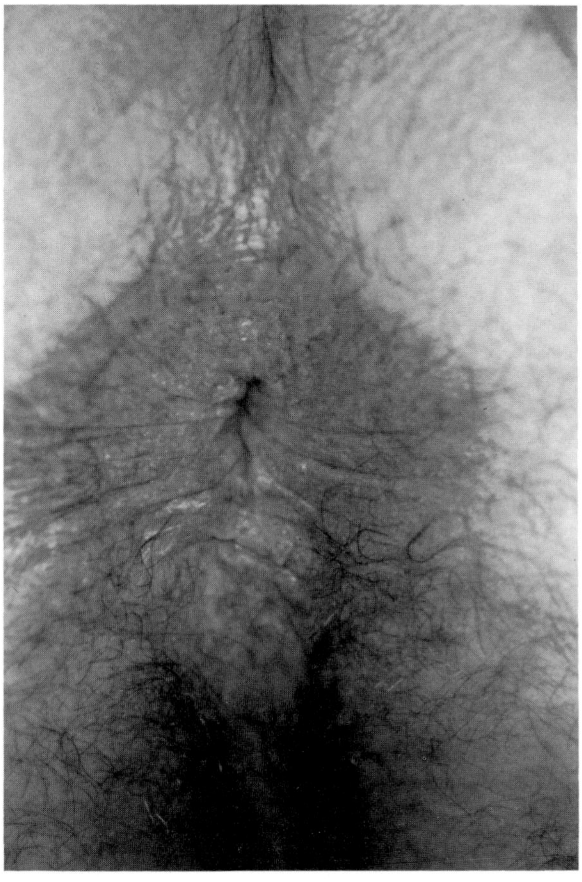

FIGURE 24–2. Topical allergy to dibucaine (Nupercainal) anesthetic cream.

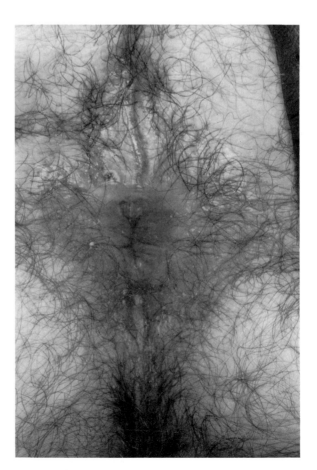

FIGURE 24–3. Perianal psoriasis with intergluteal involvement.

Malignant perianal skin conditions that present as pruritus ani require biopsy for accurate diagnosis. Paget's disease is characterized by a thickened, scaly, raised, eczematoid eruption that itches intensely and is unresponsive to topical corticosteroids.[15] This lesion should be excised with clear margins and may require split-thickness skin grafting in advanced cases. Bowen's disease is a rare, slowly progressive, indurated, erythematosquamous, intraepidermal skin cancer. It is frequently associated with unrelated distant malignancies.[25] A trial of topical fluorouracil prior to wide excision has been advocated.[21] Unilateral or multiple scattered perianal skin lesions and suspicious lesions of the anal canal that do not respond to local measures, whether pruritic or not, should be promptly biopsied under local anesthesia. Occasionally, rare lesions requiring definitive treatment may be uncovered.[17] In situ squamous carcinoma and cloacogenic cancer of the anus are being seen with increasing frequency in male homosexual and immunocompromised patients.[27,28]

Infections

In a recent study, patients with pruritus ani were found to have the same perianal bacteriologic flora as asymptomatic matched controls.[23] Thus, when seen on the perianal skin, infections are usually superimposed on a pre-existing skin condition, although rarely they may occur as primary bacterial, viral, mycotic, or parasitic infections. Erythrasma is a rare bacterial infection (due to *Corynebacterium minutissimum*) that is well demarcated, reddish, scaly, and best diagnosed by red fluorescence under a Wood's ultraviolet lamp. Erythromycin is curative. Mixed bacterial and fungal infections (intertrigo) occurring perianally are seen mostly in obese and diabetic patients. Conservative measures directed at better hygiene and skin drying usually suffice for healing without the need for antibiotics.

Viral infections are predominantly venereal: herpes simplex (HSV), condylomata acuminata caused by the human papilloma viruses (HPV), and cytomegalovirus (CMV) causing colitis. HSV infections progress over several weeks from painful, vesicular perineal or vulval eruptions to scaly, pruritic, healing eschars. Oral acyclovir taken prophylactically has been shown to reduce the frequency and severity of recurrences.[13] Condylomata acuminata (HPV) are intra-anal and perianal warty excrescences. High recurrence rates are related to inadequately fulgurated lesions (especially intra-anal) and hidden persistence of the virus in adjacent skin. Topical podophyllin is usually adequate in eliminating cutaneous lesions but cannot be used for intra-anal lesions. Immunotherapy has been employed successfully in recurrent and advanced infections.[1] Interferon-alpha injected locally has recently been used; preliminary studies show benefit over conventional treatment.[8] Viral proctitides and idiopathic anal ulceration are seen in HIV-positive patients. Excessive rectal secretions and compromise of sphincteric competence may result, respectively, from these conditions.

Mycotic infections include *Candida* and other fungi (*Dermatophyton* and *Trichophyton*). Candidiasis (*Candida albicans*) of the perineum is rarely a primary infection, occurring in about 1% of random scrapings.[2] Candidiasis does occur as a superinfection after antibiotic therapy; it also invades atrophic steroid-abused skin. The typical lesion (Fig. 24–4) is wet, ulcerated, erythematous, and has well-defined borders. These lesions require aggressive treatment with nystatin, drying (a hairdryer is useful), and a thorough search for and control of associated diabetes mellitus or vaginitis. Evidence suggests that the pruritus associated with dermatophytic infections may result from hypersensitivity to mycotic allergens.[7]

Parasitic infestation with intestinal pinworms is rare in adults in homes where there are no affected children. The 6-mm pinworms can be seen grossly in the stool or in examination of the anal canal. The eggs are identifiable microscopically on perianal skin samples taken on adhesive tape. All family members should be tested before and after antihelminthic treatment with piperazine. Chronic intestinal amebiasis is the cause of an extremely rare infestation of the perianal skin that is aggressively erosive and must be suspected in patients with proven trophozoites in the stool.

DISCUSSION

A few words of emphasis regarding treatment are important. Although there are many causes of pruritus ani,

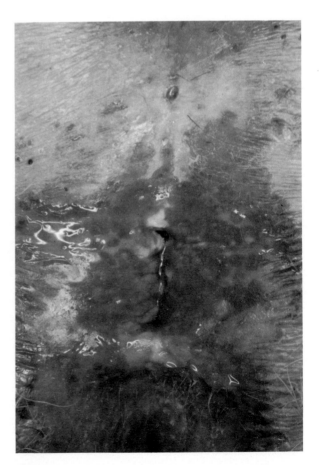

FIGURE 24–4. Acute candidal infection superimposed on chronic "steroid-abused" perianal skin.

it is clear that many, if not most, patients will be classified as "idiopathic" (Fig. 24–5) for want of a clear etiology.[16] Fortunately, the vast majority of this group of patients respond well to a vigorous, unrelenting, often long-term regimen of anal hygiene, dietary control, management of diarrhea and constipation, along with avoidance of irritating oral and topical medications. A small group of carefully selected patients (15%) will benefit from anorectal surgical procedures aimed at eradicating offending conditions such as fissures, fistulas, prolapsing hemorrhoids, anal mucosal prolapse, and a variety of isolated skin lesions.

Occasionally, short courses of topical corticosteroid creams under close medical direction may be required to treat acute exacerbations; however, the chronic, long-term use of such agents, particularly the more potent fluorinated congeners, is to be avoided. Radiation treatments, alcohol skin injections, and "undercutting" procedures are of historic interest only and are mentioned only to be condemned. A small group of patients with intractable pruritus ani treated with intramural injections of methylene blue with safety and apparent benefit[9,10] has been reported; another study indicates initial "cure" in a similar group of refractory patients. Liberal use of biopsies in all perplexing cases is encouraged. Generally, routine cultures are of marginal value.

If, after persistence and full compliance over 6 to 8 weeks, the regimens outlined here do not produce a sustainable and satisfactory improvement, dermatologic consultation should be obtained.

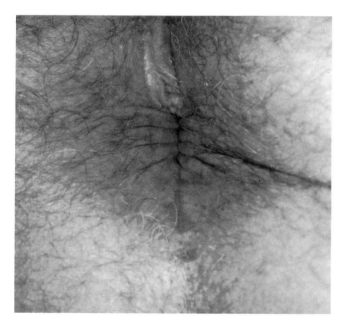

FIGURE 24–5. Common idiopathic chronic pruritus ani for which no cause could be identified.

REFERENCES

1. Abcarian, H., and Sharon, N.: The effectiveness of immunotherapy in the treatment of anal condylomata. Dis. Colon Rectum, *25:* 648, 1982.
2. Alexander, S.: Dermatological aspects of anorectal disease. Clin. Gastroenterol., *4:*651, 1975.
3. Allan, A., and Ambrose, N.S.: Physiological studies of pruritus ani. Br. J. Surg., *74:*576, 1987.
4. Alexander-Williams, C.: Pruritus ani. Postgrad. Med., *77:*56, 1985.
5. Bruynzeel, D.P.: Letter to the Editor. BMJ, *305:*955, 1992.
6. Dailey, T.H.: Pruritus ani. Pract. Gastroenterol., *4:*1, 1980.
7. Dodi, G.: The mycotic flora in proctological patients with and without pruritus ani. Br. J. Surg., *7:*967, 1985.
8. Eron, L.J., Judson, F., Tucker, S., et al.: Interferon therapy for condylomata acuminata. N. Engl. J. Med., *314:*1059, 1986.
9. Eusebio, E.B., Graham, J., and Mody, N.: Treatment of intractable pruritus ani. Dis. Colon Rectum, *33:*770, 1990.
10. Eusebio, E.B.: Letter to the Editor. Dis. Colon Rectum, *34:*289, 1991.
11. Eyers, A.A., and Thomson, J.P.: Pruritus ani: Is anal sphincter dysfunction important in aetiology? BMJ, *2*(6204):1549, 1979.
12. Friend, W.G.: The cause and treatment of idiopathic pruritus ani. Dis. Colon Rectum, *20:*40, 1977.
13. Guinan, M.E.: Oral acyclovir for treatment and suppression of genital herpes simplex viral infection. JAMA, *255*(13):1747, 1986.
14. Harrington, C.I.: Letter to the Editor. BMJ, *305:*955, 1992.
15. Helwig, E.B., and Graham, J.H.: Anogenital (extramammary) Paget's disease. Cancer, *16:*387, 1975.
16. Jones, D.J.: Pruritus ani. BMJ, *305:*575, 1992.
17. Lee, K.-C., Su, W., and Muller, S.A.: Multicentric cloacogenic cancer of the skin and vulva. J. Am. Acad. Dermatol., *23:*1005, 1990.
18. Murie, J., Andrew, J.S.W., and Mackenzie, I.: The importance of pain, pruritus and soiling as symptoms of haemorrhoids and their response to haemorrhoidectomy or rubber band ligation. Br. J. Surg., *68:*247, 1981.
19. Novak, E., Gilbertson, T.J., and Seckman, C.E.: Anorectal pruritus after intravenous hydrocortisone sodium succinate and sodium phosphate. Clin. Pharmacol. Ther., *20:*1009, 1976.
20. Oliet, E.J., and Estes, S.A.: Perianal comedones associated with chronic topical fluorinated steroid use (letter). J. Am. Acad. Dermatol., *7*(3):405, 1982.
21. Raaf, J.H., Krown, S.E., and Pinsky, C.M.: Treatment of Bowen's disease with topical dinitrochlorobenzene and 5-fluorouracil. Cancer, *37:*1633, 1976.
22. Shafir, A.: An injection technique for the treatment of idiopathic pruritus ani. Int. Surg., *75:*43, 1990.
23. Silverman, S.H., Youngs, D.J., Allan, A., et al.: The fecal microflora in pruritus ani. Dis. Colon Rectum, *32:*466, 1989.
24. Smith, L.E., Henrichs, D., and McCullay, R.D.: Prospective studies on the etiology and treatment of pruritus ani. Dis. Colon Rectum, *25:*358, 1982.
25. Strauss, R., and Fazio, V.W.: Bowen's disease of the anal and perianal area: A report and analysis of 12 cases. Am. J. Surg., *137:* 231, 1979.
26. Wexner, S., Smithy, W., Milsom, J., and Dailey, T.: The surgical management of anorectal disease in AIDS and pre-AIDS patients. Dis. Colon Rectum, *29:*719, 1986.
27. Wexner, S.W., Dailey T.H., and Milsom, J.W.: The demographics of anal cancer are changing. Dis. Colon Rectum, *30:*942, 1987.

Chapter 25

FISSURE-IN-ANO

ALAN E. TIMMCKE / TERRY C. HICKS

Anal fissure is defined as a painful, longitudinal defect in the lining (anoderm) of the anal canal. Fissures generally extend from just below the dentate line to the anal verge. They may be acute and superficial or chronic, displaying exposed muscle fibers, fibrotic undermined margins, a redundant "sentinel" skin tag, and a hypertrophied anal papilla (Fig. 25–1). Fissures are the most common cause of painful rectal bleeding and frequently produce pain out of proportion to the size of the lesion. Fissures afflict all age groups but predominantly occur in the third and fourth decades of life. Both sexes are affected equally.[3] Fissures frequently occur in infants and children and represent the most common source of rectal bleeding in this age group.[5]

Anal fissures are consistently located in the posterior midline in 99% of men and in 90% of women. The majority of the remainder are located anteriorly. Lesions found in other locations should arouse suspicion of an associated underlying disease process (e.g., inflammatory bowel disease).[15]

ETIOLOGY

The etiology of anal fissure is unclear and probably is multifactorial. It has been postulated that trauma, anal canal anatomy, sphincter dysfunction, and ischemia may be contributory.[6,39]

Trauma is believed to be the initiating factor for most fissures. Patients often relate the onset of symptoms to passing a large, hard stool. Less frequently, trauma associated with labor and delivery or the insertion of a foreign body may be implicated. Diarrhea may also cause trauma to the anus. Repeated forceful bowel movements and associated chemical burning may make the anoderm susceptible to trauma.

Conditions such as inflammatory bowel disease or previous anal surgery may predispose the patient to fissure formation. The association of anal fissure and inflammatory bowel disease is well established. Anal surgery can produce scarring and stenosis, resulting in susceptibility to tearing upon dilation.

The anatomic configuration of the anal sphincters likely predisposes the posterior and anterior locations to tearing. The superficial external anal sphincter forms an elliptic, slit-like aperture that lies in an anteroposterior plane. The superficial external sphincter fibers are fixed anteriorly, at which point they decussate, and posteriorly, at which point they join the anococcygeal ligament. It is believed that with the passage of stool, greater shearing forces occur at these points of fixation.[13,31]

The internal anal sphincter may contribute to anal fissure. The smooth muscle internal anal sphincter is predominantly responsible for the resting pressure of the anus. Nothmann and Schuster,[30] Hancock,[18] and Arabi and associates[2] all demonstrated that patients with anal fissure had elevated resting anal sphincter pressures when compared with normal control subjects.

Duthie and Bennett[7] reported conflicting findings; they were unable to demonstrate a difference in resting pressures between fissure patients and controls. Nothmann and Schuster[30] demonstrated normal reflex relaxation of the internal anal sphincter when the rectum was distended. However, in their study of patients with anal fissure, normal relaxation was followed by a contraction that exceeded the previous baseline resting pressure (Fig. 25–2). They also found that after healing of the fissure, this reflex "overshoot" disappeared. The overshoot phenomenon may play a role in perpetuating pain or delaying healing of an anal fissure.

Using Doppler laser flowmetry of the anoderm combined with anal manometry, Schouten and co-workers have demonstrated anodermal blood flow in the posterior midline to be less than in other segments of the anal canal. The higher the anal resting pressure the lower the blood flow.[39] This relative ischemia may explain the severity of the pain associated with fissures and their failure to heal.

DIAGNOSIS

Careful history-taking prior to examination of a patient usually leads to the correct diagnosis. The most common presenting symptom of anal fissure is anal pain, particularly painful defecation. Other associated symptoms include bleeding, pruritus, or discharge. The pain is frequently described as a cutting, tearing, or burning sensation that is initiated with the passage of stool and usually persists for several hours after defeca-

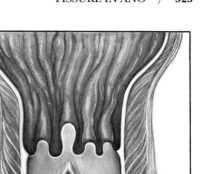

FIGURE 25-1. Acute and chronic fissure. (Modified from Hicks, T.C., and Ray, J.E.: Rectal and perianal complaints. *In* Polk, H.C., Jr., Stone, H.H., and Gardner, B. (eds.): Basic Surgery, 3rd ed. Norwalk, CT, Appleton-Century-Crofts, 1987, p. 455, with permission.)

tion. Some patients experience such severe or prolonged pain that they postpone regular bowel movements, leading to severe constipation. The subsequent passage of hard stools may lead to repeated anal trauma and associated continued spasm of the anal sphincter. This vicious cycle, once established, perpetuates the pain. The blood is usually bright red, scant, and often found only on the toilet tissue. Up to 50% of patients with anal fissure also complain of pruritus, which is most likely secondary to persistent anal discharge. Patients with severe pain from fissure may also have urinary symptoms such as dysuria, frequency, and retention.[24]

DIFFERENTIAL DIAGNOSIS

Anal fissures must be distinguished from anal ulcers that are produced by other disease processes, such as inflammatory bowel disease, infection, or malignancy. Not infrequently, anal disease represents the initial man-

ifestation of Crohn's disease or ulcerative colitis. Often, delayed healing of a fissure or its recurrence after surgical intervention suggests the possibility of inflammatory bowel disease. Up to 50% of patients with Crohn's disease experience anal fissures at some time during the course of the disease. These fissures are often multiple and atypically located. Unfortunately, proctosigmoidoscopy may not confirm the diagnosis of Crohn's disease because intestinal disease may be located in more proximal bowel. Biopsy of suspicious anal fissures is rarely helpful in confirming the presence of Crohn's disease, and complete evaluation of the upper and lower gastrointestinal tract may be necessary. Anal ulcers also can be associated with ulcerative colitis. They are usually broadbased and found off the midline. The surgeon can confirm the diagnosis of proctocolitis by sigmoidoscopy.

Chronic pruritus ani is often associated with fissure formation, but these lesions are usually superficial, externally located, and not associated with the pain and spasm seen in acute fissure-in-ano.

Infections such as herpes, syphilis, chancroid, and tuberculosis may result in anal ulcers.[15] Anal herpes can produce painful ulceration that may be confused with anal fissure. These ulcers are atypically located and typically far more painful than their superficial appearance suggests. Viral cultures can confirm the diagnosis of anal herpes. Syphilitic fissures often display mirror-image lesions, and the diagnosis can be made by darkfield examination of the lesions and confirmed by rapid plasma reagin (RPR) studies. Chancroid can produce anal ulcers, but this is unusual without prominent inguinal adenopathy. Tuberculous anal ulcer is a very rare entity that is virtually never seen without concomitant pulmonary disease.

Epidermoid carcinoma of the anus and adenocarcinoma of the rectum involving the anal canal may result in painful defecation. These lesions, however, are usually atypical in appearance and are easily recognized by the clinician. Biopsy confirms the clinical diagnosis. Leukemic anal infiltrates are often extremely painful, and adequate abscess drainage is required, though it is seldom

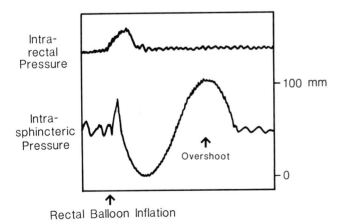

FIGURE 25-2. Rectoanal inhibitory reflex with "overshoot" phenomenon. (Modified from Nothmann, B.J., and Schuster, M.M.: Internal anal sphincter derangement with anal fissures. Gastroenterology, 67:216, 1974, with permission.)

satisfying for this late stage of malignant disease. Reports have described ulcerated lesions within the anal canal associated with acquired immunodeficiency syndrome (AIDS). These lesions may result from anal herpes, cytomegalovirus, Kaposi's sarcoma, and B-cell lymphoma. Again, the physician must be suspicious of any lesion found off the midline or any lesion that shows slow healing. These findings should lead to further diagnostic tests, including biopsy.

PHYSICAL EXAMINATION

Although a careful history often suggests the diagnosis of an anal fissure prior to physical examination, physical examination is necessary not only to confirm the diagnosis but also to eliminate other associated or contributing diseases. Patients with anal fissure often approach examination with a great deal of anxiety. It is important for the physician to demonstrate patience and gentleness. The usefulness of "vocal anesthesia" cannot be overemphasized.

The first and most important step is careful inspection of the anus. Gentle separation of the buttocks often brings the fissure into view (Fig. 25–3). Even in patients with marked spasm, gentle, forceful lateral traction generally everts the anus sufficiently to expose the fissure, making digital or anoscopic examination unnecessary. Occasionally, digital application of a topical anesthetic gel or ointment may be helpful. A patient with a chronic fissure may exhibit a sentinel pile external to the fissure, and if anoscopic examination is possible, a hypertrophied anal papilla may be seen (Fig. 25–4). It should be re-emphasized that fissures found in locations other than an anterior or posterior location may be associated with other underlying pathophysiologic conditions.

Next, the examiner should palpate the anus, which will often confirm the presence of sphincter spasm and tenderness. Digital and sigmoidoscopic examinations should be performed to rule out inflammatory bowel disease or a potential carcinoma. Frequently, the pain is

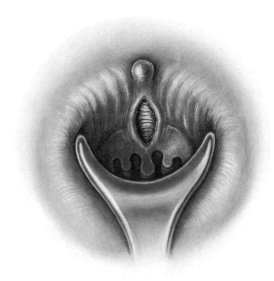

FIGURE 25–4. Physical examination of chronic fissure. (Modified from Hicks, T.C., and Ray, J.E.: Rectal and perianal complaints. *In* Polk, H.C., Jr., Stone, H.H., and Gardner, B. (eds.): Basic Surgery, 3rd ed. Norwalk, CT, Appleton-Century-Crofts, 1987, p. 455, with permission.)

so severe that these examinations must be delayed and performed under anesthesia.[20]

TREATMENT

Medical Management

A trial of medical management should be attempted in all patients. The decision to continue a trial of conservative medical management should be based on clinical judgment. An acute superficial anal fissure producing symptoms of relatively short duration generally responds symptomatically and heals following a medical regimen. Such a regimen includes bulk stool softeners (e.g., psyllium or methylcellulose preparations), a high-fiber diet including liberal use of unprocessed bran, maintenance of adequate hydration, and the use of warm sitz baths, particularly following defecation, to relax reflex anal sphincter spasm and avoid painful wiping. The bulk stool softeners and high-fiber diet produce a large, lubricated, easily passed stool that requires less time for the painful act of defecation or that induces less vigorous perianal cleansing. In addition, the large diameter of the stool may produce natural dilation of the anal sphincter, reducing spasm. Adequate hydration is required to ensure that stools remain soft and well lubricated. Patients should be reminded to maintain regular, soft stools for weeks after symptoms have subsided because it is not uncommon for a single hard stool to reopen a recently healed anal fissure.

Ointments, emollients, and creams, some containing anesthetics or anti-inflammatory agents (e.g., hydrocortisone), have been used with variable success. They require digital application within the anal canal to be of any benefit, an act that many patients find not only painful but also distasteful. The reported efficacy of these agents is perhaps due to their lubricating effect, the nat-

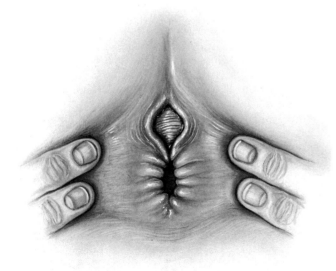

FIGURE 25–3. Inspection of fissure.

ural history of healing that many acute fissures exhibit, or possibly the placebo effect of applying an agent directly to the site of pain. Anesthetic ointments, in addition to being of little long-term benefit, can result in perianal dermatitis. The use of suppositories is to be avoided. Their insertion is frequently painful, and they have been shown to migrate high within the rectum at which point their ingredients have little or no effect on a fissure located within the anal canal. Their reported efficacy is probably due to the same factors described for ointments and creams. The use of smooth muscle relaxants and antispasmodics (e.g., dicyclomine) has been suggested, but presently no controlled clinical trials have been reported.[26]

Long-acting local anesthetics, generally suspended in oil and injected lateral to the anal sphincter to block the anal branches of the pudendal nerves, enjoyed popularity in the 1920s and 1930s. Because of associated problems with incontinence and, not infrequently, abscesses, fistulas, and sepsis attendant on injection of poorly absorbed immunogenic substances, the practice has been abandoned.[11,17,27,41]

Anal dilators for outpatient use were advocated by Gabriel in 1948.[12] They were suggested as a means of applying anesthetic ointment by Goligher.[15] It would seem, considering the pain produced by even a gentle digital examination, that all but the most unusual patient would prefer application of an anesthetic prior to insertion of a dilator. Although anal dilators are still used to some extent in Great Britain, there is little evidence to support their use.

Conservative measures rarely promote healing of a typical chronic anal fissure characterized by a prominent sentinel tag, exposed circumferential fibers of the internal anal sphincter muscle, indurated undermined margins, and an associated hypertrophied anal papilla (Fig. 25–4). Chronic fissures that respond symptomatically seldom heal completely, and symptoms frequently recur. An associated superficial fistula also strongly suggests the eventual need for surgical management. However, despite the clinical features of chronicity, it is not unusual for a fissure to be painless, producing only occasional bleeding, discharge, or pruritus. When symptoms are of insufficient severity to recommend operative treatment, conservative management is the only option.

It must be kept in mind that operative treatment and the occasional disturbance in continence that results may render symptoms of discharge or pruritus more severe. Indeed, a chronic, relatively asymptomatic, indolent fissure may represent the initial manifestation of inflammatory bowel disease. Ultimately, whether an anal fissure appears to be acute or chronic, the decision to use surgical treatment depends on the presence of persistent pain or bleeding and the lack of an acceptable response to medical management. Frequently, it is the patient who decides that attempts at conservative medical management have failed and, for reasons of intolerable pain or bleeding, requests surgery.

Surgical Management

Eisenhammer[8,10] was the first to recognize that division of the lowermost portion of the internal anal sphincter usually resulted in rapid relief of pain and subsequent healing of the fissure. Goligher[15] credits Miles as having been the first to perform internal sphincterotomy for the treatment of anal fissure in 1938, although Miles[25] referred to the structure he was dividing as the "pecten band" and failed to recognize that it was actually the lower portion of the internal anal sphincter. Gabriel, in 1948,[12] popularized excision of the fissure (fissurectomy), during the course of which he also divided a portion of muscle that he thought represented the spastic subcutaneous external anal sphincter. However, Eisenhammer,[9] supported by the subsequent anatomic studies by Goligher and associates,[16] must be given credit for recognizing the importance of the internal anal sphincter in the pathogenesis and treatment of anal fissure. All successful surgical procedures for the management of anal fissure, although varying in method, employ stretching or division of the internal anal sphincter.

Anal Sphincter Stretch

Recamier has been credited with the first use of manual stretching of the anal sphincters for the treatment of anal fissure.[23,36] More recently, Goligher[14] popularized the procedure as a surgical alternative to internal anal sphincterotomy. In 1973, Lord,[22] to whom the method has been eponymously attributed, suggested extending the use of the technique to the treatment of hemorrhoids. Although the procedure is usually successful in alleviating pain initially, it requires general anesthesia and results in only a 72% rate of fissure healing, a 16% rate of recurrent pain, and a 20% rate of fecal soiling.[14,40] The technique involves insertion of four to eight fingers in the anal orifice and exertion of either lateral or anterior and posterior pressure to produce sphincter dilation, which is sustained for several minutes. In addition to having a rather unaesthetic and uncontrolled appearance, sphincter stretch has little to recommend it in terms of results or lack of complications.

Fissure Excision

Popularized by Gabriel in 1948, it seems that the success of fissure excision was not the result of excising the fissure but of dividing or stretching the internal anal sphincter, a maneuver that Gabriel unknowingly included.[12,15] The triangular wound that he describes has its apex at the dentate line and its base nearly 4 cm distal to this line. The defect is slow to heal and frequently results in a characteristic "keyhole deformity" with consequent fecal soiling. Since the advent of lateral subcutaneous internal anal sphincterotomy, it has become apparent that the fissure rarely requires excision. Fissure excision becomes necessary only to open an associated superficial fistula, remove a large prolapsing hypertrophied papilla, or improve anal hygiene hampered by a large, redundant skin tag.

Internal Anal Sphincterotomy

Internal anal sphincterotomy has become the preferred procedure for the treatment of symptomatic anal fissure. Eisenhammer, in 1951, advocated an open technique in which the internal anal sphincter is divided in the posterior midline from the level of the dentate line distally.[8] This was usually accomplished through the fissure itself, and the wound was allowed to heal by secondary intention. Bennett and Goligher[3] reported that this technique resulted in a slowly healing wound associated with fibrosis, which produced a characteristic keyhole deformity. It was this deformity that was thought to be responsible for the rather high incidence of fecal soiling (22%) and impaired control of flatus (19%) or feces (9%) associated with the procedure. Similar results influenced Eisenhammer, in 1959, to advocate a lateral approach for dividing the sphincter, in the hope that such a wound would heal more promptly and result in a less prominent longitudinal defect.[10] Lateral internal anal sphincterotomy was originally performed using an open technique similar to that of posterior midline sphincterotomy; a later modification included closure of the skin, resulting in even more rapid healing and less postoperative pain (Fig. 25–5).

Lateral Subcutaneous Internal Anal Sphincterotomy

Parks, in 1967, advocated lateral subcutaneous internal anal sphincterotomy performed through a short circumferential incision placed laterally in the skin outside the anal verge (Fig. 25–6).[33] In this procedure, an incision in the anal canal and its associated pain are avoided. The anoderm is carefully dissected free of the underlying internal anal sphincter, and, after further dissection in the intersphincteric groove, sphincter division is accomplished under direct visualization. Meticulous

hemostatis is possible. The wound is either left open or is closed, as described by Parks,[33] with several interrupted sutures. The incision can be oriented circumferentially or radially, the latter healing more readily if left open. The addition of a subcuticular closure using an absorbable suture seems to facilitate healing and reduce discomfort.

Notaras[28,29] was the first to advocate blind lateral subcutaneous internal anal sphincterotomy. The technique lends itself very well to the use of local anesthesia in an outpatient surgical setting. In this procedure, a narrow scalpel (No. 11 Bard-Parker, a cataract blade, or a No. 52 Beaver) is inserted through a lateral stab wound at the level of the lower margin of the internal sphincter just medial to the intersphincteric groove, as shown by the hemostat in Figure 25–7A. As originally described, the blade is positioned parallel to the sphincter and is advanced beneath the anal skin until its tip is at the level of the dentate line; then, turning the knife perpendicularly and making a gentle oscillating motion outward, the sphincter is divided (Fig. 25–7, inset). A modification of the technique, advocated more recently, involves inserting the blade between the internal and external sphincters, turning it inward, and with a gentle motion severing the sphincter (Fig. 25–7A through C). The knife is then removed and, with lateral pressure, the few remaining fibers of the muscle are avulsed. Sustaining the pressure for a few moments produces hemostasis.

In both techniques, the small wound is left open. The modified technique reduces the possibility of incising fibers of the external anal sphincter, which would increase the likelihood of fecal incontinence. The modified technique can also be used with local anesthesia. With placement of a finger within the anal canal, blind

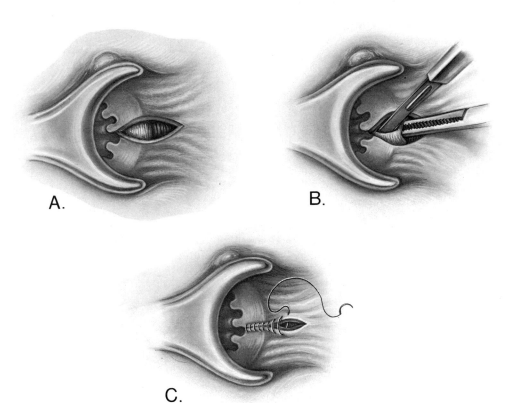

FIGURE 25-5. Lateral internal anal sphincterotomy. *A,* Internal anal sphincter visible through incision. *B,* Lateral division of internal anal sphincter. *C,* Wound closure. (Modified from Storer, E.H., Goldberg, S.M., and Nivatvongs, S.: Colon, rectum and anus. *In* Schwartz, S.I. (ed.): Principles of Surgery, 4th ed. New York, McGraw-Hill, 1984, p. 1169, with permission.)

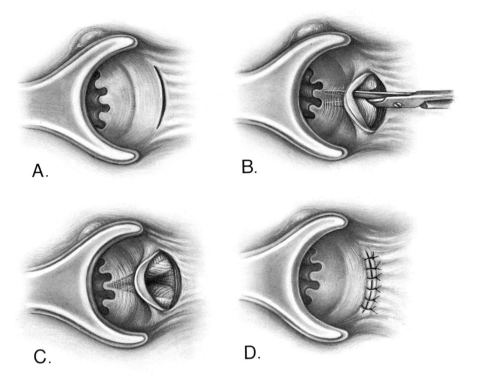

FIGURE 25-6. Lateral subcutaneous internal anal sphincterotomy. *A,* Lateral circumanal incision. *B,* Internal anal sphincter division. *C,* Divided internal anal sphincter. *D,* Wound closure. (Modified from Parks, A.G.: The management of fissure-in-ano. Hosp. Med., *1:*737, 1967, with permission.)

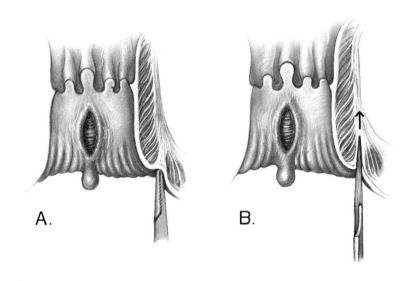

FIGURE 25-7. Blind lateral subcutaneous internal anal sphincterotomy. *A,* Hemostat demonstrating intersphincteric groove. *B,* Insertion of scalpel between internal and external sphincters. *C,* Sphincter division by inward motion of the scalpel. *Inset,* Original Notaras technique showing outward motion of scalpel. (Modified from Notaras, M.J.: The treatment of anal fissure by lateral subcutaneous internal sphincterotomy—a technique and results. Br. J. Surg., *58:*96, 1971, by permission of the publishers, Butterworth & Co., © 1971.)

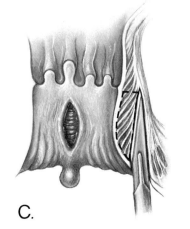

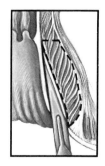

cutting of the sphincter can be guided digitally to avoid lacerating the anoderm (Fig. 25–8). A bivalve or Hill-Ferguson anal retractor can be employed to improve visibility and place the sphincter on tension and to eliminate the need for placing a finger within the anal canal. Such a retractor may be used with local anesthesia, but it necessitates a more extensive local block, and even then, rectal distention often produces discomfort and makes sedation of the patient necessary. For these reasons, most surgeons who employ a retractor reserve it for use with a general anesthetic. The technique of blind sphincterotomy can more easily be used with local anesthesia (Fig. 25–8).

This procedure can be performed in the lithotomy, prone, or left lateral position, depending on the patient's, surgeon's, and anesthetist's preferences. We prefer the prone–jackknife position. In this position, the incision is in a right lateral location for a right-handed surgeon. This avoids the left lateral hemorrhoid column, which is often the most prominent. With the patient under light sedation, a roll is placed beneath the hips, and the buttocks are spread apart using 4-inch tape straps. Using a 1.5-inch 27- or 30-gauge needle, the perianal subcutaneous tissues are injected bilaterally with 3 to 5 ml of 0.5% lidocaine containing 1:200,000 epinephrine. An additional 3 to 5 ml of this solution is then infiltrated bilaterally in the intersphincteric space. On the side on which the sphincter is to be divided, an additional 1 ml is injected into the space between the anoderm of the anal canal and the internal sphincter. Blind cutting of the sphincter, avoiding laceration of the anoderm, can then be accomplished (Fig. 25–8). Alternatively, with the degree of anesthesia and sedation provided by this technique, a medium Hill-Ferguson retractor can be used to place the sphincter on stretch and allow visualization of the overlying anoderm. If more prolonged anesthesia is desired, 0.25% bupivacaine with 1:200,000 epinephrine may be substituted.

POSTOPERATIVE MANAGEMENT

Postoperative care consists of the use of a psyllium preparation, sitz baths, and a mild analgesic. A regular diet and normal activities can generally be resumed within 24 hours. Pain is generally less intense than that

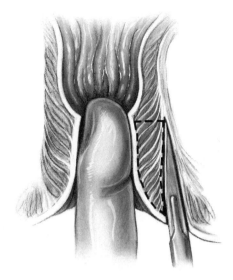

FIGURE 25–8. Digitally directed blind lateral subcutaneous internal anal sphincterotomy. (Modified from Notaras, M.J.: The treatment of anal fissure by lateral subcutaneous internal sphincterotomy—a technique and results. Br. J. Surg., 58:96, 1971, by permission of the publishers, Butterworth & Co. © 1971.)

produced by the fissure preoperatively. In fact, most patients experience complete relief of pain within 48 hours of surgery despite the fact that complete healing of the fissure may take several weeks. This observation lends support to the theory that internal anal sphincter spasm, and not the fissure itself, is responsible for the pain associated with anal fissure.

RESULTS AND COMPLICATIONS

As seen in Table 25–1, between 97 and 100% of patients with fissures who are treated with lateral subcutaneous internal anal sphincterotomy experience complete healing.[1,4,19,21,29,32,34,35,38] The majority of patients (> 90%) are free of pain within 48 hours and can return to work. Healing of the fissure is complete in 96% of patients within 1 month. Minor defects in anal control are documented following lateral subcutaneous internal anal sphincterotomy, but they generally consist only of impaired control of flatus and minor soiling. Mucus

TABLE 25–1. LATERAL SUBCUTANEOUS INTERNAL ANAL SPHINCTEROTOMY

Author	No. of Patients	% Healed	% Recurrence	Minor Defects of Anal Control (%)			% Other Complications
				Feces	Flatus	Soiling	
Hawley[19]	24	100	0	0	0	0	0
Hoffman and Goligher[21]	99	97	3	1.0	6.1	7.1	3
Notaras[29]	82	100	0	1.4	2.7	5.5	1.4
Ray et al.[35]	21	100	0	0	0	0	4.8
Rudd[38]	200	99.5	0.5	0	0	0	0.5
Abcarian[1]*	150	98.7	1.3	0	0	0	1.3
Oh[32]	550	99.6	0.4	?	?	?	6.9
Ravikumar et al.[34]	60	96.7	3.3	0	0	0	5.0
Boulos and Araujo[4]	28	100	0	0	17.9	?	7.1

*The lateral sphincterotomies in this series were not performed subcutaneously.

leakage and occasional fecal soiling are both common following lateral sphincterotomy using an incision in the anal canal or anal stretching. Of the 1,214 patients represented in Table 25–1, only 2 patients experienced any prolonged fecal incontinence. Other complications include bleeding, abscess formation, fistulization, hemorrhoidal prolapse, hematoma, perianal ecchymosis, and pruritus. These conditions are encountered rarely, and combined they account for problems in less than 7% of patients.

We believe that lateral subcutaneous internal anal sphincterotomy is the procedure of choice for the surgical management of anal fissure. The surgeon who is infrequently called upon to perform anal surgery will perhaps find the well-visualized technique described by Parks[33] most satisfactory. Those with more familiarity and experience with anal anatomy might prefer the blind technique of Notaras.[28] In either case, the results of these techniques with regard to impaired fecal continence are superior to those of sphincter stretch and posterior midline sphincterotomy, and these latter procedures should be abandoned.[37]

REFERENCES

1. Abcarian, H.: Surgical correction of chronic anal fissure: Results of lateral internal sphincterotomy vs. fissurectomy-midline sphincterotomy. Dis. Colon Rectum, 23:31, 1980.
2. Arabi, Y., Alexander-Williams, J., and Keighley, M.R.B.: Anal pressures in hemorrhoids and anal fissure. Am. J. Surg., 134:608, 1977.
3. Bennett, R.C., and Goligher, J.C.: Results of internal sphincterotomy for anal fissure. BMJ, 2:1500, 1962.
4. Boulos, P.B., and Araujo, J.G.C.: Adequate internal sphincterotomy for chronic anal fissure: Subcutaneous or open technique? Br. J. Surg., 71:360, 1984.
5. Connor, J.J.: Pediatric proctology. Dis. Colon Rectum, 18:126, 1975.
6. Corman, M.L.: Colon and Rectal Surgery. Philadelphia, J.B. Lippincott, 1984.
7. Duthie, H.L., and Bennett, R.C.: Anal sphincter pressure in fissure-in-ano. Surg. Gyncol. Obstet., 119:19, 1964.
8. Eisenhammer, S.: The surgical correction of chronic internal anal (sphincteric) contracture. S. Afr. Med. J., 25:486, 1951.
9. Eisenhammer, S.: The internal anal sphincter: Its surgical importance. S. Afr. Med. J., 27:266, 1953.
10. Eisenhammer, S.: The evaluation of the internal anal sphincterotomy operation with special reference to anal fissure. Surg. Gynecol. Obstet., 109:583, 1959.
11. Gabriel, W.B.: Treatment of pruritus ani and anal fissure: The use of anesthetic solution in oil. BMJ, 1:1070, 1929.
12. Gabriel, W.B.: Principles and Practice of Rectal Surgery, 4th ed. London, H.K. Lewis, 1948.
13. Gabriel, W.B.: Principles and Practice of Rectal Surgery, 5th ed. Springfield, IL, Charles C. Thomas, 1963.
14. Goligher, J.C.: An evaluation of internal sphincterotomy and simple sphincter stretching in the treatment of fissure-in-ano. Surg. Clin. North Am., 42:1299, 1965.
15. Goligher, J.C.: Surgery of the Anus, Rectum and Colon, 4th ed. London, Baillière Tindall, 1980.
16. Goligher, J.C., Leacock, A.G., and Brossy, J.J.: Surgical anatomy of the anal canal. Br. J. Surg., 43:51, 1955.
17. Gorsch, R.V.: Oil soluble anesthetics in proctology. Med. Rec., 139:35, 1934.
18. Hancock, B.D.: The internal sphincter and anal fissure. Br. J. Surg., 64:92, 1977.
19. Hawley, P.R.: The treatment of chronic fissure-in-ano. A trial of methods. Br. J. Surg., 56:915, 1969.
20. Hicks, T.C., and Ray, J.E.: Rectal and perianal complaints. In Polk, H.C., Jr., Stone, H.H., and Gardner, B. (eds.): Basic Surgery, 3rd ed. Norwalk, CT, Appleton-Century-Crofts, 1987, p. 455.
21. Hoffmann, D.C., and Goligher, J.C.: Lateral subcutaneous internal sphincterotomy in treatment of anal fissure. BMJ, 3:673, 1970.
22. Lord, P.H.: Diverse methods of managing hemorrhoids: Dilatation. Dis. Colon Rectum, 16:180, 1973.
23. Maisonneuve, J.G.: Du traitement de la fissure a l'anus par la dilatation forcée. Gaz d'hop, 3rd series 1:220, 1849.
24. Mazier, W.P., De Moraes, R.T., and Dignan, R.D.: Anal fissure and anal ulcers. Surg. Clin. North Am., 58:479, 1978.
25. Miles, W.E.: Rectal Surgery. London, Cassell, 1939.
26. Miller, L.G., Rogers, J.C., Brown, E.B., et al.: Dicyclomine for medical management of persistent anal fissure with associated spasm of the internal sphincter. Tex. Med., 88:65, 1992.
27. Morgan, C.N.: Oil soluble anesthetic in rectal surgery. BMJ, 2:938, 1935.
28. Notaras, M.J.: Lateral subcutaneous sphincterotomy for anal fissure—a new technique. Proc. R. Soc. Med., 62:713, 1969.
29. Notaras, M.J.: The treatment of anal fissure by lateral subcutaneous internal sphincterotomy—a technique and results. Br. J. Surg., 58:96, 1971.
30. Nothmann, B.J., and Schuster, M.M.: Internal anal sphincter derangement with anal fissures. Gastroenterology, 67:216, 1974.
31. Oh, C.: Lateral subcutaneous internal sphincterotomy for anal fissure. Mt. Sinai J. Med., 42:596, 1975.
32. Oh, C.: The role of internal sphincterotomy. Mt. Sinai J. Med., 49:484, 1982.
33. Parks, A.G.: The management of fissure-in-ano. Hosp. Med., 1:737, 1967.
34. Ravikumar, T.S., Sridhar, S., and Rao, R.N.: Subcutaneous lateral internal sphincterotomy for chronic fissure-in-ano. Dis. Colon Rectum, 25:778, 1982.
35. Ray, J.E., Penfold, J.C.B., Gathright, J.B., et al.: Lateral subcutaneous internal anal sphincterotomy for anal fissure. Dis. Colon Rectum, 17:139, 1974.
36. Récamier, J.C.A.: Extension, massage et percussion cadencée dans le traitement des contractures musculaires. Rev. Medicale Franc., 1:74, 1838 (Translated Dis. Colon Rectum, 23:362, 1980).
37. Rosen, L., Abel, M.E., Gordon, P.H., et al.: Practice parameters for the management of anal fissure. The Standards Task Force. American Society of Colon and Rectal Surgeons. Dis. Colon Rectum, 35:206, 1992.
38. Rudd, W.W.H.: Lateral subcutaneous internal sphincterotomy for chronic anal fissure, an outpatient procedure. Dis. Colon Rectum, 18:319, 1975.
39. Schouten, W.R., Briel, J.W., Auwerda, J.J.: Relationship between anal pressure and anodermal blood flow. The vascular pathogenesis of anal fissures. Dis. Colon Rectum, 37:664, 1994.
40. Watts, J.McK., Bennett, R.C., and Goligher, J.C.: Stretching of anal sphincters in treatment of fissure-in-ano. BMJ, 2:342, 1964.
41. Yeomans, F.C., Gorsch, R.V., and Mathesheimer, J.L.: Benachol in the treatment of pruritus ani (preliminary report). Trans. Am. Proct. Soc., 28:24, 1927.

Chapter 26

HEMORRHOIDAL DISEASE

EUGENE P. SALVATI / THEODORE E. EISENSTAT

Hemorrhoids have been a recognized affliction of humans for several thousand years, and through the centuries they have been dealt with both medically and surgically in many different ways. Goligher[16] states that at least 50% of people older than 50 years of age have some degree of hemorrhoid formation. New methods for the management of hemorrhoids are constantly being introduced. Some have withstood the test of time, whereas others have been discarded. We have chosen to present only those methods that are currently in use, have proved to be practical, and can be duplicated by the infrequent operator or the young surgeon.

ETIOLOGY

Anatomically, everyone has hemorrhoids. Thomson[49] first referred to hemorrhoids as cushions and described them as being composed primarily of blood vessels, elastic and connective tissue, and smooth muscle fibers. Haas and associates[19] confirmed the findings of Thomson and stated that these cushions form in utero and aid in anal continence. Stelzner[48] had previously shown that the arterial bleeding from hemorrhoids is due to arteriovenous anastomoses in the hemorrhoidal plexus. Jackson and Robertson[21] first related that the elastic tissue seen in young persons degenerates in the older individual. It appears that this breakdown in the connective tissue as one ages is responsible for the symptoms of hemorrhoids (i.e., bleeding, protrusion).

Recent studies by Deutsch and colleagues,[11] El-Gendi and Abdel-Baky,[13] and Lin,[26] measuring the anorectal pressure by manometry in symptomatic internal hemorrhoids, have all shown higher anal pressures than in control patients. This evidence of increased internal sphincter pressure may be a factor in the etiology of hemorrhoids, although it is not known whether the increased internal sphincter tone causes the hemorrhoids or is the result of their development. Other obvious contributory factors, such as constipation, increase the tendency for hemorrhoids to bulge and protrude, since the deteriorating connective tissue is no longer able to support the blood vessels. Heredity is also probably a factor, but this has not been proven.

ANATOMY

Hemorrhoids receive their blood supply from the superior hemorrhoidal artery, which is a branch of the inferior mesenteric artery. The middle hemorrhoidal artery and inferior hemorrhoidal artery anastomose with branches from the superior hemorrhoidal artery; thus, the anorectal area is richly vascularized. The superior, middle, and inferior hemorrhoidal veins correspond to each artery and drain blood from the anal tissues. Arteriovenous communications are present between the two systems. There are generally three main groups of hemorrhoids, which are located in the right anterior, right posterior, and left lateral segments. It was originally thought that this differentiation was due to the divisions of the superior hemorrhoidal artery, which terminated in these locations,[21] but Thomson[49] was unable to verify this by cadaver injection. Secondary groups can also be present, and their most common location is in the left posterior quadrant and to a lesser degree in the left anterior quadrant.

CLASSIFICATION

Hemorrhoids can be classified as external or internal, with the latter being further subdivided. External hemorrhoids arise from the inferior hemorrhoidal artery, are anatomically located distal to the dentate line, and are covered with skin. Internal hemorrhoids arise from the superior hemorrhoidal artery, are covered with mucosa, and present proximal to the dentate line. Hemorrhoids can occasionally be so large that the anatomic indentation at the dentate line is obliterated, in which case they can be referred to as mixed.

Internal hemorrhoids are divided into first, second,

third, and fourth degrees. Internal hemorrhoids that bleed but do not protrude are considered to be first-degree hemorrhoids. Second-degree hemorrhoids bleed and protrude but reduce spontaneously. Third-degree hemorrhoids bleed and protrude and require manual reduction. Fourth-degree hemorrhoids are prolapsed distal to the dentate line and cannot be reduced.

SYMPTOMS

Most hemorrhoids are asymptomatic. Symptoms that occur generally can be classified as those caused by external hemorrhoids and those caused by internal hemorrhoids. By far, the most common hemorrhoidal complaint is the sudden swelling of anal tissue resulting from the development of an external thrombosis. Probably everyone will experience this at some time. This sudden swelling can be very painful. Occasionally, it is associated with itching. The thrombosis can cause a pressure necrosis of the skin with resultant bleeding, following which discomfort is generally reduced. Internal hemorrhoids are seldom painful. They manifest themselves by painless bright red bleeding, which is noted on the toilet paper or can drip down into the toilet bowl. This can be associated with protrusion from the anal canal. The protrusion generally reduces itself spontaneously but may have to be done manually. A mucus discharge may be present, with staining of the underwear. Internal hemorrhoids seldom cause itching and may acutely prolapse and develop associated internal and external thromboses. In this situation they are extremely painful.

THROMBOSED EXTERNAL HEMORRHOIDS

Thrombosis occurs suddenly,[43] frequently after heavy physical exertion (Fig. 26–1). Examination will reveal a hard, bluish lump beneath the skin in the anal canal. This is due to thrombosis of one or more external hemorrhoidal veins or to the rupture of a vein with resultant perianal hematoma. The thrombosis or hematoma is covered with skin. It is a mistake to try to reduce it into the rectum or have the patient attempt to do so, since anatomically it does not belong in the rectum, but rather in the anal canal. Most thromboses improve with hot baths and rest. If they remain painful after 48 hours, however, they should be excised. This can be accomplished as an office procedure under local anesthesia.

The area superficial to, lateral to, and beneath the thrombosis is injected with 2 to 3 ml of 0.25% bupivacaine with 1:200,000 epinephrine. A 30-gauge needle makes the injection less painful and easier to perform. The area is then massaged thoroughly and slowly. This ensures good anesthesia and helps disperse the edema. An Allis clamp is placed in the skin at the apex of the thrombosis, and an elliptic piece of skin is excised along with the thrombosis down to the sphincter mechanism. Curved scissors are best for carrying out this maneuver. The dentate line is never crossed, as this will frequently result in a postexcisional fissure. The incision is kept as far distal in the anal canal as is technically feasible. Grosz[18] has suggested making a circumferential incision in relation to the anus, as he feels the wound will expose more clots and will heal faster. There appears to be merit in this proposal. After hemostasis is secured with an electrosurgical unit or ferric subsulfate (Monsel's solution), a dressing of cotton, followed by 4 × 4-inch gauze squares and two V pads, is used and taped in place with 1-inch plastic tape.

The patient is instructed to return home and go to bed and not remove the dressing until the following morning, at which time a hot bath is taken. The bath is repeated several times during the day and thereafter twice daily until the wound heals. Bleeding may result if baths are started the same day as the excision. Acetaminophen with oxycodone hydrochloride (Percocet) is

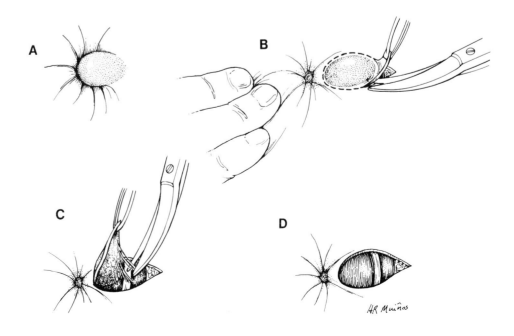

FIGURE 26-1. *A*, Thrombosed external hemorrhoid in the right lateral quadrant. *B*, Allis clamp applied to apex of thrombosis and elliptical incision made. *C*, Thrombosis dissected free of sphincter. *D*, Appearance of wound after thrombectomy.

given to the patient with instructions to take one tablet before the local anesthetic wears off and as needed thereafter. A psyllium seed preparation, such as Konsyl or Metamucil, is prescribed, 1 tsp three times daily. The patient is seen in the office in 2 weeks for anoscopy and sigmoidoscopy.

Recurrent external hemorrhoidal thromboses occurring three or more times generally require hemorrhoidectomy. Occasionally, a patient will present with an ulcerated thrombosed external hemorrhoid. This is the only situation in which an external hemorrhoid will bleed. It should always be excised, since it will continue to bleed for days if it is not. External hemorrhoidal tags will occasionally develop in the unexcised external thrombosis. If they become bothersome by making adequate cleansing difficult for the patient, they can be excised under local anesthesia.

TREATMENT OF INTERNAL HEMORRHOIDS

The treatment of internal hemorrhoids is based on their classification. Most internal hemorrhoids are asymptomatic and do not require any therapy. However, when frequent bleeding, protrusion, and soilage occur, treatment is indicated. In determining the therapy, one must realize that it is necessary only to control the symptoms, not to achieve any anatomic change. The simplest method with the least complications is the method of choice if it controls the bleeding and protrusion.

Treatment of First-Degree Internal Hemorrhoids

When the patient complains of occasional rectal bleeding, a high-fiber diet is sufficient to control the symptoms and should be prescribed. Two methods are available for the control of frequent bleeding: injection and ligation. They have been available for many years and thus have a long, favorable track record. Four other methods have become available recently: infrared coagulation, contact laser, contact coagulation, and direct current. These four methods all rely on the use of heat.

Injection

The injection method can be used safely on patients who have undergone anticoagulation with sodium warfarin (Coumadin). Injection of internal hemorrhoids using phenol solution was first described by Mitchell in 1871.[16] This method has withstood the test of time. The procedure we use is taken from Gabriel.[15] The purpose of the injection is to create submucosal fibrosis with resultant shrinkage of the internal hemorrhoids. Five per cent phenol in cottonseed oil is used. A 10-ml Luer-Lok syringe is filled with the solution, and a Frankfeldt injection needle or spinal needle is attached. A medium-sized Hirschman anoscope is inserted into the rectum, and the internal hemorrhoids are identified. Two to 3 ml of the solution is then injected at the upper pole of the hemorrhoid. (Fig. 26–2A). The injection must be given submucosally. If the mucosa blanches, the injection is being given intramucosally, and the injection should be stopped and the needle advanced further into the tissue; otherwise a slough of the tissue will occur. The submucosal injection is given until striations of the blood vessels beneath the mucosa are evident (Fig. 26–2B). All three quadrants are injected, and the tissue is then thoroughly massaged. Injections are repeated at 1- and 3- month intervals. Any site that is indurated should not receive an injection. Injections are quite successful in the management of first-degree hemorrhoids and will control bleeding effectively.

COMPLICATIONS. The major complication of hemor-

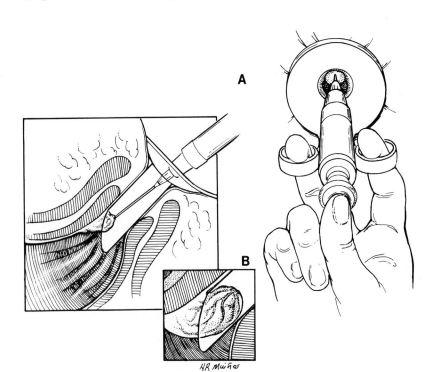

FIGURE 26-2. *A,* Injection of internal hemorrhoid. *B,* Postinjection striations.

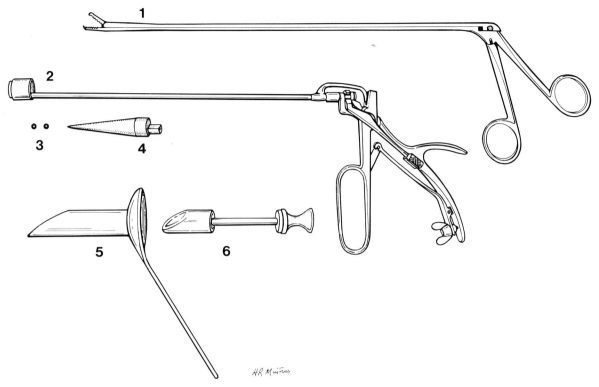

FIGURE 26-3. Ligation instruments. Alligator grasping forceps (*1*), Barron ligator (*2*), O-ring (*3*), loading cone (*4*), Hirschman's anoscope (*5*), and obturator (*6*).

rhoid injection is sloughing if the mucosa is injected, and this can easily be avoided. In men, if the needle is placed too deeply, the prostate can be injected. We have seen a liver abscess following an injection in one patient. Transient bacteremia has been reported following sclerotherapy.[1] Occasionally, an oleoma may develop, but this is harmless. Pain and sloughing of the skin can occur if the injection is placed distal to the dentate line. The injection method is quite safe, except for the complications listed, if 5% phenol in cottonseed oil is used.

RESULTS. The 5-year success rate is about 85% according to a study by Milligan.[29]

Ligation

The ligation method is applicable for first-, second-, or third-degree hemorrhoids. Ligation of internal hemorrhoids by the application of a rubber band was described by Blaisdell.[5] The principle of his method was retained, but the type of instrument and the elastic band were modified by Barron.[4] Reports by Salvati on the ligation technique appeared in 1967 and 1970.[41,42] The technique involved is simple. The instruments used are shown in Figure 26-3. A Hirschman anoscope is inserted into the anal canal and is maintained in proper position by an assistant after the dentate line is identified. The ligator has previously been loaded with an elastic band (Fig. 26-4). The internal hemorrhoid is grasped at its apex by the alligator forceps and is pulled into a double-sleeve cylinder to which is attached a long stem with a handle and pistol trigger (Fig. 26-5*A* and *B*). After the hemorrhoid has been drawn within the

inner cylinder, the trigger is pulled, forcing the elastic band around the hemorrhoid (Fig. 26-5*C* through *E*). Since the rectal mucosa is not sensitive, no anesthetic is required. The pressure exerted by the band strangulates the tissue, and it sloughs away in 48 to 72 hours, leaving a raw surface that heals gradually. One group of hemorrhoids is treated at a time, at intervals of 3 weeks. More groups may be treated at the same visit if they are only first-degree hemorrhoids; but simultaneous liga-

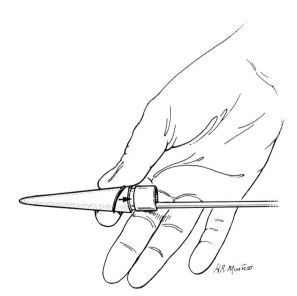

FIGURE 26-4. O-ring being applied to ligator via plastic loading cone.

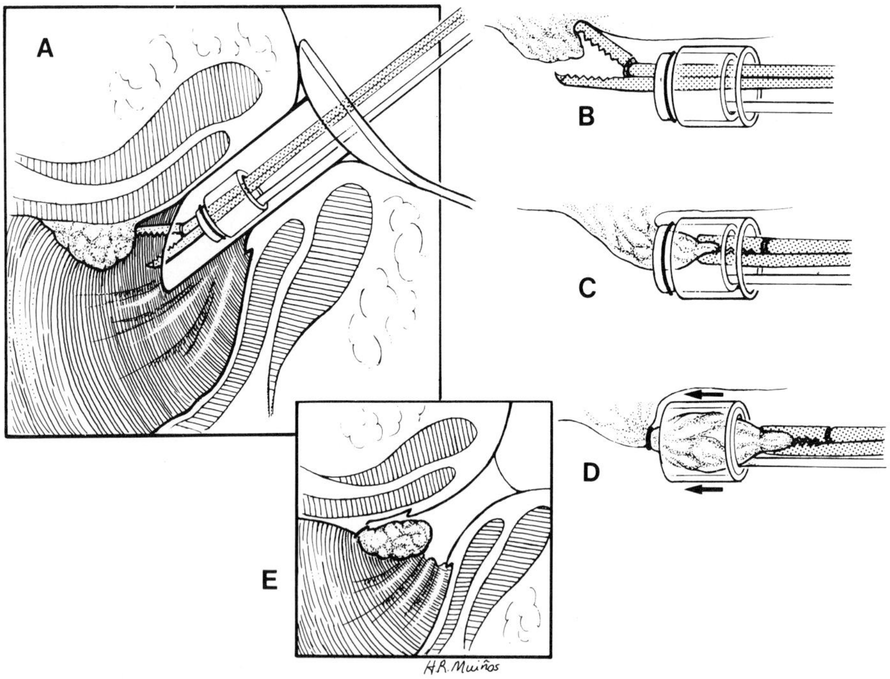

FIGURE 26-5. *A,* Ligator in Hirschman's anoscope. *B,* Internal hemorrhoid being grasped. *C,* Internal hemorrhoid pulled up into drum. *D,* O-ring applied to internal hemorrhoid. *E,* Appearance of hemorrhoid after ligation.

tions of second- and third-degree hemorrhoids can result in considerable discomfort. Generally, three to four treatments are required, as this will encompass the three major groups and a secondary group.

COMPLICATIONS. The most common complication following ligation is pain. It occurs in 6% of cases.[41] Occasionally, a band has to be removed because of pain. Bleeding is the next most common complication and occurs in 2% of cases.[41] Bleeding is generally self-limiting, but it can be life-threatening and should be treated accordingly. If a patient has three bloody bowel movements in a row, medical attention should be sought promptly. A rigid sigmoidoscope should be inserted and the blood evacuated from the rectum. The bleeding ligated site should be injected with 2 to 3 ml of 1% lidocaine with 1:200,000 epinephrine or 0.25% bupivacaine with 1:200,000 epinephrine. This will control most bleeding, but if it does not, the site can either be electrocoagulated or religated.

External thromboses occur in 0.5% of patients who undergo ligation.[41] It is sometimes necessary to remove the thrombosis if the pain persists.

Wechter and Luna[52] reviewed the complication rate in 39 studies of 8,060 patients who had rubber band ligation. They found that aside from pain or recurrence, the total complication rate was less than 6%.

The most dreaded complication of the ligation treatment is sepsis with death.[38] The ligation method was used for 20 years before this complication was ever reported or recognized. More than 40,000 bands have been applied in our practice, with only one possible incident of sepsis, which resolved with antibiotics. It is important, however, that one be aware of the possibility of sepsis even though it is extremely rare and to promptly see patients who are in pain following ligation, especially if they are having problems with voiding. All fatal cases have had persistent pain and difficulty in voiding as the

presenting symptoms. Prompt hospitalization and immediate institution of triple-antibiotic therapy will generally reverse the septic process.[8] Patients who complain of pain with their hemorrhoids should not undergo a banding procedure until a septic process is ruled out.

RESULTS. Rothberg and co-workers[37] reported on a long-term follow-up of rubber band ligation hemorrhoidectomy, reviewing 595 patients over a 5- to 15-year period. Symptomatic control was obtained overall in 80% of the patients. A third of the group required one or two subsequent bandings to completely control symptoms. Wrobleski and colleagues[55] reported similar results in 266 patients who had been followed for a median of 5 years. Of this group, 80% improved and 60% were completely free of symptoms.

Infrared Coagulation

The use of infrared coagulation to treat internal hemorrhoids was first reported by Neiger.[32] The apparatus produces infrared radiation from a 14-V Wolframhalogen projector bulb. A 1-second pulse is used, and two to six points are coagulated on each hemorrhoid (Fig. 26-6). Leicester and colleagues,[24] from St. Mark's Hospital, conducted a prospective randomized trial to evaluate infrared coagulation in comparison with injection and ligation. It was their conclusion that infrared coagulation was more effective than injections in treating first-degree hemorrhoids and was also effective in second-degree hemorrhoids, but in third-degree hemorrhoids ligation appeared better. Infrared coagulation has been used in our practice and appears to be effective with first-degree hemorrhoids and for those patients who have recurrent symptoms after ligation, but whose lack of redundancy precludes further banding. It is painless and apparently free of side effects. However, this method has not been used long enough to determine what the long-

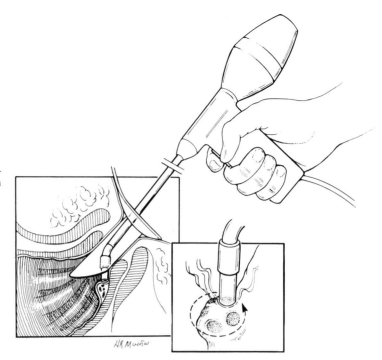

FIGURE 26-6. Infrared coagulation. *Left,* Coagulator inserted through Hirschman's anoscope. *Right,* Coagulation points.

term result will be, and its place in the treatment of internal hemorrhoids remains uncertain.

Laser Coagulation

In performing hemorrhoidectomy, both the neodymium:yttrium-aluminum-garnet (Nd:YAG) and carbon dioxide lasers have been used. First- and second-degree internal hemorrhoids are coapted by using the flat contact probe or the coagulation probe, according to Sanker and associates.[44] It is applied around the hemorrhoid in a rosette fashion and then onto it directly. Joffe[22] states that the power used is between 5 and 10 watts for a duration of 2 to 3 seconds with coaxial water flow. Care must be taken not to "vaporize" the tissue.

Wang and associates[51] randomized 88 patients into two groups. Group A received the Nd:YAG laser phototherapy for internal hemorrhoids combined with the carbon dioxide laser for external hemorrhoids. Group B was treated with a closed hemorrhoidectomy. They reported less pain and a shorter hospitalization with the laser group. A follow-up after 1 year showed 80% of the patients to be free of symptoms.

Leff[23] utilized the carbon dioxide laser as a cutting tool to perform 170 closed hemorrhoidectomies. Operative nonlaser hemorrhoidectomy was performed on 56 patients. Patients were monitored for postoperative pain, wound healing, and complications. No differences were seen between laser and nonlaser hemorrhoidectomy.

Direct Current and Contact Bipolar Diathermy

Electric direct current has been reported to be painless and effective for all grades of hemorrhoids.[33] A probe is placed into the internal hemorrhoid and a varying direct current is used to coagulate the tissue. Hinton

and colleagues[20] randomized 50 patients with either bipolar diathermy or direct current therapy with third-degree hemorrhoids. Both methods were effective in 80% of the cases. However, there was a considerable difference in the mean time for each treatment session (<1 minute for bipolar diathermy compared to 8.5 minutes for direct current therapy). Thus, patient acceptability was greater for bipolar therapy. Long-term results are not available.

Zinberg and co-workers[56] compared three nonoperative techniques using infrared coagulation in 302 patients, heater probe coagulation in 264 patients, and direct current therapy in 192 patients. Ninety per cent of the patients received intravenous sedation. Over 95% of the patients treated had first- or second-degree hemorrhoids. Good results were reported in 97% of the cases treated with infrared coagulation, in 90% of those treated with heater probe coagulation therapy, and in 95% of the direct current therapy group. Long-term results remain unknown. A contact bipolar probe called a Bicap has been manufactured by ACMI. It has been used by Griffith and colleagues[17] and by Dennison and associates[9] to treat first- and second-degree hemorrhoids. In Griffith's series, 16 of 26 patients obtained relief of their symptoms. Mild to moderate discomfort was reported in 41% of these patients. The place for these modalities in the treatment of first- and second-degree hemorrhoids remains to be seen.

Treatment of More Complex Hemorrhoids

Ligation and surgery are the only proven effective treatments for second- and third-degree internal hemorrhoids. The decision to ligate or operate can occasionally be difficult. Over the years, we have developed some guidelines. A hemorrhoidectomy is indicated if there is a history or presence of the following: (1) an associated anal pathologic condition, such as fissure, fistula, or anal stenosis, or a combination; (2) recurrent external hemorrhoidal thromboses; (3) large external hemorrhoids with a "flat" or "short" anal canal; or (4) ligation failures. Obviously, surgery is indicated for permanently prolapsed or fourth-degree internal hemorrhoids.

Surgery

Contraindications

Inflammatory bowel disease (mucosal colitis or Crohn's proctitis) is a contraindication to surgery. Endoscopic examination will rule out these two conditions. A history of three or four loose bowel movements per day should lead the surgeon to investigate the possibility of underlying Crohn's ileitis. Irritable bowel syndrome is a relative contraindication, since three to four loose bowel movements per day will fail to dilate the anal canal, and this may lead to a postoperative stricture. Symptomatic prostatic hypertrophy in men should be corrected before a hemorrhoidectomy is performed.

Preoperative Preparation

All patients should have a sigmoidoscopic examination prior to surgery. A barium enema or colonoscopy should also be performed with a history of a change in bowel habits. A disposable sodium diphosphate enema is administered the night before and the morning of surgery.

Closed Hemorrhoidectomy

We perform two types of hemorrhoidectomy. The first, and by far the most common, is the closed hemorrhoidectomy using the dissection and clamp technique. Closing the external wounds was popularized by Ferguson and co-workers.[14] Muldoon described this procedure and his experience in detail in 1981.[31] The use of a clamp to remove hemorrhoids was first described by Mitchell in Belfast.[30]

Surgery is performed with the patient in the prone–jackknife position using a local anesthesia—300 units of hyaluronidase are added to a 50-ml bottle of 0.25% bupivacaine with 1:200,000 epinephrine.[36] Injection is given subcutaneously circumferentially in the anal canal as well as submucosally (Figs. 26–7 and 26–8). Schneider[46] was the first to describe the addition of hyaluronidase to a local anesthetic for use in anorectal surgery. Hyaluronidase permits the anesthetic to diffuse rapidly through the tissues, as it breaks down the intercellular cement. The patient is given midazolam hydrochloride (Versed) slowly, intravenously, in small increments of 1 to 2 mg, up to 10 mg, as needed for sedation. Fentanyl (Sublimaze), 50 to 150 μg; and propofol (Diprivan), 10 to 30 mg in separated doses as needed or other combinations can be used, but careful monitoring is essential.

The external hemorrhoids are removed as groups; that is, from the right anterior, the right posterior, and the left lateral quadrants. Three hemostats are placed on the external components, and elliptic incisions are made on both sides up to but not crossing the dentate line (Fig. 26–9). The external hemorrhoid is dissected off the external and internal sphincters up to its upper limit, a hemorrhoidal clamp is applied to the internal

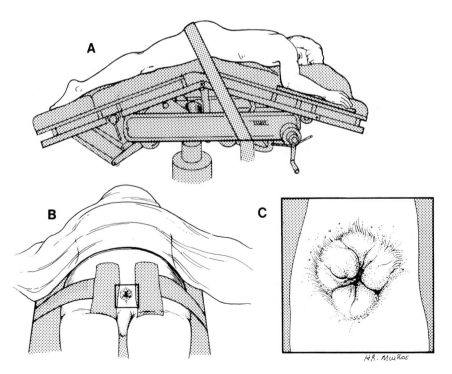

FIGURE 26-7. *A,* Prone–jackknife position. Note application of tape for retraction. *B,* Tape retraction. *C,* Hemorrhoids.

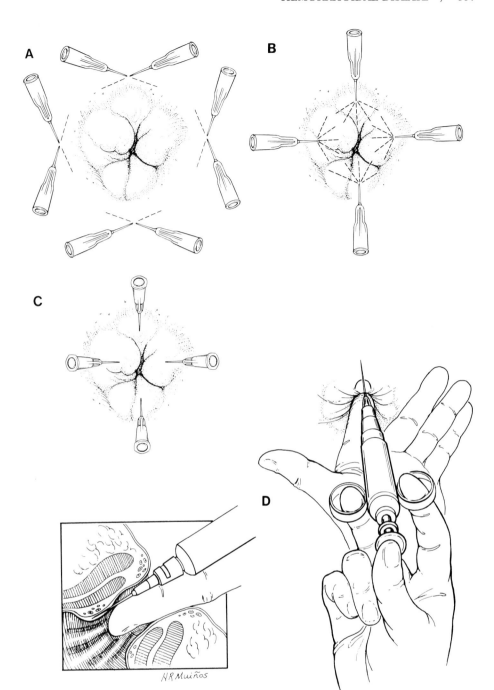

FIGURE 26-8. Local injection: perianal (*A*), intra-anal (*B*), submucosal (*C*). *D*, Technique of submucosal injection.

hemorrhoid, and the tissue superior to the clamp is removed (Fig. 26-10). A running suture of 3-0 chromic catgut is placed over the clamp beginning at the upper pole and advancing down to the dentate line. The clamp is then removed and the same suture run back over the suture line and tied. The external wound is then closed with the same suture (Fig. 26-11).

The same procedure is carried out in the right posterior and left lateral quadrants. No more than three groups should be removed in this manner in order to prevent narrowing of the anal canal. Secondary groups may be present between the primary groups; that is, the left posterior, left anterior, and right lateral quadrants. The most common secondary group is the left posterior quadrant. Secondary groups should be removed by the

amputative technique. For example, to remove a secondary group in the left posterior quadrant, an incision is made at the dentate line extending the distance occupied by the left posterior quadrant. The incision is deepened to the internal sphincter, and the internal hemorrhoid is dissected upward off the internal sphincter. When mobilized sufficiently, it is removed transversely. The mucosa is then approximated to the skin to re-establish the dentate line using interrupted 3–0 chromic catgut sutures and beginning in the midline. There should be no tension on the mucosa, and a 1-cm bite should be taken. The same procedure is carried out in the left anterior and right lateral quadrants, if necessary, although this is seldom indicated. At the completion of the procedure, the operator should be able to insert the

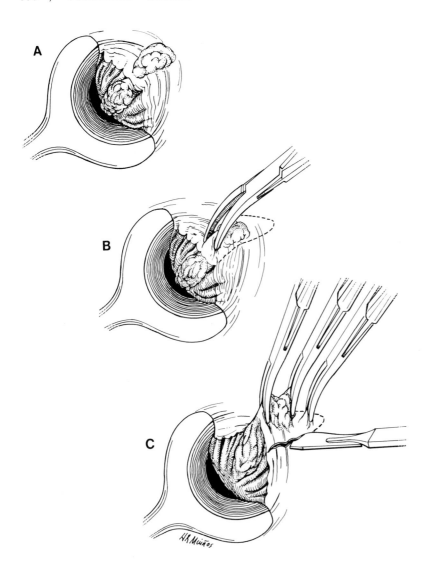

FIGURE 26-9. Closed hemorrhoidectomy. *A,* External and internal hemorrhoid. *B,* Hemostat applied. *C,* Hemostats applied and incision made.

35-mm Hill-Ferguson retractor without difficulty if the operation has been properly performed.

Amputative Hemorrhoidectomy

The amputative technique is used for patients with third- or fourth-degree hemorrhoids when the external hemorrhoids are very large or the hemorrhoids are mixed. This technique was first described by Whitehead.[53] The method has acquired a bad reputation for producing a rectal ectropion if performed incorrectly. Burchell reported on a modified Whitehead hemorrhoidectomy in 1967.[6] Wolff and Culp[54] published a report on a 3-year follow-up of 440 patients who underwent a modified Whitehead hemorrhoidectomy. They had a total morbidity rate of 12.2%, including a 7.2% flap detachment rate; however, no patient experienced an ectropion. We make an incision just at the dentate line involving one half of the circumference of the anal canal and beginning at the 12-o'clock position. The skin is freed distally, and all external hemorrhoidal tissue is dissected off the sphincters and excised. Mucosa is treated similarly, mobilizing sufficient mucosa to excise all the internal hemorrhoidal tissue transversely. The mucosa is then attached to the skin to re-establish the dentate line, and alternate sutures are taken in the internal sphincter as well (Fig. 26–12). When completed on one side, the procedure is performed on the opposite side. When done in this manner, the location of the dentate line is accurate and an ectropion will not occur.

Postoperative Care

At the completion of the operation, a crushed, rolled piece of No. 100 Gelfoam (absorbable gelatin sponge) is inserted in the rectum and a 4 × 4-inch gauze dressing is applied to the external wounds followed by a V pad taped in place with a 1-inch nonallergenic paper tape. The gelatin sponge rapidly becomes a gelatinous mass and is spontaneously passed by the patient with the first bowel movement or passage of flatus. The use of the absorbable gelatin sponge seems to reduce the incidence of hematoma, which can occur when the effect of the epinephrine wears off.

Demerol, 75 to 100 mg, or morphine, 10 to 15 mg, is used for pain and is given freely as needed. These agents are seldom required except during the first 24 hours following surgery. A psyllium seed preparation is pre-

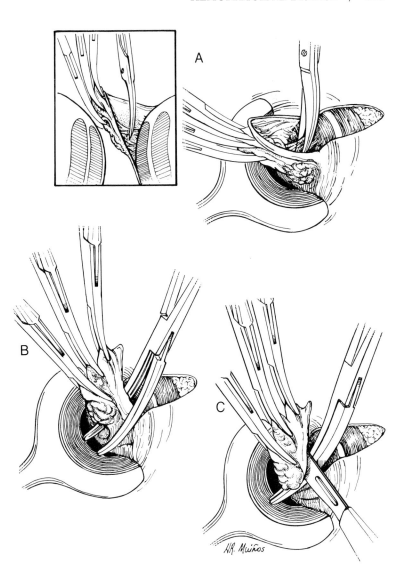

FIGURE 26-10. Closed hemorrhoidectomy. *A*, Surgical dissection off of sphincter. *B*, Application of hemorrhoidal clamp. *C*, Excision of hemorrhoid distal to clamp.

scribed three times daily in 5-ml amounts and bisacodyl, three tablets, is given the evening of the operation. If the patient has a bowel movement the following day, he or she is discharged with instructions to take hot tub baths for 20 minutes three times daily and to continue the psyllium seed preparation. Senokot (Senna) tablets are prescribed if patients miss 1 day without a bowel movement, and they are advised to take a Fleet enema if 2 days pass without a bowel movement.

The patient is seen in the office a week after discharge, and a careful distal phalanx digital rectal examination is done to ensure that there is no impaction. This is repeated every 2 weeks until the anal canal regains its elasticity over a period of 6 to 8 weeks postoperatively. Anoscopy is performed prior to discharge to be certain all wounds are healed, and the patient is advised to remain on the psyllium seed preparation for at least 3 months subsequent to surgery. This "natural" dilation of the anal canal prevents strictures and is far preferable to any type of manual dilation. Mineral oil and milk of magnesia should be avoided, as the bowel movements will become loose or too soft, resulting in failure to dilate the anal canal. It is failure to provide for regular soft but formed bowel movements in the

postoperative period that leads to anal strictures and fissures.

Complications

URINARY RETENTION. The most common complication following hemorrhoidectomy is urinary retention. Generally, caudal and spinal anesthesia produce a higher incidence of urinary retention. The use of a local anesthetic with intravenous sedation lessens the incidence of urinary retention.[39] Scoma[47] has shown that limiting the use of intravenous fluids during and following the operation will definitely lower the incidence of urinary retention, since a bladder rapidly filled with urine is less likely to be emptied immediately following the surgery, when the patient's discomfort is the greatest. The patient should always be gotten out of bed to void and catheterized only after 12 hours have elapsed if fluid restriction has been practiced. When a patient requires a second catheterization, it should be done with a No. 18 Foley catheter, which is left in place for 48 hours.

PAIN. Excessive pain can be prevented by avoiding placement of sutures in the sphincter. The use of a long-acting local anesthetic, such as 0.25% bupivacaine, will

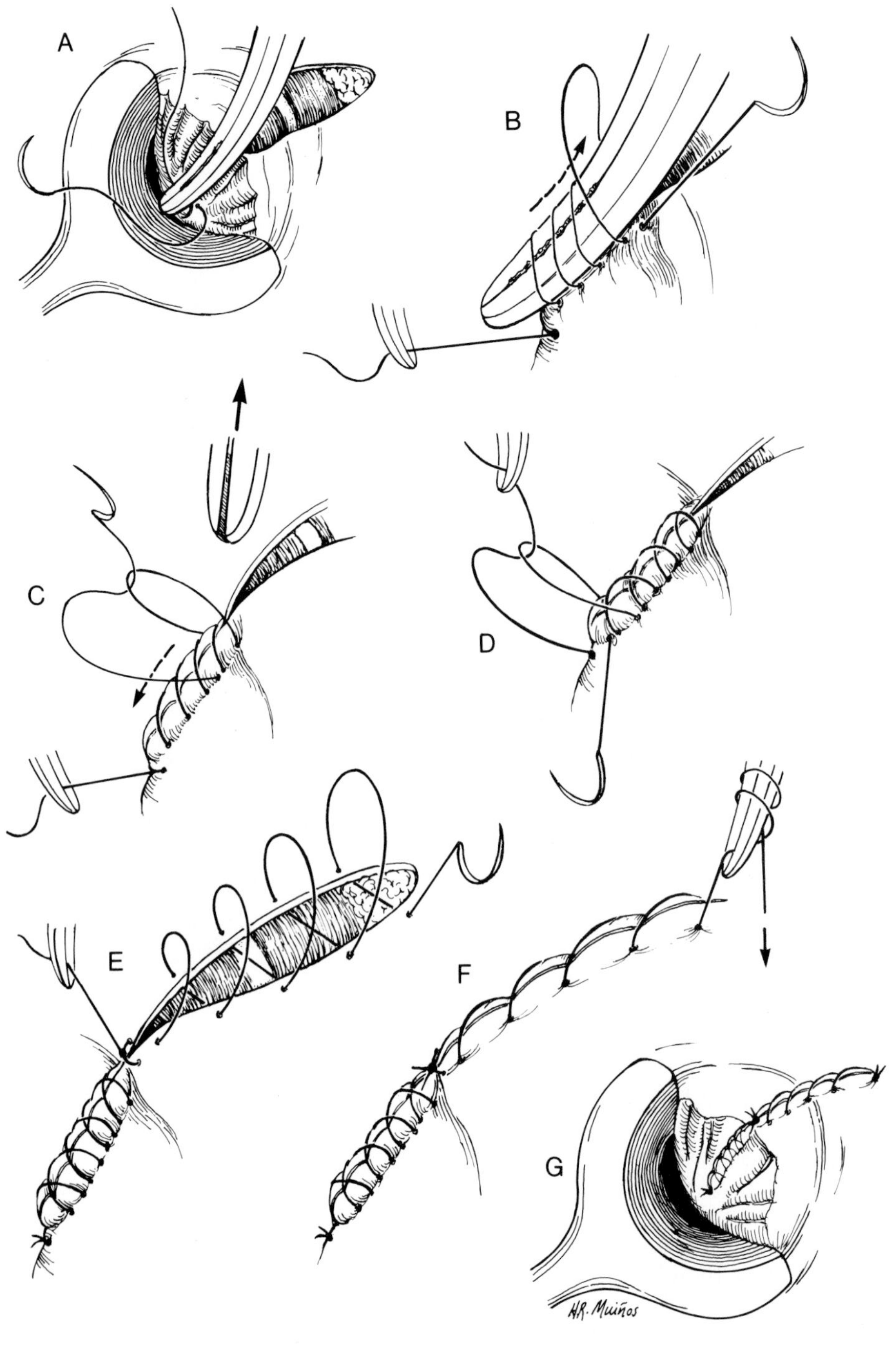

FIGURE 26-11. Closed hemorrhoidectomy. *A*, First suture placed. *B*, Loops around clamp only. *C*, Clamp removed and returning lock stitch. *D*, Returning suture tied to proximal knot. *E*, External wound closed. *F*, Suture ended with single knot. *G*, Appearance after excision of external and internal hemorrhoid.

reduce the postoperative pain considerably, whereas the use of lidocaine will not because it wears off quite rapidly, lasting only about 60 minutes.

BLEEDING. Bleeding may occur early or late. Early bleeding is very rare and is generally due to technical error. Late bleeding can occur anytime between the eighth and fourteenth days after the operation, when the sutures separate. The incidence of bleeding is about 1% and is frequently precipitated by early vigorous activity by the patient. When severe, it can be controlled by giving another local anesthetic, removing all the blood from the rectum, and using electrocautery to coagulate the bleeding site. Suturing of the bleeding site can be difficult and is not recommended. The most common hemorrhoid group to manifest delayed bleeding is that of the right anterior quadrant.

STRICTURE. Stricture is a delayed complication that usually is the result of overzealous removal of hemorrhoidal tissue. Skin bridges among the main groups should always be generous. It should be possible to place a 35-mm Hill-Ferguson retractor comfortably in the anal canal following completion of the procedure. Proper bowel management postoperatively will aid in the prevention of strictures. If a stricture does occur, it can be relieved with a lateral internal sphincterotomy if the preceding precautions have been observed.

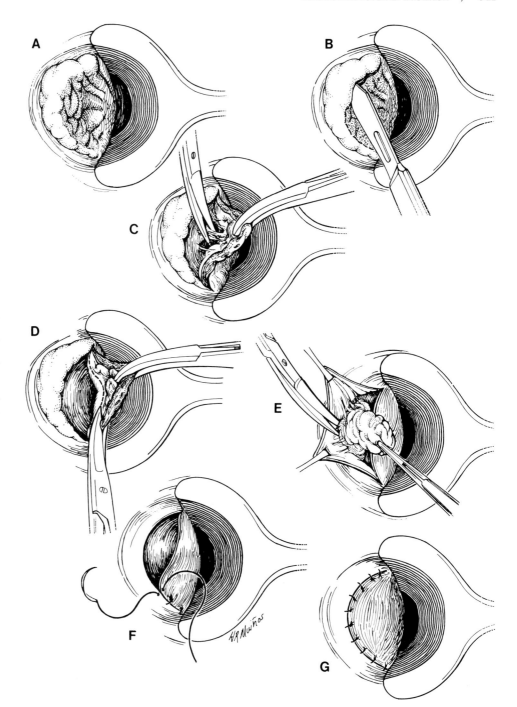

FIGURE 26-12. Amputative hemorrhoidectomy. *A*, Hemorrhoids. *B*, Incision at dentate line. *C*, Dissection of internal hemorrhoid off of internal sphincter. *D*, Transection of internal hemorrhoid. *E*, Excision of external hemorrhoid subcutaneously. *F*, Reapproximation of skin to mucosa. *G*, Completion of left-side amputative hemorrhoidectomy.

FISSURE. A fissure generally develops secondary to a stricture. The use of an emollient suppository twice daily and a psyllium seed preparation will cure most postoperative fissures. Occasionally, a lateral internal sphincterotomy is necessary.

ANAL TAGS. Anal tags will develop no matter how carefully an operation is performed. They can be excised under local anesthesia, but none should be excised prior to 3 months after surgery, since most will become smaller and prove to be more inconsequential after a sufficient time.

UNHEALED WOUNDS. Occasionally, a wound fails to heal. Vigorous cauterization with 10% silver nitrate and the use of an emollient suppository will frequently bring about final healing. Some unhealed wounds, however, are due to stricturing and fissuring of the anal canal from the removal of too much tissue. Lateral internal sphincterotomy, and occasionally anoplasty, may be necessary if the wounds fail to heal after 3 to 4 months. When anoplasty is necessary, the use of the "diamond" graft as described by Caplin and Kodner[7] is advocated. It is simple, based on sound surgical principles, and works well.

INCONTINENCE. Incontinence should be a rare complication. However, if the external or internal sphincter is damaged, or a posterior sphincterotomy or rectal divulsion is performed, incontinence of a major or minor degree can occur. The value of local anesthesia is that

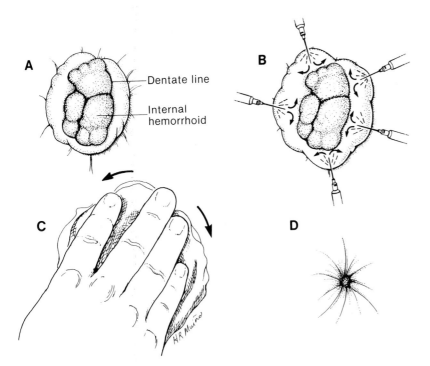

FIGURE 26–13. Acute hemorrhoidal disease. *A*, External hemorrhoidal edema with fourth-degree internal hemorrhoids. *B*, Injection of hyaluronidase–0.25% bupivacaine solution with 30-gauge needle. *C*, Massage of edematous prolapsed hemorrhoidal tissue. *D*, Appearance following massage and reduction.

it gives a dry field and permits accurate delineating of the sphincters. A rectal divulsion is not indicated and should not be done in association with a hemorrhoidectomy. If there is difficulty inserting the Hill-Ferguson retractor into the anal canal, the proper maneuver is a partial lateral internal sphincterotomy.

ECTROPION. This complication should not occur when a closed hemorrhoidectomy is performed as described. Amputative hemorrhoidectomy has a reputation for causing ectropion, but it will not occur if the procedure is performed as described.

ACUTE HEMORRHOIDAL DISEASE

Acute hemorrhoidal disease is commonly referred to as strangulated or gangrenous hemorrhoids. There is massive prolapse of the internal hemorrhoids with associated external and internal edema and thromboses to a varying degree. The edema and prolapse can be reduced immediately, the thromboses excised, and the internal hemorrhoids ligated. This is accomplished by adding 150 units (1 ml) of hyaluronidase to 9 ml of 0.25% bupivacaine with 1:200,000 epinephrine.[12,40] A 10-ml Luer-Lok syringe with a 30-gauge needle attached is used to inject the solution directly into the edematous prolapsed mass. Thorough massage of the edematous prolapsed hemorrhoidal mass is then carried out, following which the prolapsed internal hemorrhoids will be reduced back into the rectum and all external and internal edema will disappear (Fig. 26–13). Any large thromboses, both external and internal, are removed, and all the internal hemorrhoids that were prolapsed are ligated. If ligation is not performed, prolapse will recur. Treatment is permanent in most instances.

CRYOTHERAPY

The management of hemorrhoids would not be complete without mention of cryotherapy, a technique first described by Lewis and co-workers[25] and popularized by Savin,[45] Detrano,[10] and Oh and Dressling.[34] A more recent article and the largest series to be reported using this technique was by Oh.[34,35] In a review of 1,000 cases, Oh concluded that cryotherapy should not be used for external hemorrhoids or for fourth-degree internal hemorrhoids. Cryohemorrhoidectomy is rarely performed today because of its associated postoperative problems of pain, profuse anal discharge, and failure to control external hemorrhoids.

ANAL DILATION

Anal dilation was recommended by Lord.[27] The anus is dilated gradually up to eight fingers under general anesthesia until the subcutaneous fibrous bands are ruptured. It was Lord's feeling that these bands led to increased intrarectal pressure, causing engorgement of the hemorrhoids. The technique is used to some degree in England but has been abandoned in the United States, as anal incontinence, especially in older patients, can occur and the long-term results leave something to be desired.[50] It appears to be effective only for first- or second-degree hemorrhoids.

REFERENCES

1. Adami, B., Echardt, V.F., Suermann, R.B., et al.: Bacteremia after proctoscopy and hemorrhoidal injection sclerotherapy. Dis. Colon Rectum, *24*:373, 1981.
2. Arabi, Y., Alexander-Williams, J., and Keighley, M.R.B.: Anal pres-

sure in hemorrhoids and anal fissure. Am. J. Surg., *134*:608, 1977.

3. Barron, J.: Office ligation of internal hemorrhoids. Am. J. Surg., *105*:563, 1963.

4. Barron, J.: Office ligation treatment of hemorrhoids. Dis. Colon Rectum, *6*:109, 1963.

5. Blaisdell, P.: Scientific Exhibit. American Medical Association, San Francisco, June, 1954.

6. Burchell, M.C., Thow, G.B., and Mason, R.R.: A modified White-head hemorrhoidectomy. Dis. Colon Rectum, *19*:225, 1976.

7. Caplin, D.A., and Kodner, I.J.: Repair of anal stricture and mucosal ectropion by simple flap procedure. Dis. Colon Rectum, *29*:92, 1986.

8. Clay, L., White, J.J., Davidson, J.T., and Chandler, J.J.: Early recognition and successful management of pelvic cellulitis following hemorrhoidal banding. Dis. Colon Rectum, *29*:579, 1986.

9. Dennison, A., Whiston, R.J., Rooney, S., et al.: A randomized comparison for infrared photocoagulation with bipolar diathermy for the outpatient treatment of hemorrhoids. Dis. Colon Rectum, *33*:32, 1990.

10. Detrano, S.J.: The role of cryosurgery in management of anorectal disease: Three hundred and fifty cases. Dis. Colon Rectum, *18:* 284, 1975.

11. Deutsch, A.A., and Moshkovitz, M., Nudelman, I., et al.: Anal pressure measurements in the study of hemorrhoid etiology and their relation to treatment. Dis. Colon Rectum, *30*:855, 1987.

12. Eisenstat, T.E., Salvati, E.P., and Rubin, R.J.: The outpatient management of acute hemorrhoidal disease. Dis. Colon Rectum, *22:* 315, 1979.

13. El-Gendi, M.A., and Abdel-Baky, N.: Anorectal pressures in patients with symptomatic hemorrhoids. Dis. Colon Rectum, *29*:388, 1986.

14. Ferguson, J.A., Mazier, W.R., Granchrow, M.I., and Frend, W.G.: The closed technique of hemorrhoidectomy. Surgery, *70*:480, 1971.

15. Gabriel, W.B.: The Principles and Practice of Rectal Surgery, 5th ed. Springfield, IL, Charles C Thomas, 1963, p. 132.

16. Goligher, J.: Surgery of the Anus, Rectum and Colon, 5th ed. London, Balliere Tindall, 1984, p. 98.

17. Griffith, C.D.M., Morris, D.L., Ellis, I., et al.: Outpatient treatment of hemorrhoids with bipolar diathermy coagulation. Br. J. Surg., *74*:827, 1987.

18. Grosz, C.R.: A surgical treatment of thrombosed external hemorrhoids. Dis. Colon Rectum, *33*:49, 1990.

19. Haas, P., Fox, T.A., and Haas, G.P.: The pathogenesis of hemorrhoids. Dis. Colon Rectum, *27*:442, 1984.

20. Hinton, C.P., and Morris, D.L.: A randomized trial comparing direct current therapy and bipolar diathermy in the outpatient treatment of third-degree hemorrhoids. Dis. Colon Rectum, *33:* 931, 1990.

21. Jackson, C.C., and Robertson, E.: Etiologic aspects of hemorrhoidal disease. Dis. Colon Rectum, *8*:185, 1965.

22. Joffe, S.N.: Contact neodymium: YAG laser surgery in gastroenterology: A preliminary report. Lasers Surg. Med., *6*:155, 1986.

23. Leff, E.I.: Hemorrhoidectomy-laser vs. nonlaser: Outpatient surgical experience. Dis. Colon Rectum, *35*:743, 1992.

24. Leicester, R.J., Nicholls, R.J., and Mann, C.U.: Infrared coagulation: A new treatment for hemorrhoids. Dis. Colon Rectum, *24:* 602, 1981.

25. Lewis, M.I., Cruz, T.D.L., Gazzaniga, D.A., and Ball, T.L.: Cryosurgical hemorrhoidectomy: Preliminary report. Dis. Colon Rectum, *12*:371, 1969.

26. Lin, J.K.: Anal manometric studies in hemorrhoids and anal fissures. Dis. Colon Rectum, *32*:839, 1989.

27. Lord, P.H.: A new regime for the treatment of hemorrhoids. Proc. R. Soc. Med., *61*:935, 1968.

28. Miles, W.E.: Observations upon internal piles. Surg. Gynecol. Obstet., *29*:497, 1919.

29. Milligan, E.T.C.: Hemorrhoids. BMJ, *2*:412, 1939.

30. Mitchell, A.B.: A simple method of operating on piles. BMJ, *1*:482, 1903.

31. Muldoon, J.P.: The completely closed hemorrhoidectomy: A reliable and trusted friend for 25 years. Dis. Colon Rectum, *24*:211, 1981.

32. Neiger, A.: Hemorrhoids in everyday practice. Proctology, *2*:22, 1979.

33. Norman, D.A., Newton, R., and Nicholas, G.U.: Management of Hemorrhoidal Disease: An Effective, Safe and Painless Outpatient Approach Utilizing D.C. Current. So. Lake Tahoe, CA, Gastroenterology Division Bunton University Hospital, 1986.

34. Oh, C., and Dresling, D.A.: Cryohemorrhoidectomy. Mt. Sinai J. Med., *42*:179, 1974.

35. Oh, C.: Problems of cryohemorrhoidectomy. Cryobiology, *19*:283, 1982.

36. Ramalho, L.D., Salvati, E.P., and Rubin, R.J.: Bupivacaine, a long acting local anesthetic in anorectal surgery. Dis. Colon Rectum, *19*:144, 1976.

37. Rothberg, R., Rubin, R.J., Eisenstat, T.E., and Salvati, E.P.: Rubber band ligation hemorrhoidectomy. Long term results. Am. Surg., *49*:167, 1983.

38. Russell, T.R., and Donohue, J.H.: Banding a warning, Dis. Colon Rectum, *5*:291, 1985.

39. Salvati, E.P.: Urinary retention in anorectal and colonic surgery. Am. J. Surg., *94*:114, 1957.

40. Salvati, E.P., Harmondi, W.J., and Kratzer, G.L.: Acute hemorrhoidal disease. J. Int. Coll. Surg., *34*:662, 1960.

41. Salvati, E.P., Evaluation of ligation of hemorrhoids as an office procedure. Dis. Colon Rectum, *10*:53, 1967.

42. Salvati, E.P.: Ligation of internal hemorrhoids. Proc. R. Soc. Med., *63*:111, 1970.

43. Salvati, E.P.: Hemorrhoids, anal fissure, anal abscess and fistula. *In* Conn, H. (ed.): Current Therapy. Philadelphia, W.B. Saunders, 1980, p. 366.

44. Sanker, M.Y., and Joffe, C.S.: Technique of contact laser hemorrhoidectomy: An ambulatory surgical procedure. Contemp. Surg., *30*:9, 1987.

45. Savin, S.: Hemorrhoidectomy—how I do it: Results of 444 cryorectal surgical operations. Dis. Colon Rectum, *22*:10, 1977.

46. Schneider, H.C.: Hyaluronidase with local anesthesia in anorectal surgery. Am. J. Surg., *88*:703, 1954.

47. Scoma, J.A.: Hemorrhoidectomy with urinary retention and catheterization. Conn. Med., *40*:751, 1976.

48. Stelzner, F.: Die Hamorroiden und andere Kreukheiten des Corpus cavernosum recto und des Analkanals. Dtsch. Med. Wochenschr., *88*:698, 1963.

49. Thomson, W.H.F.: The nature of hemorrhoids. Br. J. Surg., *62*:542, 1975.

50. Walls, A.D.F., and Ruckley, C.V.: A five year followup of Lords dilatation for hemorrhoids. Lancet, *1*:1212, 1976.

51. Wang, J.Y., Chang-Chien, C.R., Chen, J.-S., et al.: The role of lasers in hemorrhoidectomy. Dis. Colon Rectum, *34*:78, 1991.

52. Wechter, D.G., and Luna, G.K.: An unusual complication of rubber band ligation of hemorrhoids. Dis. Colon Rectum, *30*:137, 1987.

53. Whitehead, W.: Surgical treatment of hemorrhoids. BMJ, *1*:149, 1882.

54. Wolff, B.G., and Culp, C.E.: The Whitehead hemorrhoidectomy: An unjustly maligned procedure. Dis. Colon Rectum, *31*:587, 1988.

55. Wrobleski, D.E., Corman, M.L., Veidenheimer, M.C., and Coller, J.A.: Long term evaluation of rubber ring ligation in hemorrhoidal disease. Dis. Colon Rectum, *23*:478, 1980.

56. Zinberg, S.S., Stern, D.H., Furman, D.S., and Wittles, J.M.: A personal experience of comparing three nonoperative techniques for treating internal hemorrhoids. Am. J. Gastroenterol., *84*:5, 1989.

Chapter 27

ANORECTAL ABSCESSES AND FISTULA-IN-ANO

PHILIP H. GORDON

Anorectal abscesses and fistula-in-ano have a common cause. Indeed, the term fistulous abscess has been used to describe this problem. The abscess is an acute situation, whereas the fistula is chronic.

Understanding the anatomy of the pelvic floor is critical to appreciate the origin and ramifications of abscesses and fistulas. The pelvic floor consists of two funnel-shaped structures, one situated within the other. The inner structure is the lower end of the circular muscle of the rectum, which becomes thick and rounded and is referred to as the internal sphincter. Surrounding this is a funnel of pelvic floor muscle formed by the levator ani, puborectalis, and external sphincter. Between the two structures is the intersphincteric plane. In the midportion of the anal canal at the level of the dentate line, the ducts of the anal glands empty into the crypts.

Numerous conditions may play an etiologic role in the formation of a fistulous abscess. Infection of the anal glands is probably the most common cause of fistulous abscess.[29] Parks and Morson demonstrated infected anal glands in 70% of cases and histologic evidence suggestive of this origin in another 20%, bringing the total that may be attributed to infection of the anal glands to 90% (Fig. 27-1).[29] Obstruction of these ducts, whether secondary to fecal material, foreign bodies, or trauma results in stasis and infection. Goligher and co-workers found intersphincteric abscesses in only 23% of anorectal abscesses, suggesting that this cause is less often the precursor.[12] The theory of cryptoglandular origin, however, is supported by the fact that the primary internal orifice is found at the level of the pectinate line.

The most common course for a fistula to pursue is from the mid anal canal downward in the intersphincteric plane to the anal verge. Infection may overcome the barrier of the external sphincter muscles, thereby penetrating the ischioanal fossa, or it may extend upward in the intersphincteric plane, either remaining in the rectal wall or extending extrarectally (Fig. 27-2). In addition to tracking upward and downward, pus may pass circumferentially around the anus. This passage can occur in one of three tissue planes, the most common of which is the ischioanal fossa. This course commences in the posterior midline of the anal canal, penetrates the sphincter mass, and then descends with two limbs, one in each ischioanal fossa. Such circumferential spread is referred to as a horseshoe abscess. In addition, circumferential spread may occur in the intersphincteric plane or in the pararectal tissues above the levator muscles (Fig. 27-3).

DIAGNOSIS

History

A fistulous abscess may be either acute or chronic. The patient with an abscess presents with acute pain and swelling in the anal region. The pain occurs with sitting or moving and is usually aggravated by defecating and even by coughing or sneezing. The clinical history may reveal a preceding bout of diarrhea. General symptomatology includes malaise and pyrexia. In patients with anorectal suppuration, the most common presenting symptoms include pain (93%), swelling (50%), and bleeding via the rectum (16%).[43] Other symptoms include purulent anal discharge, diarrhea, and fever. The pain of an intersphincteric abscess is generally throbbing and remains continuous throughout the day and night. It is aggravated by defecation but lasts longer than the pain resulting from fissures. Minor anal bleeding may occur. Discharge, when present, is due to small amounts of pus discharging into the anal canal.

In the chronic state, the patient will give a history of an abscess that either burst spontaneously or required drainage. The patient will notice a small discharging si-

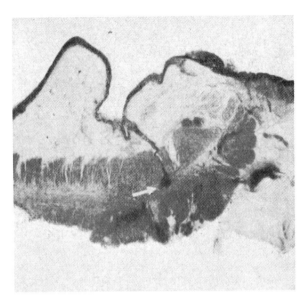

FIGURE 27-1. Thick section (500 μm) through the anal canal that shows an anal gland (*arrow*) penetrating the internal sphincter. It breaks up into short terminal branches in the longitudinal layer; surrounding these is a darkly staining area of lymphoid tissue. (×4.) (From Parks, A.G.: Pathogenesis and treatment of fistula-in-ano. BMJ, *1*:463, 1961, with permission.)

nus, or the discharge may cause skin excoriation and pruritus. There may be pain with defecation, as well as bleeding due to granulation tissue in the region of the internal opening. In decreasing order of frequency, presenting symptoms in patients with fistula-in-ano are discharge (65%), pain (34%), swelling (24%), bleeding (12%), and diarrhea (5%).[42]

Physical Examination

In the acute phase of a fistulous abscess, the cardinal signs of inflammation are present with rubor, calor, tumor, dolor, and functio laesa (redness, heat, swelling, pain, loss of function). There may be no swelling with an intersphincteric abscess. Anal examination will be exquisitely painful or impossible, but in some cases the

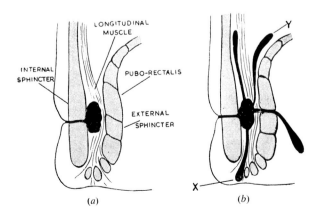

FIGURE 27-2. Spread of infection from the primary anal-gland abscess (*a*) into the surrounding tissues (*b*). The most common course is that marked X; the most rare, Y. (From Parks, A.G.: Pathogenesis and treatment of fistula-in-ano. BMJ, *1*:463, 1961, with permission.)

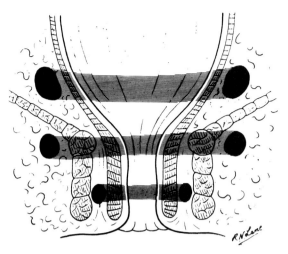

FIGURE 27-3. Diagram illustrating the three planes in which circumferential spread, or "horseshoeing," can occur. (From Parks, A.G., Gordon, P.H., and Hardcastle, J.F.: A classification of fistula-in-ano. Br. J. Surg., *63*:1, 1976, with permission.)

suggestion of a mass is present. A point that might be helpful in the differentiation between an intersphincteric abscess and an acute fissure-in-ano is that inguinal lymph nodes may be enlarged and painful with an abscess. When pain is severe but the cause is unknown, examination under anesthesia is not only justified but indicated. Neglect allows extension of the abscess. With the supralevator abscess, a tender mass in the pelvis may be diagnosed by rectal or vaginal examination. Abdominal examination may reveal signs of peritoneal irritation because the pelvic peritoneum forms the roof of the supralevator space.

In the chronic state, an external opening can usually be seen as a red elevation of granulation tissue with purulent serosanguinous discharge. The number of external openings and their relationship to the anal canal may reveal considerable information. According to Goodsall's rule, if there is an opening posterior to the coronal plane, the fistula probably originates from the dorsal midline, but if the opening is anterior, the fistula probably runs directly to the nearest crypt. Openings seen on both sides of the anal canal are likely to arise from a midline posterior crypt with a horseshoe-type fistula (Fig. 27–4). Most primary openings (58%) are found in either the posterior or anterior aspects of the anal canal.[42] An external opening adjacent to the anal margin may suggest an intersphincteric track, whereas a more laterally located opening would suggest a transsphincteric track. The further the distance of the external opening from the anal margin, the greater the probability of a complicated upward extension.

A cord-like structure may be felt just beneath the skin, leading from the secondary opening to the anal canal. Further palpation may reveal circumferential extension, which would be recognized by a ring of induration hugging the puborectalis sling in a horseshoe fashion. In the anal canal, one might be able to palpate a pit indicative of an internal opening. Rarely, one is able to feel a nodule resulting from a chronic intersphincteric abscess.

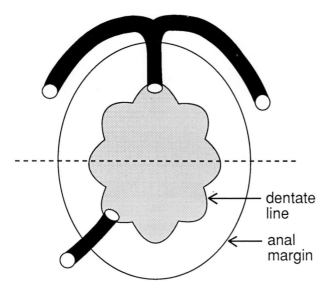

FIGURE 27-4. Diagram of Goodsall's rule. Secondary fistulous openings anterior to a transverse anal line usually lead directly to the anal canal, whereas openings posterior to this line generally follow a curved course to the midline posteriorly at the level of the dentate line.

Probing, when done, must be performed with a feather-like touch in order to prevent false channels; it is best avoided outside the operating room. Following the gentle introduction of a probe into the track, a low fistula will pass toward the anus at an angle of approximately 30 degrees to the skin. Passage of the probe at an 80-degree angle to the skin or almost parallel to the anal canal indicates the presence of a "high" fistula, or at least a supralevator or ischioanal extension of a "low" fistula. Primary openings are successfully located by a probe in two thirds of patients; in the remainder, methylene blue dye or pursuit of the granulation tissue is employed.

Anoscopy and Sigmoidoscopy

Anoscopy and sigmoidoscopy must be performed for at least three reasons. First, anoscopy may help to identify the internal opening in the anal canal. Second, endoscopy may help distinguish between a rectal and anal canal opening. Third, sigmoidoscopy allows examination of the rectal mucosa in order to determine the presence of an underlying proctocolitis, if one exists.

Radiography

In the majority of patients who present with a fistula-in-ano, radiologic examination is of limited value. A barium enema, however, is indicated in patients with a history of bowel symptoms or in anyone with a recurrent fistula-in-ano. Fistulography may be helpful in the delineation of an extrasphincteric fistula of pelvic origin or in the evaluation of patients with recurrent fistulas.[27] Weisman and colleagues found that fistulograms revealed unexpected pathology or altered operative management in 48% of 27 patients studied.[45] They concluded that fistulography in properly selected patients

may add useful information for the definitive management of fistula-in-ano. Law and co-workers used anal endosonography in the evaluation of perianal sepsis and fistula-in-ano and believe knowledge may be gained that influences operative treatment.[19] For patients with difficult fistulas that recur despite skilled attention, Lunniss and co-workers conducted a study to determine the value of magnetic resonance imaging (MRI).[22] They found MRI scan interpretations agreed precisely with independently documented operative findings in 14 of 16 patients.

ANORECTAL ABSCESSES

Microbiologic Features

Many surgeons believe that identification of offending organisms in anorectal sepsis is a waste of time, effort, and money. However, Grace and associates believe the importance of cultures is the prognosis with respect to fistula development.[14] In their study, none of the patients from whom the pus cultures grew skin-derived organisms was found to have fistula-in-ano; in contrast, 54% of patients from whom pus cultures grew bowel-derived organisms had fistula-in-ano. Once the fistula-in-ano is established, the chronic inflammation does not seem to be maintained by either excessive numbers of organisms or organisms of an unusual type.[38]

Incidence and Classification

Anorectal abscesses are more common in men than in women by a ratio of 2:1[13,33] to 3:1.[43] Since different authors use different classifications, it is difficult to know the exact incidence of each kind. I use the following classification: (1) perianal, (2) ischioanal, (3) intersphincteric, and (4) supralevator.

In most series, perianal abscesses constitute the predominant type of abscess, but in a review of 117 consecutive patients with anorectal suppuration, the distribution of abscesses encountered was as follows: perianal, 19%; ischiorectal, 61%; intersphincteric, 18%; and supralevator, 2%.[42] In a review by Ellis[9] of 200 abscesses, the types quoted were perianal, 54.5%; ischiorectal, 39%; submucous (or high intermuscular), 0%; pelvirectal, 0%; and atypical, 6.5%. In a study of the anatomic locations of anorectal suppuration in 506 patients, Prasad and co-workers found the following distribution: perianal, 48%; ischiorectal, 22%; intersphincteric, 12%; supralevator, 9%; intermuscular, 5%; and submucosal, 4%.[31] The distribution of perianal and ischiorectal abscesses reported by Ellis and by Prasad and co-workers was an almost complete reversal of that seen by Vasilevsky and Gordon. No satisfactory explanation can be offered for this observed difference.

Role of Antibiotics

There is little, if any, role for the use of antibiotics in the primary management of para-anal suppuration. Adjunctive antibiotic therapy may be indicated in special circumstances—namely, in patients with rheumatic or

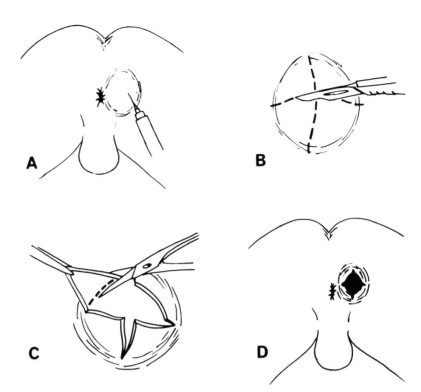

FIGURE 27–5. Incision and drainage of a perianal or ischioanal abscess. *A,* Infiltration of local anesthetic. *B,* Cruciate incision over abscess. *C,* Excision of skin edges. *D,* Opened abscess cavity.

acquired valvular heart disease; in patients who are immunosuppressed; when soft tissue infection is unusually extensive, as with involvement of the perineum, groin, thigh, or abdominal wall; and in diabetics with extensive adjacent cellulitis. It is neither necessary nor wise to wait until fluctuation can be demonstrated, as delay simply affords the inflammatory process an opportunity to extend and cause damage to the adjacent tissue, or more specifically, to the anal sphincter mechanism.

Treatment

Abscesses in the perineum are treated in the same manner as are abscesses in other parts of the body; that is, they must be adequately drained. This usually consists of making a cruciate incision or removing an ellipse of skin over the abscess.

Perianal Abscess

A simple perianal abscess can almost always be drained under local anesthesia in the office or in the outpatient department. The skin is usually prepared with an antiseptic solution. The most tender point is determined, and a 2-cm area of skin in this region is anesthesized with 0.5% lidocaine with 1:200,000 epinephrine. A cruciate incision is made that will readily allow free drainage of the pus. Skin edges must be excised because if only an incision is made, edges will readily fall together and seal, and the abscess may recur. In general, no packing is inserted, as this only impedes the drainage of pus. Minor bleeding can easily be controlled by electrocoagulation. If cautery is unavailable, packing for a few hours may be necessary to control bleeding (Fig. 27–5).

Ischioanal Abscess

The majority of ischioanal abscesses may also be incised and drained under local anesthesia as an outpatient procedure. Extensive abscesses might better be drained under general anesthesia. One or more counterincisions liberally used may drain the cavity satisfactorily.

Intersphincteric Abscess

A general or regional anesthetic is required for an intersphincteric abscess. Treatment consists of laying open the abscess, with division of the internal sphincter from its lower end up to the level of the dentate line,

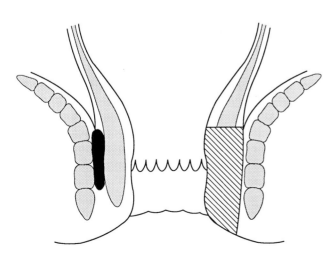

FIGURE 27–6. Treatment of an intersphincteric abscess.

or higher if the cavity extends higher (Fig. 27–6). Simply draining the abscess is inadequate therapy. This was clearly demonstrated by Chrabot and colleagues who, in reviewing recurrent anorectal abscesses, found that all patients with intersphincteric abscesses had fistulas.[6]

Supralevator Abscess

Of the various forms of anorectal suppuration, supralevator abscess is the least common and most difficult to recognize. Because there is no external evidence of disease, the diagnosis may be unduly delayed. Severe pain in the perianal and gluteal regions is the predominant feature. Such an abscess may arise in one of three ways. It may be due to the upward extension of an intersphincteric abscess; it may be caused by an upward extension of an ischioanal abscess; or it may result from pelvic disease such as perforated diverticulitis, Crohn's disease, or appendicitis.

Therapy depends on the presumed origin of this abscess. If the supralevator abscess is secondary to an upward extension of an intersphincteric abscess, it should be drained into the rectum by division of the internal sphincter (Fig. 27–7). The cut edges are run with an absorbable suture such as 3-0 chromic catgut to control bleeding. No packing is used. This abscess should not be drained through the ischioanal fossa because a suprasphincteric fistula may result and become difficult to manage (Fig. 27–7). If a supralevator abscess arises secondary to the upward extension of an ischioanal abscess, it should be drained through the ischioanal fossa. Attempts at draining this kind of abscess into the rectum will result in an extrasphincteric fistula becoming much more difficult to handle (Fig. 27–7). When draining supralevator abscesses of pelvic origin, one must take into consideration the original disease. These abscesses can be drained by three routes: (1) into the rectal lumen, (2) through the ischioanal fossa, or (3) through the abdominal wall. The choice of procedure depends on the area to which the abscess points most closely and on the general condition of the patient.

Horseshoe Abscess

Horseshoe extensions of anorectal abscesses may occur in the intersphincteric plane, the ischioanal fossa, or the supralevator plane. A general or regional anesthetic is usually necessary to treat sepsis of this nature. The level of circumferential spread will determine the manner of therapy. Horseshoe abscesses in the intersphincteric plane can usually be managed quite satisfactorily by dividing the internal sphincter for the height of the abscess cavity in the portion of the circumference where the abscess is bulging, thus, hopefully, exposing the crypt of origin (Fig. 27–6).

For horseshoeing in the ischioanal fossa, posterior drainage and the liberal use of counterincisions in both ischioanal fossae is an ideal treatment. Fortunately, horseshoeing in the supralevator plane is exceedingly rare. If the abscess arises because of an upward extension of an ischioanal abscess, bilateral drainage in each ischioanal fossa may be required.

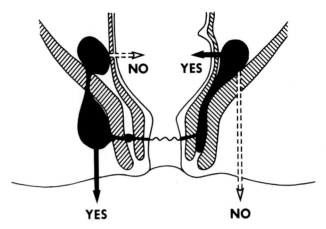

FIGURE 27-7. Drainage methods for supralevator abscesses.

Primary Versus Secondary Fistulotomy

Controversy continues over whether a primary fistulotomy should be employed in the treatment of anorectal abscesses. Some authorities favor a one-stage procedure in which incision and drainage are combined with fistulotomy.[1,8,11,25] They believe that this procedure will eradicate the origin of the infectious process, thereby almost eliminating the development of recurrent abscesses and anal fistulas, which they believe are otherwise inevitable. Proponents of a more conservative approach prefer a two-stage procedure, whereby incision and drainage are performed initially, followed by fistulotomy at a later date only if necessary. They argue that an operation might not be needed, and patients should not be exposed needlessly to the potential risk of incontinence, a dreaded possible consequence of fistulotomy, especially in the presence of acute inflammation.[21,30,35,36,43] In a prospective randomized trial, Schouten and Van Vroonhoven compared definitive operation with drainage alone.[35] Patients with a definitive operation had a recurrence or persistence rate of only 2.9% compared with 40.6% for those who had drainage alone, but assessment of anal continence preoperatively and postoperatively provided a telling story. Disturbance of anal function developed in 39.4% of patients who underwent definitive operation, almost double the 21.4% in those who underwent drainage alone. They concluded that since 60% of patients will have no further problem with abscess formation and with the increased disturbance of anal continence after definitive operation, a staged procedure should be recommended.

I found that following the drainage of anorectal abscesses, 11% of patients experienced recurrent abscesses, and 37% of patients were left with an anal fistula, for an overall recurrence or persistence rate of 48%.[43] It is interesting to note that when looking at the subset of patients in that study who were having their abscesses drained for the first time, a recurrent abscess developed in only 5% of them, and 31% of these patients later experienced an anal fistula. Thus only 36% of this subset of patients in this study required a definitive operation. It would appear that primary fistulotomy is not necessary, especially for patients with an anorectal abscess who are being treated for the first time. In addition, the majority of perianal and ischioanal abscesses can be drained using local anesthesia, which obviates the need for a general or spinal anesthetic. The use of local anesthetics also removes the temptation to perform a fistulotomy. Since one third to two thirds of patients will never have a further problem, a primary lay-open technique would be unnecessary.[34,43]

Necrotizing Soft Tissue Infection

In rare instances, anorectal suppuration may assume life-threatening proportions. Abcarian has pointed out that this may be attributed to delay in diagnosis and management; virulence of the organism, especially gas-forming anaerobic bacteria; bacteremia and occurrence of metastatic infections; and underlying disorders (e.g., diabetes mellitus, blood dyscrasias).[1] The lethal potential of this disease was well described by Marks and associates in their report of 11 deaths related to fistula-in-ano with abscess.[23] To prevent death, they recommend immediate incision and drainage; complete débridement, ignoring form and function; adequate anesthesia; and preoperative broad-spectrum antibiotic loading. Heppel and Benard have also stressed the importance of aggressive management of life-threatening perineal sepsis.[15]

Bode and co-workers addressed three controversial areas in the management of necrotizing perineal infections.[4] They identified fecal diversion, suprapubic cystostomy, and orchiectomy. They consider fecal diversion unnecessary because whole gut lavage and "medical colostomy" with total parenteral nutrition or enteral feeding will prevent the morbidity and mortality associated with colostomy and colostomy closure. These measures afford the same advantages as fecal diversion (limitation of perineal soiling) and maintain the patient's nutritional status. They believe suprapubic catheters are indicated only if urinary tract disease is the source of the sepsis. Because blood supply and venous drainage of the testicles occur via the spermatic vessels, testicular necrosis resulting from a fulminant perineal infection is rare. Although scrotal débridement is often necessary, the testicles may be "banked" with their intact blood supply in normal abdominal wall or thigh pockets.

The Leukemic Patient

Injudicious incision and drainage procedures in patients with acute leukemia or uncontrolled chronic leukemia can result in necrosis of the perineal area accompanied by uncontrolled septicemia and hemorrhage; sloughing of the whole buttock area and fecal incontinence may result.

At Memorial Hospital, New York, for those extremely ill patients, two methods of treatment are used.[37] The first combines radiation therapy consisting of 300 to 400 rads over 1 to 3 days (with repetition a week later if induration persists or recurs) and symptomatic care consisting of sitz baths or warm compresses, stool softeners, analgesics, and broad-spectrum antibiotics. This form of therapy is used in patients who have extremely de-pressed polymorphonuclear leukocyte counts, who are moribund, or in patients whose lesions have established spontaneous drainage. The second mode of treatment combines radiation therapy, surgery, and symptomatic care. The most suitable candidates for surgical treatment are patients suffering from chronic forms of leukemia or those with acute leukemia that is in remission. Barnes and associates, in a review of the literature, reported that perianal infection in patients with acute leukemia has been associated with mortality rates of 45 to 78%.[3] Lesions were painful, indurated, and associated with urinary retention, peritoneal signs, and extension to the genitals in some cases. They believed their policy of early incision and débridement contributed to their patients' improved survival. Shaked and co-workers showed that surgical drainage during agranulocytosis resulted in slow wound healing, prolonged hospitalization, and a higher mortality rate when compared with the group that received antibiotics alone (28% versus 18%).[39] They found that when the incision and drainage were performed after the granulocyte count increased to greater than 1,000 cells/mm^3, the postoperative course was uncomplicated with subsequent good healing. Patients who are operated on while they still have granulocytopenia showed no noticeable improvement in their general condition.

Postoperative Care

Patients who have had abscesses drained under local anesthesia should be advised to continue a regular diet, to take sitz baths three or four times daily, and to take a stool softener such as a psyllium seed preparation. Analgesics should be prescribed as necessary. These patients should be given a follow-up appointment in 1 month but be advised to return promptly if the pain does not diminish. Patients with intersphincteric abscesses drained under general anesthesia are discharged after the first bowel movement. They are followed weekly or biweekly until the wound is completely healed.

FISTULA-IN-ANO

Indications for Operation

The presence of a symptomatic fistula-in-ano is an indication for operation. Spontaneous healing of fistula-in-ano is very rare. Neglected fistulas may result in repeated abscesses and persistent drainage with its concomitant morbidity. Very rarely, malignancy may supervene in a long-standing fistula. Patients with compromised anal continence present a relative contraindication, since the further division of muscle required in the treatment of the fistula might render the patient totally incontinent.

Principles of Treatment

The objective of fistula surgery is to cure the fistula with the lowest possible recurrence rate and with minimal, if any, alteration in continence, and to do so in the shortest time possible. To approximate this ideal, a number of principles should be observed: (1) the primary opening of a track must be identified; (2) the relationship of the track to the puborectalis must be established; and (3) division of the least amount of muscle in keeping with cure of the fistula should be practiced.

Classification

The classification that I have adopted is the one described by Parks and associates.[30] Although very detailed, it gives an accurate description of the anatomic course of the fistulous tracks. This knowledge then acts as a guide to the operative treatment.

Parks' classification of fistula-in-ano is as follows:

1. Intersphincteric
   a. Simple low track
   b. High blind track
   c. High track with rectal opening
   d. Rectal opening without a perineal opening
   e. Extrarectal extension
   f. Secondary to pelvic disease

2. Transsphincteric
   a. Uncomplicated
   b. High blind track

3. Suprasphincteric
   a. Uncomplicated
   b. High blind track

4. Extrasphincteric
   a. Secondary to anal fistula
   b. Secondary to trauma
   c. Secondary to anorectal disease
   d. Due to pelvic inflammation

The courses of these tracks are depicted in Figure 27–8.

In a review of 400 fistulas by Parks and associates, the following distribution was found: intersphincteric, 45%; transsphincteric, 30%; suprasphincteric, 20%; and extrasphincteric, 5%.[30] Because of the highly selected patient population in this series, Parks estimated that a more representative incidence of the disease in the general population would be: intersphincteric, 70%; transsphincteric, 23%; suprasphincteric, 5%; and extrasphincteric, 2%. In an analysis of 160 consecutive patients who were classified at the time of operation by me, the distribution of fistulas was as follows: intersphincteric, 41.9%; transsphincteric, 52.1%; suprasphincteric, 1.9%; and extrasphincteric, 0%.[42] A horseshoe extension occurred in 8.8% of fistulas and 3.8% did not exactly conform to the classification, as they were either complex or combinations of more than one type of fistula.

Technique

Prior to any operative treatment of fistula-in-ano, it is wise to ascertain whether the patient has normal continence. Fistula surgery has an unenviable reputation because of the risks of recurrence and impairment of anal continence. Therefore, extreme care must be exercised

to minimize these problems. It would seem wise to alert patients to this possibility.

Simple Low-Level Fistula

With the patient under a light general anesthetic, preferably in the prone–jackknife position, the perianal region is prepared and infiltrated with a local anesthetic such as 0.5% lidocaine with 1:200,000 epinephrine. An anal speculum such as a Pratt bivalve is inserted in the anal canal, and any obvious internal opening is identified. A grooved, directional probe is then inserted into the external orifice and is passed along the distance of the track. In simple intersphincteric and low transsphincteric fistulas, the tissue over the track is divided by sliding the scalpel along the grooved probe director. Granulation tissue is then curetted and sent for biopsy. Careful examination is made by inspection and probing of the granulating tracks to uncover side or cephalad branches of the fistula tracks. Hemostasis is obtained using electrocoagulation. Marsupialization is then accomplished by approximating the skin edges to the edge of the track with a running absorbable suture, such as 3–0 chromic. This technique is preferred over trimming large amounts of skin and subcutaneous tissue, because it is our impression that the wounds heal more quickly. No packing is inserted. A loose cotton dressing is applied to prevent soiling of clothes, and a T-binder (or even underpants alone) is used rather than tape because the latter is uncomfortable to remove, especially in hirsute individuals.

When the probe cannot be advanced along the full distance of the track, as was the case in 40% of Parks' cases, a weak solution of 1:10 methylene blue is injected. This additional method reduced the number of cases in which the internal opening could not be demonstrated to 10%. When no such opening can be found, the general direction of the fistulous tracks as shown by probing from the external opening will indicate fairly clearly where the connection with the lining of the anal canal is located. Patients with multiple secondary openings generally have tracks that communicate with one another and with a single crypt of origin. Probing usually demonstrates this condition.

Horseshoe Fistula

The operation for a horseshoe fistula commences by laying open a lateral limb of the horseshoe track. This procedure is followed by exposing the posterior extremity of the track, and then the other lateral limb is unroofed. A search is made for the opening into the posterior wall of the anal canal at the level of the dentate line so that the primary source of the fistula is exposed. It is important not to miss such an opening, for to do so inevitably results in recurrence, despite the wide unroofing of the secondary limbs. If no primary internal opening is discovered, but the tracks lead to the posterior midline, it is probably wise, based on the assumption that the initiating factor is infection of cryptoglandular origin, to divide the lower half of the internal sphincter posteriorly to expose any such gland. All

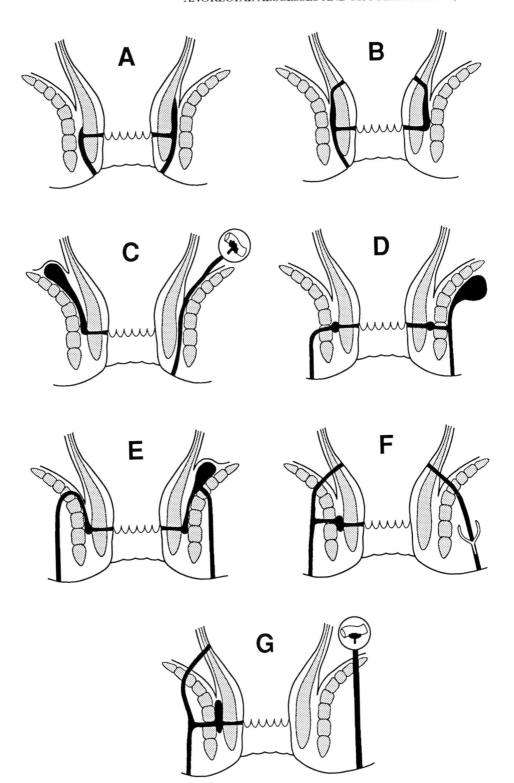

FIGURE 27-8. Diagrammatic representation of Parks' classification of fistula-in-ano. *A*, types 1a, 1b. *B*, types 1c, 1d. *C*, types 1e, 1f. *D*, types 2a, 2b. *E*, types 3a, 3b. *F*, types 4a, 4b. *G*, types 4c, 4d. (See text for further discussion.)

tracks are curetted of their granulation tissue and carefully examined for further side tracks. Marsupialization is effected, as this will markedly decrease the size of the wound and expedite healing.

Anterior horseshoe abscesses or fistulas are uncommon, but when they occur they are very difficult to manage, especially in women. The process may arise in a crypt in the anterior midline, and after penetrating the

internal and external sphincter, it lies deep to the transverse perineal muscle. In planning treatment, one must remember that there is no puborectalis anteriorly, and therefore the patient would be rendered incontinent more readily by an immediate fistulotomy. In the acute stage, the abscess should only be drained. In the fistulous stage, the primary source is handled in the anal canal by division of the lower half of the internal sphincter. Adequate drainage of the secondary track is then established and a seton is inserted. If the track traverses only the lower portion of the external sphincter, repair can be accomplished as described for posterior horseshoe fistulas.

Advancement Rectal Flaps

For patients whose fistula crosses the sphincter muscle at a high level (e.g., high transsphincteric and suprasphincteric fistulas), there is always concern that division of the muscle below the track will result in significant alteration in continence. In these circumstances, the advancement rectal flap technique is appealing and the subject of renewed interest.[2,5,7,10,20,26,44] Principles of repair include excision of the internal opening in the anal canal, excision or curettage of the main tracks, advancement of a flap of mucosa and submucosa or full thickness of rectum beyond the original internal opening, and suture of the flap to the anal canal distal to the original opening. The attractive features of this repair include the fact that no sphincter division is required, contour defects are avoided, there is less pain because there is no perineal wound, and there is more rapid healing.

Fistulotomy Versus Fistulectomy

Controversy still exists over whether a fistulotomy or a fistulectomy is the more appropriate operative treatment for a patient with an anal fistula. This point will not be belabored because there are a number of reasons to strongly recommend fistulotomy. First, removal of the complete track and adjacent scar tissue will only result in an appreciably larger wound. Second, there would be a larger separation of the ends of the sphincter after fistulectomy that would lead to a longer healing time and a greater chance of incontinence. For these reasons, it would appear that this topic should not be controversial.

Setons

When a track crosses the sphincter at a high level, it may be deemed safer not to divide all the muscle beneath the track. Only a portion of the muscle is cut, and a seton is inserted. The rationale for this maneuver is threefold. The first aim is to stimulate fibrosis adjacent to the sphincter muscle so that when the second stage, which involves laying open the track, is completed, the sphincter will not gape. After insertion of a seton, it is anticipated that division of the sphincter will be followed by scar formation proximal to the ligature, thus holding the muscle fibers together. This may, in fact, already have been accomplished by fibrosis of the fistulous tract. Another benefit of the seton is that it allows the surgeon to better delineate the amount of muscle beneath the fistulous tract. With the patient anesthetized, the operator cannot always be certain of the amount of muscle caudal to the track. Re-examination in an awake patient may reveal adequate muscle re-

maining above the level of the fistulous track. The third advantage of using the seton is that it acts as a drain (Fig. 27–9).

Actual insertion of the seton through the fistulous track is usually a simple matter. However, based on the belief that the pathogenesis of most anal fistulas originates from cryptoglandular disease, the internal sphincter should be divided from the level of the internal opening at the dentate line to its distal end to eradicate the source. Of course, the overlying skin is divided from this point to the secondary fistulous opening. A nonabsorbable suture is then threaded through the fistulous tract. I have employed heavy silk loosely tied with many knots so that a handle is created for manipulation. Occasionally, because of repeated handling during cleansing, the seton will eventually "saw" through the muscle. Usually, however, the muscle is divided at a second stage 6 to 8 weeks later. If the wound does heal well, consideration can be given to removal of the seton without division of the contained muscle.[41] In one series, primary healing occurred in 78% of 32 patients after removal of the seton.[18]

There are a number of clinical situations in which a seton should be considered. These include the presence of high-level fistulas, anterior fistulas in women, patients with coexistent inflammatory bowel disease (especially Crohn's disease), elderly individuals with a markedly weakened sphincter, individuals who have had previous operations and in whom extensive scarring is present, when there is uncertainty of the height of the track or the amount of muscle previously cut, and in the presence of simultaneous fistulas.

Parks and Stitz assessed function in 68 patients in whom a seton was employed.[28] Of those patients who had a seton inserted but removed without further division of muscle, 17% complained of partial loss of control, whereas 39% of patients who later had division of the seton-contained muscle experienced problems with control. Ramanujam and co-workers used setons in patients who had suprasphincteric fistulas.[32] Only one patient (2.2%) suffered permanent incontinence for flatus, none to feces, and the recurrence rate was only 2.2%.

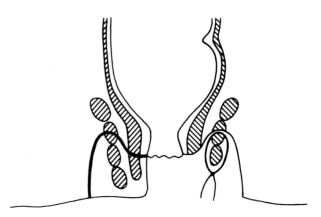

FIGURE 27-9. Placement of the seton.

Anal Fistula Associated With Crohn's Disease

A major controversy is the management of patients with an anal fistula in the presence of Crohn's disease. These fistulas may be very complex and may involve varying degrees of the sphincter mechanism. Extensive procedures expose these patients to the risk of non-healing fistulas, as well as to inducing or worsening anal incontinence. At the same time it must be emphasized that other patients with Crohn's disease have fairly simple fistulas, which nonetheless severely trouble them. In these cases, a fistulotomy for relief of symptoms is indicated. If no rectal disease exists, the risk of worsening the situation is minimal. Simple intersphincteric fistulas may be easily handled, and transsphincteric fistulas may be treated with or without the use of a seton. For patients with anovaginal fistulas, an anocutaneous flap was used successfully in seven of ten patients.[16] A protective stoma was established for the seven patients with proctitis. Extrasphincteric fistulas, however, invariably indicate active rectal involvement, and proctectomy usually provides the only chance for control.

Although operations on the anal canal of patients with Crohn's disease have been considered a relative contraindication, excellent results have been reported.[17,40] Notwithstanding the good results reported in these studies, plus gratifying results in patients I have treated, a general word of caution must be issued to counsel against the radical treatment of a fistulous abscess in Crohn's disease. Healing in some patients tends to be prolonged; therefore, removal of large amounts of tissue may result in inordinate healing times.

Complications of Operation for Fistulous Abscess

A long list of potential complications may ensue following operations for a fistulous abscess. Excluding urinary retention, which occurred in 25% of his patients, Mazier found that 5.4% of patients developed complications that included hemorrhage, incontinence, acute external thrombosed hemorrhoids, cellulitis, inadequate drainage and pocketing, fecal impaction, recurrent fistulas, rectovaginal fistulas, persistent sinus, bridging, and stricture.[24] However, with caution, these complications can be reduced to a minimum. It is my impression that avoiding primary fistulotomy surgery will help reduce such untoward events.

Postoperative Care

The postoperative care of the wound may be as important as the operative procedure. The prime goals are sound healing from the depths of the wound and prevention of contact leading to premature healing of opposing skin edges. Patients are placed on a regular diet, and non–codeine containing analgesics are administered as needed. Warm baths are taken three times a day for perineal toilet and patient comfort. A gentle laxative is given orally until the first bowel movement, and a bulk-forming agent is administered until wound healing has been completed.

Because of the operative trauma and division of some muscle, patients may experience fecal leaks in the immediate postoperative period, especially if stools are liquid. However, if the anorectal ring has been preserved, after a week or 10 days control approximates normalcy.

The healing time required depends on the complexity of the fistula. Simple fistulotomy may heal in 4 to 5 weeks, whereas complex fistulas may take several months to heal. Most uncomplicated fistulas heal within 12 weeks of operation.[42] A number of factors were noted to be associated with prolonged healing. Healing time was increased with increasing complexity of the fistula. Fistulas characterized by extrarectal extensions or high blind tracks take a long time to heal, as do suprasphincteric or horseshoe fistulas. Delayed healing also occurs in patients with inflammatory bowel disease. This may not necessarily be attributable to the presence of inflammatory bowel disease per se, since some of these patients had more complex types of fistulas.

Results

Reported results of fistula surgery vary considerably. Clearly, results will depend upon the complexity of the fistula treated. A review of the literature reveals recurrence rates between 0 and 26% with a reasonable expectation of 4 to 7%. Disturbances of continence from 0 to 40% have been reported with reasonable expectations in the 4 to 9% range. It might be noted that there is often a reciprocal relationship in the incidence of recurrence and incontinence. Reports with low recurrence rates not infrequently cite a higher incidence of incontinence, whereas reports with higher recurrence rates may describe a low rate of incontinence. It is extremely difficult to compare the results of these often very different series of patients. Many large series have inadequate follow-up, with many patients being lost to follow-up, whereas others have very short follow-up. Most authors do not define incontinence, and the reader is unaware of whether the problems are temporary or permanent; whether the patient was incontinent for flatus, liquid stool, or solid stool; or whether there was soiling. In a series of 160 patients upon whom I operated, the sole immediate postoperative complication was bleeding, which occurred 1 week postoperatively and ceased spontaneously (0.7%).[42] Alteration in continence occurred in 6% of patients, with 2.6% experiencing temporary incontinence to flatus, 1.3% experiencing incontinence to liquid stool, and 0.7% experiencing incontinence to solid stool. Permanent loss of control for flatus occurred in one patient (0.7%) and for liquid stool in one patient (0.7%). No patients experienced loss of control for solid stool. Recurrence developed in 6.3% of patients, all instances occurring between 5 and 25 months postoperatively.

REFERENCES

1. Abcarian, H.: Acute suppurations of the anorectum. *In* Nyhus, L.M. (ed.): Surgery Annual, Vol. 8. Norwalk, CT, Appleton-Century-Crofts, 1976, p. 305.

2. Aguilar, P.S., Plasencia, G., Hardy, T.G., et al.: Mucosal advancement in the treatment of anal fistula. Dis. Colon Rectum, *28:* 496, 1985.

3. Barnes, S.G., Sattler, F.R., and Ballard, J.O.: Perirectal infections in acute leukemia. Improved survival after incision and debridement. Ann. Intern. Med., *100:*515, 1984.

4. Bode, W.E., Ramos, R., and Page, C.P.: Invasive necrotizing infection secondary to anorectal abscess. Dis. Colon Rectum, *25:*416, 1982.

5. Buchmann, P., and Klotz, H.: Anal advancement flap for the treatment of fistula-in-ano: An ongoing prospective study. Br. J. Surg., *79*(Suppl.):S129, 1992.

6. Chrabot, C.M., Prasad, M.L., and Abcarian, H.: Recurrent anorectal abscesses. Dis. Colon Rectum, *26:*105, 1983.

7. Detry, R., Remacle, G., and Kartheuser, A.: Treatment of deep anal fistula by the flap advancement technique. Br. J. Surg., *79*(Suppl.):S129, 1992.

8. Eisenhammer, S.: A final evaluation and classification of the surgical treatment of the primary anorectal cryptoglandular intermuscular (intersphincteric) fistulous abscess and fistula. Dis. Colon Rectum, *21:*237, 1978.

9. Ellis, M.: 1955 quoted in Goligher, J.C.: Surgery of the Anus, Rectum and Colon, 3rd ed. London, Balliere Tindall, 1975.

10. Fazio, V.W.: Complex anal fistulas. Gastroenterol. Clin. North Am., *16:*93, 1987.

11. Fucini, C.: One-stage treatment of anal abscess and fistulas. A clinical appraisal on the basis of two different classifications. Int. J. Colorectal Dis., *6:*12, 1991.

12. Goligher, J.C., Ellis, M., and Pissidis, A.G.: A critique of anal glandular infection in the etiology and treatment of idiopathic anorectal abscesses and fistulas. Br. J. Surg. *54:*977, 1967.

13. Goligher, J.C.: Surgery of the Anus, Rectum and Colon, 3rd ed. London, Balliere Tindall, 1975.

14. Grace, R.H., Harper, I.A., and Thompson, R.G.: Anorectal sepsis: Microbiology in relation to fistula-in-ano. Br. J. Surg., *69:*401, 1982.

15. Heppell, J., and Benard, F.: Life-threatening perineal sepsis. Perspect. Colorectal Surg., *4:*1, 1991.

16. Hesterberg, R., Schmidt, W.U., Muller, F., and Roher, H.D.: Treatment of anovaginal fistulas with an anocutaneous flap in patients with Crohn's disease. Int. J. Colorectal Dis., *8:*51, 1993.

17. Hobbiss, J.H., and Schofield, P.F.: Management of perianal Crohn's disease. J. R. Soc. Med., *75:*414, 1982.

18. Kennedy, H.L., and Zegarra, J.P.: Fistulotomy without external sphincter division for high anal fistulae. Br. J. Surg., *77:*898, 1990.

19. Law, P.J., Talbot, R.W., Bartram, C.I., and Northover, J.M.A.: Anal endosonography in the evaluation of perianal sepsis and fistula-in-ano. Br. J. Surg., *76:*752, 1989.

20. Lewis, P., and Bartolo, D.C.C.: Treatment of trans-sphincteric fistula by full thickness anorectal advancement flaps. Br. J. Surg., *77:*1187, 1990.

21. Lockhart-Mummery, H.E.: Treatment of abscesses. Dis. Colon Rectum, *18:*650, 1975.

22. Lunnis, P.J., Armstrong, P., Barker, P.G., et al: Magnetic resonance imaging of anal fistulae. Lancet, *340:*394, 1992.

23. Marks, G., Chase, W.V., and Mervine, T.B.: The fatal potential of fistula-in-ano with abscess: Analysis of 11 deaths. Dis. Colon Rectum, *16:*224, 1973.

24. Mazier, W.P.: The treatment and care of anal fistulas: A study of 1000 patients. Dis. Colon Rectum, *14:*134, 1971.

25. McElwain, J.W., MacLean, M.D., Alexander, R.M., et al.: Experience with primary fistulectomy for anorectal abscess; a report of 1,000 cases. Dis. Colon Rectum, *18:*646, 1975.

26. Oh, C.: Management of high recurrent anal fistulae. Surgery, *93:* 330, 1983.

27. Parks, A.G., and Gordon, P.H.: Perineal fistula of intraabdominal or intra pelvic origin simulating fistula-in-ano: Report of seven cases. Dis. Colon Rectum, *19:*500, 1976.

28. Parks, A.G., and Stitz, R.W.: The treatment of high fistula-in-ano. Dis. Colon Rectum, *19:*487, 1976.

29. Parks, A.G.: Pathogenesis and treatment of fistula-in-ano. BMJ, *1:* 463, 1961.

30. Parks, A.G., Gordon, P.H., and Hardcastle, J.E.: A classification of fistula-in-ano. Br. J. Surg., *63:*1, 1976.

31. Prasad, M.L., Read, D.R., and Abcarian, H.: Supralevator abscesses: Diagnosis and treatment. Dis. Colon Rectum, *24:*456, 1981.

32. Ramanujam, P.S., Prasad, M.L., and Abcarian, H.: The role of seton in fistulotomy of the anus. Surg. Gynecol. Obstet., *157:*419, 1983.

33. Ramanujam, P.S., Prasad, M.L., Abcarian, H., and Tan, A.B.: Perianal abscesses and fistulas. Dis. Colon Rectum, *27:*593, 1984.

34. Sainio, P.: Fistula-in-ano in a defined population; incidence and epidemiological aspects. Ann. Chir. Gynaecol., *73:*219, 1984.

35. Schouten, W.R., and Van Vroonhoven, Th.J.M.V.: Treatment of anorectal abscess with or without primary fistulectomy. Results of a prospective randomized trial. Dis. Colon Rectum, *34:*60, 1991.

36. Scoma, J.A., Salvati, E.P., and Rubin, R.J.: Incidence of fistulas subsequent to anal abscesses. Dis. Colon Rectum, *17:*357, 1974.

37. Sehdev, M.R., Dowling, M.D., Seal, S.H., Stearns, M.W.: Perianal and anorectal complications in leukemia. Cancer, *31:*149, 1973.

38. Seow-Choen, E., Hay, A.J., Heard, S., and Phillips, R.K.S.: Bacteriology of anal fistulae. Br. J. Surg., *79:*27, 1992.

39. Shaked, A.A., Shinar, E., and Freund, H.: Managing the granulocytopenic patient with acute perianal inflammatory disease. Am. J. Surg., *152:*510, 1986.

40. Sohn, N., Korelitz, B.I., and Weinstein, M.A.: Anorectal Crohn's disease: Definitive surgery for fistulas and recurrent abscesses. Am. J. Surg., *139:*394, 1981.

41. Thomson, J.P.S., and Ross, A.H.M.: Can the external anal sphincter be preserved in the treatment of trans-sphincteric fistula-in-ano. Int. J. Colorectal Dis., *4:*247, 1989.

42. Vasilevsky, C.A., and Gordon, P.H.: Results of treatment of fistula-in-ano. Dis. Colon Rectum, *28:*225, 1985.

43. Vasilevsky, C.A., and Gordon, P.H.: The incidence of recurrent abscess or fistula-in-ano following anorectal suppuration. Dis. Colon Rectum, *27:*126, 1984.

44. Wedell, J., Meier zu Eissen, P., Banzhaf, G., and Kleine, L.: Sliding flap advancement for the treatment of high level fistulae. Br. J. Surg., *74:*390, 1987.

45. Weisman, R.I., Orsay, C.P., Pearl, R.K., and Abcarian, H.: The role of fistulography in fistula-in-ano. Report of five cases. Dis. Colon Rectum, *34:*181, 1991.

Chapter 28

NEOPLASMS OF THE ANUS AND ANAL CANAL

NORMAN D. NIGRO

This chapter deals with cancers of the anal region, which include those in the perianal skin, an area referred to as the anal margin, and those that develop in the epithelium of the anal canal. Histologically, cancers of the anal margin are like skin cancers elsewhere. Consequently, their management is not often a problem, and the prognosis generally is good. Conversely, cancers of the anal canal consist of invasive squamous cells or one of several variants of squamous cells. These tumors are more aggressive, and management is more complex and more radical than it is with anal margin cancers. Since the treatment is the same regardless of cell type, it is more convenient to use an all-inclusive, single term such as squamous cell or epidermoid cancer of the anal canal. Either of these terms includes all varieties of squamous cell tumors, including those that are called cloacogenic.

Very rarely, adenocarcinoma and melanoma also occur in the anal region. Adenocarcinoma can develop in the rectal mucosa of the proximal part of the anal canal, in an anal gland located around the canal, or in an apocrine gland of the perianal skin. These cancers are similar to adenocarcinoma of the rectum, and they should be treated in the same way. Melanoma will be mentioned only briefly because the treatment of this lesion in the anal canal has been uniformly ineffective. However, recent investigations by Rosenberg and associates at the National Cancer Institute (NCI) of methods that enhance the immune system are encouraging.[47]

Surgery has been the treatment of choice for anal margin cancer, and for the most part, this is true today. In contrast, the therapy for anal canal cancer has changed over the past decade. Traditionally, the treatment was a radical operation, although a few radiotherapists have used radiation as the primary therapy for years. Recently, there has been a trend in favor of the combined modality approach to cancer therapy in general, and this applies to cancer of the anal canal as well.

In fact, radiation, chemotherapy, and surgery in various combinations are being investigated rather extensively. There is considerable evidence already that some combination of radiation and chemotherapy alone is quite effective in dealing with the local lesion and that abdominoperineal resection of the rectum is not generally necessary. This rather recent development justifies a discussion of all aspects of the problem in order to establish the rationale for the best current treatment for squamous cell cancer of the anal canal.

ANATOMY

The word anus is defined as "the anal orifice; the lower opening of the digestive tract,"[55] but surgeons frequently use it to indicate the general region and call the orifice itself the anal verge. The anal region is divided into an internal part, the anal canal; and an external component, the skin of the anal margin. Although the gross anatomy was first described several centuries ago and the microscopic features studied for more than 100 years, confusion still exists as to definitions, nomenclature, and boundaries. This is due to the complexity of anatomic structures placed so close together and the lack of some identifiable boundary lines. An important structure that can be identified on anoscopic examination is the mucocutaneus junction, most often called the dentate line (Fig. 28–1). It is the place where the entoderm and ectoderm joined during embryonic development. Anal papillae, varying in number up to six or eight, are thought to be remnants of the proctodeal membrane. They are small, saw tooth–like triangular projections that encircle the area and are located at the base of the longitudinal mucosal columns of Morgagni. Presumably, these columns result from the downsizing of the hindgut to meet the anal canal. The anal valves are a series of semilunar folds that are located between

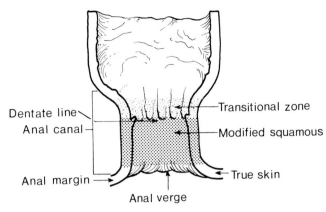

FIGURE 28-1. Important anatomic landmarks in the anal area. The perianal skin area for about 6 cm in all directions from the anal verge is called the anal margin.

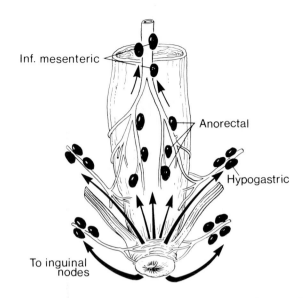

FIGURE 28-2. Direction of lymphatic spread from anal cancer. Lesions in the upper third of the canal spread to the mesenteric system, those in the middle third of the canal spread to the hypogastric nodes, and those in the distal third of the canal and in the anal margin spread to the inguinal area. Owing to overlap, spread often occurs in more than one direction.

the bases of the vertical columns. Behind each one is a recess or anal crypt, and the anal glands empty into them. All these structures help identify the dentate line. In addition, the tissue above it looks like mucosa, whereas the surface distal to it looks more like skin.[57]

The anal margin refers to the perianal area extending from the anal verge for a distance of 5 or 6 cm around it. As already mentioned, the anal verge refers to the opening itself. There is no line to mark it either grossly or microscopically. In fact, the precise level of the opening varies slightly, depending upon the degree of muscle contraction around it. Just inside the opening, the skin is a lighter color and lacks hair. Outside the anal verge, the skin appears more normal. Microscopically, there is a gradual change from skin containing hair follicles and sweat glands on the outside to modified skin without these structures on the inside. The term anal canal is defined in two ways. One is called the anatomic anal canal, which is based on the ectodermally derived part. Hence, it extends from the dentate line to the anal verge. It is about 2 cm in length. The other is called the surgical anal canal. It is the part of the channel that is within the grasp of the anorectal sphincter musculature, so it extends from the pelvic floor to the anal verge. It is about 5 cm in length. Recently, Fenger, in an excellent review of the anatomy of the anal canal, defined it more simply by saying that it extends from the top to the bottom of the internal sphincter.[9] Today, the surgical anal canal is the version used most frequently.

The anal canal and the perianal area contain a profuse supply of blood vessels and lymphatics. The middle rectal blood vessels help supply the lower part of the rectum and the upper part of the anal canal. The inferior rectal vessels supply the lower part of the canal as well as the surrounding muscles and skin in the anal margin. There is a profuse network of lymphatic vessels under the lining of the anal canal. Spread of cancer through this system is common and occurs in all directions (Fig. 28-2). In general, lesions in the upper third of the anal canal spread primarily to the mesenteric system, those in the midportion spread to the pelvic nodes, and tumors in the lower part of the canal and in the anal margin spread to the inguinal node system. Since

there are extensive communications among the three lymphatic systems in the anal region, a lesion in any location may spread in more than one direction.

ANAL MARGIN CANCER

Because tumors of the anal margin are located in the skin outside the anal verge, they can be examined directly and do not require the aid of an endoscope. However, when tumors develop close to the anal verge, they may spread into the lower part of the canal, in which case it is necessary to use an anoscope to determine the proximal extent. Anal margin cancers differ from anal canal cancer significantly in cell characteristics, prognosis, and treatment. Therefore, it is important that they be considered separately. This point is emphasized because the two are combined in some published reports. This is a source of confusion with regard to the prognosis and therapy of anal cancers.

Anal margin cancers are not nearly as common as cancers of the anal canal. Morson analyzed the experience of 157 patients with epithelial cancer of the anal region at St. Mark's Hospital, London, during the period 1928 to 1956.[33] Of these cancers, 38 were anal margin cancers, 103 were anal canal cancers, and the location was not specified in 16 patients. McConnell reviewed 96 patients from the Liverpool Cancer Registry.[30] He found that 41 patients had anal margin cancer, whereas 55 patients had anal canal cancer. More recently, Hintz and co-workers suggested that about 25% of anal tumors are located in the anal margin, whereas 75% occur in the anal canal.[21]

In contrast to adenocarcinoma of the rectum, which occurs more often in men, cancer of the anal region has an equal distribution in men and women. However, there is a striking difference in sex incidence between cancer of the anal margin and cancer of the anal canal. Anal margin cancer is more common in men, whereas anal canal cancer is more frequent in women. The age incidence is the same in both groups, as it is in adenocarcinoma of the rectum.

Unlike neoplasms of the anal canal, the pathologic classification of anal margin cancer is straightforward. The types, as listed in the International Classification of Tumors,[32] are widely accepted and are listed in Table 28–1. Since they are generally similar to those occurring in the skin elsewhere, it is rather easy to classify them and to assess the degree of differentiation. There is a tumor, node, metastasis (TNM) staging system designed for anal margin cancer.[22] It is not difficult to apply and is of value in the management of these patients.[23]

Symptoms are minimal—generally there is the presence of a lump or a "sore" that persists and is unresponsive to simple measures. Sometimes there is associated discharge, irritation, and itching. Diagnosis is made by biopsy.

Squamous Cell Cancer

The most frequent type of malignant tumor of the perianal skin is the squamous cell cancer. It is usually a well-differentiated, highly keratinized tumor of relatively small size. These cancers are superficial and are more often exophytic than ulcerative. Symptoms are minor, namely the presence of a lump or small ulcer that is not especially painful or tender. It does not heal even after several months of local therapy with ointments, baths, and so on. Surgical excision is the treatment of choice. The lesion should be removed with a wide margin of skin around it. In most cases, the wound should be left open because it will heal quickly with satisfactory results. Skin grafts may be applied to prevent stricture when the lesion spreads to a significant degree from the outside into the anal canal. Recurrence is uncommon, but sometimes the lesion is not completely removed. In this case, surgical excision should be repeated. Inguinal nodes are not often involved.

Large, highly invasive ulcerative squamous cancers have been observed in the anal margin and in the perineum. These invasive cancers may spread to the inguinal nodes and beyond. They require extensive therapy

TABLE 28–1. CLASSIFICATION OF EPITHELIAL CANCERS OF THE ANAL REGION*

ANAL MARGIN	ANAL CANAL
Squamous cell carcinoma	Squamous cell carcinoma
Basal cell carcinoma	Variants
Bowen's disease	Basaloid
Paget's disease	Cloacogenic
Tumor-like lesions	Mucoepidermoid
Condyloma acuminatum	Miscellaneous Lesions
	Adenocarcinoma
	Carcinoma associated with fistula
	Malignant melanoma

*Modified from Morson, B.C., and Sobin, L.H.: International Histological Classification of Tumors, #15: 62, 1976, with permission.

similar to that for invasive cancer of the anal canal, which is described later in this chapter.

Basal Cell Cancer

Only ten patients with basal cell cancer of the anal margin were seen at St. Mark's Hospital in a 25-year period.[33] Similarly, Grodsky, in a review of the literature in 1965, found that only 50 cases had been reported up to that time.[17] The lesion is similar to "rodent ulcers" seen on exposed skin: the average patient age is 60 years. This cancer should not be confused with basaloid cancer of the anal canal. Symptoms are nonspecific, but any indurated swelling that has been present for months, especially if it is ulcerated, should be suspected as representing a possible low-grade cancer. A wide excisional biopsy should be done not only for diagnosis but also for therapy.

Bowen's Disease

Bowen's disease is a chronic, intradermal, squamous cell cancer that has a tendency to remain intradermal for years. Clinically, it resembles perianal skin typical of pruritus ani. Microscopically, Bowen's disease is a squamous cell carcinoma confined to the epidermis. The basement membrane is intact and the basal layer is orderly and appears normal. However, there is a loss of normal cell polarity and stratification in the superficial layers of the skin. A highly characteristic feature is a large, atypical cell with a haloed, hyperchromatic nucleus. These bowenoid cells are scattered throughout the epidermis.[33] Wide local excision is the accepted therapy and is generally curative. Recently, Marfing and associates reviewed a series of 106 patients with Bowen's disease of the anal margin.[28] Eighty-four per cent of these patients were treated by local excision, and nearly half had been followed for more than 5 years. Recurrent Bowen's disease developed in 9% of the patients; some had as many as four recurrences. Nearly 6% experienced subsequent invasive squamous cell cancer requiring radical surgery. Only five patients (4.7%) experienced cancers of other organs. This evidence, plus that of Anderson and co-workers,[1] suggests that there is no significant relationship between Bowen's disease and internal malignancies. Consequently, frequent extensive examinations in search of such cancers are unnecessary. However, long-term follow-up for recurrence of Bowen's disease or for the development of invasive squamous cell cancer of the anal margin is recommended. If the latter occurs, chemoradiation therapy similar to that used for anal canal tumors is indicated in most patients.

Paget's Disease

Extramammary Paget's disease of the anal margin is a rare malignant lesion. Clinically, the disease is a progressively spreading, eczematoid condition of the perianal skin associated with intractable itching. It is usually present for many months or even years before the correct diagnosis is made.[18] The condition cannot be distinguished clinically from the nonmalignant forms of skin diseases that cause itching or from Bowen's disease. The diagnosis can be made only by biopsy. It is an adenocarcinoma of an apocrine skin gland. Microscopically, the lesion is characterized by the presence of large, pale-staining, ovoid, vacuolated cells with a single large nucleus. They look like the signet ring cells seen in mucinous adenocarcinoma, and the clear spaces contain mucin, which is not present in Bowen's disease. Quite often there is an underlying infiltrating adenocarcinoma. This occurred in 13 of 38 patients studied by Helwig and Graham[20] and in five of seven patients reported by Williams and co-workers.[60]

Treatment and prognosis depend on the presence of underlying invasive adenocarcinoma. If invasive cancer is not present, local excision with clear margins is sufficient. Multiple excisions are often required for complete removal of the lesion. In one study, all patients with invasive cancer that had already spread to the inguinal lymph nodes died despite radical operation.[20,60] However, patients with early invasive cancer do well with abdominoperineal resection.[60] The use of chemoradiation therapy as a preoperative measure followed routinely by abdominoperineal resection in 4 weeks may be worthwhile in patients with underlying infiltrative cancer of this variety.

Tumor-like Lesions

Condyloma acuminatum of the anal margin is nearly always a benign disease. However, on rare occasions it is associated with squamous cell cancer. Friedberg and Serlin reviewed the association of these two lesions and also suggested that although giant condyloma does not undergo malignant change, it sometimes behaves like carcinoma.[12] More recent articles by Lee and associates and Prasad and co-workers cite additional case reports and advise abdominoperineal resection as the treatment of choice.[26,43]

We have seen a 32-year-old man with a superficial perineal fistula associated with condyloma acuminatum. Cancer was not suspected, but after operation the specimen showed the condyloma mixed with moderately well-differentiated squamous cell cancer. After the wound healed, the patient was given radiation and chemotherapy according to the regimen described under "Squamous Cell Cancer of the Anal Canal" (see further on). Abdominoperineal resection was not done, and the patient was free of disease 5 years following therapy.

A second patient had a large mass of perianal condyloma excised in the routine manner. Early squamous cell cancer was found in the specimen, but no further therapy was given. Two years later, the patient returned with a large recurrent mass covering the entire perianal area. On biopsy, the tissue contained a mixture of condyloma and squamous cell cancer. The mass was not excised. Instead, the patient was given the chemoradiation therapy regimen described later in this chapter. In 3 months, the lesion disappeared and there has been no recurrence for 4 years.

On the basis of this experience, we advocate the administration of radiation and chemotherapy for condyloma acuminatum associated with squamous cell cancer.

If the lesion disappears, radical operation is not required. If the lesion persists, abdominoperineal resection may be indicated.

Discussion

A recent review of the management of anal margin cancer by Papillon and Chassard suggests that these neoplasms are more often invasive than the above discussion indicates.[38] Their clinic is a cancer treatment center for a wide area in France. Thus, it is quite likely that most patients referred to them have advanced disease. It is clear that the treatment for anal margin cancer has to be individualized. It varies from simple excision to chemoradiation and to radical surgery.

SQUAMOUS CELL CANCER OF THE ANAL CANAL

The majority of cancers of the anal region occur in the anal canal. These lesions are far more aggressive and more lethal than anal margin cancer. Consequently, the major portion of this chapter deals with these tumors. Another very important element is that although the treatment for anal canal lesions traditionally has been surgery, it now has changed to combined simultaneous radiation and chemotherapy, with operation reserved for special circumstances. This new trend calls for a review of all aspects of the subject to help clarify the current management of this disease.

The tissues of the anal canal are best divided into three zones. The most proximal is simply normal rectal mucosa. The middle part is called the transitional zone, formerly referred to as the cloacogenic zone. It is a narrow strip that extends 1 to 2 cm above the dentate line, although Fenger has shown that it can involve any part of the area from 0.6 cm below to 2 cm above the dentate line.[9] This area contains a complex mixture of cells of varying size and shape, with a predominance of cuboidal or polygonal cells. Interspersed between them are islands of rectal mucosal cells, which migrate into the area from above, and normal squamous cells, which come from below. A few endocrine and some melanin-containing cells are also present in this area. Mucin histochemical studies suggest that the pattern of mucin secretion of cells in this zone differs from that of rectal mucosal cells. Fenger suggests that mucin histochemical information may be useful in classifying the numerous malignant epithelial tumors that occur in the anal canal.[9] The surface covering the lower third of the canal is modified skin that has no hair follicles and no skin glands. For a more detailed description of the histologic features of this area, see the recent review by Fenger.[9]

Etiology

The cause of the disease is unknown, although its association with other conditions has led to speculation regarding some predisposing conditions, at least in some patients. There has long been an impression that anal margin cancer is due in part to constant irritation of the perianal skin from conditions such as anal fissure, fistulas, anal pruritus, and even to poor anal hygiene. However, these are common problems, so their association may be merely coincidental. There is now somewhat better evidence to suggest that the association of squamous cell cancer with condyloma acuminatum in genital and perianal areas is significant. These soft, wartlike lesions have been found to be due to human papillomaviruses. Early in the twentieth century, there were several papers published suggesting an association between carcinoma of the vulva and condylomata. Siegal described their association in the perianal area, and other reports followed.[49] In a series of 35 patients with anal cancer, Brennan and Stewart found five associated with condylomata.[3]

Recent case reports of anal cancer in male homosexuals, and the suggestion from such studies that they may be at increased risk for the disease, has initiated considerable interest in this aspect of the problem. Peters and Mack investigated the association of anal cancer and marital status in 970 patients with the disease in Los Angeles County.[42] They found that anal carcinomas are more common in women than in men and that single men and divorced persons of both sexes have a higher risk for this form of cancer. It seems reasonable from such information to theorize that the increased risk for anal cancer is due to sexual behavior, specifically anal intercourse. It appears that the pattern of anal cancer in women is consistent with that hypothesis.

Among the possible mechanisms that may promote cancer formation by anal intercourse is infection with one or more viral agents. As already mentioned, the papillomavirus has been found in condyloma acuminatum tissue. Furthermore, Northover stated in a recent editorial that HPV-16 DNA is incorporated into the genome of anal cancer tissue in at least 50% of patients in the United Kingdom.[36] Obviously, more evidence is needed to implicate viral infection resulting from sexual activity in the etiology of anal cancer. It is also quite possible that there are several predisposing factors in the etiology of the disease and that not all are sexually related.

Pathologic Features

It is not surprising, considering the variation in the epithelial surfaces of the anal region, that carcinomas developing in the area vary from well-differentiated, keratinized squamous cell cancer to very undifferentiated carcinoma. Most, if not all, tumors of the anal canal develop from cells located in the transitional zone. Normal cells in the area vary considerably and, naturally, so do the cancers that develop from them. Accordingly, pathologists classify these tumors as basaloid, transitional, epidermoid, cloacogenic, squamous cell, and undifferentiated. Boman and associates, in a report from the Mayo Clinic, identified another variation, a small cell type.[2] They found it to be highly lethal. On rare occasions, adenocarcinomas develop in the anal canal either from the rectal mucosa in the most proximal part of the canal or from the anal glands located in the tissues around the canal at the level of the dentate line. Malignant melanoma may occur in the same location.

Routes of Spread

Like gastrointestinal cancer in general, anal cancer spreads by direct extension, through the lymphatic system, and via the bloodstream. The tumors often spread directly to adjacent tissues, including the sphincter muscles and the vagina, or to the capsule of the prostate then to the urethra. Wolfe and Bussey found that tumors occasionally spread along tissue planes, particularly in the submucosal space, and upward for 5 or 6 cm before ulcerating into the rectum.[61]

There is an extensive lymphatic plexus in the area, and spread through this system is most common. It occurs in all directions, upward through the superior hemorrhoidal and inferior mesenteric vessels and nodes, laterally though the pelvic system, and downward to the inguinal nodes. In general, lesions in the upper third of the anal canal spread primarily to the mesenteric system, those in the midportion spread to the pelvic nodes, and tumors in the lower part of the canal and those in the anal margin spread to the inguinal node system. Since there are extensive communications between the three lymphatic systems in the anal region, a lesion in any location may spread in more than one direction. Bloodstream metastases in patients with squamous cell cancer of the anus are not nearly as common as in patients with adenocarcinoma of the rectum or colon. In a review by Kuehn and colleagues, 13 of 189 patients had metastases to the liver, whereas six patients had metastases to the lungs.[25] The primary lesion in these 19 patients was located in the area above the dentate line. Stearns and associates found four patients with liver metastases out of 180 patients who were explored. Three others developed metastases at a later date. In that series, only two patients had pulmonary metastases diagnosed before death.[53] Papillon and Montbarbon have found that distant metastases occur in about 10% of patients.[40]

Staging

The ability to objectively categorize the extent of disease in cancer patients in a precise way permits an accurate assessment of the prognosis in an individual patient. Furthermore, it is helpful for comparing the effect of different therapeutic measures. The classic method for staging cancer is the Dukes classification of colorectal cancer. Richards and associates of the Mayo Clinic applied it to cancer of the anal canal, but this staging system is difficult in these lesions because the anatomic features of the area do not lend themselves to precise localization of the extent of disease as they do in the rectum or colon.[46] In addition, a surgical specimen is very helpful in applying the Dukes classification. The TNM system, based in part on the extent of tumor spread, is unsatisfactory for the same reason. Variations have been proposed by Frost and associates,[13] Boman and colleagues,[2] Singh and associates,[50] and Papillon and Montbarbon.[40] All include the size of the primary lesion and the involvement of regional lymph nodes. However, none has been widely accepted as yet.

Patterns of Failure and Prognosis

The establishment of objective criteria to estimate prognosis is hampered in this disease by the relatively few patients available for study and by the difficulty in assessing the degree of tumor invasion. However, in the past decade or so, some aspects of this problem have become clearer because of increased interest in the disease, resulting in a greater number of published reports. There is general agreement that the size of the primary lesion correlates very well with survival, and the grave prognostic sign of regional lymph node metastases has been confirmed.

Frost and co-workers reviewed the records of 192 patients treated between 1954 and 1979 at the M.D. Anderson Hospital.[13] In a subgroup of 132 patients who had abdominoperineal resection, they found that the survival rate was related to tumor size, extent of local invasion, and the status of regional lymph nodes. The 5-year survival rate for early lesions (superficial invasion only) was 76%, whereas for late lesions (deep invasion or lymph node involvement), it was 29%. Broken down according to size, it was 78% for small tumors (1 to 2 cm), 55% for medium-sized tumors (3 to 5 cm), and 40% for large cancers (6 cm). Cell type was not a factor; in fact, survival rates for squamous cell and cloacogenic cancer were virtually the same. Some patients had radiation therapy either before or after operation. The gross tumor disappeared in 11 patients who had preoperative radiation, but three of these patients were found to have involved lymph nodes in the operative specimen. For the entire group, the survival rate was 83%. The fixed primary lesions of ten patients became operable after radiation therapy. Thirty-one patients who experienced local recurrences were treated with surgery or radiation alone, or a combination of the two. Retreatment resulted in a 38% 5-year survival rate in that group. Twenty-nine patients had inguinal node involvement at the time the primary lesion was diagnosed, and 29% survived 5 years after treatment. Eleven of 16 of these patients who had abdominoperineal resection were found to have other involved lymph nodes in addition to those in the inguinal area. There were 20 patients who experienced inguinal node metastases after the original therapy but who still had a chance for cure. Eighteen of these patients underwent groin dissection, and 42% survived at least 5 years.

Boman and associates analyzed the Mayo Clinic experience.[2] The records of 188 patients with anal cancer were reviewed. Among 114 who had abdominoperineal resection and who were followed for at least 5 years, 71% were long-term survivors. They found that tumor size, depth invasion, regional lymph node involvement, and histologic grading were predictive of survival. Forty per cent of the patients in the entire series experienced recurrences. The exact site of recurrence after abdominoperineal resection was documented in 38 patients. Twenty-seven lesions recurred locally (i.e., in the pelvis or groin); five patients had both local and distant metastases, and six patients had developed only distant metastatic disease. The incidence of failure by stage of the initial lesion was as follows: patients with extension of disease to but not beyond the external sphincter had a 23% failure rate, while in those with extension beyond the sphincter it was 48%, and patients with lymph node involvement had a 36% failure rate. Recurrent disease was treated with surgery or radiation, or a combination of both. Only two patients survived more than 5 years after treatment of the recurrence. The authors described a highly aggressive small cell carcinoma of the anal canal that they suggest is a separate entity. There were 13 such patients, five of whom had distant metastases at the time of diagnosis, and only one of seven of these patients who could be treated surgically survived 5 years.

Papillon and Montbarbon recently updated their series, among which were 272 patients with anal canal cancer who had a chance for cure, of whom 159 were followed for at least 5 years after treatment.[40] The survival rate was 65.4%. Treatment failure occurred in 47 patients. In their investigation of the role of tumor size in prognosis, the authors found that among patients with tumors less than 4 cm, the long-term survival rate was 76.2%, but among those with larger lesions, it was 58.3%. In addition, there were 19 patients with synchronous inguinal node metastases. In a 3-year follow-up, eight had died of their disease. The authors concluded that tumor size and involvement of inguinal lymph nodes correlated best with survival.

Symptoms and Diagnosis

Unfortunately, early symptoms of anal canal cancer are minimal and usually consist of slight bleeding and discomfort following defecation. Patients assume they have hemorrhoids or a fissure. This leads to self-medication and delay in seeking medical care. As the size of the growth increases, the complaints, especially pain, become severe enough to cause the patient to seek medical care. Loss of weight is not common, but when present it suggests advanced disease. Sometimes patients voluntarily reduce food intake because defecation is so painful. In rare situations, patients will notice a lump in the groin as the first indication of anal canal cancer.

The diagnosis is made on examination and biopsy. The long duration of continuous symptoms plus the induration characteristic of cancer suggest the possibility of malignancy and the need for biopsy. The lesion may extend proximally into the rectum or distally to and even outside the anal verge. The cancer is generally ulcerative and the size varies. Some cancers are elongated, elliptical, fissure-like lesions, whereas others encircle the anal canal to varying degrees. Advanced cancers may completely encircle it and may extend upward or distally to involve tissues beyond the anal canal. An important point, however, is that most if not all anal canal cancers, whatever their size, involve the area of the dentate line.

In general, adequate appraisal of the location, measurement of the size, and some estimate of the depth of invasion is best done under anesthesia, usually caudal or spinal. Biopsy is done at the same time. Generally, only a portion of the lesion should be removed for biopsy. Complete removal is unwise because it will not be possible to estimate the effect of the treatment; hence, the decision for further therapy may be more difficult.

Therapy

Anal canal cancers are of the squamous cell variety and the majority are aggressive neoplasms that tend to recur or have regional extensions that are difficult to remove surgically (Fig. 28–3). Consequently, surgery alone is often insufficient therapy. Therefore, radiation has been combined with the operation, since the area of maximum effect of the two modalities is complementary. Furthermore, in recent years it has become generally recognized that some drugs potentiate the effect of radiation. It seems reasonable, therefore, to combine all three methods of treatment for patients with squamous cell cancer of the anal canal. Such an approach was initiated by Nigro and associates, and a preliminary report was published in 1974.[35] Radiation and chemotherapy were given preoperatively in an attempt to contract the area of disease for more effective removal by operation. It soon became apparent that the preoperative therapy itself was effective in eradicating the local lesion in many patients. Others have confirmed this observation. A brief discussion of each of these modes of therapy will help clarify the rationale for their combined use in the treatment of this disease.

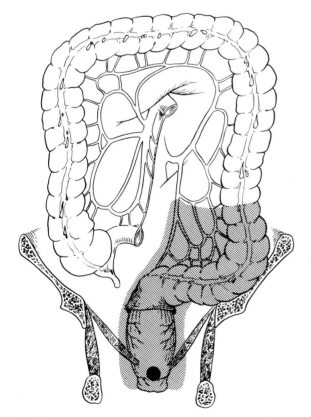

FIGURE 28–3. Abdominoperineal resection is not as good a cancer operation for lesions in the anal canal as it is for those in the rectum because anatomic constraints prevent adequate local excision of the primary tumor and its lymphatic extensions.

Surgery

For at least three quarters of a century, surgery has been the treatment of choice for cancer of the anal canal. Local excision was performed for anal canal cancers less than 2 cm, whereas abdominoperineal resection of the rectum with an extensive perineal phase was the operation commonly used for all cancers larger than 2 cm, regardless of cell type. Groin dissection was indicated only when the tumor had spread to the lymph nodes.

Boman and associates recently reported their results after operation alone in 114 patients followed for at least 5 years.[2] Forty per cent of these patients experienced recurrent disease; nevertheless, 71% of the entire group survived 5 years or more. Frost and co-workers reported 76% long-term survival for early lesions and 29% for patients with deeply invasive primary cancers.[13] Greenall and associates reported a 55% 5-year survival rate for patients treated by abdominoperineal resection for anal canal cancer.[16] Others have reported long-term survival rates ranging from a low of 20% to a high of more than 70%. In a large series of patients treated by surgery with a median observation time of 10 years, Jensen and associates found a 67% recurrence rate.[23] This wide variation in results is primarily due to differences in patient characteristics among the studies and to many short-term follow-ups. It is clear, however, that radical operation is effective in patients with early lesions but not in those with more advanced disease. To deal with the latter problem, some surgeons have combined operation and radiotherapy.

Radiation Therapy

Radiation was used as a definitive therapy for anal canal cancer in the early part of the twentieth century. Gordon-Watson and Dukes reported their experience using interstitial radium implants.[15] These results were quite good, especially in patients with localized cancers. They made the obvious point that the treatment avoided the permanent colostomy that is a part of abdominoperineal resection. Later, Gabriel reported the results in a series of 57 patients with anal cancer treated at St. Mark's Hospital from 1922 to 1935.[14] Some were managed with radium implants, whereas others had radical surgery. Both methods appeared to be effective for early lesions, but Gabriel felt that radium therapy was not as reliable in the treatment of more advanced disease. The radium had little or no effect on involved regional lymph nodes, and the complications of the therapy itself were also a negative factor. Consequently, he advocated surgical treatment for all patients with this disease. This had considerable influence in initiating the trend toward surgery alone for this disease in Britain and America. Nevertheless, some investigators continued to use radiation therapy.

Dalby and Pointon published a report on the use of radium implants in 59 patients with anal canal cancer.[7] Thirty-nine per cent survived 5 years without recurrence, but ten patients experienced severe anal strictures, six of whom required colostomy. In 1974, Papillon reported his results in 98 patients treated from 1949 to

1968.[39] Most patients were treated with interstitial radium, although a few treated toward the end of that period also had external beam radiation. Of 64 patients followed for 5 years, 44 were alive and free of cancer. Of those 44 patients, 40 had only radiation, whereas four had radical surgery following the radiation treatment.

Modern megavoltage external beam equipment came into general use about 1960. It constituted a significant advance, improving effectiveness and at the same time reducing the incidence of serious complications. Cantril and associates reported its use in a series of 47 patients with anal canal cancer treated from 1966 to 1981.[5] Thirty-nine patients were treated with curative intent. Eight of these patients had involved lymph nodes that were either inguinal or pelvic. In 35 patients, the radiation was the only planned therapy, but four patients required surgery for serious complications of the radiotherapy. The 5-year survival rate for the 47 patients was 79.3%. The authors concluded that external beam radiation using modern equipment can control anal cancer with an acceptable degree of morbidity.

Papillon and Montbarbon more recently used external beam and interstitial radiation, a combination that permits the administration of a high dose of radiation to the primary tumor and to the regional lymph nodes as well.[40] It is a split-course protocol with the external beam radiation given first followed in 2 months by ^{192}Ir implant in the residual tumor. Of 97 patients, 74 were followed for more than 3 years and were free of cancer. The therapy was not successful in 18 patients who then had radical surgery. Five other patients required colostomy because of radiation disease.

The effectiveness of radiation therapy in the management of anal cancer as reported in the literature is not uniform. This results from several factors among which are the variation in radiation dosage and technique of administration, the limited number of patients available for study by any single group of investigators, and the variation in patient characteristics, some including anal margin cancer. However, it is clear that radiation therapy is far more effective in the management of squamous cell cancer of the anal canal than it is in adenocarcinoma of the rectum. Nonetheless, it has not been widely accepted as definitive therapy because the incidence of serious complications is unacceptable.

Combined Therapy

The initial attempt of combining 5-fluorouracil (5-FU) with mitomycin C and radiation given preoperatively in the management of anal canal cancer by Nigro and associates at Wayne State University was intended to increase the effectiveness of the operation.[35] Therefore, a rather modest dose of radiation (3,000 Gy over 3 weeks) was selected. The duration of 5-FU infusion, originally 5 days, was reduced to 4 days to avoid toxicity. Because of the observation by Vietti and co-workers that in vitro 5-FU given with radiation acts as a radiation protector, and because it has a marked radioenhancing effect when given immediately after radiation, the infusion was started concurrently with radiotherapy.[58] The infusion was repeated 4 weeks later, usually 1 week after radiation was completed. Mitomycin C was selected from the many cytotoxic bone marrow–suppressing drugs because experience had shown that it had activity against other squamous carcinomas. In addition, it was observed in in vitro studies that mitomycin C is particularly effective in anoxic tissues. Recently, the advantages of using mitomycin C with radiotherapy in the treatment of tumors containing anoxic cells was reviewed by Sartorelli.[48]

The therapy for squamous cell cancer of the anal canal used by our group at Wayne State University beginning in January 1972 is given in Table 28–2. Chemotherapy and radiation therapy are begun jointly on day 1 of the treatment. 5-FU is given via a central venous catheter in a dosage of 1,000 mg/m^2/24 hours for 4 days as a continuous infusion. This 96-hour infusion is repeated in 1 month even in the presence of mild bone marrow depression, since 5-FU infusions have been shown to be nonmyelosuppressive. Mitomycin C is given on day 1 as a single-bolus intravenous injection at a dose of 15 mg/m^2. Radiation therapy is given as 3,000 Gy, calculated at the midplane of the pelvis, at 1,000 Gy/wk starting on day 1. The radiation portal includes the primary lesion with margin, the true pelvis, and the inguinal lymphatics. The lower edge of the radiation field should include the ischial tuberosities and the perineum. An abdominoperineal resection of the rectum was performed 4 to 6 weeks later.

A review of the results in a series of 44 patients treated by us from January 1972 to July 1983 will serve to illustrate our experience with combined therapy. Forty-four patients, all with biopsy-proven squamous cell cancer of the anal canal, were included, with the exception of patients with in situ cancer and those with metastases to distant organs. Twenty-one patients had small lesions (2 to 3 cm), 14 patients had moderate-sized growths (4 to 5 cm), and nine patients had large cancers (5 to 8 cm). Two patients had inguinal node involvement. All patients, except one who had extensive bilateral inguinal node disease, were judged to be candidates for radical surgery. The protocol was changed in the latter part of 1975 when we found that five of our first six patients had no cancer in the operative specimen after abdominoperineal resection. Subsequently, the operation was

TABLE 28–2. TREATMENT OF SQUAMOUS CELL CANCER OF THE ANAL CANAL

I. Preoperative
  A. External radiation
    1. 3,000 Gy to the primary tumor and pelvic and inguinal nodes
    Start: Day 1—200 cGy/day
  B. Systemic chemotherapy
    1. 5-FU: 1,000 mg/m^2/24 hours as a continuous infusion for 4 days
    Start: Day 1
    2. Mitomycin C: 15 mg/m^2 intravenous bolus
    Day 1 only
    3. 5-FU: Repeat 4-day infusion
    Start: Day 28
II. Abdominoperineal resection*
  A. 4 to 6 weeks after radiation therapy

*Routine use stopped after 1975 (see text).

not done unless cancer remained following chemoradiation therapy. There were exceptions because some colleagues did not make the change until later. In patients whose lesion disappeared grossly, the scar was excised for biopsy purposes 4 to 6 weeks after radiation treatment. A few patients refused to have this done. Abdominoperineal resection was performed routinely according to the original protocol for some patients, for residual cancer remaining after chemoradiation therapy, and for recurrent disease.

After chemoradiation therapy, there was no gross tumor remaining in 40 patients, whereas visible cancer was present in four patients. Thirteen patients had radical operations done routinely after the preoperative therapy, whereas four other radical operations were done because gross cancer remained. The operative specimens were free of tumor in 12 patients; the specimens contained microscopic cancer in one patient, and there was gross cancer in four patients. Twenty-two patients had excision of the scar following chemoradiation therapy. There was no tumor in any of the 22 specimens. Five patients, whose cancer disappeared grossly, refused to have the scar excised for biopsy purposes. One of these patients died of disease, whereas the other four are alive without evidence of disease after 5 to 9 years. We no longer biopsy scars that appear normal clinically. Our experience suggests that it is unnecessary. Furthermore, it often causes some degree of incontinence. There were three recurrences in the patients treated conservatively after chemoradiation therapy. The recurrences became apparent 5 to 18 months after negative biopsy results following chemoradiation treatment. Abdominoperineal resection of the rectum was performed on one of these three patients, making a total of 18 patients who had radical surgery in this series of 44 patients.

Inguinal node metastases were present in only two patients. Both instances were found at the time of diagnosis of the primary lesion; one patient had extensive bilateral involvement, whereas the other had only one involved node on one side. The patient with bilateral disease had a small primary lesion that disappeared but recurred a year later: it was then excised locally. He was treated with more radiation to the inguinal areas but died 2 years later. The other patient with unilateral involvement had chemoradiation therapy followed by abdominoperineal resection of the rectum plus groin dissection on the one side. All tissue removed from these two operative procedures was free of cancer, and the patient had no evidence of disease 6 years after therapy.

The chemoradiation treatment is not without danger. Nearly all patients experience mild symptoms such as stomatitis, diarrhea, temporary loss of hair, irritation of the perineal skin, and depression of the white blood cell count. All symptoms are temporary. More severe problems may develop if the therapy is not given carefully with attention to detail. The infusion must be given evenly throughout the 24-hour period, and it should be interrupted if signs of toxicity develop. In our patients, the infusion was stopped on the fourth day in seven patients. All patients received the full radiation dose.

There were 12 deaths, seven of which were due to squamous cell cancer, whereas five others were due to other causes. Of the seven patients who died of their disease, six had abdominoperineal resection following completion of chemoradiation therapy, whereas the other patient, who had bilateral inguinal node involvement, had only additional radiation therapy to the inguinal areas. One patient who had delayed radical operation after negative results of biopsy following chemoradiation therapy was found to have a pelvic recurrence 5 years after the operation. She received periodic chemotherapy for 2 years then died of cardiac decompensation. Autopsy showed that she had minimal pelvic cancer. Although she survived 9 years, she is considered a treatment failure. However, it does not alter the 5-year survival rate. The actual 5-year survival rate for the 44 patients is 73%, and the corrected rate is 84%.

During the past decade or so, several investigators have published the results of their experience using some combination of chemoradiation therapy and operation for patients with squamous cell cancer of the anal canal. Meeker and associates reviewed a series of 19 patients treated with the protocol given in Table 28–2.[31] Nine patients had abdominoperineal resection, but seven patients had no cancer in the operative specimen. The scar in seven other patients was biopsied, and all tissue was free of cancer. Three others refused biopsy: one died of cancer, the other two are long-term survivors. There were two other deaths in patients who had abdominoperineal resection, but all tissue removed was free of cancer. Three patients with unilateral inguinal lymph node involvement had groin dissection after preoperative therapy. All tissue was free of cancer. Disease-free survival at 40 months was 87.5%.

Sischy reviewed the results in 33 patients treated with a similar protocol except for some minor variation in the amount of radiation and drugs given.[51] The first four patients had routine abdominoperineal resection, but since all tissue was free of cancer, routine operation was discontinued. Of the other 29 patients, 26 had local control. Three patients died of cancer and one is alive with cancer. The crude survival rate was 81%, with a follow-up of 1 to 8 years.

Cummings and associates had treated patients with radiation alone and with at least two variations of combined chemoradiation therapy.[6] The first combined therapy protocol consisted of 5-FU and mitomycin C plus 5,000 Gy. However, toxicity was excessive so the protocol was changed to a split-course regimen. The group that received radiation only consisted of 25 patients, whereas there were 30 in the chemoradiation treatment groups. Control of the primary lesion was achieved in 60% of the radiation-only group, whereas it was more than 90% in both the combined continuous and split-treatment groups. Surgical therapy (abdominoperineal resection) salvaged seven patients after failure of radiation therapy alone; there were three other failures, but the disease in these patients was inoperable. With the help of surgery, radiation therapy achieved an 88% long-term survival rate, practically the same as in the combined therapy groups.

Papillon and associates have treated patients with anal canal cancer for many years with radiation therapy.[39] It consisted of external beam radiation followed after a 2-month rest with ^{192}Ir implants. The 5-year survival rate was 65.4%. Patients with advanced local disease had surgical therapy (abdominoperineal resection) following the radiation treatment. Later, Papillon and Montbarbon added chemotherapy, but at a lower dose than in the Wayne State protocol, for patients with advanced local disease.[40] The results improved significantly so that since 1985 chemotherapy has been given with the radiation to all patients with carcinoma of the anal canal regardless of the stage of disease or the size of the lesion. In comparing patients treated by radiation alone to those combined with chemotherapy, the local failure rate was reduced from 26% to 13%.

Enker and co-workers updated the Memorial Hospital series of patients treated with combined therapy including surgery.[8] The protocol was similar to the Wayne State therapy except that the radiation was given several days after completion of the chemotherapy. There were 44 patients, 24 of whom had abdominoperineal resection, whereas 20 had the scar excised after the chemoradiation treatment. There was no cancer in the operative specimen in 26 patients. Ten patients experienced recurrences, either local or pelvic. Thirty-two patients were alive without evidence of disease, four were alive with disease, and eight died of cancer. The median follow-up was 39 months with a range of 1 to 89 months.

Flam and associates reviewed their experience with 30 patients treated from 1979 to 1986 with chemoradiation only.[11] The protocol consisted of two cycles of 5-FU and mitomycin C plus pelvic radiation therapy. The amount of radiation ranged from 4,000 to 4,500 Gy, and an additional amount (900 Gy) was given to the perineum if the primary lesions were large, or to the inguinal area if the lymph nodes were involved. When this treatment failed, more chemoradiation therapy was given, rather than resorting to operation. Twenty-six of the 30 patients were free of cancer after the initial round of therapy. The other four patients had residual local disease but were rendered free of cancer by additional chemoradiation therapy. Toxicity was a problem in four patients, who required hospitalization, but all recovered. Twenty-seven patients are alive and free of disease after 9 to 76 months, whereas three died of other causes.

In summary, there is little doubt that the most effective combination of radiation and chemotherapy for the treatment of squamous cell cancer of the anal canal has not been devised as yet. Certainly there is potential for improvement, which is sure to come. The therapy initiated by Nigro and associates has had the longest trial.[35] It has been shown by Leichman and colleagues[27] and by Nigro[34] to be quite effective in a series of patients with long-term follow-up, and there is confirmation by others. However, some investigators have used variations of the original treatment, including different amounts of radiation and different doses of drugs. Moreover, the number of patients in each of the studies and the short length of follow-up do not as yet establish any of the variations published so far as being superior to the original. Nevertheless, it is clear that a combination of pelvic radiation and two cycles of 5-FU infusion plus one dose of mitomycin C is at least as effective in the treatment of anal canal cancer as is radical surgery.

Current Therapy

There is sufficient evidence now to justify the choice of a combination of radiotherapy and chemotherapy as the initial treatment for all macroscopic squamous cell cancers of the anal canal. This, of course, includes those less than 2 cm in size. Furthermore, it is clear that the chemotherapy must be given concomitantly with the radiation for maximum effect. The protocol devised at Wayne State University in 1972 has had the longest trial thus far; although various combinations of these modalities have been reported, the optimal regimen has not been established as yet. Consequently, we advocate the use of the same protocol (see Table 28–2) for the initial treatment. It is relatively simple to give, has minimal side effects, and the results are at least comparable to radical surgery. The condition of the patient is evaluated 6 to 8 weeks after completion of the radiation therapy. If the primary lesion has disappeared clinically and if the original lesion was less than 5 cm in greatest diameter, the patient is followed frequently at least for the first year. Conversely, additional chemoradiation therapy is given to patients whose primary tumor was 5 cm or greater, because these patients are at high risk for recurrence. Likewise, patients whose cancers do not disappear or which recur are given more chemoradiation treatment.[34] Currently, for the second course of treatment we prefer to give 2,000 Gy in 2 weeks to the local lesion together with an infusion of 5-FU, 1,000 mg/m^2, for 4 days, and on the first day a single-bolus injection of mitomycin C, 5 mg/m^2 (Table 28–3). Cisplatin (100 mg/m^2) may be substituted for the mitomycin C. It is given as a bolus injection after appropriate hydration on three occasions a month apart, and the 4-day infusion of 5-FU is included on each occasion. The effectiveness of this second course of therapy is as yet unknown, although preliminary evidence by Flam and co-workers is encouraging.[11] Patients in whom recurrent disease develops or those who continue to have residual cancer after two courses of chemoradiation therapy should be treated on an individual basis. The possibilities are surgery, more radiation if possible, and second-line chemotherapy, or any combination of these treatments. Experience under these circumstances is so limited that we cannot be more specific.

TABLE 28–3. CHEMORADIATION THERAPY—COURSE 2

I. External radiation
  A. 2,000 Gy to the primary tumor, pelvic and inguinal nodes
    Start: Day 1—200 cGy/day
II. Systemic chemotherapy
  A. 5-FU: 1,000 mg/m^2/24 hours as a continuous infusion for 4 days
    Start: Day 1
  B. Mitomycin C: 5 mg/m^2 intravenous bolus on day 1
    Start: Day 1 only
  C. 5-FU: repeat 4-day infusion
    Start: Day 28

Treatment of metastatic inguinal lymph nodes has been surgical. In the past, groin dissection was done at the time of abdominoperineal resection or shortly after in patients with initial involvement. When involved nodes were found later, operation was done as soon as possible after their discovery. At present, the role of radiation therapy in the management of this problem is not clearly defined. Although the general feeling in the past was that metastatic lymph node disease does not respond well to radiation therapy, Papillon maintains that radiotherapy is effective in the management of nodal disease in patients with squamous cell cancer, and our experience tends to support this.[40] The trend now is to use a combination of surgery and radiotherapy, and no doubt variations of this combination are being investigated. We treat all patients with squamous cell cancer of the anal canal, including those with inguinal node metastases, with the chemoradiation therapy protocol. As has been stated, the radiation field includes the inguinal areas. In 6 weeks, a superficial groin dissection is done on the affected side if the node has not returned to normal clinically. Some surgeons would perform the operation in any event. It is quite clear, however, that patients with extensive bilateral inguinal lymph node involvement should be treated with additional radiation to the groin areas as soon as convenient after the first course of chemoradiation therapy. In our experience, this is only a palliative measure.

The development of concomitant chemoradiation therapy for epidermoid cancer of the anal canal is an important advance in cancer treatment. It not only enhances survival but also preserves structure and function through organ preservation.

MISCELLANEOUS LESIONS

Rarely, adenocarcinoma of the anal canal develops in the mucosa in the most proximal part of the surgical anal canal. This lesion is treated in the same manner as is adenocarcinoma of the rectum, a subject discussed elsewhere in this volume (see Chapter 19). Another infrequent lesion is carcinoma associated with anorectal fistula. McAnally and Dockerty estimated that cancer is present in approximately 0.1% of all anorectal fistulas.[29] Cancer appears to be associated with fistulas in one of two ways. In the first instance, an adenocarcinoma forms in an anal gland in the area of the dentate line. Eventually, the gland ruptures into the tissues surrounding the anal canal and lower rectum, forming a fistula. The patient is unaware of the condition until the fistula forms, causing symptoms that progress until surgery is required. At the time of operation, cancer may be suspected because the sinus tract contains a great deal of mucus and the lining has a mucosal appearance. Either the diagnosis is confirmed on frozen section or the pathologist finds it during the routine examination of the operative specimen. The second situation is quite the reverse. A patient who has had a fistula for many years with minimal symptoms suddenly finds the symptoms worsening. At operation, a fistulectomy is performed. Generally, the surgeon has no reason to suspect malig-

nant degeneration, but the cancer is found in the tissues removed at operation. It is almost always a squamous cell cancer.[4]

In the first type, the cancer causes fistula formation, whereas in the second type, a fistula of long duration degenerates into malignancy. It appears that the first type, adenocarcinoma-fistula, is the more common variety. By the time the diagnosis is made, the cancer in both situations has invaded the tissues around the anus, rectum, and even into the buttocks. Occasionally, inguinal lymph nodes are involved. The prognosis in the adenocarcinoma-fistula lesion is poor.

Abdominoperineal resection with an extensive perineal phase is indicated. An inguinal groin dissection is included as needed. Following recovery from the operation, radiation therapy should be given, since recurrences are so common; according to Jensen and colleagues,[24] the 5-year survival rate is less than 5%. Another approach in an attempt to improve results would be to give chemoradiation therapy preoperatively followed in 2 to 4 weeks with abdominoperineal resection of the rectum. Continued therapy postoperatively should also be considered on an individual basis. The situation is not so lethal with squamous cell carcinoma–fistula lesions. After the diagnosis is made, radiation and chemotherapy, as outlined for squamous cell cancer of the anal canal, should be given. Abdominoperineal resection may or may not be necessary depending upon circumstances.

MELANOMA OF THE ANAL REGION

Melanoma is the most lethal form of cancer that occurs in the anal canal. Fortunately, it is exceedingly rare, with a frequency ranging from 0.25 to 1.25% of all cancers of the anal region, and it is only one eighth as common as squamous cell cancer of the anal canal.[37] A series was reported recently by Wanebo and co-workers.[59] They reviewed the records of 51 patients treated at Memorial Sloan-Kettering Cancer Center during the past 50 years. Only six patients survived 5 years in spite of the fact that two thirds of these patients had radical surgery.

The symptoms of anal melanoma are similar to many benign and malignant lesions of the anal canal. According to Quan and associates, the symptoms consist of a feeling of fullness, bleeding, and discomfort.[44] Rarely, the first sign of disease is the presence of an inguinal mass. Loss of weight and pelvic neurologic complaints are late signs of the disease.[54] Diagnosis naturally is made on biopsy of the mass, which only rarely is ulcerated. If there is pigmentation, the diagnosis is suspected, but more often the primary tumor is not pigmented, in which case the lesion is thought to be a squamous cell cancer. Pack and Oropeza, in discussing biopsy, warn against incising a suspected melanoma.[37] If the lesion is small, it should be excised widely, and if it is ulcerated, a fragment should be removed with a cautery knife. Since these cancers are in the anal canal, biopsy is done under anesthesia.

The lesion is so aggressive that spread occurs early through both venous and lymphatic routes. In fact, the disease is generally a systemic problem by the time the diagnosis is made. Hence, radical surgery is of little long-term value. Quinn reported on 107 patients with long-term follow-up in the literature.[45] Seventy-four patients had radical surgery, and only five patients survived 5 years. There were four long-term survivors in another 29 patients treated by local excision. It follows from this that when local excision can be done adequately, it is probably as useful as abdominoperineal resection. Nevertheless, radical surgery is indicated at times in a faint hope for long-term survival in patients with small lesions or for palliation when the lesion is too large to remove by local means. Radiation and chemotherapy do not appear to have any role in the management of the primary lesion.

Current research, especially animal experimentation, is directed to new approaches for systemic cancer therapy. For example, the combination of interferon and difluoromethylornithine, a chemical that inhibits cell proliferation especially in cancer tissue, demonstrated suppression of a transplantable mouse melanoma.[56] Another, perhaps more encouraging, approach being investigated in animals is the use of liposome-delivered drugs to activate cells of the immune system.[10] Successful management of this disease in humans awaits the development of effective therapy along these lines for systemic cancer. As mentioned earlier, Rosenberg's investigations of methods that enhance the immune system are encouraging.[44]

REFERENCES

1. Anderson, S.L., Nielsen, A., and Reymann, F.: Relationship between Bowen's disease and internal malignant tumors. Arch. Dermatol., 108:367, 1973.
2. Boman, B.M., Moertez, C.G., and O'Connez, M.J.: Carcinoma of the anal canal: A clinical and pathologic study of 188 cases. Cancer, 54:114, 1984.
3. Brennan, J.T., and Stewart, C.F.: Epidermoid carcinoma of the anus. Ann. Surg., 176:787, 1972.
4. Bretlau, P.: Carcinoma arising in anal fistula. Acta Chir. Scand., 133:496, 1967.
5. Cantril, S.T., Green, J.P., Schall, G.L., et al.: Primary radiation therapy in the treatment of anal carcinoma. Int. J. Radiat. Oncol. Biol. Phys., 9:1271, 1983.
6. Cummings, B.J., Keane, T., Thomas, G., et al.: Results and toxicity of the treatment of anal canal carcinoma by radiation therapy or radiation therapy and chemotherapy. Cancer, 54:2062, 1984.
7. Dalby, J.E., and Pointon, R.S.: The treatment of anal carcinoma by interstitial irradiation. Am. J. Roentgenol., 85:515, 1961.
8. Enker, W.E., Heilwell, M., Janov, A.J., et al.: Improved survival in epidermoid carcinoma of the anus in association with preoperative multidisciplinary therapy. Arch. Surg., 121:1386, 1986.
9. Fenger, C.: Histology of the anal canal. Am. J. Surg. Pathol., 12:41, 1988.
10. Fidler, I.J., and Balch, C.M.: The biology of cancer metastasis and implications for therapy. Curr. Probl. Surg., 24:129, 1987.
11. Flam, M.S., Hohn, M.J., Mowry, P.A., et al.: Definitive combined modality therapy of carcinoma of the anus. Dis. Colon Rectum, 30:495, 1987.
12. Friedberg, M.J., and Serlin, O.: Condyloma acuminatum: Its association with malignancy. Dis. Colon Rectum, 6:352, 1963.
13. Frost, D., Richards, P., Montague, E., et al.: Epidermoid cancer of the anorectum. Cancer, 53:1285, 1984.
14. Gabriel, W.B.: Squamous-cell carcinoma of anus and anal canal: Analysis of 55 cases. Proc. R. Soc. Med., 34:139, 1941.
15. Gordon-Watson, D., and Dukes, C.E.: The treatment of carcinoma

16. Greenall, M.J., Ivan, S.H., Urmacher, C., et al: Treatment of epidermoid carcinoma of the anal canal. Surg. Gynecol. Obstet., 161:509, 1985.
17. Grodsky, L.: Rare nonkeratinizing malignancies of anal region. Arch. Surg., 90:216, 1965.
18. Grodsky, L.: Extramammary Paget's disease of the perianal region. Dis. Colon Rectum, 3:502, 1960.
19. Grodsky, L.: Leukoplakia of the anus. Calif. Med., 84:420, 1956.
20. Helwig, E.G., and Graham, J.H.: Anogenital (extramammary) Paget's disease: A clinicopathological study. Cancer, 16:387, 1963.
21. Hintz, B.L., Charyulu, D.D.N., and Sudarsanam, A.: Anal carcinoma: Basic concepts and management. J. Surg. Oncol., 10:141, 1978.
22. International Union Against Cancer (UICC): In Hermanek, P., and Sobin, I.M. (eds.): TNM Classification of Malignant Tumors. New York, Springer-Verlag, 1987.
23. Jensen, S.L., Hagen, K., Harling, H., et al.: Long-term prognosis after radical treatment for squamous-cell carcinoma of the anal canal and anal margin. Dis. Colon Rectum, 31:273, 1988.
24. Jensen, S.L., Shokouh-Amiri, M.H., Hagen, K., et al.: Adenocarcinoma of anal ducts: A series of 21 cases. Dis. Colon Rectum, 31:268, 1988.
25. Kuehn, P.G., Eisenberg, H., and Reed, J.F.: Epidermoid carcinoma of the perianal skin and anal canal. Cancer, 22:932, 1968.
26. Lee, S.H., McGregor, D.H., and Duziez, M.N.: Malignant transformation of perianal condyloma acuminatum. Dis. Colon Rectum, 24:462, 1981.
27. Leichman, L., Nigro, N.D., Vaitkevicius, V.K., et al.: Cancer of the anal canal: Model for preoperative adjuvant combined modality therapy. Am. J. Med., 78:211, 1985.
28. Marfing, T.E., Abel, M.E., and Gallagher, D.M.: Perianal Bowen's disease and associated malignancies. Dis. Colon Rectum, 30:782, 1987.
29. McAnally, A.K., and Dockerty, M.B.: Carcinoma developing in chronic draining cutaneous sinuses and fistulas. Surg. Gynecol. Obstet., 88:87, 1949.
30. McConnell, E.M.: Squamous cell carcinoma of the anus—a review of 96 cases. Br. J. Surg., 57:89, 1970.
31. Meeker, W.R., Sickle-Santanello, B.J., Philpott, G., et al.: Combined chemotherapy, radiation, and surgery for epithelial cancer of the anal canal. Cancer, 57:525, 1986.
32. Morson, B.C.: Histological typing of intestinal tumors. In Morson, B.C., and Sobin, L.H.: International Histologic Classification of Tumors, 15:62, 1976.
33. Morson, B.C.: The pathology and results of treatment of cancer of the anal region. Proc. R. Soc. Med., 52(Suppl.):117, 1959.
34. Nigro, N.D.: Multidisciplinary management of cancer of the anus. World J. Surg., 11:446, 1987.
35. Nigro, N.D., Considine, B., and Vaitkevicius, V.K.: Combined therapy for cancer of the anal canal. Dis. Colon Rectum, 17:354, 1974.
36. Northover, J.M.A.: Epidermoid cancer of the anus—the surgeon retreats. J. R. Soc. Med., 84:389, 1991.
37. Pack, G.T., and Oropeza, R.: A comparative study of melanoma and epidermoid carcinoma of the anal canal: A review of 20 melanomas and 29 epidermoid carcinomas (1930–1965). Dis. Colon Rectum, 10:161, 1967.
38. Papillon, J., and Chassard, J.L.: Respective roles of radiotherapy and surgery in the management of epidermoid cancer of the anal margin. Dis. Colon Rectum, 35:422, 1992.
39. Papillon, J., Mayer, M., Montbarbon, J.F., et al.: A new approach to the management of epidermoid carcinoma. Cancer, 51:1830, 1983.
40. Papillon, J., and Montbarbon, J.F.: Epidermoid carcinoma of the anal canal: A series of 276 cases. Dis. Colon Rectum, 30:324, 1987.
41. Papillon, J.: Radiation therapy in the management of epidermoid cancer of the anal region. Dis. Colon Rectum, 17:181, 1974.
42. Peters, R.K., and Mack. T.M.: Patterns of anal carcinoma by gender and marital status in Los Angeles County. Br. J. Cancer, 48:629, 1983.
43. Prasad, M.L., and Abcarian, H.: Malignant potential of perianal condyloma acuminatum. Dis. Colon Rectum, 23:191, 1980.

44. Quan, S.H.Q., White, J.E., and Deddish, M.R.: Malignant melanoma of the anorectum. Dis. Colon Rectum, *2*:275, 1959.
45. Quinn, D., and Selah, C.: Malignant melanoma of the anus in a Negro: Report of a case and review of literature. Dis. Colon Rectum, *20*:627, 1977.
46. Richards, J.C., Beahrs, O.H., and Woolner, L.B.: Squamous cell carcinoma of the anus, anal canal and rectum in 109 patients. Surg. Gynecol. Obstet., *114*:475, 1962.
47. Rosenberg, S.A., Lotze, M.T., Yang, J.C., et al.: Prospective randomized trial of high-dose interleukin-2 alone or in conjunction with lymphokine-activated killer cells for the treatment of patients with advanced cancer. J. Natl. Cancer Inst., *85*:622, 1993.
48. Sartorelli, A.C.: Therapeutic attack of hypoxic cells of solid tumors: Presidential address. Cancer Res., *48*:775, 1988.
49. Siegal, A.: Malignant transformation of condyloma acuminatum. Am. J. Surg., *103*:613, 1962.
50. Singh, R., Nime, F., and Mittelman, A.: Malignant epithelial tumors of the anal canal. Cancer, *48*:411, 1981.
51. Sischy, B.: The use of radiation therapy combined with chemotherapy in the management of squamous cell carcinoma of the anus and marginally resectable adenocarcinoma of the rectum. Int. J. Radiat. Oncol. Biol. Phys., *11*:1587, 1985.
52. Stearns, M.W., Jr.: Epidermoid carcinoma of the anal region. Am. J. Surg., *90*:727, 1955.
53. Stearns, M.W., Jr., and Quan, S.H.Q.: Epidermoid carcinoma of the anorectum. Surg. Gynecol. Obstet., *131*:953, 1970.
54. Stearns, M.W., Jr., Urmacher, C., Sternberg, S.S., et al.: Cancer of the anal canal. Curr. Probl. Cancer, *4*:1, 1980.
55. Stedman, T.L.: Stedman's Medical Dictionary. Baltimore and London, Williams & Wilkins, 1982.
56. Sunkara, P.S., Prakash, N.J., Rosenberger, A.L., et al.: Potentiation of antitumor and antimetastatic activities of difluoromethylornithine by interferon inducers. Cancer Res., *44*:2799, 1984.
57. Thorek, P.: Anatomy in Surgery. Philadelphia, J.B. Lippincott, 1951.
58. Vietti, T., Eggerding, F., and Valeriate, F.: Combined effect of X radiation and 5-fluorouracil on survival of transplanted leukemia cell. J. Natl. Cancer Inst., *47*:865, 1971.
59. Wanebo, H.J., Woodruff, J.M., Farr, G.H., et al.: Anorectal melanoma. Cancer, *47*:1891, 1981.
60. Williams, S.L., Rogers, L.W., and Quan, S.H.Q.: Perianal Paget's disease: Report of seven cases. Dis. Colon Rectum, *19*:30, 1976.
61. Wolfe, H.R.I., and Bussey, H.J.R.: Squamous cell carcinoma of the anus. Br. J. Surg., *55*:295, 1968.

Chapter 29

PROLAPSE AND PROCIDENTIA

HERAND ABCARIAN

Rectal prolapse is a relatively common condition. Its treatment relies on the accuracy of diagnosis and a rational therapeutic plan. The following definitions should help clarify the various protrusions encountered in the rectal area.

Prolapse of rectal mucosa (partial rectal prolapse) is the abnormal descent of the rectal mucosa with or without protrusion through the anus (Fig. 29–1B).

Rectal prolapse or procidentia is the abnormal descent of all layers of the rectal wall with or without protrusion through the anus (Fig. 29–1D). The term *hidden or internal prolapse* is used to describe rectal prolapse in a nonprotruding state, whereas *procidentia* is usually used to describe a protruding rectal prolapse.

Intussusception of the rectum occurring at the rectosigmoid junction or below is perhaps an early phase of complete rectal prolapse. In contrast to other intussusceptions, it carries no pathologic lesions at its leading point (Fig. 29–1C).

Perineal hernia originates in the cul-de-sac of Douglas and protrudes as an intussusception through the anal canal.

PROLAPSE OF THE RECTAL MUCOSA (PARTIAL RECTAL PROLAPSE)

When prolapse is only partial, the rectal mucosa descends to an abnormal location; depending on whether it protrudes from the anus, it can be considered internal or external. *Internal mucosal prolapse* consists of redundant rectal mucosa felt during rectal examination. It may involve only a portion or all of the bowel circumference. *External mucosal prolapse* consists of protruding redundant mucosal folds from the anus.

Etiology

Prolapse of the rectal mucosa is more common in children than is procidentia. It is seen most frequently between the ages of 1 and 5 years. It is also common in

old, debilitated individuals and is seen more often in women than in men.

The exact cause of mucosal prolapse is unknown. An alteration in the attachment of the mucosa to the submucosal layer of the lower rectum is believed to be the fundamental factor. Prolapse of the rectal mucosa is often associated with conditions involving an increase in intra-abdominal pressure from straining during defecation, such as occurs in diarrhea, constipation, benign prostatic hypertrophy, or chronic obstructive lung disease. It may also follow large internal hemorrhoids or low rectal polyps. Occasionally, mucosal prolapse occurs after anal fistulotomy or following obstetric perineal tears in which the sphincter mechanism has been divided or lacerated.

In children, lack of the sacral curve and loose fixation of the rectum to the pelvic walls have been suggested as possible causes. Malnutrition and wasting diseases may play an important contributory role.

Symptoms and Diagnosis

Internal mucosal prolapse seldom causes symptoms, is diagnosed incidentally during proctosigmoidoscopy, and requires no treatment. However, in a few patients, symptoms of bleeding, mucous drainage, or progression to external prolapse may require treatment. At proctoscopy, the mucosa appears normal, but long-standing prolapsing rectal mucosa may appear congested or even ulcerated.

External mucosal prolapse causes protrusion from the anus, which in the early stages is small, occurs only after defecation, and reduces spontaneously. Later, the protrusion occurs more frequently, becomes larger, and has to be reduced manually. Finally, mucosa protrudes with the slightest effort (even with standing), remains irreducible, causes seepage of mucus, and stains the underclothes. Erosion and ulceration of the protruding mucosa leads to frequent bleeding. Continuous relaxation of the anal sphincters leads to varying degrees of incontinence.

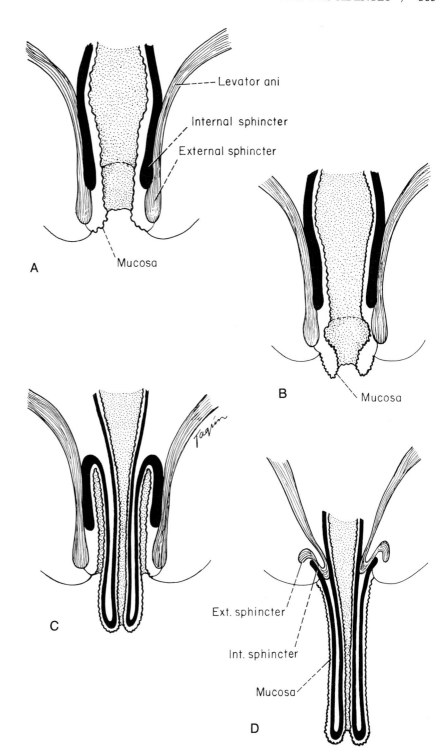

FIGURE 29-1. Variations of rectal prolapse. *A,* Normal anatomy. *B,* Mucosal prolapse. *C,* Intussusception of the rectum through the anus. *D,* Eversion of the rectal wall. (From Ottinger, L.W.: Fundamentals of Colon Surgery. Boston, Little, Brown, 1974, with permission.)

Severe pain is rare and occurs only if the prolapsed mucosa becomes strangulated or severely edematous.

The protruding mass has radiating furrows, which are often associated with and arranged along the typical location of internal hemorrhoids—in the right posterior, right anterior, and left lateral positions (Fig. 29–2*A*). This pattern helps distinguish it from a true procidentia, in which the protruding mass has circular furrows (Fig. 29–2*B*). Even in older individuals, rectal examination demonstrates a good sphincter tone, and the size rarely

exceeds 3 cm. The criteria differentiating the two types of rectal prolapse are listed in Table 29–1.

Palpation of the prolapse, with the index finger in the anal canal and the thumb gently squeezing the mass, reveals only the thickness of the doubled mucosal layer. The protrusion should be reduced gently, and anoscopic and proctosigmoidoscopic examination should be carried out to exclude the presence of tumor, polyps, intussusception, or procidentia before the appropriate treatment is determined.

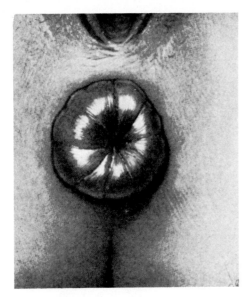 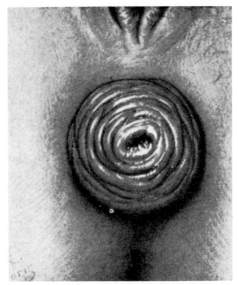

A

B

FIGURE 29-2. *A,* Prolapse showing radiating furrows. *B,* Procidentia showing striations circularly arranged. (From Bacon, H.E.: The Anus, Rectum and Sigmoid Colon, Vol. 1, 3rd ed. Philadelphia, J.B. Lippincott, 1949, with permission.)

Treatment

Medical Treatment

Treating prolapse of the rectal mucosa includes the removal of any obvious contributing factor such as polyps, diarrhea, constipation, malnutrition, and obstructive uropathy. Following this, the treatment of mucosal rectal prolapse depends on the age of the patient and the severity of the condition.

Nonsurgical Treatment

Nonsurgical treatment is frequently successful in younger children and should always be tried first. It is less effective in older children, however, and is often ineffective in adults. Therefore, definitive surgical treatment should not be delayed if nonoperative methods are unsuccessful. In infants, the prolapse should be reduced after each defecation and held in place by a gauze or cotton roll placed on the anus. The buttocks are then strapped together with adhesive or Montgomery tapes. As the child grows older, the size and frequency of the prolapse will decrease until it subsides spontaneously.

Injection Sclerotherapy

A solution of 5% phenol in oil or 5% quinine and urea hydrochloride can be used for sclerotherapy. The

child is sedated and the prolapse is reduced. Using an anoscope, 0.25 to 0.5 ml of the solution is injected submucosally in each quadrant of the prolapse proximal to the level of the dentate line. Adults require no sedation or anesthesia. If the injection is too superficial, the mucosa will blanch and might subsequently slough. As a rule, the prolapse responds to one treatment, but occasionally two or more series of injections may be necessary.

Rubber Band Ligation

An effective method in the treatment of prolapsing mucosa not responsive to medical management or injection sclerotherapy is rubber band ligation. Using a McGivney or Barron hemorrhoidal ligator, a rubber band is placed at the apex of the prolapsing mucosa. Additional quadrants may be ligated in 1- to 2-week intervals until the prolapse is eliminated. For details of the technique and complications of the procedure, see Chapter 26.

Surgical Treatment

Mucosal prolapse in adults is almost always associated with prolapsing hemorrhoids. If anal sphincter function is adequate, hemorrhoidectomy yields excellent results. At the time of hemorrhoidectomy, the redundant rectal mucosa is excised, and the area is fixed to the internal sphincter with a running absorbable suture. With attention to technical detail, excellent functional results can be achieved, with no stricture, mucosal ectropion, or incontinence (see Chapter 26).

The results of hemorrhoidectomy in the presence of anorectal incontinence are unsatisfactory. In patients with significant sphincter injury or in women with a traumatic cloaca, anal sphincteroplasty combined with excision of prolapsing rectal mucosa often yields excellent results.

In elderly patients with generalized weakness of the

TABLE 29-1. DIFFERENTIAL DIAGNOSIS OF RECTAL MUCOSA PROLAPSE AND PROCIDENTIA

	RECTAL MUCOSAL PROLAPSE	RECTAL PROCIDENTIA
Size	<5 cm	>5–10 cm
Bowel lumen	Central	Posterior
Folds	Radial	Circular
Hemorrhoids	Readily visible	Not seen
Thickness	Only mucosa	All layers
Sphincter tone	Maintained	Diminished

sphincter mechanism, incontinence, and mucosal prolapse, the Thiersch operation may be applicable (see further on).

RECTAL PROCIDENTIA (COMPLETE RECTAL PROLAPSE)

Rectal procidentia is rather uncommon but has been recognized for centuries. A description of rectal procidentia is present in both the Ebers and Chester Beatty papyri from ancient Egypt. Ancient Greek literature also describes rectal prolapse and, like the Egyptian writings, recommends therapy with suppositories containing honey.

Substantial series of patients from all western countries, as well as from developing nations, recount the disabling and therapeutically challenging nature of procidentia.[1] Because of the extensive historic and geographic epidemiology of procidentia, as well as the phylogenic dispersion of the disease (seen in horses, pigs, and dogs as well as in humans), procidentia is not considered one of the colorectal diseases associated with a modern western lifestyle.

Rectal procidentia is rare in men older than 45 years of age and in women less than 20 years of age.[29] Most patients requiring an operation are elderly women. Forty to 50% of these women are nulliparous, a number far in excess of that found randomly in women of the same age. Therefore, birth trauma can be ruled out as a cause of rectal prolapse. A high percentage of younger patients have neurologic or mental disorders. Goligher[9] noted in his practice that 3% of the patients were frankly psychotic and 30% were "rather odd."

Other conditions causally associated with procidentia include pelvic neuropathies such as tabes dorsalis and multiple sclerosis and pelvic trauma. Patients with dysenteric infections also have been noted to have procidentia.[4] Procidentia is more frequent among children prior to the development of the normal toddler's lordosis and acquisition of a normal anorectal angle. Spontaneous resolution of the prolapse is the rule when these children begin normal ambulation. In the elderly population, excessive straining at stool appears to be the most common denominator. This type of behavior is frequently seen in residents of mental institutions with severe psychoneurosis and in acutely ill patients with dysenteric infections and wasting.

Etiology

The anatomic features of rectal procidentia include abnormally low descent of the peritoneum covering the anterior rectal wall, loss of posterior fixation of the rectum to the sacral curve, and lengthening and downward displacement of the sigmoid and rectum. Other changes, possibly resulting from the descent of a full-thickness rectal prolapse, include diastasis of the levator ani and an incompetent anal sphincter mechanism.

There are two theories concerning the cause of rectal procidentia—that it is a sliding perineal hernia and that it is an intussusception.

Sliding Perineal Hernia

Moschowitz proposed that rectal procidentia is in reality a sliding perineal hernia, which develops at a weak point in the transversalis fascia and is secondary to increased intra-abdominal pressure.[16] He concluded that procidentia originates as a hernia in the pouch of Douglas and that because of adherence of peritoneal reflections to the rectum and relative fixation of the anus, the hernia protrudes as an intussusception through the anal canal. This theory is supported by the clinical observation of a posteriorly placed lumen seen in procidentia and the occasional presence of small bowel anteriorly in the hernia sac included in the prolapse (Fig. 29–3). Moschowitz, therefore, proposed that apposition of transversalis fascia anteriorly through the pouch of Douglas should correct the problem. This procedure has been abandoned because of recurrence rates as high as 50%, and attempts have been made to develop other causative theories.

Intussusception

Devadhar[6] suggested a new concept; that is, intussusception as a mechanism for development of rectal procidentia. Broden and Snellman,[5] using cineradiography, demonstrated that the initial step in the genesis of procidentia was circumferential intussusception of the rectum and pointed out that the leading edge of the in-

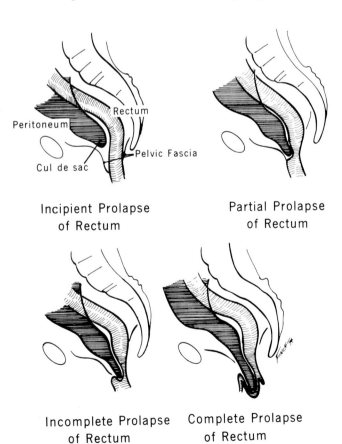

FIGURE 29-3. Rectal procidentia as conceived by Moschowitz. (After Goldberg, S.M., and Gordon, P.H.: Clin. Gastroenterol., *4*:490, 1975, with permission.)

tussusception was 6 to 8 cm from the anal verge. This theory was confirmed by Theuerkauf and colleagues,[27] who demonstrated intussusception of the rectosigmoid by cineradiographic defecography as patients strained at stool. In this study, however, the leading edge of the intussusception was thought to be higher, at the pelvic brim, 15 to 18 cm from the anal verge (Fig. 29–4).

Ripstein and Lanter[20] believed that the intussusception arose secondary to failure of either development or fixation of the mesorectum, together with straightening of the anorectal angle (Fig. 29–5). The basis could be congenital, since the rectum in utero is located intra-

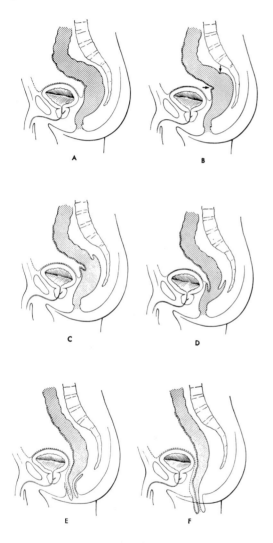

FIGURE 29-4. *A,* Normal relationship of rectum to pelvic structures. *B,* Earliest stage of intussusception (prolapse) just proximal to upper-most normal fixed point of rectum. *C,* Fixed point lowers. Upper rectum separated from sacrum. Intussusception commencement assumes lower position. Sigmoid mesentery elongates. Pseudomesorectum may develop. Rectosigmoid begins to straighten. *D,* Further lowering of fixed point. Previous changes become exaggerated. Cul-de-sac deepens. Rectum may or may not protrude. *E,* Area of hesitation (variable time lengths). Rectum may or may not protrude. *F,* Final stage of intussusception (prolapse). Commencement occurs at muco-cutaneous border. Deep cul-de-sac (may contain small bowel). Elongated sigmoid mesentery. Straight rectosigmoid. Rectum and sacrum separated. Rectum protruded completely. (From Theuerkauf, F.J., Beahrs, O.H., and Hill, J.R.: Rectal prolapse: Causation and surgical treatment. Ann. Surg., *171*:819, 1970, with permission.)

peritoneally throughout its entire length and is attached to the sacrum and coccyx by a long mesorectum. Conversely, if the abnormality is acquired when the rectum has no mesentery but is separated from the sacrum by loose areolar tissue, the cause might be trauma, obstetric injury, or surgical mobilization of the rectum.

Altemeier and colleagues[2] proposed a classification of rectal prolapse that takes into consideration both the aforementioned theories: type I prolapse of redundant rectal mucosa (false prolapse usually associated with hemorrhoids), type II intussusception without a sliding hernia, and type III sliding hernia of the cul-de-sac, which they believe occurs in the majority of cases.

Finally, it is important to point out that physiologic studies of the pelvic floor by Porter[18] have demonstrated that a nonrelaxing puborectalis muscle may have a role in the development of rectal prolapse. The fact that the intussusception begins well above the pelvic floor points out that the nonrelaxing puborectalis muscle may contribute to the development of procidentia only by causing severe constipation and excessive straining at stool.

Symptoms and Diagnosis

The most significant complaint is prolapse of the rectum. After some time, the prolapse occurs with the least effort, even with assuming the erect position, and must be reduced manually, but often with no difficulty. There is usually a feeling of bearing down or tenesmus and of incomplete evacuation. The majority of patients have severe difficulty managing their bowels and complain of constipation, incontinence, or both. Passage of mucus and bleeding may be seen in occult or overt rectal prolapse. Occasionally, uterine prolapse accompanies rectal procidentia.

Physical examination may reveal the prolapsed rectum with thick concentric folds and a posteriorly placed lumen (see Fig. 29–2*B*). Palpation of the prolapse reveals that the entire thickness of the rectal wall is involved. At times, the presence of small bowel in the anterior hernia sac can be diagnosed by observing the peristaltic movements or by eliciting a tympanitic note or auscultating peristaltic sounds over the anterior wall of the procidentia. If the protruding mass is reduced, the sphincter mechanism appears patulous, and the sphincter is decidedly weaker than usual when the patient is asked to contract the anus (see Table 29–1).

If the history suggests a rectal prolapse but the procidentia cannot be seen during a routine physical examination, the patient should be asked to squat and strain, and visual or digital examination of the patient's rectum can confirm the diagnosis. Proctosigmoidoscopy reveals congestion and edema of the distal 8 to 10 cm of the rectal mucosa. At times, ulceration and bleeding can be seen easily, but on other occasions a small mucosal ulceration on the anterior wall of the rectum may be the only sign of hidden or occult rectal prolapse.

Associated Conditions

Solitary rectal ulcer is an uncommon pathologic lesion described in detail by Madigan and Morson in 1969.[14]

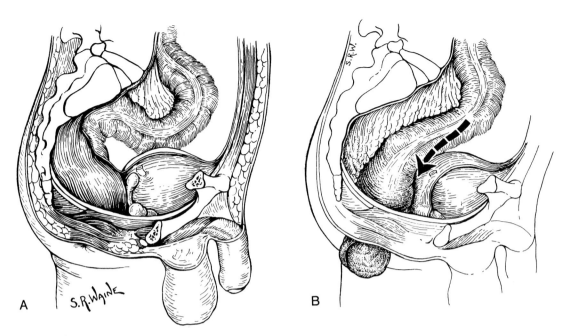

FIGURE 29-5. *A*, Sagittal view of normal rectum illustrating backward displacement into the hollow of the sacrum. *B*, Typical lesion in massive prolapse following displacement of rectum with a mesorectum extending from the sacrum. Intra-abdominal pressure acts in the long axis of the rectum. (From Ripstein, C.B., and Lanter, B.: Etiology and surgical treatment of massive prolapse of the rectum. Ann. Surg., *156*:259, 1963, with permission.)

Although this entity was thought to be idiopathic, Schweiger and Alexander-Williams[24] reported that in their experience, solitary rectal ulcers were almost always associated with rectal prolapse. In a series reported by Biehl and co-workers,[3] two thirds of patients with prolapse also complained of urgency, frequency, and straining, symptoms commonly associated with solitary rectal ulcer syndrome; yet in that series, only one patient had a demonstrable ulcer. In another series of 33 patients reported by Keighley and Shouler,[12] six patients had procidentia, 11 patients had anterior wall prolapse, and 12 patients were noted to have perineal descensus. Of 33 ulcers, 23 were seen anteriorly.

Proctitis cystica profunda is a rectal erythematous lesion that on biopsy shows cystic glandular structures deep to the mucosa and in the submucosa and muscularis. This is a benign lesion that causes bleeding, mucous drainage, tenesmus, and constipation. Lesions are usually located anteriorly; 15 of 28 patients with proctitis cystica profunda were found to have rectal prolapse by Stuart.[26] The association of solitary rectal ulcer and proctitis cystica profunda with rectal procidentia is so strong that the presence of these lesions in the anterior wall of the rectum led Ihre and Seligson[11] to believe that these patients have "internal procidentia." However, only 25 of their 40 patients improved after a Ripstein procedure.

Complications of Procidentia

Anal incontinence may be due to continuous stretch of the anal sphincter by the prolapsing mass, or it could be due to pudendal neuropraxis secondary to downward displacement of the pelvic floor. These complications necessitate operation on the prolapse as soon as an accurate diagnosis is established.

Ulceration and bleeding of the prolapsed mass are common, but excessive hemorrhage is rare. Strangulation and gangrene may result from incarceration. If the prolapse is irreducible and the bowel is nonviable, emergency rectosigmoidectomy is the procedure of choice. Rupture of the prolapse with evisceration is exceedingly rare and requires an emergency operation.

Operative Treatment

Prolapse in Children

Prolapse in children is often mucosal and should be managed by elimination of contributing factors (e.g., constipation, diarrhea, or laxative use). Careful examination will reveal the prolapse and exclude the presence of a juvenile polyp, which should be removed. As discussed earlier, taping of the buttocks can be effective. If not, submucosal injection of a sclerosing solution should be the next step.

In cases in which injection sclerotherapy is ineffective, Stephens[25] has recommended insertion of a subcutaneous suture of catgut, which is in essence a temporary Thiersch operation. Finally, Goligher[10] has reported emergency resection of rectosigmoid on rare occasions for large irreducible prolapse in children.

Prolapse in Adults

The treatment of rectal procidentia is always surgical. The multiplicity of operations and the recurrence rate seen after each of the procedures point to the lack of a uniformly successful operation. Moreover, none of the more popular operations addresses or solves the incontinence commonly seen in patients. Parks and associates described a decrease in rectal sensation with a loss of normal sampling response. This results in uncoordinated defecation, which is manifested by incontinence, constipation, or both.[17]

The choice of operative procedures depends not only on the severity of the illness and the patient's risk because of age, cardiovascular disease, and neurologic or psychiatric disorders, but also on the surgeon's experience with a specific technique. For many surgeons, abdominal approaches—that is, anterior resection, with or without rectopexy—or transabdominal rectopexy as popularized by Ripstein[22] and Wells[30] are easier to master.

The perineal operation popularized by Altemeier and associates[2] and modified by Prasad and co-workers[19] has been shown to have low morbidity and mortality even in poor-risk elderly patients. This method is also ideal for irreducible or gangrenous prolapse. However, this approach is unfamiliar to most general surgeons.

The Thiersch operation, and its modification by Lomas and Cooperman,[13] is a palliative procedure chiefly reserved for poor-risk, bedridden individuals with limited life expectancy. The procedure, although simple, is often followed by breakage or erosion of the wire or synthetic material through the overlying skin.

Finally, residual incontinence after initial operation must be addressed. On the average, 40% of patients do not regain continence after abdominal proctopexy or anterior resection. Many patients are so relieved by not having to deal with the procidentia every day that they do not mind dealing with incontinence by wearing a pad or curtailing their social activities. However, almost 10% of patients will require a further operative procedure if their continence does not improve by the first postoperative procedure year. Only the operation of Prasad and co-workers addresses the issue of incontinence and attempts to correct the sphincter abnormalities at the time of the initial procedure.[19]

All operations are performed with full mechanical bowel cleansing, oral antibiotics, and single-dose preoperative intravenous cephalosporin administration.

Posterior Rectopexy

Patients with complete rectal prolapse should undergo posterior rectopexy. Patients must be able to tolerate laparotomy. The operation results in intractable constipation in patients who have had chronic constipation preoperatively. Regional and general anesthesia are equally satisfactory.

Technique of Ripstein[22]

With the patient in the Trendelenburg position, the abdomen is entered through a low vertical or transverse incision. The rectum is mobilized by incising the lateral peritoneal reflections, with care taken to avoid ureteral injury. The rectum is mobilized posteriorly by blunt dissection, care being taken to avoid injury to the presacral veins underneath Waldeyer's fascia. A 5-cm-wide T-shaped polytetrafluoroethylene (Teflon) sling is sutured with nonabsorbable sutures to the anterior sacral fascia

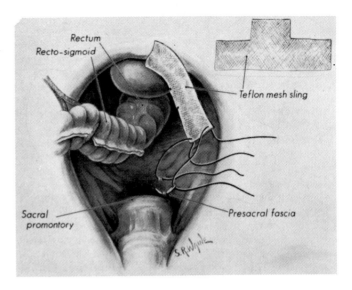

FIGURE 29–6. Surgical repair of rectal prolapse. Rectum is mobilized and Teflon mesh sling is sutured to presacral fascia with interrupted nonabsorbable sutures. (From Ripstein, C.B.: Surgical care of massive rectal prolapse. Dis. Colon Rectum, 8:34, 1965, with permission.)

and periosteum approximately 5 cm below the sacral promontory. The sling should be loose enough to allow one finger to be passed under the sling alongside the rectum. After pulling the rectum cephalad, the sling is sutured to the seromuscular layers of the rectum below the peritoneal reflection (Figs. 29–6 through 29–8). The peritoneal floor is not tightly sutured. Ripstein advocated suction drainage of the presacral area with a large-bore drain, but this is not always necessary, especially when complete hemostatis is ensured.

The majority of nonseptic complications of the Ripstein procedure (i.e., stricture, fecal impaction, intrac-

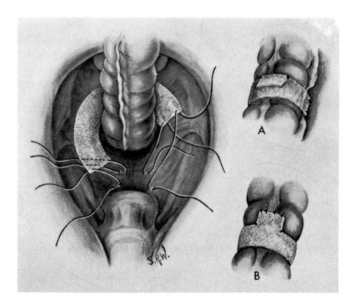

FIGURE 29–7. Surgical repair of rectal prolapse. Teflon sling encircles rectum, holding it posteriorly. (From Ripstein, C.B.: Surgical care of massive rectal prolapse. Dis. Colon Rectum, 8:34, 1965, with permission.)

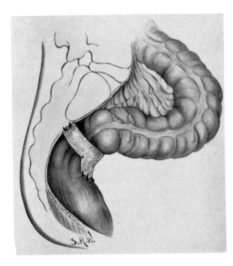

FIGURE 29-8. Lateral view of complete operation. Rectum is fixed posteriorly into hollow sacrum. (From Ripstein, C.B.: Surgical care of massive rectal prolapse. Dis. Colon Rectum, *8:*34, 1965, with permission.)

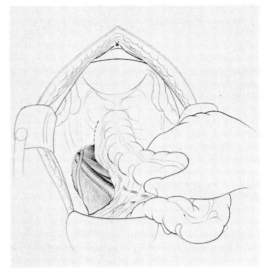

FIGURE 29-10. Incision through base of sigmoid mesentery—left ureter identified. (From Morgan, C.N.: Operation for complete prolapse of the rectum. *In* Maingot, R. [ed.]: Abdominal Operations, Vol. 2, 6th ed. New York, Appleton-Century-Crofts, 1974, with permission.)

table constipation) are related to the tightness of the sling around the rectum. This can be avoided by the Wells[27] procedure of fixing the polytetrafluoroethylene mesh to the sacrum at its midpoint, wrapping the mesh around the rectum, and suturing it to the seromuscular layer loosely, leaving a 2-cm area of the anterior rectum bare to expand if necessary.

Technique of Morgan[15]

The rectum is approached through a lower abdominal incision in the Morgan technique. The uterus is retracted anteriorly by means of a suture passed along the round ligaments (Figs. 29–9 through 29–11). The rectum is mobilized posteriorly, with special care to avoid

the presacral veins, from the level of the promontory to the coccyx (Figs. 29–12 through 29–15).

A polyvinyl alcohol (Ivalon) sponge, 3-mm thick and 22 × 11 cm, is autoclaved, punctured with a needle before use, and softened in saline. The sponge is then fixed to the presacral fascia with a series of nonabsorbable mattress sutures, with its long axis parallel to the rectum and its lower edge placed as low as possible posteriorly (Figs. 29–16 and 29–17). With cephalad traction on the rectum, the two lower corners of the sponge are approximated with a single nonabsorbable suture

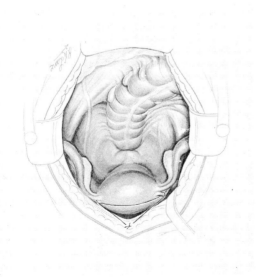

FIGURE 29-9. Uterus fixed anteriorly by a suture. (From Morgan, C.N.: Operation for complete prolapse of the rectum. *In* Maingot, R. [ed.]: Abdominal Operations, Vol. 2, 6th ed. New York, Appleton-Century-Crofts, 1974, with permission.)

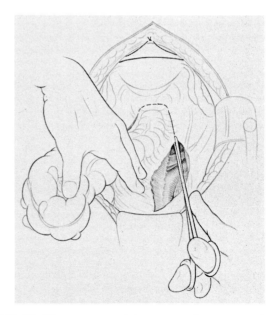

FIGURE 29-11. Extension of the peritoneal incisions at base of mesentery into the pelvis. (From Morgan, C.N.: Operation for complete prolapse of the rectum. *In* Maingot, R. [ed.]: Abdominal Operations, Vol. 2, 6th ed. New York, Appleton-Century-Crofts, 1974, with permission.)

passed through the perirectal tissue anterior to the rectum (Fig. 29–18). The stitch is then tied loosely, leaving a 1-cm area between the edges of the sponge. The upper end of the sponge is approximated with a similar corner suture. One or two "hitch" sutures are placed between the rectosigmoid peritoneum and are fixed to the sacral promontory (Fig. 29–19). The pelvic peritoneum is then closed with a continuous suture to cover the sponge completely, and after placing the omentum in the pelvis, the abdomen is closed in routine fashion.

Technique of Effron[7]

In the method devised by Effron, no synthetic material is used. Instead, a series of pursestring sutures approximate the mesorectum into the hollow of the sacrum (Fig. 29–20). These horizontal pursestring sutures are placed in the posterior third of the rectal circumference and the mesorectum and are then passed through the periosteum of the sacrum, avoiding the presacral vessels. A total of four or five sutures are taken 1 cm apart up to the sacral promontory and are tied in serial fashion. The peritoneum is closed on one side and is left open on the opposite side to provide drainage (Fig. 29–21). Goligher[9] has reported a similar procedure carried out in 40 patients with no complications and excellent short-term results.

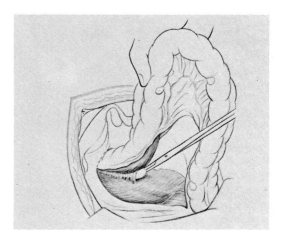

FIGURE 29–13. Mobilization of the rectum from the front of the sacrum. (From Morgan, C.N.: Operation for complete prolapse of the rectum. *In* Maingot, R. [ed.]: Abdominal Operations, Vol. 2, 6th ed. New York, Appleton-Century-Crofts, 1974, with permission.)

Anterior Resection of the Rectum

Anterior resection (method of Theuerkauf and co-workers[27]) effectively eliminates the redundant bowel. Mobilization of the rectum all the way down to the level of the coccyx is necessary to take up all the slack. Placing the anastomosis at the level of the third sacral vertebra fixes the rectum to the sacrum by scar formation. Resection of 20 to 30 cm of the redundant sigmoid is accomplished in standard fashion. The splenic flexure need not be mobilized.

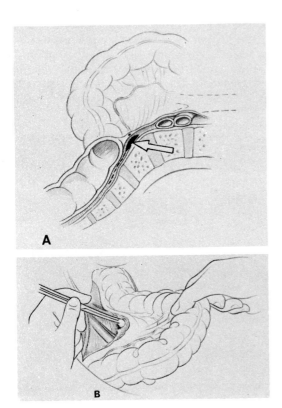

FIGURE 29–12. *A,* Blunt dissection demonstrating extraperitoneal space behind sigmoid mesentery at the level of the sacral promontory. *B,* Extraperitoneal space identified in left side and base of mesocolon lifted forward. (From Morgan, C.N.: Operation for complete prolapse of the rectum. *In* Maingot, R. [ed.]: Abdominal Operations, Vol. 2, 6th ed. New York, Appleton-Century-Crofts, 1974, with permission.)

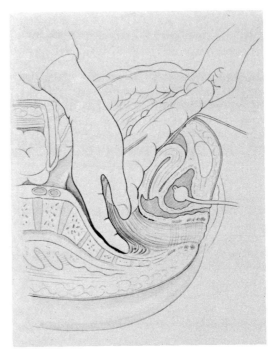

FIGURE 29–14. Final mobilization of the rectum posteriorly from the sacrum to the level of the coccyx. (From Morgan, C.N.: Operation for complete prolapse of the rectum. *In* Maingot, R. [ed.]: Abdominal Operations, Vol. 2, 6th ed. New York, Appleton-Century-Crofts, 1974, with permission.)

Theuerkauf and associates[27] suggested additional fixation of the bowel by suspending the rectum to the parietal peritoneum of the pelvic brim and anchoring the left colon to the left parietal peritoneum whenever feasible (Fig. 29–22). Newer data from the Mayo Clinic suggest that there is very little difference in the long-term recurrence rate between anterior resection and low anterior resection of the rectum.[23] However, the operative morbidity is considerably less with the former operation.

Abdominal Proctopexy and Sigmoid Resection

Frykman[8] originally described abdominal proctopexy and sigmoid resection in 1955. The technique includes complete mobilization of the rectum down to the level of the levators without dividing the lateral stalks. With cepahalad traction on the rectum, the lateral stalks are sutured to the presacral fascia with nonabsorbable sutures. The sigmoid and descending colon is then mobilized, and after resection of all the redundant sigmoid, a tension-free anastomosis is placed just below the pelvic brim (Fig. 29–23).

The rationale of this operation is that posterior fixation of the rectum will prevent recurrent intussusception, and resection of the redundant sigmoid will ameliorate many of the bowel management problems frequently seen after a Ripstein rectopexy. In a 30-year experience with this operation, Watts and colleagues[28] reported only two recurrences in 138 patients. Also, 77% of the patients reported perfect continence, while 40% of the patients were incontinent preoperatively with 24% reporting total incontinence.

PERINEAL OPERATIONS

The five major anatomic alterations in rectal prolapse are illustrated in Figure 29–24. Each method of peri-

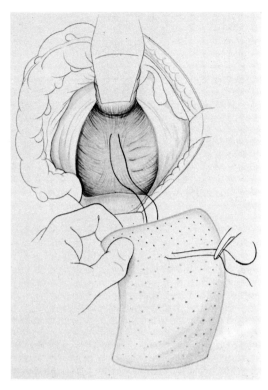

FIGURE 29-16. Insertion of the posterior fixation suture. (Morgan, C.N.: Operation for complete prolapse of the rectum. *In* Maingot, R. [ed.]: Abdominal Operations, Vol. 2, 6th ed. New York, Appleton-Century-Crofts, 1974, with permission.)

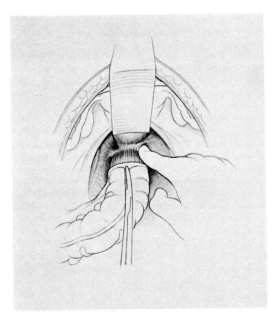

FIGURE 29-15. Exposure of the vaginal vault of the seminal vesicles. (From Morgan, C.N.: Operation for complete prolapse of the rectum. *In* Maingot, R. [ed.]: Abdominal Operations, Vol. 2, 6th ed. New York, Appleton-Century-Crofts, 1974, with permission.)

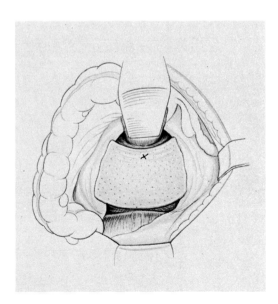

FIGURE 29-17. Fixation of Ivalon to the connective tissue on the front of the sacrum as low as possible (the suture is placed through the middle of the Ivalon higher than as shown in Figs. 29–16 and 29–17). (From Morgan, C.N.: Operation for complete prolapse of the rectum. *In* Maingot, R. [ed.]: Abdominal Operations, Vol. 2, 6th ed. New York, Appleton-Century-Crofts, 1974, with permission.)

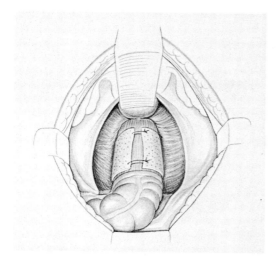

FIGURE 29-18. Upper and lower edges of implant approximated by linen sutures. Note 1-cm gap anteriorly and the formation of a gutter. (From Morgan, C.N.: Operation for complete prolapse of the rectum. *In* Maingot, R. [ed.]: Abdominal Operations, Vol. 2, 6th ed. New York, Appleton-Century-Crofts, 1974, with permission.)

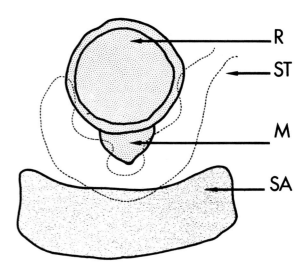

FIGURE 29-20. Cross section of rectum, mesorectum, and sacrum, demonstrating the placement of the pursestring suture. (*R* = rectum, St = stitch, M = mesorectum, SA = sacrum.) (From Efron, G.: A simple method of posterior rectopexy for rectal procidentia. Surg. Gynecol. Obstet., *145:*75, 1977. By permission of Surgery, Gynecology and Obstetrics.)

neal, as well as of abdominal, repair attempts correction of each of these abnormalities.

METHOD OF ALTEMEIER[2]. This operation approaches the entire problem though the perineum and includes excision of the redundant bowel, obliteration of the hernia sac, and approximation of the levator ani in front of the rectum.

The procedure is done in the dorsal lithotomy–Trendelenburg position under spinal or general anesthesia. The prolapse is grasped with Allis clamps and is placed on gentle traction to expose the dentate line. An initial circumferential incision is made 3 mm from the

dentate line (Figs. 29–25 through 29–27). The sac of the sliding hernia on the anterior surface of the bowel is opened, trimmed, and obliterated with a continuous 3-0 chromic catgut suture making an inverted Y-closure (Fig. 29–28). The thickened mesosigmoid is clamped and cut, and bleeders are secured with 0 chromic catgut. The levator ani muscles are then exposed anterior to the bowel and are grasped with Allis clamps. Three to five 0 chromic catgut sutures are used to approximate the edges of the muscle, thus closing the defect in the

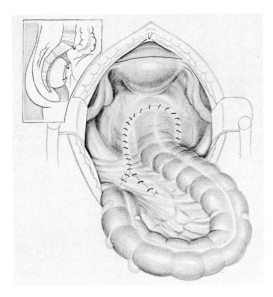

FIGURE 29-19. Repair of peritoneal edges in the pelvis anteriorly and those of the mesosigmoid on both sides. (From Morgan, C.N.: Operation for complete prolapse of the rectum. *In* Maingot, R. [ed.]: Abdominal Operations, Vol. 2, 6th ed. New York, Appleton-Century-Crofts, 1974, with permission.)

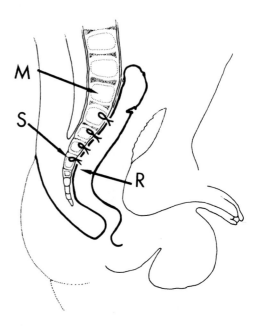

FIGURE 29-21. Sagittal section of the pelvis demonstrating the completed rectopexy with the tied sutures. (M = sacrum, S = sutures, R = rectum.) (From Efron, G.: A simple method of posterior rectopexy for rectal procidentia. Surg. Gynecol. Obstet., *145:*75, 1977. By permission of Surgery, Gynecology and Obstetrics.)

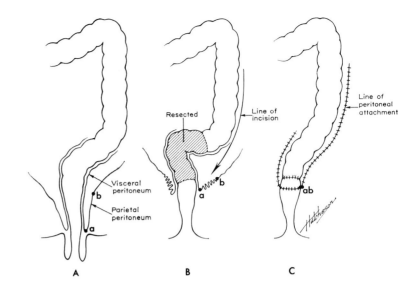

FIGURE 29-22. *A*, Prolapsed rectum completely protruded. *Point a* (visceral peritoneum of the rectum) and *point b* (area of parietal peritoneum for proposed rectal attachment) widely separated. *B*, Prolapsed rectum replaced, showing rectum in advanced position, proposed incision, and bowel to be resected. *C*, Subsequent suspension and fixation produced by joining visceral and parietal peritoneum after rectal advancement, bowel resection, excision of excess cul-de-sac, and anastomosis. (*Point a* and *point b* approximated and joined.) (From Theuerkauf, F.J., Beahrs, O.H., and Hill, J.R.: Rectal prolapse: Causation and surgical treatment. Ann. Surg., *171:*819, 1970, with permission.)

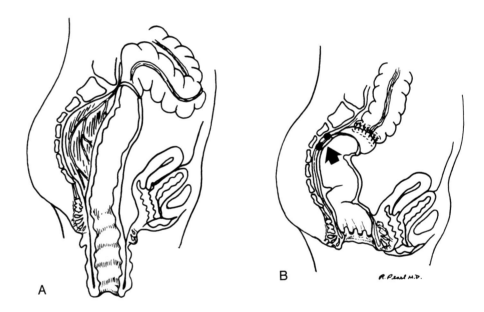

FIGURE 29-23. Abdominal sigmoidectomy with rectal fixation. *A*, Prolapsed rectum demonstrating loss of sacralization and redundancy of sigmoid colon. *B*, Redundant sigmoid colon resected. Rectum sutured to presacral fascia (*arrow*).

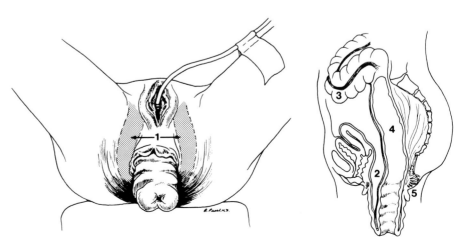

FIGURE 29-24. Anatomic features of rectal prolapse. *1*, Diastasis of levator ani muscle; *2*, deep pouch of Douglas; *3*, redundant sigmoid colon; *4*, straightening of the rectum; *5*, patulous anus.

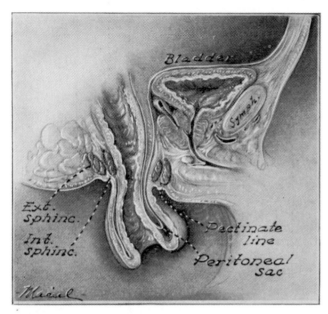

FIGURE 29–25. Diagrammatic illustration of a true rectal prolapse indicating the presence of herniation of the cul-de-sac through the anterior rectal wall. (From Altemeier, W.A., Hoxworth, P.I., and Giuseffi, J.: Further experiences with the treatment of prolapse of the rectum. Surg. Clin. North Am., *35*:1437, 1955, with permission.)

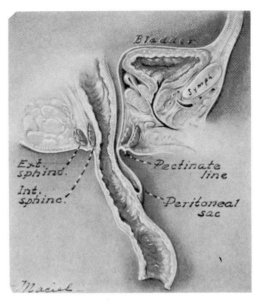

FIGURE 29–27. Half-tone drawing of prolapse after circumferential incision of outer loop and conversion into a single loop of redundant rectum and rectosigmoid. Note relationship of hernia sac to anterior wall of rectosigmoid. (From Altemeier, W.A., Hoxworth, P.I., and Giuseffi, J.: Further experiences with the treatment of prolapse of the rectum. Surg. Clin. North Am., *35*:1437, 1955, with permission.)

pelvic floor (Fig. 29–29). The redundant bowel is then divided into two lateral halves, and holding sutures are placed in each quadrant at the level of the proposed anastomosis, which is then completed circumferentially with 3-0 chromic catgut (Figs. 29–30 and 29–31). A petrolatum gauze wick is inserted into the anal canal.

PERINEAL PROCTECTOMY, POSTERIOR RECTOPEXY, AND POSTANAL LEVATOR REPAIR TECHNIQUE OF PRASAD AND CO-WORKERS[9]. This method modifies the original Altemeier procedure by incising the rectum 2 cm above the dentate line to avoid dividing the internal sphincter, fixing the bowel to the anterior sacrococcygeal fascia, and approximating the levator ani *behind* the bowel in order to re-create the normal anatomic anterior angulation at this level.

The patient is operated on in the dorsal lithotomy–Trendelenburg position under spinal anesthesia. A dilute (1:200,000) solution of epinephrine is infiltrated circumferentially 2 cm above the dentate line (Fig. 29–32A). The circumferential incision is then made at this level to avoid division of the internal sphincter (Fig. 29–32B). The straightened rectosigmoid is then skeletonized (Fig. 29–32C). The pouch of Douglas is obliterated with a 2-0 polyglactin suture just as in the Altemeier procedure.

Drawing the bowel anteriorly, the sacrococcygeal fascia is exposed posteriorly, and the rectum is fixed to the fascia with one or two 2-0 polypropylene sutures (Fig. 29–33). The pubococcygeus muscle is identified at its

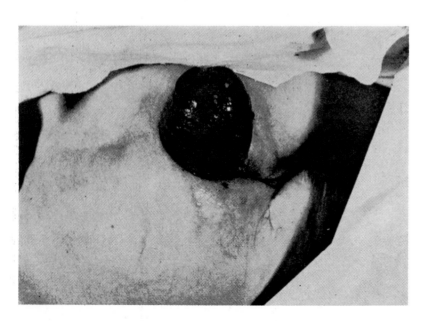

FIGURE 29–26. Photograph of complete or true rectal prolapse that protruded 6 inches beyond the anal orifice. Note the superficial ulceration. (From Altemeier, W.A., Hoxworth, P.I., and Giuseffi, J.: Further experiences with the treatment of prolapse of the rectum. Surg. Clin. North Am., *35*:1437, 1955, with permission.)

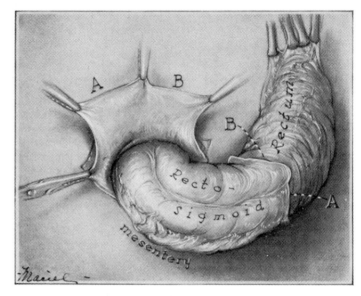

FIGURE 29-28. Illustration of opened hernial sac and elongated loop of rectosigmoid, mesentery, and rectum falling through hernial orifice. (From Altemeier, W.A., Hoxworth, P.I., and Giuseffi, J.: Further experiences with the treatment of prolapse of the rectum. Surg. Clin. North Am., *35*:1437, 1955, with permission.)

attachment to the coccyx. Using three to five 2-0 polypropylene sutures, the puborectalis muscle is approximated in the midline. This closes the widened pelvic outlet and at the same time acutely angles the rectum anteriorly, re-creating the anorectal angle, which had become obtuse preoperatively (Fig. 29–34A). If necessary, one or two sutures can be used to approximate the levators anterior to the rectum to reinforce the pelvic floor (Fig. 29–34B). The protruding bowel is then excised, and a single-layer full-thickness coloanal anastomosis is performed with 2-0 polyglactin sutures (Fig. 29–35).

This operation corrects all five anatomic abnormalities of the procidentia; namely, the redundant rectosigmoid, lack of posterior fixation, straightening of the rectum and the anorectal angle, the deep cul-de-sac of Douglas, and the diastasis of the pelvic diaphragm (Figs. 29–24 and 29–36). Therefore, it is not surprising that continence is improved in about 80% of the patients postoperatively.

DELORME PROCEDURE. (Technique of Uhlig and Sulli-

van[28]). This procedure involves stripping of the mucosa from the prolapsed bowel, plicating the denuded muscularis layer, and reanastomosing the mucosal ring. Under spinal anesthesia and in the lithotomy position, the submucosal plane of the prolapse is infiltrated with 1: 200,000 epinephrine solution to facilitate dissection. A circular incision is made 1 cm cephalad to the dentate line (Fig. 29–37A). The mucosa is dissected free, and with repeated infiltration and sharp dissection, a sleeve of mucosa and submucosa is separated from the muscularis layer up to the apex of the prolapse (Fig. 29–37B). The denuded muscularis is then plicated longitudinally using 2-0 polyglactin sutures in each quadrant. Additional sutures can be placed in between the gradient sutures to facilitate reduction of the prolapse (Fig. 29–37C). After meticulous hemostatis, the prolapsed bowel is reduced and the sutures are tied. The redundant stripped mucosa is then excised and the proximal and distal mucosa are reapproximated with absorbable sutures (Fig. 29–37D).

This procedure can be performed in poor-risk pa-

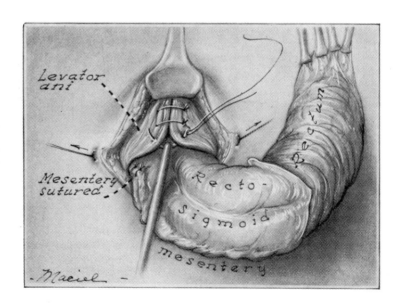

FIGURE 29-29. Demonstration of closure of levator muscles anterior to the rectosigmoid after high ligation of the hernial sac. (From Altemeier, W.I., Hoxworth, P.I., and Giuseffi, J.: Further experiences with the treatment of prolapse of the rectum. Surg. Clin. North Am., *35*:1437, 1955, with permission.)

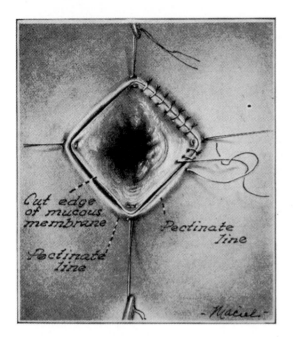

FIGURE 29-30. Completion of anastomosis of divided bowel to mucous membrane at pectinate line. (From Altemeier, W.A., Hoxworth, P.I., and Giuseffi, J.: Further experiences with the treatment of prolapse of the rectum. Surg. Clin. North Am., *35*:1437, 1955, with permission.)

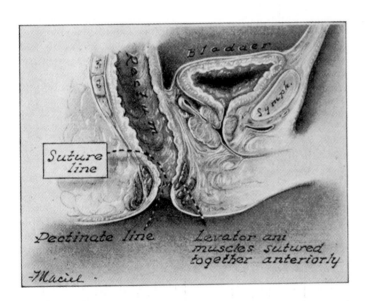

FIGURE 29-31. Sagittal section drawing showing position of anastomosis at completion of operation and reconstruction of pelvic floor. (From Altemeier, W.A., Hoxworth, P.I., and Giuseffi, J.: Further experiences with the treatment of prolapse of the rectum. Surg. Clin. North Am., *35*:1437, 1955, with permission.)

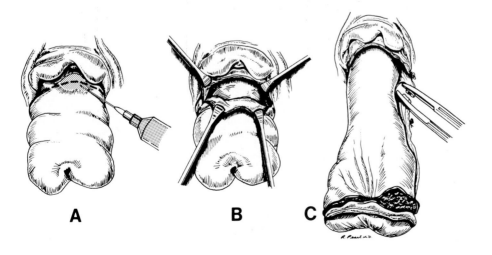

FIGURE 29-32. *A*, With the patient in the lithotomy position, gentle traction is applied on the rectal wall, after which a diluted epinephrine solution is injected into the outer layer of the prolapsed rectal wall. *B*, A circular incision is made through the full thickness of the outer layer of the prolapsed segment just proximal to the everted dentate line. *C*, The rectal prolapse has been completely unfolded. The mesenteric vessels are carefully ligated close to the bowel wall.

FIGURE 29-33. *A*, The rectum is elevated anteriorly to expose the presacral space. A posterior rectopexy is performed (*arrow*) by approximating the seromuscular layers of the bowel wall to the precoccygeal fascia above the levator ani muscles. *B*, Lateral view showing the completed posterior rectopexy (*arrow*). Note that the fixation is above the levator ani muscles (*shaded area*).

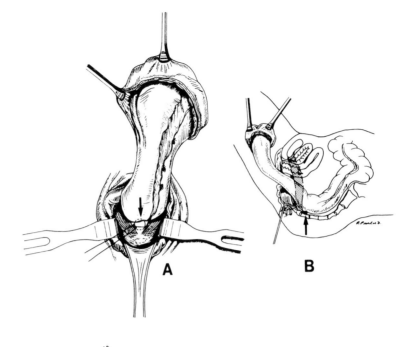

FIGURE 29-34. *A*, The levator ani muscles are approximated posteriorly (*arrow*). This repair pushes the bowel anteriorly to help recreate the anorectal angle. *B*, One or two sutures are used to approximate the levators anterior to the rectum to reinforce the pelvic floor (*arrow*).

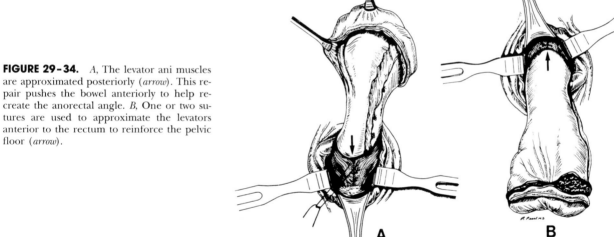

FIGURE 29-35. *A*, Technique of coloanal anastomosis. The prolapse is amputated and the colon is sutured to the dentate line in a circumferential fashion (*dotted line*). *B*, Completed anastomosis. *C*, Appearance of anus after reducing suture line.

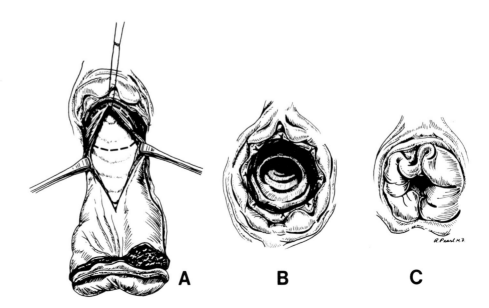

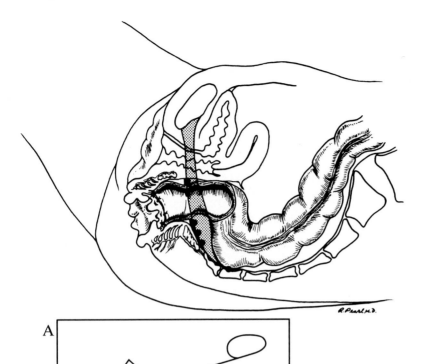

FIGURE 29-36. Summary of repair illustrating posterior rectopexy and postanal levator repair (*black dots*). Notice how the anorectal angle has been re-established.

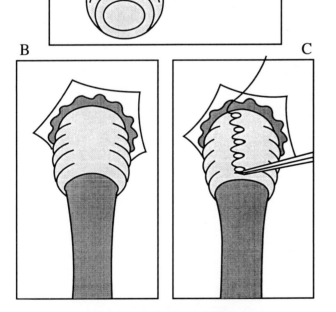

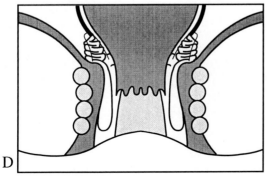

FIGURE 29-37. Delorme operation. *A,* After submucosal injection of 1:200,000 epinephrine solution, a circular incision is made 1 cm above the dentate line. *B,* A sleeve of mucosa and submucosa is stripped from underlying muscularis layer until tension is encountered. *C,* The muscularis layer is plicated longitudinally using multiple rows of 2/0 polyglactin sutures. *D,* The stripped mucosa is excised and the cut edges of proximal and distal mucosa are approximated with 3/0 polyglactin sutures. (From Gordon P.H.: Rectal procidentia. *In* Gordon, P.H. and Nivatvongs, S. (eds.): Principles and Practice of Surgery for the Colon, Rectum, and Anus. St. Louis, Quality Medical Publishing, Inc., p. 472, 1992, with permission.)

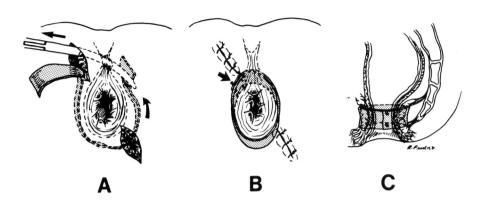

FIGURE 29-38. Anal circlage procedure. *A,* Superficial and deep portions of the external sphincter are encircled by a strip of synthetic material tunneled through left posterior and right anterior skin incisions. *B,* Anal circlage completed. The ends of the strip are either sutured or stapled to each other (*arrow*). *C,* Lateral view showing position of the band. Notice how it passes through the deep postanal space.

tients under local anesthesia. It is well tolerated and associated with few complications. The major disadvantage is the high recurrence rate and the tedious dissection needed in larger prolapses.

THIERSCH OPERATION. (Lomas and Cooperman Modification, 1972[13]). Because of the frequent breakage of the malleable wire used to encircle the anus in the Thiersch method, Lomas and Cooperman suggested the use of polypropylene mesh (Marlex). A 1.5-cm four-fold thickness of mesh is used to encircle the anus. Two perianal incisions are made in opposite quadrants (right posterior and left anterior). A tunnel is created deep to the external sphincter, taking care not to perforate the posterior vaginal wall. The mesh is passed around the anus and sutured with polypropylene sutures or staples, allowing only one finger in the anus (Fig. 29–38). After irrigation of the wound and careful hemostasis, the subcutaneous tissue and skin are closed in layers.

Major complications of this procedure include infection, migration of the mesh to the subcutaneous plane, or its erosion into the anorectum. However, because of the simplicity of the procedure and its suitability for even the patient who is an extremely poor risk, it can be ideal for bedridden, elderly, or senile patients, or for patients with persistent postoperative incontinence after another definitive procedure for rectal procidentia.

REFERENCES

1. Ajao, O.G., and Adekeunle, O.O.: Rectal prolapse in Ibadan, Nigeria. Trop. Doct., *9:*117, 1979.
2. Altemeier, W.A., Culbertson, W.R., Schowengerdt, C., et al.: Nineteen years' experience with the one stage perineal repair of rectal prolapse. Ann. Surg., *173:*993, 1971.
3. Biehl, A.G., Ray, J.E., and Gathright, J.B.: Repair of rectal prolapse: Experience with the Ripstein sling. South. Med. J., *71:*923, 1978.
4. Boutsis, C., and Ellis, H.: The Ivalon sponge-wrap operation for rectal prolapse. Dis. Colon Rectum, *17:*21, 1974.
5. Broden, B., and Snellman, B.: Procidentia of the rectum studied with cineradiography: A contribution to the discussion of causative mechanism. Dis. Colon Rectum, *11:*330, 1968.
6. Devadhar, D.S.C.: A new concept of mechanism and treatment of rectal procidentia. Dis. Colon Rectum, *8:*75, 1965.
7. Efron, G.: A simple method of posterior rectopexy for rectal procidentia. Surg. Gynecol. Obstet., *145:*75, 1977.
8. Frykman, H.M.: Abdominal rectopexy and primary sigmoid resection for rectal procidentia. Am. J. Surg., *90:*780, 1955.
9. Goligher, J.C.: Prolapse of the rectum. *In* Nyhus L.M., and Condon, R.E. (eds.): Hernia, 2nd ed. Philadelphia, J.B. Lippincott, 1978.
10. Goligher, J.C.: Surgery of the Anus, Rectum and Colon, 4 ed. London, Balliere Tindall, 1980, p. 224.
11. Ihre, T., and Seligson, U.: Intussusception of the rectum—internal procidentia: Treatment and results in 90 patients. Dis. Colon Rectum, *18:*391, 1975.
12. Keighley, M.R.B., and Shouler, P.: Clinical and manometric features of the solitary rectal ulcer syndrome. Dis. Colon Rectum, *27:*502, 1984.
13. Lomas, M.I., and Cooperman, H.: Correction of rectal procidentia by use of polypropylene mesh (Marlex®). Dis. Colon Rectum, *15:*416, 1972.
14. Madigan, M.R., and Morson, B.C.: Solitary ulcer of the rectum. Gut, *10:*871, 1969.
15. Morgan, C.N.: Operation for complete prolapse of the rectum. *In* Maingot, R. (ed.): Abdominal Operations, Vol. 2, 6th ed. New York, Appleton-Century-Crofts, 1969.
16. Moschowitz, A.V.: The pathogenesis, anatomy, and cure of prolapse of the rectum. Surg. Gynecol. Obstet., *15:*7, 1912.
17. Parks, A.G.: Anorectal incontinence. Proc. R. Soc. Med., *68:*21, 1976.
18. Porter, N.H.: A physiologic study of the pelvic floor in rectal prolapse. Ann. R. Coll. Surg., *31:*379, 1962.
19. Prasad, M.L., Pearl, R.K., Abcarian, H., et al.: Perineal proctectomy, posterior rectopexy, and postanal levator repair for the treatment of rectal prolapse. Dis. Colon Rectum, *29:*547, 1986.
20. Ripstein, C.B., and Lanter, B.: Etiology and surgical therapy of massive prolapse of the rectum. Ann. Surg., *157:*259, 1963.
21. Ripstein, C.B.: Surgical care of massive rectal prolapse. Dis. Colon Rectum, *8:*34, 1965.
22. Ripstein, C.B.: Definitive corrective surgery of massive rectal prolapse. Dis. Colon Rectum, *15:*334, 1972.
23. Schlinkert, R.T., Beart, R.W.J., Wolff, B.G., and Pemberton, J.H.: Anterior resection for complete rectal prolapse. Dis. Colon Rectum, *28:*409, 1985.
24. Schweiger, M., and Alexander-Williams, J.: Solitary ulcer syndrome of the rectum. Lancet, *1:*170, 1977.
25. Stephens, F.D.: Minor surgical conditions of the anus and perineum (in pediatrics). Med. J. Aust., *1:*224, 1958.
26. Stuart, M.: Proctitis cystia profunda: Incidence, etiology, and treatment. Dis. Colon Rectum, *27:*153, 1984.
27. Theuerkauf, F.T., Beahrs, O.H., and Hill, J.R.: Rectal prolapse, causation and surgical treatment. Ann. Surg., *171:*819, 1970.
28. Uhlig, B.E., Sullivan, E.S.: The modified Delorme operation: Its place in surgical treatment of massive rectal prolapse. Dis. Colon Rectum, *22:*513, 1979.
29. Watts, J.D., Rothenberger, D.A., Bulls, J.G., et al.: The management of procidentia: 30 year experience. Dis. Colon Rectum, *28:*96, 1985.
30. Wells, C.: New operations for rectal prolapse. Proc. R. Soc. Med., *52:*602, 1959.

Chapter 30

ANAL INCONTINENCE

JAMES W. FLESHMAN / IRA J. KODNER / ROBERT D. FRY /
ELISA H. BIRNBAUM

Fecal continence is the controlled elimination of feces at a socially acceptable time and place. There are degrees of anal incontinence, which vary with the consistency of material that must be controlled by the anal sphincter. A simple method of defining anal incontinence is to state the material that cannot be controlled by the anal sphincter mechanism. This includes incontinence of flatus only; incontinence of liquid stool and flatus; and incontinence of solid stool, liquid stool, and flatus. Incontinence also varies with the nature of the impaired control—from uncomfortable urgency to complete lack of sensation during the passage of feces. Grading systems for incontinence are more complicated. The frequency of incontinence episodes, type of incontinence, and degree of incontinence are combined to give a numerical value. One such system proposed by Miller and associates is seen in Table 30-1.[29] Understanding the mechanism of continence and the physiologic defects responsible for incontinence has been confusing because of the incomplete knowledge of the anatomy and physiology of defecation.

ANATOMY

Anal continence depends on several factors, which include (1) the internal anal sphincter, (2) the external anal sphincter, (3) the puborectalis muscle, (4) the maintenance of an acute anorectal angle, (5) adequate rectal capacity, (6) consistency of stool, and (7) normal anal sensation. It is the synchronized function of each of these components that results in normal control of defecation.

The anal canal has been defined anatomically and surgically.[13,32] The anatomic anal canal begins at the anal verge, at which point anoderm meets the perianal skin (Fig. 30-1). The anoderm contains numerous sensory nerve endings and lacks hair follicles and sebaceous or sweat glands. The canal extends to the dentate or pectinate line, at which point the mucosa of the rectum meets the anoderm. The anatomic anal canal extends a distance of approximately 1 to 1.5 cm. Above the dentate line there is a transition from a squamous epidermoid cell type, arising from embryologic ectoderm, to a cuboidal and then columnar epithelium, arising from embryologic endodermal gut. As the transitional zone merges into the mucosal lining of the rectum, the normal glandular pattern of rectal mucosa becomes apparent. There are 8 to 12 columns of rectal mucosa, which extend to the dentate line (Fig. 30-1). Each column of mucosa meets an upward extension of anoderm. Between each pair of columns is an intervening crypt at the dentate line. Anal glands that reside in the intersphincteric plane open into some but not all of these crypts. These glands are believed to secrete mucus and lubricate the anal canal. They are the source of abscess-fistula disease in the anal canal.

The surgical anal canal includes the entire muscular mechanism of the sphincter and extends cephalad to the anorectal ring, which is the palpable sling of the puborectalis muscle where it joins the other components of the levator muscle complex of the pelvis (Fig. 30-1). The sphincter mechanism consists of the voluntary puborectalis and external anal sphincter muscles and the involuntary internal anal sphincter muscle (Fig. 30-2).

The puborectalis and the external anal sphincter muscles have different innervation, but they must be thought of as a functional unit.[36,48] These muscles function as an extension of the levator mechanism of the pelvic floor. The internal anal sphincter is an autonomically innervated muscle that is responsive to sympathetic and parasympathetic control. The internal anal sphincter maintains resting basal pressure and normally relaxes when the rectal ampulla is distended. This reflex has been shown to depend on a local intramural nerve reflex that can be obliterated by circular transmural incision of the rectum above the anal canal.[22]

PHYSIOLOGY

The rectum serves as a reservoir for the storage of stool. The compliance, distensibility, and capacity of this reservoir contribute to normal anal continence. The rectum can normally hold at least 1,500 ml of infused saline before the anal sphincters lose control.[42] This volume is reduced in patients with anal incontinence. The

386

TABLE 30-1. THE INCONTINENCE SCORE SYSTEM*

Grade	Flatus	Fluid	Solid
I[†]	1	4	7
II[‡]	2	5	8
III[§]	3	6	9

*From Miller, R., Bartolo, D.C.C., Locke-Edmunds, J.C., and Mortensen, N.J.: Prospective study of conservative and operative treatment for faecal incontinence. Br. J. Surg., 75:101, 1988, with permission.
[†]Incontinence less frequent than once a month.
[‡]Incontinence between once a month and once a week.
[§]Incontinence more than once a week.

rate of infusion into the rectum also influences the tolerable capacity. This may explain the incontinence seen in patients with diseases affecting rectal distensibility such as scleroderma, radiation fibrosis, or recent low colorectal anastomosis. The rectal capacity can be abnormally high in patients with constipation in whom overflow incontinence of liquid stool develops around a solid mass of stool that distends and distorts the rectum and anus.

Anal sensation also plays an important role in maintaining continence.[42] This sensory function is related to the density of nerve endings in the anoderm. The anal canal has been shown to be extremely sensitive to temperature change, constant current electrical stimulation, and fine touch.[26,28] The sensory function of the rectum is minimal and contributes little to the maintenance of continence. The sensation of rectal distention does not seem to be as important, even though studies have shown improved continence after sensory retraining in patients with delayed rectal sensation.[1] Patients who have had a proctocolectomy with ileal reservoir and ileoanal anastomosis maintain continence despite the loss of the rectum.

A physiologic phenomenon known as the sampling reflex uses reflex internal anal sphincter relaxation in response to rectal distention to allow anal resting pressure to equilibrate with rectal pressure. Thus, the contents of the rectum can be evaluated by the anoderm to differentiate gas from stool, which is followed by appropriate external sphincter contraction to prevent soilage. The nature of the sensory input responsible for this mechanism has not been determined. Studies on ambulatory patients show the sampling mechanism to occur several times an hour throughout the day.[27] This mechanism allows discrimination among gas, solid, and liquid to maintain continence of stool and timely elimination of flatus.

The rectoanal inhibitory reflex is lost when the muscle is incised circumferentially around the upper anal canal. The distal mucosectomy and proximal proctectomy performed during a pelvic pouch procedure for ulcerative colitis eliminates the rectoanal inhibitory reflex. However, this reflex has recently been shown to recover after 12 months of follow-up, either by regeneration of intramural fibers or recruitment of pelvic floor muscle nerve fibers.[33]

The maintenance of an acute anorectal angle may be the major mechanism of continence of solid stool and requires a functioning puborectalis muscle. Defecography and balloon topography confirm the straightening of this angle during normal defecation (Fig. 30–3A) and the sharpening of the angle to maintain continence during maneuvers such as the Valsalva and cough (Fig. 30–3B).[17] A group of patients with chronic constipation has been defined as having severe difficulty emptying the rectum because the puborectalis and external sphincter do not relax during defecation.[21] The physiology of the puborectalis is unusual in that it maintains

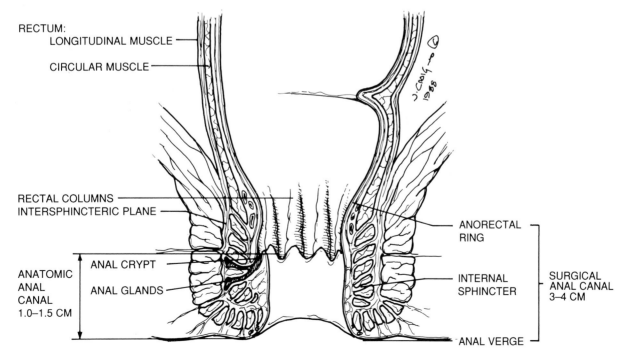

FIGURE 30-1. The anal canal. Anatomic and surgical features.

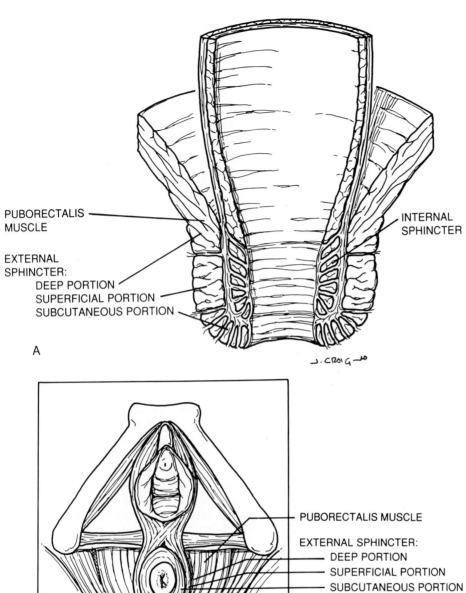

PUBORECTALIS
MUSCLE

EXTERNAL
SPHINCTER:
  DEEP PORTION
  SUPERFICIAL PORTION
  SUBCUTANEOUS PORTION

INTERNAL
SPHINCTER

A

J. CRAIG

FIGURE 30-2. Anal canal musculature. *A.* Cross section. *B.* Perineal view.

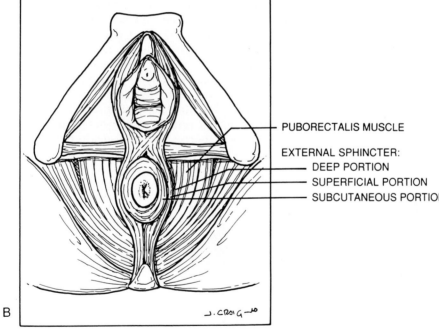

PUBORECTALIS MUSCLE

EXTERNAL SPHINCTER:
  DEEP PORTION
  SUPERFICIAL PORTION
  SUBCUTANEOUS PORTION

B

J. CRAIG

a normal state of contraction and must be voluntarily relaxed to allow defecation.

The exact contribution of each of the muscles of the sphincter to anal continence is not known. The internal anal sphincter maintains resting pressure and must play some role in the maintenance of continence. However, normal resting pressure does not provide adequate continence for liquid and gas when the external sphincter has been damaged and voluntary squeeze is abolished. There have been reports that a normal squeeze effort by the external sphincter is required to maintain continence of solids and liquids, and only a normal resting pressure is necessary to maintain continence of liquids only.[40] This would suggest that the function of the external sphincter is maintenance of control of solid stool. However, a recent study at our institution on patients who had repair of anterior sphincter injuries showed that restoration of the anterior sphincter length and resting basal pressure to normal levels was adequate for maintenance of solid stool continence; a normal external sphincter voluntary effort was required for maintenance of liquid and gas continence.[10] Thus, the understanding of the mechanism of anal continence is increasing, but it is still incomplete. The techniques for

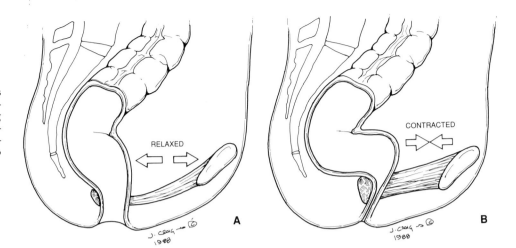

FIGURE 30-3. The puborectalis muscle maintains the anorectal angle. *A.* Relaxation and straightening of the anorectal angle during defecation. *B.* Contraction and sharpening of the anorectal angle to maintain continence.

evaluating sphincter function, both clinically and on an investigational level, have become much more sophisticated in recent years and will be described in this chapter.

ETIOLOGY

Anal incontinence can be attributed to a mechanical defect in the muscle, inadequate innervation of the sphincter mechanism, or idiopathic causes. Mechanical defects in the sphincter can be caused by obstetric trauma; a fistulotomy for either cryptogenic abscess-fistula disease or Crohn's disease; or injury to the pelvic floor and anal sphincter from blunt trauma, impalement, gunshot wounds, or foreign body insertion.

The most frequent mechanical injuries to the anal sphincter seen at our institution are obstetric injuries after a midline episiotomy. The obstetric literature has long debated the justification for routine use of midline or mediolateral episiotomy. Anal incontinence or rectovaginal fistula after a midline episiotomy and primary repair is uncommon, but it does represent a major source of anal sphincter injuries in some institutions.[3,5,38] Studies have shown little impairment of function after primary repair of a midline episiotomy.[14] This may be related to the initial length of the perineal body and normal healing after the primary repair.

Sphincter injury after fistulotomy has been shown to correlate with the amount of sphincter cut during the fistulotomy and with the location of the fistula being treated.[16] Transection of the internal anal sphincter in the treatment of posterior or posterolateral fistulas of the low anal canal causes minimal loss of continence. A large amount of the external sphincter must be cut in the posterior quadrant to cause incontinence. As long as some of the puborectalis muscle is maintained, continence of solid stool will be preserved. Transection of the external anal sphincter and internal sphincter in the posterior midline may result in minimal leakage of liquid and gas caused by the resultant keyhole deformity. The puborectalis sling is not present in the anterior aspect of the anal canal. The anterior sphincter mechanism is also shorter in women.[25] Injury to the anterior portion of the sphincter mechanism in women carries a high risk of incontinence. Even the use of a seton can result in significant incontinence.[36] To alleviate this risk, techniques have been developed that treat a fistula without requiring a fistulotomy, such as the sliding flap repair for low rectovaginal and anal perineal fistulas.[43] Approximately 35% of patients with Crohn's disease will have anal manifestations, often resulting in fistula formation.[12] Of 63 patients treated for low anterior anal or rectovaginal fistulas at the Jewish Hospital of St. Louis, ten patients had Crohn's disease. All ten of these patients were treated successfully with a sliding flap repair. Management of these fistulas requires strict preservation of the sphincter mechanism because of the high incidence of liquid stool in these patients. The sliding endorectal flap with adequate counterdrainage has been shown to be a safer technique (Fig. 30-4). In this method, a flap of mucosa and some internal sphincter is advanced over the fistula to close the internal opening.

Blunt trauma with a fracture of the pelvis may result in sphincter disruption or nerve injury. Impalement of the rectum frequently results in anal sphincter injury as well. If the sphincter can be repaired and sepsis controlled, a good result can usually be expected.[24] Bilateral disruption of the nerve supply to the external sphincter or puborectalis muscle usually results in incontinence despite reconstruction of the sphincter muscle. The insertion of foreign bodies into the rectum for sexual stimulation may cause stretching or laceration of the anal canal with resultant sphincter injury and incontinence.[7] Suppurative disease and ulceration due to cytomegalovirus are more frequently seen now in patients with acquired immunodeficiency syndrome (AIDS). The local effects of these conditions may present initially as loss of continence. Local therapy is only occasionally successful in controlling these problems.

Neurogenic or neuromuscular causes of anal incontinence are now more frequently diagnosed. The incontinence previously classified as idiopathic in many patients is now found to have neurologic causes.[20] Electromyographic evaluation of the anal sphincter mechanism and nerve conduction studies of the pudendal and spinal nerves are responsible for proper diagnosis in these patients. Patients with spinal cord injuries

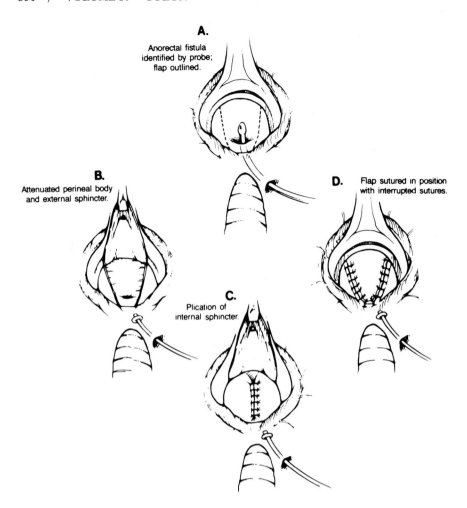

A.
Anorectal fistula
identified by probe;
flap outlined.

B.
Attenuated perineal body
and external sphincter.

C.
Plication of
internal sphincter.

D.
Flap sutured in position
with interrupted sutures.

FIGURE 30-4. Sliding endorectal flap repair of anal canal fistula. *A.* Anal canal fistula. *B.* Creation of mucosal flap and counter drainage of fistula. *C.* Closure of fistula through muscle. *D.* Mucosal flap sutured over fistula closure site. (From Shemesh, E.I., Kodner, I.J., Fry, R.D., and Neufeld, D.M.: Endorectal sliding flap repair of complicated anterior anoperineal fistulas. Dis. Colon Rectum, *31:*22, 1988.)

experience anal incontinence in several ways. Pelvic floor spasm and loss of anal sensation can cause constipation and "overflow" incontinence. The loss of a complete reflex arc prevents a normal "sampling" mechanism. Although the internal anal sphincter relaxes in response to rectal distention, the external sphincter does not contract appropriately to prevent soilage. The degree of dysfunction depends on the level of injury. Cauda equina injuries result in an overall decreased tone of the anal canal. Upper-level spinal cord or central nervous system problems result in spasm of the external sphincter with no voluntary contraction at appropriate times and subsequent incontinence.

Urogenital exstrophy and imperforate anus are the major congenital causes of anal incontinence. Children with low imperforate anus in whom the rectal tube has passed through the pelvic floor sling but has failed to connect with the perineal skin or the ectodermal sinus generally have a good result after creation of an anal opening. Even if they have a mild residual defect, they may be trained to have improved control. The upper-level imperforate anal defect, in which the endodermal tube terminates above the pelvic floor, does not allow as good a result. However, the sagittal dissection technique, which identifies the sphincter mechanism and pulls the rectal tube through the pelvic floor opening, has resulted in an improved outcome in these children.[8] Hirschsprung's disease may also present as overflow anal

incontinence. This is easily treated and should always be considered when a youngster complains of incontinence.

Acquired neurogenic or neuromuscular defects include systemic diseases such as diabetes, multiple sclerosis, myotonic dystrophy, scleroderma, or any disorder that results in dysfunction of nerves, neuromuscular junctions, and muscle fibers themselves. Electromyographic techniques have facilitated the diagnosis and definition of these problems.

A large number of patients experience anal incontinence as a result of pudendal nerve injury. Only recently has electromyography allowed the demonstration of these pudendal nerve injuries. The causes of pudendal nerve injury include obstetric trauma to the nerve during childbirth, stretching of the nerve from chronic perineal descent related to straining during defecation, and complete rectal prolapse. Nerve injury in patients with perineal descent has been correlated with the degree of descent and the chronicity of the problem.[18] The nerve injury from childbirth is partially reversible. A study at St. Mark's Hospital has prospectively shown that vaginal delivery causes stretching of the pudendal nerve and a temporary delay in pudendal nerve terminal motor conduction. In the majority of cases, conduction returns to normal, but there is a subgroup of patients who have a persistent defect[47]

Patients with rectal prolapse and anal incontinence

have been studied to identify the group with nerve injury who will remain incontinent after repair of the prolapse. Electromyography using single-fiber densities and pudendal nerve latency has documented pudendal nerve damage in patients who remain incontinent.[30] Full rectal prolapse is associated with anal incontinence in almost two thirds of patients. Repair of the prolapse results in recovery of anal continence in half of those patients who initially had incontinence. Operative approaches to rectal prolapse using a perineal proctectomy and anterior and posterior sphincter reconstruction as described by Prasad and associates[39] may improve the recovery of continence in most patients. However, bilateral pudendal nerve dysfunction is usually associated with less than complete improvement.

Patients with idiopathic incontinence probably also have a neurogenic defect. However, in some patients a mechanical or neurologic defect cannot be documented. In this group of patients, the major associated factors appear to be increasing age, psychologic problems, or overflow incontinence from idiopathic constipation (especially in children).

Other causes of anal incontinence include irritable bowel syndrome, acute and chronic diarrheal states, radiation proctitis, and chronic inflammatory disease of the rectum (Crohn's and ulcerative colitis). A reduced rectal capacity or a condition overwhelming the rectal capacity is most likely responsible for the incontinence in these instances. Incontinence after a low anterior resection of the rectosigmoid for rectal cancer is also an example of this phenomenon. Preoperative radiation of the rectum has been shown not to affect the anal sphincter.[2] Rectal prolapse repair may actually uncover anal incontinence when the obstructing prolapse is removed. The incontinence may then be responsible for a reduction in rectal vault capacity (after low anterior resection) or chronic pudendal nerve and internal anal sphincter stretch.

INVESTIGATIVE TECHNIQUES

The presence of anal incontinence is generally easy to establish. Recently, numerous techniques have been developed that allow a more objective approach to the diagnosis, categorization, and management of anal incontinence.

The patient who presents with any degree of anal incontinence requires a physical examination to determine the severity of the problem and to identify any underlying medical problems that may predispose to the incontinence. Anoscopy or proctosigmoidoscopy to inspect the anal canal and rectum is essential. Other sources of a colorectal pathologic condition that mimic anal incontinence must be sought using either double-contrast barium enema or colonoscopy. Excessive mucous discharge by a villous tumor or overflow incontinence from an obstructing rectal cancer may mimic anal incontinence. After these basic studies are completed, a more detailed investigation will be required to determine the nature of the incontinence.

Defecography

Defecography (videofluoroscopy of the barium-filled rectum during defecation) will identify rectal prolapse or intussusception.[17] The technique requires an arrangement in the radiology department that allows fluoroscopic examination of the patient in the sitting position. Usually patients will know if they have rectal prolapse. However, some patients will complain only of mucous discharge, bleeding, or incontinence; the prolapse will be discovered only during defecography.

Anal Manometry

There are numerous manometry systems used to evaluate the anal sphincter, and they are becoming more available as a diagnostic modality. Anal manometry can be performed using stationary pressure measurements or with a continuous catheter pullout to produce a sphincter profile. The sphincter has longitudinal and radial variation.[49] The maximum resting pressure and maximum squeeze pressure can be documented with reproducible and reasonable accuracy. A sphincter profile is useful but is generally meaningless unless it can be related to the quadrants of the sphincter mechanism. Anal manometry also provides information about the minimal volume that can be detected by the rectum and anal canal, and it establishes the presence of a normal rectoanal inhibitory reflex. The presence of this reflex has several implications, including the differentiation of Hirschsprung's disease from overflow incontinence caused by idiopathic constipation.

Anal manometry in our institution, using a hydraulic capillary infusion technique, routinely provides a sphincter profile (Fig. 30–5A). The manometry catheter measures the pressure in each of the four quadrants in the anal canal using radially positioned side ports located 4 cm from the tip of the catheter (Fig. 30–5B). Patients with a mechanical sphincter defect will have a shortened sphincter length, low resting pressure, or low squeeze pressure in the area of the sphincter muscle injury. A rapid pullout technique, withdrawing the catheter at 5 mm/sec during maximal squeeze, will provide a squeeze profile that is useful in detecting external sphincter injury.

Electromyography

The ability to diagnose neurogenic anal incontinence has improved as methods for investigating the nerves of the anal sphincter and pelvic floor have improved. Concentric needle electromyographic mapping of the external anal sphincter in patients with imperforate anus and mechanical injuries has been used for a number of years. However, single-fiber needle techniques developed by Swash at St. Mark's Hospital in London[31] allow better documentation of nerve injury to the external anal sphincter muscle. A special fine-needle electrode is used to record motor unit potentials in an area 270 μm in diameter arising from the external anal sphincter muscle at rest. This area is small enough that a single nerve fiber will control the surrounding muscle fibers.

A

HYDRAULIC CAPILLARY INFUSION SYSTEM

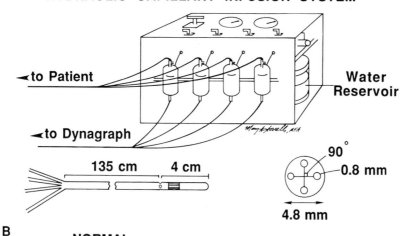

◄ to Patient

◄ to Dynagraph

Water Reservoir

135 cm   4 cm

90°
0.8 mm
4.8 mm

FIGURE 30-5. Anal manometry. *A.* Hydraulic capillary infusion system and multiport polyvinyl catheter; *B.* Sphincter pressures—resting profile and maximal squeeze.

B

NORMAL

Resting Pressure   Squeeze Pressure

mm Hg

175 L 75 0

175 R 75 0

175 A 75 0

175 P 75 0

A single-phase motor unit potential will be recorded in a normal muscle (Fig. 30–6). In the event of nerve injury and subsequent reinnervation by ingrowth of multiple adjacent nerve fibers, a multiphasic motor unit potential will be recorded. The fiber density is obtained by taking the average number of phases in 20 motor units recorded around the circumference of the sphincter. The range of normal is 1.5 ± 0.16 phases. The puborectalis muscle has been shown to respond to nerve injury and reinnervation in a manner similar to the external sphincter, and documentation of nerve injury to one muscle is almost always reflected in the other.[45]

Measurement of pudendal nerve terminal motor latency allows documentation of peripheral nerve injury in patients with suspected neurogenic anal incontinence. The technique requires stimulation of the pudendal nerve in its course through Alcock's canal beneath the ischial spine. The motor unit potential produced in the external anal sphincter is recorded in the anal canal. A stimulating electrode is placed on the tip of the examiner's gloved finger and a recording electrode is positioned over the ventral surface of the proximal phalanx (Fig. 30–7A). Transanal stimulation of the pudendal nerve using 50 volts in 0.1-msec square waves is generally not uncomfortable to the patient and allows measurement of the pudendal nerve terminal motor la-

tency in the majority of patients tested. A current of 8 to 10 mA is required. The normal range of latency is 2 ± 0.2 msec (Fig. 30–7B). Clinical correlation has shown that a delay in terminal motor latency correlates well with anal incontinence from neurogenic causes.[20] Delays in nerve conduction have been documented in women after vaginal delivery; in patients who have perineal descent or rectal prolapse; and in patients with a peripheral neuropathy such as diabetes, multiple sclerosis, or scleroderma. The nerve conduction delay is caused by demyelination of the fast-conducting fibers of the pudendal nerve from stretch or entrapment of the nerve or from involvement of the nerve by a systemic disease.

Determination of delays in spinal nerve conduction from levels L1 and L4 is useful in evaluating patients with nerve root injury caused by a herniated disk, spinal stenosis, arthritis, or trauma.[45]

Saline infusion tests evaluate rectal capacity as well as sphincter control. Warm saline can be infused at a constant rate and to a standard volume. Patients with anal incontinence will have lower controlled volumes than will patients with normal function.[41] Microelectrical stimulation and thermal probe techniques may be useful in documenting sensory deficits in the anal canal that contribute to incontinence.[26–28] A stimulating electrode that delivers microvoltage stimulation to the tissue is

A
Fiber Density

B
Fiber Density

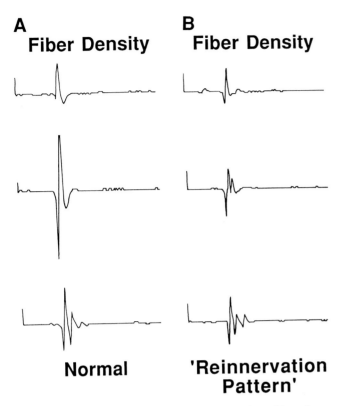

Normal

'Reinnervation Pattern'

FIGURE 30-6. Single-fiber needle electromyography. *A.* Normal pattern of motor unit potentials. *B.* Nerve injury patterns of motor unit potentials.

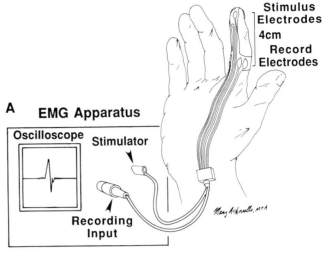

A EMG Apparatus

Oscilloscope Stimulator

Recording Input

Stimulus Electrodes
4cm
Record Electrodes

B
TERMINAL MOTOR LATENCY

2.0 ms

Motor Unit Potential

μV

200
100
0

Time (ms)

Stimulus
50 V
0.1 ms

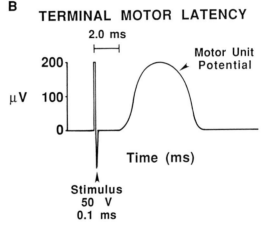

FIGURE 30-7. Pudendal nerve terminal motor latency. *A.* Equipment. *B.* Normal tracing.

placed in the anal canal, and the threshold of sensation is determined. The anoderm is also very sensitive to small changes in temperature.

Transanal Ultrasound

Transanal ultrasound is rapidly becoming the most accurate method of detecting a defect in the anal sphincter mechanism. A 360-degree rotating 10-mHz transducer (Bruel & Kjaer Model #1846, Marlboro, MA) covered by an anal cap is used in our lab.[50] The layers of the anal sphincter are easily seen. A thickened hypoechoic ring represents the internal anal sphincter (Fig. 30-8). The external sphincter appears as a less hypoechoic area encircling the internal sphincter with dense white lines throughout representing interfaces between fascicles of the skeletal muscle (Fig. 30-8). The puborectalis muscle appears as a horseshoe-shaped sweep of the upper portion of the external sphincter with anteriorly stretching arms on either side of the upper vagina and/or cervix (Fig. 30-9).

In the patient with a sphincter defect, the hypoechoic scar is seen to replace the concentric layers of the internal and external sphincter (Fig. 30-10). The anatomy of the anal canal and pelvic floor can be defined. The thickness of the muscle and scar in the area of injury can be measured. The thickness of the perineal tissue between rectum and vagina is also obtainable. Fistulas can be traced, abscesses identified, and sphincter defects documented using the transanal ultrasound. A combination of transanal ultrasound and pudendal

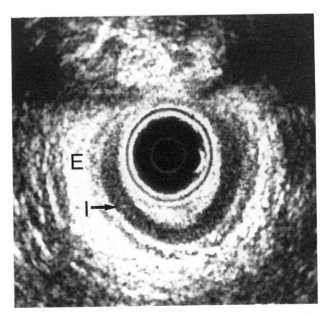

FIGURE 30-8. Transanal ultrasound demonstrating a normal hypoechoic internal sphincter (*I*) surrounded by the external sphincter (*E*).

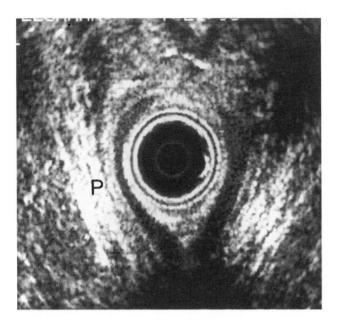

FIGURE 30-9. Transanal ultrasound demonstrating a normal puborectalis muscle (*P*).

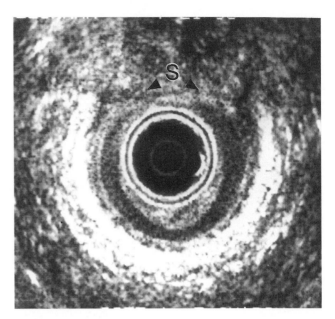

FIGURE 30-10. Transanal ultrasound demonstrating replacement by scar (*S*) of the normal sphincters in a patient with a sphincter defect.

nerve latency determination may become the working colorectal surgeon's preferred method of evaluating anal incontinence in the future.

As more effort is directed to understanding the physiology of anal sphincter function and the pathophysiology of anal incontinence, new techniques will be developed to evaluate and manage anal incontinence. At the present time, no single technique gives all the information needed to adequately assess anal sphincter function. A combination of investigative procedures is probably necessary to fully evaluate the cause of anal incontinence and to plan management.

TREATMENT

After the nature of the incontinence has been determined, a plan of therapy must be formulated. A medical regimen is started in most patients to improve their situation with minimal risk. If there is no muscle defect, muscle retraining may allow the patient to better use the existing sphincter mechanism. If these measures fail, or if there is a demonstrated defect in the muscle, surgical correction is recommended. The surgeon must use caution when reconstructing a sphincter that has inadequate innervation or when operating on a patient with psychologic problems or severe irritable bowel syndrome with no clearly demonstrated muscular defect. Continence in these patients will not significantly improve. Muscle retraining is also used in order to improve function after a surgical repair.

Medical Therapy

Patients may benefit from simple measures that slow the colonic transit, prevent diarrhea, or increase the bulk in the stool. The medications available to the phy-

sician are myriad. If the rectal vault is empty, there can be no leakage of material through an incompetent anal sphincter; therefore, part of an effective bowel control regimen must be the periodic complete emptying of the rectum. This is usually best accomplished by use of a small enema, a suppository, or a laxative. The use of a cone-tip irrigating device, as used routinely for colostomy irrigation, has been very helpful. The establishment of a successful regimen requires adaptability by both physician and patient.

Muscle Retraining

Schuster was the first to describe the use of double-balloon manometry to retrain and strengthen the anal canal musculature.[9] He reported an improvement in 75% of his patients, even in those with neurogenic anal incontinence. His technique is based on sensory retraining. As a rectal balloon is progressively inflated, the patient is taught to contract the anal sphincter while monitoring the pressure generated on the anal balloon. With time, a smaller and smaller volume of inflation can be detected, and higher squeeze pressures can be generated. The most consistent success was described in patients with a mechanical defect who had residual functioning muscle. Even some patients with a neurogenic cause of incontinence have responded to this treatment. It is difficult to identify the impact of psychologic factors in these circumstances. Since his original report, numerous other techniques have been described using surface electromyography[23] and rectal balloons.[51] MacLeod demonstrated good results in patients with mechanical defects in the anal sphincter using an anal plug surface electrode to document muscle activity during contraction of the external anal sphincter. However, he has not shown good results in patients with a neurogenic cause of incontinence (25% success rate).

A review of 37 patients treated for anal incontinence with muscle sensory retraining in our institution revealed success in approximately 50% of patients. A combination of manometric-documented squeeze and gradually reduced balloon inflation within the rectum provided both improved squeeze pressures and more normal sensory thresholds in those patients who were improved. Successful biofeedback was seen in 57% of patients with mechanical defects, 60% of patients with neurogenic defects, 71% of patients with a combined defect, but in none of the patients with idiopathic anal incontinence. A clear definition of the degree of incontinence as well as the cause is needed to predict a patient's response to biofeedback.

Surgical Treatment

Early techniques of sphincter repair gave variable results and were associated with complications of infection and breakdown of the repair. Until recent improvement in techniques, it was not uncommon that a colostomy was required to ultimately achieve an adequate repair. The technique that we recommend was popularized by Goldberg and involves extensive mobilization of the

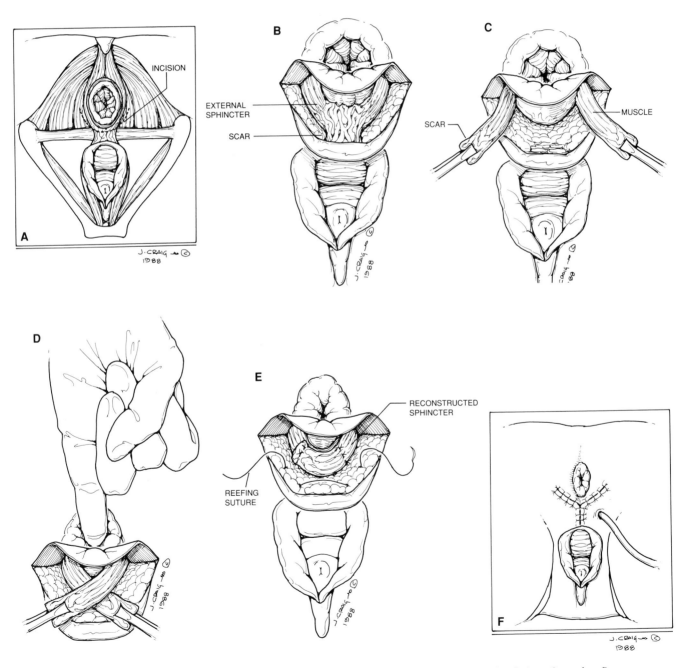

FIGURE 30–11. Anal sphincter overlapping muscle repair. *A,* Anterior incision and perineal view of muscles. *B,* Rectal flap is created and sphincter muscles are isolated. *C,* Muscle flaps are fully mobilized. *D,* Muscle flaps are overlapped around a 15-mm rubber dilator or fingertip. *E,* Muscle flaps are sutured in place and perineal body repaired. *F,* Drain is placed behind vaginal wall and closed.

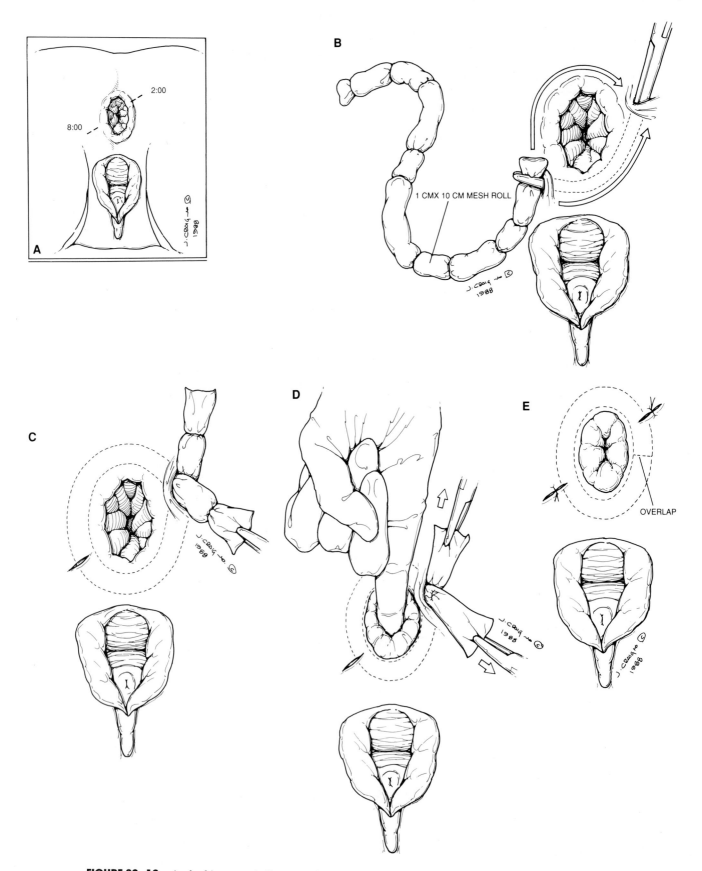

FIGURE 30–12. Anal sphincter encircling procedure. *A,* Perineal skin incisions placed at the 2-o'clock and 8-o'clock positions outside external sphincter. *B,* Mesh roll tunneled outside of external sphincter through posterior wound. *C,* Mesh is overlapped and tightened to draw in external sphincter muscle. *D,* Anal opening is calibrated and sutured with mesh. *E,* Mesh is trimmed and rotated to protect suture line.

components of the sphincter mechanism, and overlapping repair using the existing scar tissue, and meticulous pre- and postoperative care to avoid performing a colostomy.[15]

If anal incontinence is a result of severe muscle injury, surgical reconstruction is required. The overlapping muscle repair can be used to repair a muscle defect in any quadrant of the external anal sphincter. The repair of an anterior defect in women, which is the lesion we encounter most frequently, will be described. The patient undergoes complete bowel preparation including mechanical cleansing followed by oral and intravenous antibiotics perioperatively. The patient is placed in a prone, flexed position after general or, preferably, spinal anesthesia. The perianal tissue is infiltrated with saline and epinephrine solution to improve hemostasis during the procedure.

An anterior circumanal incision is made approximately 1 cm external to the mucocutaneous junction, if any skin remains between the anus and the vagina, and is extended halfway around the anus (Fig. 30–11A). A flap of skin and rectal wall is elevated from the scar tissue and underlying sphincter (Fig. 30–11B). The outer edge of the external sphincter muscle is identified on both sides at the lateral aspect of the anus. The neurovascular bundles must be protected at the point at which they penetrate the external sphincter posterolaterally. A second flap of skin and vaginal wall is then elevated from the midline scar. The sphincter mechanism is preserved by identifying the ischiorectal fat and dissecting in the plane just outside the muscle. The anterior dense scar is divided in the midline and retained to be used in the repair (Fig 30–11C). Each component of the sphincter is fully mobilized by further dissection until the muscle flaps can be overlapped (Fig. 30–11D) and secured without tension. Nonabsorbable horizontal mattress sutures are placed from the scarred end of one muscle to the base of the other (Fig. 30–11E). The tightness of the muscle repair should be calibrated by using the tip of the small finger or a 15-mm rubber dilator placed in the anal canal during the overlapping repair. The perineal body is then reconstructed with additional sutures anterior and deep to the muscle reconstruction. Sometimes the reconstruction is simplified if the perineal repair is done first. A suction drain should be placed behind the vagina and brought out through a separate incision in the perineal skin (Fig. 30–11F). This prevents accumulation of serum and blood. The skin will usually close vertically across the perineal body, which is now much wider than before. The incision will form a T shape because of the vertical closure of the perineal skin. An alternative method involves sewing the trimmed muscle flaps end to end to prevent overlapping and avoid wide lateral dissection needed for the overlapping repair. The perineal body and skin closures are the same as in the above-described technique.

After surgery, patients are kept constipated for approximately 48 hours to avoid early contamination of the wound. They are maintained on intravenous fluids and antibiotics before resuming a regular diet, stool softeners, and bulk-forming agents. Perianal hygiene must be meticulous, using warm sitz baths and dry pads for cleansing and drying. The suction catheter drain can be removed when the drainage is less than 5 ml in a 24-hour period.

A review of our experience with this procedure in 55 women revealed return of complete continence in 70% of patients treated with overlapping repair of anterior sphincter defects. Partial success was achieved in 24%; these patients remained incontinent of either liquid and gas or gas only. Only three patients (6%) did not improve after surgery. These results are consistent with other reported series using a similar technique. Patients who remain partially incontinent after surgery often have a component of nerve injury. The majority of patients in our series had an obstetric injury to the anterior external anal sphincter. The remainder had trauma to the sphincter after a fistulotomy for abscess-fistula or Crohn's disease.

A prospective manometric evaluation of 28 patients undergoing muscle repair for anal incontinence due to obstetric injury confirmed our initial results.[11] The restoration of complete continence depended on restoration of rest pressure, sphincter length and, most importantly, squeeze pressure to normal levels. A prospective manometric and electromyographic evaluation of elderly women undergoing overlapping muscle repair revealed the necessity of at least one functioning pudendal nerve to achieve complete control of continence.[44] Normal pudendal nerve function allows normal squeeze pressure to be achieved.

Patients who have incontinence resulting from partial or complete denervation of the sphincter or who have massive destruction of the muscle will not benefit from the muscle repair just described. They may be treated with an encircling procedure, using either synthetic material or gracilis muscle, or a Park's posterior repair. It should be emphasized that, if necessary, a good end colostomy can return a patient to normal life. The majority of patients with denervation of the sphincter in our series have had years of rectal prolapse.

The simplest techniques for controlling anal sphincter incontinence include placement of bands of synthetic mesh, polymeric silicone (Silastic), or silver wire around the sphincter mechanism. These materials all serve to constrict the anal canal. After a complete bowel preparation, the patient is placed in a prone flexed position (Fig. 30–12A). Small skin incisions are made at the 2-o'clock and the 8-o'clock positions just outside the external sphincter (Fig. 30–12B). The encircling material is then bluntly tunneled around the sphincter deep in the ischiorectal fat encompassing the external sphincter mechanism (Fig. 30–12C). Our current technique uses a rolled 10-cm length of either Marlex or Mersiline mesh, which is passed around the sphincter and sutured to itself to complete the circle. The band is tightened around the operator's small fingertip to determine the size of the anal orifice (Fig. 30–12 D). The ring is closed with sutures, excess mesh is trimmed, the wound is irrigated with antibiotic solution, and the band of mesh is positioned so that the point of overlap and closure of the ring is away from the skin incision (Fig. 30–12E). The skin incisions are closed. The patient usually requires a bowel control regimen to avoid constipation.

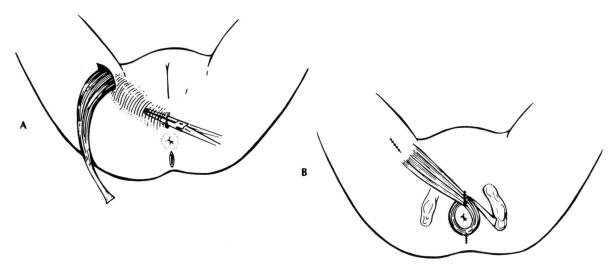

FIGURE 30-13. Gracilis muscle transfer. *A.* Gracilis muscle is harvested and tunneled subcutaneously. *B,* Anal canal is encircled and tendon is sutured to opposite ischial spine. (From Herman, F.N., Nivatvongs, S., and Goldberg, S.M.: Anal sphincter reconstruction. *In* Kodner, I.J., Fry, R.D., and Roe, J.P. [eds.]: Colon, Rectal and Anal Surgery. Current Techniques and Controversies. St. Louis, C.V. Mosby, 1985, p. 32, with permission.)

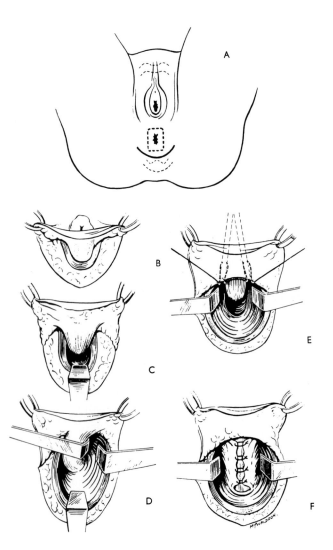

FIGURE 30-14. Parks' postanal sphincter reconstruction. *A.* Posterior circumanal incision. *B* through *D,* Intersphincteric plane dissection to level of pelvic floor. *E* and *F,* Plication of puborectalis across the midline behind the anal canal. (From Parks, A.G.: Anorectal disorders. *In* Scott, R.B., and Walker, R.M. [eds.]: The Medical Annual 1971. Bristol, John Wright and Sons, Ltd., 1971, with permission.)

An occasional suppository or enema may be all that is needed to re-establish function. The major complications of this procedure are infection and erosion of the band through the skin. In both instances, the band must be removed, and the patient returns to the preoperative status.

The encirclement of the anus with synthetic material is not often used in young patients because of long-term complications from the synthetic material. An alternative is the more extensive procedure that uses a muscle transfer to encircle the anal canal. The most popular is the gracilis muscle sling popularized by Corman.[6] The gracilis muscle is harvested from the medial aspect of the thigh, protecting its neurovascular supply (Fig. 30–13A). It is then tunneled through the subcutaneous tissue under the groin to the perineum. The muscle is looped around the anal canal and is then secured to the ischial spine on the opposite side of the anus (Fig. 30–13B). The muscle may retain function after this procedure and, with voluntary contraction, continence is maintained. The results have been variable using this technique, and it has been reserved for cases in which other techniques have failed.

Recently, a technique for combining the gracilis muscle transposition and an implantable tetanic stimulator has been described by Williams and associates.[52] The potential for avoiding a colostomy after abdominoperineal resection or in the setting of intractable neurogenic anal incontinence is very attractive. Early results are encouraging. An implantable artificial sphincter has also been used in a limited group of patients with variable success.[4] The potential for infection, erosion, and malfunction of the reservoir-type mechanism used in urologic procedures is high. Manufacturers have been reluctant to continue production as a result.

Parks first described a procedure to re-establish a long posterior anal canal and recreate an acute anorectal angle in patients with idiopathic anal incontinence.[34] The "postanal repair" is performed through a posterior circumanal incision at the anal verge (Fig. 30–14A). The intersphincteric groove is entered and the external sphincter is dissected from the internal sphincter to the level of puborectalis muscle and pelvic floor (Fig. 30–14B through D). The external sphincter and puborectalis muscle are then plicated across the midline using interrupted sutures to push the anal canal anteriorly (Fig. 30–14E and F). The repair is begun at the puborectalis, which is the deepest point of the dissection, and is extended in layers out along the external sphincter. The success of the postanal repair seems to depend on the extent of the nerve injury causing the incontinence. There was an improvement of 80% in a series of patients from St. Mark's treated for idiopathic anal incontinence using this technique.[35] Restoration of anal continence does not seem to depend on the restored anorectal angle, since there is minimal change in this portion of the sphincter when these patients are studied using defecography.[53] The effect may indeed be to increase the length of the anal canal and afford more muscle bulk and resistance to elimination. Postanal repair can improve continence in patients who have been treated for rectal prolapse if the incontinence persists after rectopexy. Complete control after combined rectopexy and postanal repair has been reported in 87% of patients with prolapse and incontinence.[19]

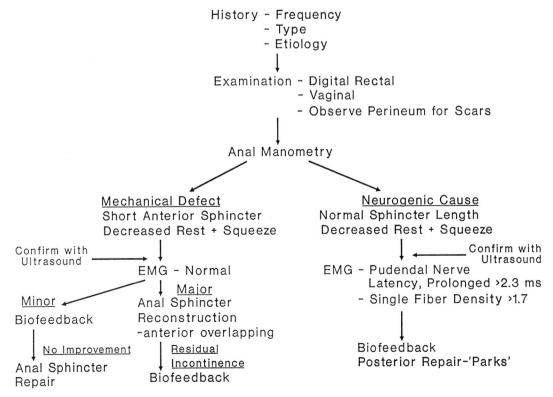

FIGURE 30-15. Algorithm for evaluation and management of anal incontinence.

CONCLUSION

The problem of anal incontinence has stimulated the investigation of anal and pelvic floor physiology. New techniques for investigation are available that allow better definition of normal and pathologic function. The causes of incontinence can be divided into three main categories: mechanical injury, neurogenic, and idiopathic. Incontinence can probably be avoided by restricted use of the midline episiotomy, cautious anterior fistulotomy (especially in women), early diagnosis of intussusception and prolapse, and limiting sphincter injury during surgical procedures in the presence of nerve injury. There are numerous techniques to retrain and repair the sphincter. The patient should be investigated thoroughly in order to evolve the best plan for management. After treatment, an objective means of following these patients is needed, and the use of manometry and electromyography should accomplish this. It is sometimes helpful to see an algorithm to begin the evaluation and plan treatment for a patient with anal incontinence. Figure 30–15 provides a suggested flow of decisions making use of available physiologic tests and viable treatment options to best treat the patient with anal incontinence.

REFERENCES

1. Buser, W., and Miner, P.B.: Delayed rectal sensation with fecal incontinence. Successful treatment using anal manometry. Gastroenterology, 91:1186, 1986.
2. Birnbaum, E.H., Dreznik, Z., Myerson, R.J., et al.: Early effect of external beam radiation therapy on the anal sphincter: A study using anal manometry and transrectal ultrasound. Dis. Colon Rectum, 35:757, 1992.
3. Browning, G.G.P., and Motson, R.W.: Anal sphincter injury, management and results of Parks sphincter repair. Ann. Surg., 199(3):351, 1984.
4. Christiansen, J., and Lorentzen, M.: Implantation of artificial sphincter for anal incontinence: Report of five cases. Dis. Colon Rectum, 32:432, 1989.
5. Christiansen, J., and Pedersen, I.K.: Traumatic anal incontinence. Results of surgical repair. Dis. Colon Rectum, 30:189, 1987.
6. Corman, M.L.: Gracilis muscle transposition. In Henry, M.M., and Swash, M. (eds.): Coloproctology and the Pelvic Floor. London, Butterworth's, 1985.
7. Critchlow, J.F., Houlihan, M.J., Landolt, C.C., and Weinstein, M.E.: Primary sphincter repair in anorectal trauma. Dis. Colon Rectum, 28:945, 1985.
8. deVries, P.A., and Pena, A.: Posterior sagittal anoplasty. J. Pediatr. Surg., 17:638, 1982.
9. Engel, B.T., Nikoomanesh, P., and Schuster, M.M.: Operant conditioning of rectosphincteric responses in the treatment of fecal incontinence. N. Engl. J. Med., 290:646, 1974.
10. Fleshman, J.W., Peters, W.R., Shemesh, E.I., et al.: Anal sphincter reconstruction: Overlapping muscle repair. Dis. Colon Rectum, 34:739, 1991.
11. Fleshman, J.W., Dreznik, Z., Fry, R.D., and Kodner, I.J.: Anal sphincter repair for obstetric injury: Manometric evaluation of functional results. Dis. Colon Rectum, 34:1061, 1991.
12. Fry, R.D., Shemesh, E.I., Kodner, I.J., and Timmcke, A.E.: Techniques and results in the management of anal and perianal Crohn's disease. Surg. Gynecol. Obstet., 168:42, 1989.
13. Fry, R.D., and Kodner, I.J.: CIBA Clinical Symposia, 37(6):2, 1985.
14. Go, P.M.N.Y.H., and Dunselman, G.A.J.: Anatomic and functional results of surgical repair after perineal rupture at delivery. Surg. Gynecol. Obstet., 166:121, 1988.
15. Goldberg, S.M., Gordon, P.H., and Nivatvong, S.: Essentials of Anorectal Surgery. Philadelphia, J.B. Lippincott, 1980.
16. Gordon, P.H.: Management of anorectal abscess and fistulas disease. In Kodner, I.J., Fry, R.D., and Roe, J.P. (eds.): Colon Rectal and Anal Surgery. St. Louis, C.V. Mosby, 1985, p. 91.
17. Hoffman, M.J., Kodner, I.J., and Fry, R.D.: Internal intussusception of the rectum. Diagnosis and surgical management. Dis. Colon Rectum, 27:435, 1984.
18. Jones, P.N., Lubowski, D.Z., Swash, M., and Henry, M.M.: Relation between perineal descent and pudendal nerve damage in idiopathic fecal incontinence. Int. J. Colorectal Dis., 2:93, 1987.
19. Keighley, M.R.B., and Matheson, D.M.: Results of treatment for rectal prolapse and fecal incontinence. Dis. Colon Rectum, 24:449, 1981.
20. Kiff, E.S., and Swash, M.: Slowed conduction in the pudendal nerves in idiopathic (neurogenic) fecal incontinence. Br. J. Surg., 71:614, 1984.
21. Kuijpers, H.C., Bleijenberg, G., and deMorree, H.: The spastic pelvic floor syndrome. Large bowel outlet obstruction caused by pelvic floor obstruction. A radiological study. Int. J. Colorectal Dis., 1:44, 1986.
22. Lubowski, D.Z., Nicholls, R.J., Swash, M., and Jordan, M.J.: Neural control of internal anal sphincter function. Br. J. Surg., 74:668, 1987.
23. MacLeod, J.H.: Biofeedback in the management of partial anal incontinence: A preliminary report. Dis. Colon Rectum, 22:169, 1979.
24. Marti, M.D., Morel, P., and Rohner, A.: Traumatic lesions of the rectum. Int. J. Colorectal Dis., 1:152, 1986.
25. McHugh, S.M., and Diamant, N.E.: Anal canal pressure profile: A reappraisal as determined by rapid pullthrough technique. Gut, 28:1234, 1987.
26. Miller, R., Bartolo, D.C.C., Roe, A., et al.: Anal sensation and the continence mechanism. Dis. Colon Rectum, 31:433, 1988.
27. Miller, R. Bartolo, D.C.C., Cervero, F., and Mortensen, N.J.McC.: Anorectal sampling: A comparison of normal and incontinent patients. Br. J. Surg., 75:44, 1988.
28. Miller, R., Bartolo, D.C.C., Cervero, F., and Mortensen, N.J.McC.: Anorectal temperature sensation—a comparison of normal and incontinent patients. Br. J. Surg., 74:511, 1987.
29. Miller, R., Bartolo, D.C.C., Lock-Edmunds, J.C., and Mortensen, N.J.: Prospective study of conservative and operative treatment for faecal incontinence. Br. J. Surg., 75:101, 1988.
30. Neill, M.E., Parks, A.G., and Swash, M.: Physiological studies of the anal musculature in fecal incontinence and rectal prolapse. Br. J. Surg., 68:531, 1981.
31. Neill, M.E., and Swash, M.: Increased motor unit fiber density in the external anal sphincter in ano-rectal incontinence: A single fiber EMG study. J. Neurol. Neurosurg. Psychiatry, 43:343, 1980.
32. Nivatvong, S., Stern, H.S., and Fryd, D.S.: The length of the anal canal. Dis. Colon Rectum, 24(8):600, 1981.
33. O'Riordan, M.G., Molloy, R.G., Gillen, P., et al.: Rectoanal inhibitory reflex following low stapled anterior resection of the rectum. Dis. Colon Rectum, 35:874, 1992.
34. Parks, A.G.: Anorectal disorders. In Scott, R.B., and Walker, R.M. (eds.): The Medical Annual. Bristol, John Wright & Sons, 1971.
35. Parks, A.G.: Anorectal incontinence. Proc. R. Soc. Med., 6:681, 1975.
36. Parks, A.G., and Stitz, R.W.: The treatment of high fistula-in-ano. Dis. Colon Rectum, 19:487, 1976.
37. Percy, J.P., Neill, M.E., Swash, M., and Parks, A.: Electrophysiological study of motor nerve supply of pelvic floor. Lancet, i:16, 1981.
38. Pezim, M.E., Spencer, J.R., Stanhope, C.R., et al.: Sphincter repair for fecal incontinence after obstetrical and iatrogenic injury. Dis. Colon Rectum, 30:521, 1987.
39. Prasad, M.L., Pearl, R.K., Abcarian, H., et al.: Perineal proctectomy, posterior rectopexy, and postanal levator repair for the treatment of rectal prolapse. Dis. Colon Rectum, 29(9):547, 1986.
40. Read, N.W., Bartolo, D.C.C., and Read, M.D.: Differences in anal function in patients with incontinence to solids and in patients with incontinence to liquids. Br. J. Surg., 71:39, 1984.
41. Read, N.W., Haynes, W.G., Bartolo, D.C.C., et al.: Use of anorectal manometry during rectal infusion of saline to investigate sphincter function in incontinent patients. Gastroenterology, 85:105, 1983.
42. Rogers, J., Henry, M.M., and Misieurcz, J.J.: Combined sensory and motor deficit in primary neuropathic anal incontinence. Gut, 29:5, 1988.

43. Shemesh, E.I., Kodner, I.J., Fry, R.D., and Neufeld, D.M.: Endorectal sliding flap repair of complicated anterior anoperineal fistulas, Dis. Colon Rectum, *31:*22, 1988.

44. Simmang, C.L., Birnbaum, E.H., Fry, R.D., Kodner, I.J., and Fleshman, J.W.: Anal sphincter reconstruction in the elderly: Does advancing age affect outcome? Dis. Colon Rectum, *37:*1065, 1994.

45. Snooks, S.J., Henry, M.M., and Swash, M.: Anorectal incontinence and rectal prolapse: Differential assessment of the innervation to puborectalis and external anal sphincter muscles. Gut, *26:*470, 1985.

46. Snooks, S.J., and Swash, M.: Nerve stimulation techniques. Pudendal nerve terminal motor latency, and spinal stimulation. *In* Henry, M.M., and Swash, M. (eds.): Coloproctology and the Pelvic Floor. Pathophysiology and Management. London, Butterworth's, 1985, p. 112.

47. Snooks, S.J., Swash, M., Henry, M.M., and Setchell, M.: Risk factors in childbirth causing damage to the pelvic floor innervation. Int. J. Colorectal Dis., *1:*20, 1986.

48. Swash, M., Snooks, S.J., and Henry, M.M.: Unifying concepts of pelvic floor disorders and incontinence. J. R. Soc. Med., *78:*906, 1985.

49. Taylor, B.M., Beart, R.W., and Phillips, S.F.: Longitudinal and radial variations of pressure in the human anal sphincter. Gastroenterology, *86:*693, 1984.

50. Tjandra, J.J., Milsom, J.W., Stolfi, V.M., et al.: Endoluminal ultrasound defines anatomy of the anal canal and pelvic floor. Dis. Colon Rectum, *35:*465, 1992.

51. Wald, A.: Biofeedback for neurogenic fecal incontinence: Rectal sensation is a determinant of outcome. J. Pediatr. Gastroenterol. Nutr., *2:*302, 1983.

52. Williams, N.S., Hallan, R.I., Koeze, T.H., and Watkens, E.S.: Restoration of gastrointestinal continuity and continence after abdominoperineal excision of the rectum using an electrically stimulated neoanal sphincter. Dis. Colon Rectum, *33:*561, 1990.

53. Womack, N.R., Morrison, J.F.B., and Williams, N.S.: Prospective study of the effects of postanal repair in neurogenic fecal incontinence. Br. J. Surg., *75:*48, 1988.

Chapter 31

BENIGN ANAL STRICTURES

JOHN G. BULS

Nonmalignant stricture of the anal canal is a relatively uncommon but debilitating condition. Patients with this problem have anal pain, obstipation, and frequent bleeding. Most experience chronic anal ulceration and fissures, and virtually all depend on various regimens of laxatives, stool softeners, enemas, and suppositories to initiate and promote defecation. When the stricture is caused by physical trauma, particularly previous anal surgery, most patients also complain of incontinence secondary to the dense inflexible band of scar tissue that forms in the anal canal.

Although previous anal surgery is the most common cause of anal stricturization, it is by no means the only cause of this problem. Idiopathic anal strictures are occasionally seen in older individuals in particular. In this situation, no obvious underlying local pathologic problem is encountered. Usually, the cause is protracted laxative abuse, especially abuse of mineral oil. These patients experience stricturization because of anal disuse. The abuse of mineral oil and other cathartics that produce liquid stools prevents the normal dilation of the anal canal with formed stool. This leads to a contracted, shortened, and inflexible anal canal.[8,9]

In other situations, congenital malformations of the anal tract may produce anal stricturization and stenosis. Specific inflammatory processes, such as Crohn's disease, can also produce this problem. Specific infections, particularly lymphogranuloma venereum, tuberculosis, and actinomycosis, all of which are uncommon in the general population, can also result in this problem.[2] Uncommon nonspecific inflammatory processes such as chronic perianal sepsis with fistula and chronic proctitis may also cause stricturization. Trauma, particularly physical trauma resulting from injury or operation, or trauma caused by chemical, thermal, or radiation damage, may also cause stricturization. One must also consider anoeroticism as a possible cause of repeated anal trauma with concomitant scar formation and stricturization.[9]

Diagnosis of anal stricture is simple, with the patient vividly describing the sensation of anal canal obstruction at the time of defecation. The degree of stricturization will be evident to the examiner at the time of digital examination. Very often it will not be possible to insert a well-lubricated index finger into such an anal canal. It may be necessary to use a well-lubricated fifth digit to complete the digital examination or to defer this procedure until examination is conducted under anesthesia. Endoscopic visualization of the anal canal is similarly difficult, as it is unlikely that the physician could pass even the medium-sized (15-mm) proctoscope in someone with significant stricture. The use of an 11-mm stricturoscope is an alternative. Most patients will not have had an anorectal examination for many years because of dread of the pain and discomfort of the procedure and because of the difficulty that previous examiners have encountered in doing an examination.

INFLAMMATORY BOWEL DISEASE

Crohn's disease, which can involve both the rectum and anal canal, may result in stricturization of the anus. In some instances, it is associated with perianal abscesses and fistulas, which in themselves can aggravate the problem. Strictures usually are situated in the rectum proper above the dentate line, but they can also involve the lower anal canal. This problem is diagnosed by inspection of the anal canal, which will reveal the characteristic perianal features of Crohn's disease. Digital examination reveals a tubular inflammatory stricture unlike that caused by congenital stenosis or trauma, which is usually short and annular. Inflammatory strictures are less well demarcated and taper off gradually into the rectum.[9]

A conservative approach to the management of these strictures is best. Gentle dilation at intervals with the patient under general anesthesia is the procedure of choice. Forceful stretching of the sphincters and operative approaches involving sphincterotomy, fistulotomy, and other aggressive treatments are to be avoided because of the likelihood of producing anal incontinence, which would markedly aggravate the problem and might precipitate the need for rectal removal when none existed previously.

INFLAMMATORY STRICTURES FROM OTHER CAUSES

Other specific inflammatory strictures are relatively uncommon. Most are directly identified by biopsy, bacteriologic culture, or other laboratory examinations. Specific anorectal infections such as tuberculosis, actinomycosis, and lymphogranuloma have become very rare in the United States. It must be remembered that gonorrheal infection of the rectum is still quite frequent. Stricturization as a consequence of these infections is rare because most of these conditions can now be controlled with effective medical therapy.

A pronounced tendency for the development of anal stenosis is seen in patients who have undergone a jejunoileal bypass operation for morbid obesity. These patients have persistent diarrhea and also often manifest the symptoms of chronic anal fissure. Treatment by multiple internal sphincterotomy procedures without sacrifice of the anal canal lining, together with efforts to control diarrhea, has been beneficial in these cases.[9]

TRAUMATIC STRICTURE

The majority of patients seen with significant anal stricturization are those in whom the stricture has resulted from some form of physical trauma, particularly previous anorectal surgery. The procedure most likely to result in this problem is hemorrhoidectomy.[4,10] It has been estimated that 5 to 10% of patients who have undergone hemorrhoidectomy will experience some form of anal stenosis. Few of these patients will have strictures severe enough to require subsequent plastic repair.[3] It appears that operations using a circumanal incisions, such as the Whitehead and Buie procedures, are more prone to stricture formation. It is rare for this complication to follow a procedure in which radial incision, such as the Fergusson and Fansler techniques, are used. Hopefully, with better training and more attention to surgical technique, the incidence of stricture and stenosis will decrease. Any hemorrhoidectomy in which excessive amounts of anoderm and perianal skin are excised will result in scar formation, contracture, and ultimate stricture.[10]

Traumatic strictures may also result from thermal or chemical burns or radiation damage. Sclerotherapy of hemorrhoids is a rare cause of stricture and results from extrarectal injection of the phenol in vegetable oil sclerosant. Electrocautery may cause stricture when used repeatedly for the removal of polyps, as in the treatment of adenomatous polyposis or Gardner's syndrome.

Treatment of Traumatic Stricture

Early after hemorrhoidectomy or any anal operation, edema from postoperative inflammation results in a functional stenosis of the anal canal.[3,10] If left untreated, particularly in a patient with erratic, irregular bowel habits, it may result in a true fibrotic stricture. This condition can be prevented in all cases by immediate postoperative use of bulk-forming stool softeners. It is not necessary to undertake any form of deliberate dilation of the anal canal with the digit or instruments. Routine dilation of the anal canal at certain set intervals after an anorectal operation is painful and unnecessary and usually results in more rectal trauma, which ultimately may produce a stricture, rather than prevent one. The most physiologic way of dilating the anal canal, particularly in situations in which there is postoperative pain, is to ensure that the patient has regular, soft, formed, bulky stools. Persisting diarrhea with frequent watery stools results in nondilation of the anal canal and aggravates the potential for permanent stricture formation.

Patients who experience significant stricturization in the early postoperative period after hemorrhoidectomy and who do not respond to increased stool bulk are best treated by anal dilation. This procedure should be initiated under anesthesia so that the anal canal can be adequately inspected to rule out an underlying problem. In many such patients, an unhealed anal wound that produces the same pathologic condition as an anal fissure will be found. This results in subcutaneous stricture formation and stenosis of the internal anal sphincter. In such circumstances, a partial internal sphincterotomy is indicated for permanent treatment of this problem and it usually results in healing of the previously unhealed wound and correction of the anal stenosis and fissure. Repeated dilations under such circumstances are usually not necessary and are to be condemned.

OPERATIVE REPAIR

All operations for the relief of benign anorectal stricture or stenosis are performed under anesthesia. At the patient's request or the anesthesiologist's preference, it can be general inhalational anesthesia or regional block anesthesia. Direct local anesthesia is not recommended, as it will not provide satisfactory pain relief and relaxation of this area to enable the operative procedure to be performed. In all instances, local anesthetic agents containing dilute epinephrine solutions are used to supplement postoperative pain relief and to provide better hemostatic control at the time of surgery. Patients are admitted to the hospital the day of operation. Bowel preparation is difficult for these patients because of the stenosis; hence, no formal bowel preparation is used. Antibiotics, oral or parenteral, are not routinely used.

The prone–jackknife position—a firm roll under the hips, a pillow under the feet, and the buttocks taped apart—is the operative position of choice. It allows perfect visualization of the perineum and anal canal.

Division of Anal Stricture with Internal Sphincterotomy (Fig. 31-1)

Patients with mild anorectal stenosis caused by a relatively narrow annular band that is within easy reach of the examining finger or anoscope should undergo division of the stricture with internal sphincterotomy. This is the usual situation after stricture formation from an unhealed hemorrhoidectomy wound or with a chronic anal fissure.[10]

With the patient in the prone–jackknife position and under anesthesia, the perineum is cleansed and draped. The area is inspected to confirm the presence of stricture. The anal canal is exposed using a bivalve anal speculum. The presence of a fissure, usually in the midline and most likely posteriorly, is confirmed along with the anal stenosis. A lateral quadrant of the anal canal is then exposed and a linear incision is made to divide skin and anoderm along with any subcutaneous stricture. This exposes the lower part of the internal sphincter muscle, which is invariably stenotic. Varying degrees of this muscle are divided. In most cases, the full thickness of the internal sphincter is transected inferior to the dentate line. This incision and sphincterotomy successfully relieves the stenosis. The small wound is closed with absorbable sutures after hemostasis has been achieved with electrocautery. This procedure is usually conducted on an outpatient basis, and the patient can be discharged once recovery from the anesthesia is complete. It is imperative for the patient to continue with a bowel regimen to ensure that soft, formed, bulky stools are passed on a regular basis commencing immediately after surgery. The wounds heal rapidly and recurrence is rare.

Subcutaneous division of the internal sphincter can be performed.[9] This results in a much smaller perianal wound and has the theoretic advantage of more rapid healing. This technique cannot be used in patients who have significant scar formation, as delineation of the internal sphincter is not possible until the subcutaneous stricture has been divided (Fig. 31-2).

Y-V Anoplasty (Fig. 31-3)

In some patients with strictures, particularly when they are caused by anal fissure or posthemorrhoidectomy problems, it is necessary to use an advancement flap of perianal skin to reline the anal canal in order to correct the stenosis.[1] This technique should not be used in older patients, particularly those with thin perianal skin, as the blood supply to the flap cannot be ensured. This technique is particularly useful in a more muscular, thick-skinned man. The procedure is performed with the patient in the prone–jackknife position. The buttocks are taped apart, with wide placement of the tape to ensure free access to all of the perianal skin. Use of local anesthesia with complete perianal and anal canal block is performed to supplement the general anesthesia. The V-shaped flap is outlined. The anal fissure, usually located in the midline posteriorly, is excised along with the thick band of fibrotic scar. The internal sphincter is incised to perform a sphincterotomy in this area. The apex of the V commences at the exterior excision line for the fissure, incising laterally in a V-shape. It is important that the base of the flap be broad. Excision of the fissure and scar tissue may sometimes be difficult, as the stenosis may be so severe that the use of a standard anal speculum is precluded. Under such circumstances, a nasal speculum may be substituted.

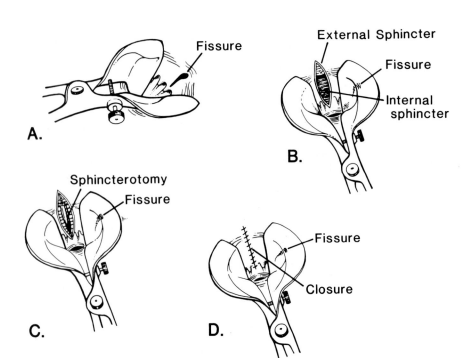

FIGURE 31-1. Internal sphincterotomy using direct exposure. *A,* The anal fissure is identified using a bivalve anal speculum. *B,* A lateral anal quadrant is exposed; a linear incision identified the internal sphincter. *C,* The lower half of the internal sphincter is divided. *D,* The incision is closed with absorbable suture.

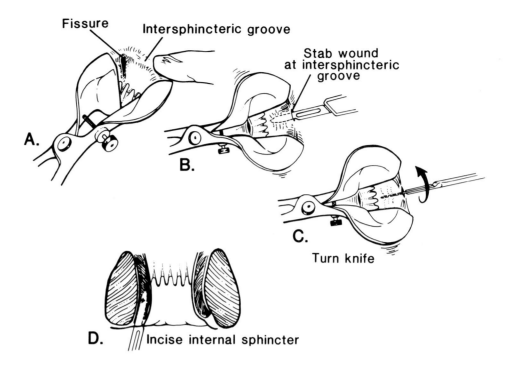

FIGURE 31–2. Internal sphincterotomy using a closed method. *A,* The anal fissure is identified using a bivalve anal speculum, and the intersphincteric groove is palpated. *B,* A stab incision is made in a lateral quadrant through the intersphincteric groove. *C,* The knife is turned. *D,* The lower half of the internal sphincter is completely divided.

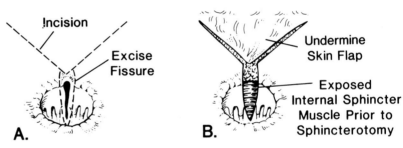

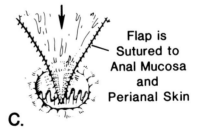

FIGURE 31–3. Y-V anoplasty. *A,* The anal fissure and stenotic area is excised. A V flap of posterior perianal skin is outlined, ensuring a broad base. *B,* The flap is raised and a partial internal sphincterotomy is performed. *C,* The mobilized flap is advanced to the dentate line and sutured with absorbable sutures.

The flap is deeply incised to ensure that subcutaneous fat is elevated with it. To preserve viability, the fascia over the subcutaneous external sphincter muscle determines the depth necessary. This flap is raised for a distance sufficient to enable the skin and subcutaneous fat to be advanced without tension to the dentate line or above. Perfect hemostasis is critical in the subcutaneous tissues. After verification of good viability, the apex of the mobilized flap is anchored to the anal canal wound at or slightly above the dentate line. Absorbable polyglycolic acid sutures, usually 3-0, are used. The lateral components of the flap are sutured to the anoderm and perianal skin with absorbable sutures of a similar material. If bleeding is a problem, a small Penrose

drain can be brought out through one of the lateral suture lines.[11]

Postoperatively, a normal diet is begun and the patient is positioned to avoid any undue or prolonged pressure on the graft. Sitz baths are not used until 24 hours have elapsed. Bulk-forming stool softeners are given after the procedure and the patient can be discharged after having had a bowel movement.

Diamond Flap (Fig. 31–4)

An alternative method of providing soft perianal skin for a flap is the diamond flap. The preparation for this

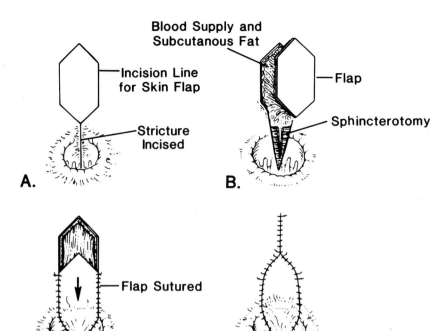

FIGURE 31-4. Diamond flap. *A*, The anal stricture is incised in the lateral quadrant of the anal canal. A diamond-shaped flap is outlined in the adjacent perianal skin. *B*, A partial internal sphincterotomy is performed. The flap is mobilized by deep incision into the subcutaneous tissues, but the blood supply to the isolated skin island is preserved. *C*, The mobilized flap is advanced into the anal canal and sutured to the dentate line with absorbable sutures. *D*, The remainder of the skin wounds are closed.

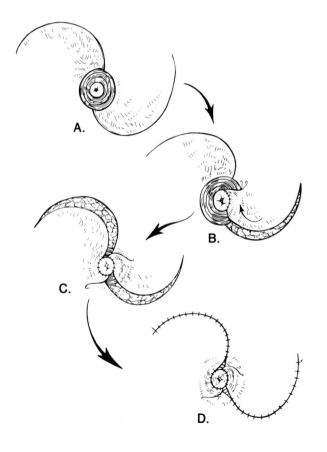

FIGURE 31-5. S flap technique. *A*, The anoderm or mucosal ectropion, along with the stricture, has been excised to the dentate line, exposing the internal sphincter. The S flaps are outlined in the buttock skin. *B*, The flaps are mobilized by deep undercutting. The mobilized flap is sutured at the level of the dentate line to completely cover the lower anal canal with skin. *C*, A similar procedure is performed on the other side if required. The large wounds are closed completely.

procedure and the position and anesthetic used are identical to those used for the Y-V flap. In this procedure, the stricture is incised and a sphincterotomy is performed. Excess scar tissue is removed. The flap will be an island of perianal skin along with its undisturbed subcutaneous fat containing the blood and nerve supplies. Such a technique can be used anywhere in the circumference of the anal canal, although it is best performed in the lateral quadrants. This technique can also be used for patients with thin skin, particularly older individuals. With a deep enough incision into the subcutaneous fat, the perianal skin can be advanced for a distance of several centimeters into the anal canal.[5] The flap is sutured as in the Y-V anoplasty, using absorbable sutures. This diamond island flap technique provides a very satisfactory alternative to the Y-V anoplasty and has proved to be a safe and effective method of treating strictures.

S Flaps (Fig. 31–5)

S flaps are used in situations in which the anoderm has been removed or will require removal for treatment of some specific condition such as Paget's disease or Bowen's disease of the anal area. This is a much more extensive operation and requires complete mechanical and antibiotic bowel preparation along with a period of bowel rest immediately after the procedure. This is a method of substituting perianal and buttock skin for anoderm and reconstituting a new dentate line high in the anal canal. It can be constructed bilaterally in certain circumstances, particularly when severe ectropion following an amputative hemorrhoidectomy has resulted in incontinence, mucous discharge, and stricturization. The S flap technique should be used with caution in older individuals because of poor blood supply to the skin. The wide mobilization necessary for this technique may result in sloughing of one or more of the flaps.[6,7]

REFERENCES

1. Angelchik, P.D., Harms, B.A., and Starling, J.R.: Repair of anal stricture and mucosal ectropion with Y-V or pedical flap anoplasty. Am. J. Surg., *166*:55, 1993.
2. Annamunthodo, H.: Rectal lymphogranuloma venereum in Jamaica. Dis. Colon Rectum, *4*:17, 1961.
3. Buls, J.G., and Goldberg, S.M.: Modern management of hemorrhoids. Surg. Clin. North Am., *58*:469, 1978.
4. Carver, N., Desai, S.N., and Gelister, J.: Skin grafting to the anal canal for the treatment of mucocutaneous anal stricture. J. R. Coll. Surg. Edinb., *38*:46, 1993.
5. Christensen, M.A., PItsch, R.M.N., Jr., Cali, R.L., et al.: "House" advancement pedical flap for anal stenosis. Dis. Colon Rectum, *35*:201, 1992.
6. Corman, M.L., Veidenheimer, M.C., and Coller, J.A.: Anoplasty for anal stricture. Surg. Clin. North Am., *56*:727, 1976.
7. Ferguson, J.A.: Repair of "Whitehead deformity" of the anus. Surg. Gynecol. Obstet., *108*:115, 1959.
8. Goldberg, S.M., Gordon, P.H., and Nivatvongs, S.: Essentials of Anorectal Surgery. Philadelphia, J.B. Lippincott, 1980, p. 333.
9. Mazier, W.P., Demoraes, R.T., and Dignan, R.D.: Anal fissure and anal ulcers. Surg. Clin. North. Am., *58*:479, 1978.
10. Milsom, J.W., and Mazier, W.P.: Classification and management of post-surgical anal stenosis. Surg. Gynecol. Obstet., *163*:64, 1986.
11. Ramanujam, P.S., Venkatesh, K.S., and Cohen, M.: Y-V anoplasty for severe anal stenosis. Contemp. Surg., *33*:62, 1988.

Chapter 32

RADIATION INJURY OF THE RECTUM

SCOTT D. GOLDSTEIN

Radiation has been used with increasing frequency as a primary or adjuvant form of therapy. Tumors of the uterine cervix, bladder, prostate, and more recently of the rectum have been treated with adjuvant radiation. Refinement of radiation delivery systems has allowed higher doses to be utilized, and surgeons must anticipate encountering greater numbers of patients with radiation damage to the rectum.

Several factors put the rectum at risk for injury in those patients receiving radiation to the pelvic area. Its anatomic proximity to other structures,[20] its relatively fixed position in the pelvis, and significantly less peristaltic activity cause the rectum to be subjected to entire doses of radiation given through particular ports.[31] The fixation that results from pelvic surgery or pelvic inflammatory disease further increases the susceptibility of the rectum to significant radiation injury.[3,15,28]

The chronic pathophysiologic alterations observed in the radiation-injured rectum stem from a progressive obliterative endarteritis that results in ischemia. Any condition or disorder that results in poor tissue perfusion may be regarded as a risk factor. Hypertension, diabetes, and atherosclerotic vascular disease are among those diseases that put the rectum at greater risk for radiation injury,[12,44] although this is a controversial issue.[3,28]

It is of paramount importance for surgeons to understand the time, dose, and volume effects of radiation when treating patients with complications of radiation therapy.[23,26,27,31,34,36,43] A collaborative effort with a radiation therapist may help predict the potential for significant rectal complications. Tables 32–1 through 32–3 illustrate the significance of the time, dose, and volume values. The ability of normal tissues to repair radiation damage more extensively and rapidly than malignant tumors forms the biologic basis for fractionated radiation therapy. This concept allows higher tumoricidal doses to be administered without damage to normal tissues.[4,47]

Two phases of radiation injury to the gastrointestinal tract are encountered and differ in their pathogenesis.[11,23,31] The early acute phase represents the toxic ef-

fect of ionizing radiation on the actively dividing mucosal cells. Radiation disrupts cellular deoxyribonucleic acid (DNA), thereby impeding cell division. Mucosal edema, inflammatory cell infiltration, hemorrhage, and possibly ulceration may follow. These manifestations usually appear within weeks or months of irradiation and are reversible. Symptoms observed are a result of the described changes in cellular activity. Diarrhea, tenesmus, and rectal bleeding are the most frequently encountered complaints.

The late or chronic phase of radiation damage is the result of an aggressive obliterative endarteritis and ischemia. This phase is progressive and irreversible. The onset of symptoms occurs several months to years after radiation therapy. Unlike the damage seen in the acute phase, which is usually limited to the mucosa, chronic or late-stage injury often involves the full thickness of the rectum. Fibrosis, rigidity, and mucosal atrophy are noted. Rectal stricture formation is the clinical result of the ischemic process, and is the most frequent initial complication of chronic radiation injury[22] (Fig. 32–1). Fistulization stemming from ischemic damage coupled with poor tissue healing secondary to DNA disruption is a more severe injury seen on occasion with complete necrosis of the rectum. Symptoms frequently encountered are bleeding, tenesmus, and diarrhea. These chronic difficulties are not reversible, and when the symptoms are significant, a surgical approach may offer the only cure.[30]

TREATMENT OF RADIATION INJURY

Acute or Early Radiation Injury

Symptoms of acute radiation injury present during or after completion of radiation therapy, and are not unlike those seen in idiopathic proctitis. Diarrhea, tenesmus, and a bloody mucoid discharge are frequently encountered problems. In the vast majority of cases, no active treatment is required, and the symptoms subside spontaneously. In the more severe cases of acute radia-

TABLE 32-1. RELATIONSHIP OF FRACTION SIZE ON BIOLOGIC EFFECT*

TOTAL DOSE (RAD)	FRACTION SIZE	NO. OF FRACTIONS	TDF
4,500	180	25	73
4,400	200	22	73
4,500	250	18	84
4,500	300	15	92
4,400	400	11	106

*From Marks, G.: The surgical management of the radiation-injured intestine. Surg. Clin. North Am., *63*:81, 1983, with permission.
TDF = measurement of normal tissue damage.

TABLE 32-3. RELATIONSHIP OF VOLUME AND DOSE (IN RAD) FOR SMALL BOWEL INJURY*

	RADIATION INJURY	
	1-5%	25-50%
True pelvis	5,000	7,000
Total pelvis	4,500	6,000
Whole abdomen	2,500	3,500

*From Marks, G.: The surgical management of the radiation-injured intestine. Surg. Clin. North Am., *63*:81, 1983, with permission.
TDF = measurement of normal tissue damage.

tion proctitis, a more thorough work-up is warranted. First, information about the radiation dose and method of delivery should be obtained to adequately assess matters. Sometimes a short break of several days in the radiation schedule is all that is required to relieve the symptoms. If this does not prove to be successful, a flexible sigmoidoscopic evaluation should be carried out to determine the extent of the injury.

Numerous supportive measures may be tried. Diarrhea and abdominal cramping respond well to bowel rest and antidiarrheal agents such as loperamide (Imodium) or diphenoxylate (Lomotil). Low-fat, low-residue, lactose-free diets offer a reasonable hope for success. For refractory cases, asulfadine or topical steroid enemas may be tried. It must be remembered that these early injuries usually resolve with time, although there appears to be some correlation between the severity of the acute injury and the development of a late rectal injury.[9,39,41]

Chronic or Late Injury

Late radiation-induced rectal injury differs from acute rectal injury in that chronic ischemia rather than mucosal sloughing is the pathophysiologic mechanism. Conservative management described for acute injury is of little value. At this stage, which may be seen as early as 6 months or as late as 30 years after radiation therapy, surgical considerations must be entertained.[2,12,13,34,48] Indications for surgical intervention are intractable proctitis, physiologically significant bleeding, severe symptomatic strictures, radiation necrosis and perforation, and rectovaginal fistulas.

Preoperative Evaluation

When considering operative intervention, a detailed preoperative evaluation is mandatory. The initial step is

TABLE 32-2. EQUIVALENT NORMAL TISSUE EFFECTS (5 FRACTIONS/WEEK)*

FRACTION SIZE	NO. OF FRACTIONS	TOTAL DOSE (RAD)	TDF
180	25	4,500	73
200	22	4,400	73
250	16	4,000	74
300	12	3,600	74
400	8	3,200	77

*From Marks, G.: The surgical management of the radiation-injured intestine. Surg. Clin. North Am., *63*:81, 1983, with permission.
TDF = measurement of normal tissue damage.

to determine the reason for which radiation therapy was administered, as well as the field radiated and the delivery technique, in an effort to ascertain as accurately as possible the full extent of the injury. Recurrent cancers may frequently mimic chronic radiation injury, and this possibility must always be considered.[21] The extent of the radiation injury is frequently greater than anticipated, and there may well be multiorgan involvement.[30,35] Digital evaluation of the rectum and vagina will give the surgeon an appreciation of the relative compliance of these structures. Recurrent tumors may also be palpated in this manner. Contrast studies of the colon and small bowel are mandatory. The small intestine, particularly the terminal ileum, which is fixed in the pelvis, is the most radiosensitive of all the intra-abdominal organs. Twenty per cent of all patients undergoing operation for radiation injury to the rectum and sigmoid colon will have a significant small bowel injury.[3,18] A barium enema must be performed in addition to a colonoscopic evaluation to completely delineate the extent of the injury.[37] Colonoscopy alone may not fully disclose small colonenteric fistulas and mild strictures. Intravenous pyelography will reveal any ureteral changes that may occur following pelvic irradiation. Cystoscopy is mandatory if the radiation therapy was directed toward a bladder cancer, or if bladder

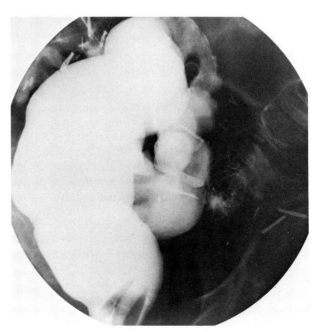

FIGURE 32-1. Radiation stricture of the rectosigmoid.

symptoms are present. Computed tomography of the abdomen will aid in the detection of recurrent cancer or metastatic disease, which would certainly alter the surgical decision-making process.

BASIC OPERATIVE STRATEGY

Regardless of the operative indications, several important technical features have general applicability.

Temporary colonic diversion prior to definitive rectal reconstructive surgery should utilize a proximal transverse loop stoma. This segment of colon is not usually involved in the irradiated field and the stoma is easily constructed. Following the reconstructive phase, the colostomy should be maintained to protect the repair. Sigmoid colostomies performed in the irradiated field carry with them a significant risk of peristomal complications[3,12,13,18,20] and require a lower abdominal entry to construct, which could interfere with the more important later definitive reconstruction stage. At the time of laparotomy, all bowel with significant injury should be removed, thereby minimizing postoperative complications as well as preventing additional late radiation injury complications.[29,30] Only healthy, nonirradiated bowel should be used for anastomosis. This requires mobilization of the splenic flexure in order to utilize the nonirradiated, tension-free mid-descending colon for the proximal portion of an anastomosis (Fig. 32–2). This ensures that at least one end of the anastomosis is created in normal, well-vascularized tissue. Because the postirradiated pelvis may be fibrotic and inflamed at the time of surgery, there is a real danger of inflicting an inadvertent ureteral injury. For this reason, ureteral catheters are inserted prior to laparotomy to identify these structures and aid the surgeon in avoiding such an occurrence.

SURGERY FOR INTRACTABLE PROCTITIS OR BLEEDING

Severe intractable proctitis and bleeding associated with a chronic radiation injury will not respond to local or supportive measures.[41] In the surgical decision-making process, the overall condition of the patient and their ability to undergo a major procedure must be carefully considered. Occasionally, blood transfusions or oral iron supplementation may be all that is required. Topical formalin has shown promise in controlling hemorrhage as has endoscopic laser photocoagulation.[29,33,38,40] These procedures are safe and certainly preclude the risks associated with major surgical procedures and probably should be attempted as a first step. Where the symptoms persist and are severe in nature, abdominoperineal resection with an end-descending colostomy or an extended sphincter-saving procedure must be considered. Simple diversion by a proximal stoma will not control these chronically severe symptoms.[19]

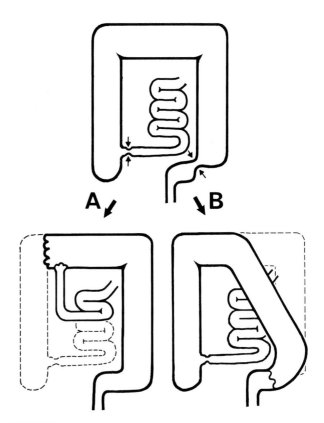

FIGURE 32–2. Terminal ileal lesions treated by right hemicolectomy and ileotransverse anastomosis (A) and rectosigmoid lesions treated by left hemicolectomy, bringing the splenic flexure down for anastomosis (B). (From Galland, R.B.: Surgical management of radiation enteritis. Surgery, 99:133, 1986, with permission.)

SURGERY FOR RECTAL STRICTURE, NECROSIS, PERFORATION, AND UPPER RECTOVAGINAL FISTULAS

Newer surgical techniques allow severe complications such as rectal stricture, necrosis, perforation, and rectovaginal fistula to be treated with a high degree of success. It should be remembered that a diverting colostomy in nonirradiated colon provides excellent palliation for these complications in poor-risk patients. If the decision is made to resect the rectum, several surgical options are available allowing the surgeon to tailor the approach to the particular circumstances encountered.

Abdominal perineal resection will remove all involved tissue, and will avoid many of the complications associated with an extremely low rectal anastomosis. This single-stage operation may well suit many patients who are too ill to undergo multistage procedures. Potential perineal wound healing difficulties can be minimized by starting the perineal phase of the dissection in an intersphincteric plane. This technique also provides viable muscle for wound closure.[17]

Most rectal injuries can be handled simply by low anterior resection. Utilizing the intraluminal mechanical circular stapler, an extremely distal anastomosis can be created successfully. The use of this approach allows the surgeon to satisfactorily manage most complications. When rectal mobilization presents a significant problem, it is best to use a proximal sigmoid patch repair with a side-to-side or an end-to-side anastomosis. This technique is particularly useful to manage mid and upper rectal strictures and fistulas in a densely fixed and immobile rectum.[6,42] Rectal resection with distal mucusectomy and coloanal anastomosis is a mandatory component of the surgeon's operative armamentarium when dealing with the radiation-injured rectum.[14,16,19,32] It is applicable for all rectal complications and can be relied upon when other reconstructive techniques fail. It carries with it two attractive advantages: that of providing well-vascularized tissue for both ends of the anastomosis, and of decreasing the possibility of further radiation complications. The success of this procedure requires only that the sphincter mechanism be of good functional quality. The impaired healing that results from radiation as well as the serious consequences of an anastomotic disruption make it necessary to create a temporary transverse colostomy in each instance. Contrast studies administered via the distal limb of the colostomy allow the anastomosis to be evaluated prior to closing the colostomy, which is usually carried out 6 to 8 weeks after initial surgery. Anastomotic strictures can be dilated transanally using an esophageal (Maloney) dilator or an endoscopic balloon dilator.

SURGERY FOR DISTAL RECTOVAGINAL FISTULA

The patients who present with radiation-induced rectovaginal fistulas are usually elderly and frequently are high-risk candidates for major abdominal surgery. When the fistula is located in the distal 6 cm of the rectum and is quite small (<1 cm), tissue interposition repair can be achieved.[1,46] The bulbocavernosus muscle is most often used for such repairs, and if successful, major abdominal surgery can be avoided (Figs. 32–3 through 32–8). A great disadvantage to the interposition repairs lies in the fact that the irradiated bowel is not resected, which puts the patient at risk for developing other complications. A temporary diverting colostomy is required if local tissues are inflamed and indurated, and should be performed to allow any complicating local condition to improve prior to attempting this repair. It must be kept in mind that a fecal diverting left-sided colostomy may well be the operation of choice in the elderly or compromised patient.

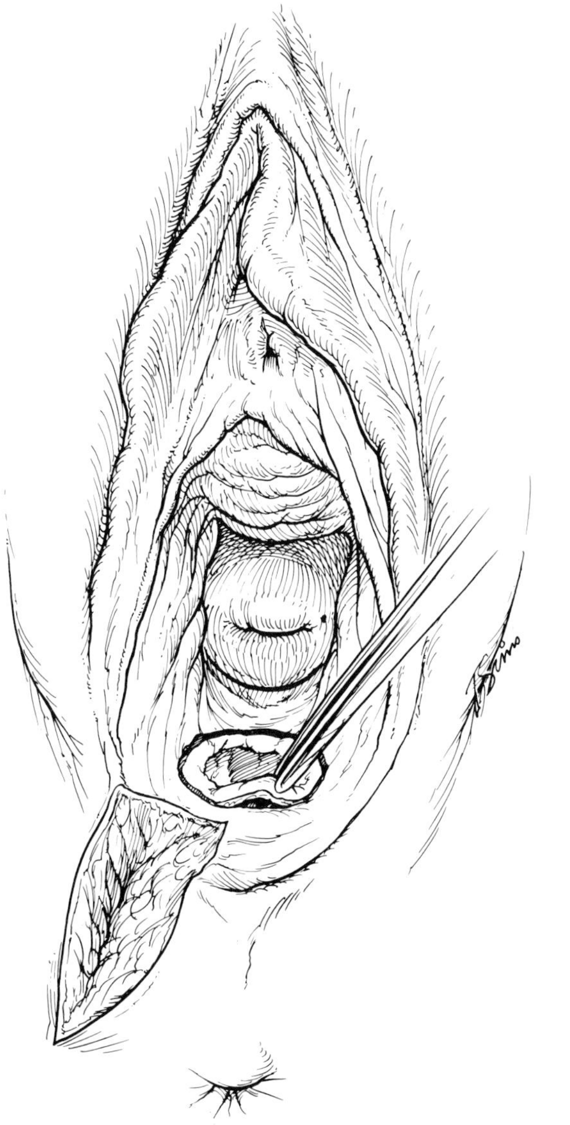

FIGURE 32-3. Bulbocavernosus flap repair of a rectovaginal fistula: incision of vaginal mucosa around the fistula. A perineotomy aids exposure. (From White, A.J.: Use of the bulbocavernosus muscle [Martius procedure] for repair of radiation induced rectovaginal fistulas. Obstet. Gynecol., *60*:114, 1982. Reprinted with permission from the American College of Obstetricians and Gynecologists.)

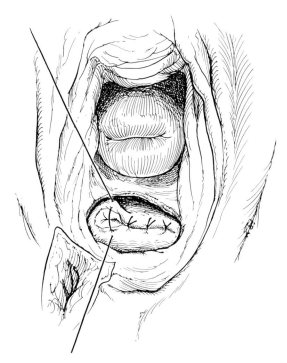

FIGURE 32-4. Transverse closure of the rectal defect. (From White, A.J.: Use of the bulbocavernosus muscle [Martius procedure] for repair of radiation induced rectovaginal fistulas. Obstet. Gynecol., *60*: 114, 118, 1982. Reprinted with permission from the American College of Obstetricians and Gynecologists.)

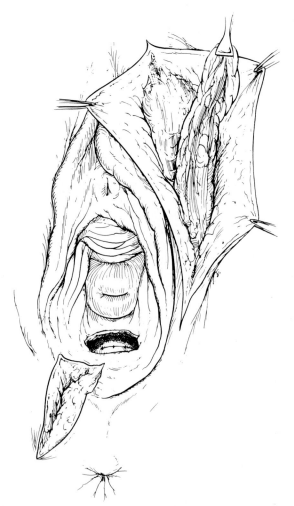

FIGURE 32-5. Mobilization of the bulbocavernosus muscle and labial fat pad. (From White, A.J.: Use of the bulbocavernosus muscle [Martius procedure] for repair of radiation induced rectovaginal fistulas. Obstet. Gynecol., *60*:114, 1982. Reprinted with permission from the American College of Obstetricians and Gynecologists.)

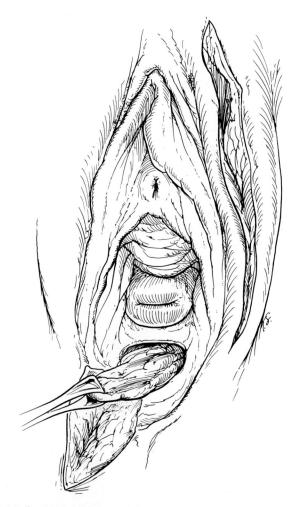

FIGURE 32-6. Pedicled bulbocavernosus placed over rectal closure. (From White, A.J.: Use of the bulbocavernosus muscle [Martius procedure] for repair of radiation induced rectovaginal fistulas. Obstet. Gynecol., *60*:114, 1982. Reprinted with permission from the American College of Obstetricians and Gynecologists.)

SURGICAL TECHNIQUES

Low Anterior Resection of the Rectum

While standard low anterior resection techniques are familiar to surgeons, there are important rules to be observed when treating irradiated bowel. A proximal transverse loop colostomy is usually performed prior to resection to permit distal inflammation to subside and to aid in achieving a more thorough evaluation of the disease process. In addition, it allows perfect mechanical bowel cleansing. The patient is placed in the supine position with the legs in stirrups to allow access to the abdomen and perineum. A balloon-tip rectal catheter is inserted into the rectum, which is then irrigated with antibiotic solution to remove residual debris. The large balloon-tip catheter should be left in place to help the surgeon identify the distal rectum during pelvic dissection. Retrograde ureteral catheters are also put in place at this time. A generous midline incision is made, allowing access to the entire colon, particularly the splenic flexure, which must be completely mobilized. Upon en-

tering the abdomen, the descending sigmoid colon junction is marked with a suture to indicate the proximal site of bowel transection. The rectum is completely mobilized posteriorly from the presacral fascia to the proximal anal canal musculature. The bladder and vagina are completely separated from the rectum anteriorly. When the rectal mobilization is completed, the rectal catheter is removed. The superior rectal and inferior mesenteric vessels are transected to allow greater mobility of the proximal colon. The rectum and sigmoid colon are then removed and a curved stapling device is applied to create the anastomosis.[24,25] Short rectal stumps are recommended because of the superior blood supply provided by the systemic circulation in the distal area. The rectal tube is reinserted and the integrity of the anastomosis is checked by insufflating air or saline with the bowel gently occluded just proximal to the anastomosis. A pelvic drain is carefully placed and the omentum is interposed between the colon and vagina. The anastomosis must be free of any tension, and the mobilized left colon should rest comfortably in the pelvis. A transverse loop colostomy must be constructed if not already present.

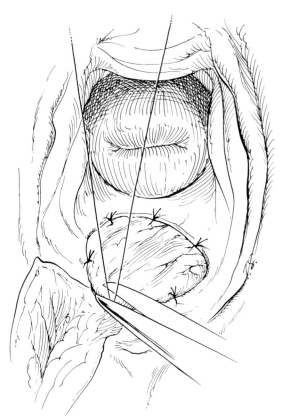

FIGURE 32-7. Pedicled bulbocavernosus sutured in place. (From White, A.J.: Use of the bulbocavernosus muscle [Martius procedure] for the repair of radiation induced rectovaginal fistulas. Obstet. Gynecol., *60*:114, 1982. Reproduced with permission from the American College of Obstetricians and Gynecologists.)

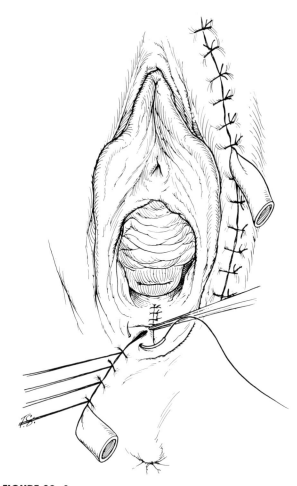

FIGURE 32-8. Closure of vagina, labium, and perineotomy. (From White, A.J.: Use of the bulbocavernosus muscle [Martius procedure] for the repair of radiation induced rectovaginal fistulas. Obstet. Gynecol., *60*:114, 1982. Reproduced with permission from the American College of Obstetricians and Gynecologists.)

ABDOMINAL TRANSANAL RESECTION WITH SUTURED COLOANAL ANASTOMOSIS

The intra-abdominal phase of this operation is performed in the same manner as that described for the low anterior resection. Special attention to complete mobilization of the left colon, splenic flexure, and transverse colon is required. The distal descending colon must reach the site of the anastomosis in the anal canal without tension. The rectum is mobilized to a point just beyond the fistula or stricture and divided at that point. The operation is continued from a perineal position. The mucosa is stripped from the sphincteric musculature with the aid of a submucosal injection of epinephrine solution (1:200,000), which helps to maintain the proper plane and assists with hemostasis. The normal nonirradiated descending colon is then passed through the muscular tube and sutured with polyglactin (Vicryl) or polyglycolic acid (Dexon) sutures in an interrupted fashion. The proximal sutures incorporate the full thickness of the descending colonic wall and the distal sutures incorporate anoderm and the internal sphincter (Figs. 32–9 through 32–14). A diverting transverse colostomy is constructed if not already present. Six to 8 weeks postoperatively, a contrast study via the distal limb of the colostomy is performed. The colostomy is then closed if no anastomotic leaks are present. Good functional results can be achieved in approximately 60 to 80% of patients. Three to six bowel movements a day are reported in most patients. Anastomotic stricture develops in 13 to 40% of patients, and usually responds to dilation.[2,8,10,14,16,32,45]

PROXIMAL SIGMOID FLAP PROCTOPLASTY

Bricker[5,6] has described another approach for the correction of a radiation-induced rectovaginal fistula or stricture that utilizes an onlay vascular sigmoid colon graft. This approach is appropriate for a select group of patients who have an otherwise normal rectum. If there is a significant degree of radiation proctitis or hemorrhage, it may be necessary to perform a rectal excision as described earlier. The Bricker technique begins with complete mobilization of the sigmoid colon and anterior rectum to expose the rectovaginal fistula or stricture. The posterior rectum need not be manipulated and the presacral space is not entered, thereby avoiding potential injury to the posterior rectum and presacral vascular plexus. The proximal sigmoid colon is divided and turned on itself, enabling the opened end to be anastomosed to the fistulous opening in the rectum af-

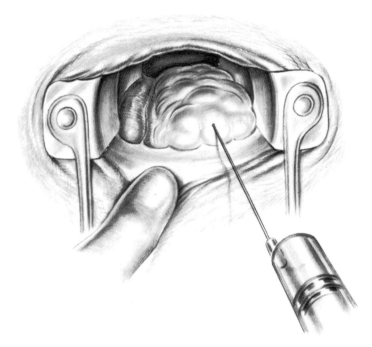

FIGURE 32-9. Rectal mucosal proctectomy and coloanal anastomosis: submucosal injection of epinephrine solution using an anal speculum. (From Parks, A.G.: Endoanal technique of low colonic anastomosis. *In* Surgical Techniques Illustrated, Vol. 2. Philadelphia, W.B. Saunders, 1985, p. 63, with permission.)

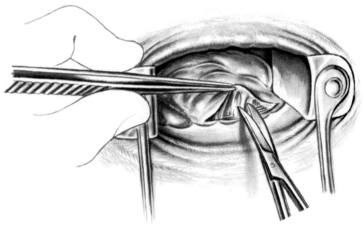

FIGURE 32-10. Dissection of the rectal mucosa off the underlying internal sphincter muscle. (From Parks, A.G.: Endoanal technique of low colonic anastomosis. *In* Surgical Techniques Illustrated, Vol. 2. Philadelphia, W.B. Saunders, 1985, p. 63, with permission.)

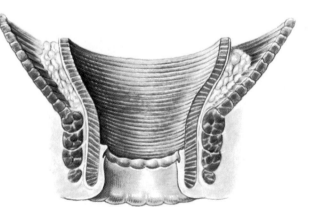

FIGURE 32-11. Mucosal proctectomy completed. (From Parks, A.G.: Endoanal technique of low colonic anastomosis. *In* Surgical Techniques Illustrated, Vol. 2. Philadelphia, W.B. Saunders, 1985, p. 63, with permission.)

ter adequate separation from the vagina. The distal descending colon is anastomosed end-to-side to the apex of the sigmoid flap (Figs. 32–15 and 32–16). A transverse colostomy is fashioned to complete the reconstruction. Steichen[42] has recently reported on his use of a modified Bricker sigmoid colon graft repair. He has in-

corporated the use of mechanical sutures for the reconstruction (Figs. 32–17 through 32–22). The benefits of this modification result from the fact that mechanical stapling devices facilitate the placement of sutures in the deep and narrow pelvis. The rectal reservoir created by either technique may alleviate the frequency and ur-

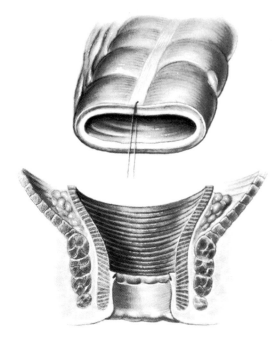

FIGURE 32-12. Cut end of descending colon pulled through rectal muscle cuff. (From Parks, A.G.: Endoanal technique of low colonic anastomosis. *In* Surgical Techniques Illustrated, Vol. 2. Philadelphia, W.B. Saunders, 1985, p. 63, with permission.)

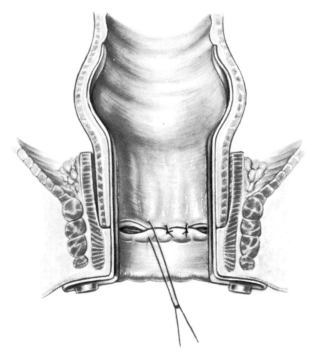

FIGURE 32-13. Coloanal anastomosis. (From Parks, A.G.: Endoanal technique of low colonic anastomosis. *In* Surgical Techniques Illustrated, Vol. 2. Philadelphia, W.B. Saunders, 1985, p. 63, with permission.)

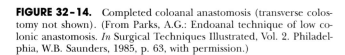

FIGURE 32-14. Completed coloanal anastomosis (transverse colostomy not shown). (From Parks, A.G.: Endoanal technique of low colonic anastomosis. *In* Surgical Techniques Illustrated, Vol. 2. Philadelphia, W.B. Saunders, 1985, p. 63, with permission.)

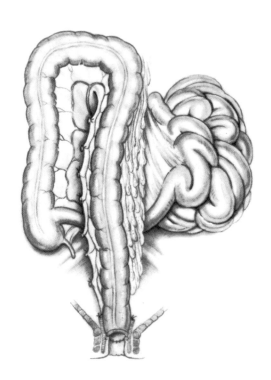

gency of evacuation so characteristic in patients with irradiated rectums.

The disadvantages of using any sigmoid colon graft repair are several, and must be carefully considered in the decision-making process. Retaining the irradiated rectum carries the potential for future problems such as bleeding and proctitis. The proximal sigmoid colon needed to accomplish the anastomosis has most often received some amount of radiation, which can result in poor healing. The divided end of the sigmoid colon may not be sufficiently long to reach deep enough into the pelvis without tension while retaining an adequate blood supply.

The procedure is also associated with significant complications. The reported rate of pelvic abscess is 9.5%; anastomotic stricture, 5.0%; sloughing or flap dehis-

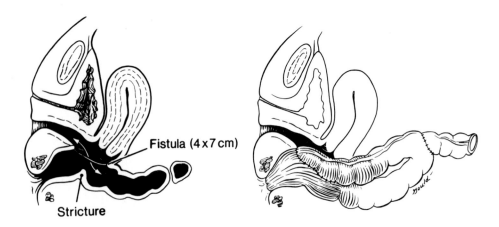

Fistula (4×7 cm)

Stricture

FIGURE 32-15. Proximal sigmoid flap proctoplasty. (From Bricker, E.M.: Repair of postirradiation rectovaginal fistula and stricture. Surg. Gynecol. Obstet., *148*:449, 1979. By permission of Surgery, Gynecology and Obstetrics.)

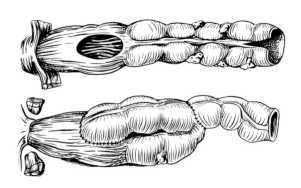

FIGURE 32-16. Proximal sigmoid flap proctoplasty; continuity is restored by suturing end of descending colon to side of the sigmoid flap (proximal diverting colostomy not shown). (From Bricker, E.M.: Repair of postirradiation rectovaginal fistula and stricture. Surg. Gynecol. Obstet., *148*:449, 1979. By permission of Surgery, Gynecology and Obstetrics.)

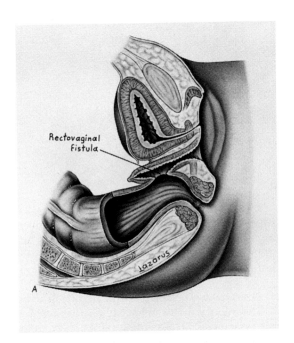

Rectovaginal Fistula

FIGURE 32-17. A rectovaginal fistula at the 4-cm level. (From Steichen, F.M.: Bricker-Johnston sigmoid colon graft for repair of postradiation rectovaginal fistula and stricture performed with mechanical sutures. Dis. Colon Rectum, *35*:599, 1992, with permission.)

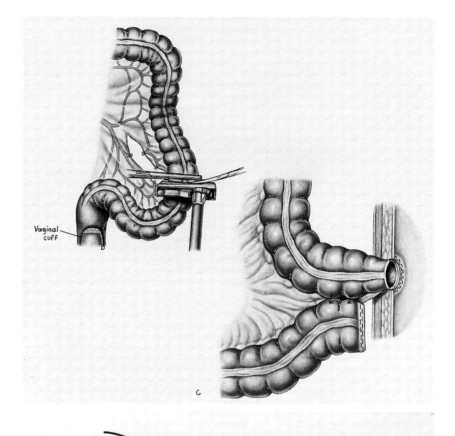

FIGURE 32-18. Hartmann's procedure performed as a first stage at the junction of the descending and sigmoid colon. (From Steichen, F.M.: Bricker-Johnston sigmoid colon graft for repair of postradiation rectovaginal fistula and stricture performed with mechanical sutures. Dis. Colon Rectum, *35:* 599, 1992, with permission.)

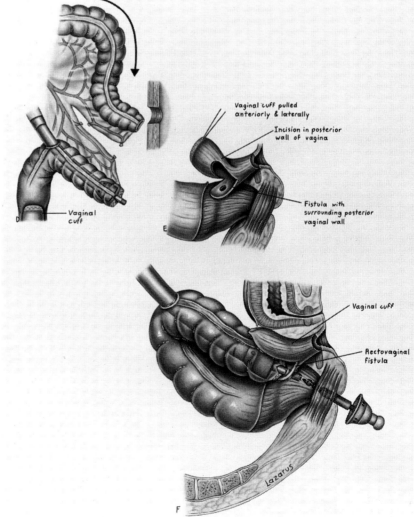

FIGURE 32-19. *3A,* Second stage: Hartmann's sigmoid pouch and descending colostomy are separated. The apex of the arch formed by the posterior rectosigmoid and anterior onlay graft of the mid and proximal sigmoid colon is incised through its antemesosigmoid wall for later placement of the CEEA instrument without anvil. *3B,* The posterior vaginal wall is elevated from the rectum by incision above and on both sides of the fistula and the fibrous rim of the fistula is exposed. *3C,* The central rod of the CEEA instrument is advanced through the linear closure of the proximal sigmoid colon and through the fistula into the rectum and is joined by the shift of the anvil advanced transanally and activated. (From Steichen, F.M.: Bricker-Johnston sigmoid colon graft for repair of postradiation rectovaginal fistula and stricture performed with mechanical sutures. Dis. Colon Rectum, *35:*599, 1992, with permission.)

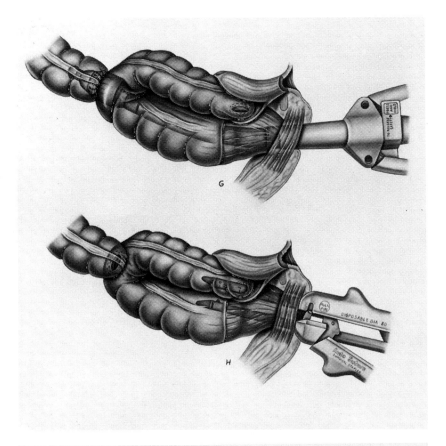

FIGURE 32-20. 4A, The CEEA 28 or 31 instrument is then advanced through the anus to accomplish an anastomosis between the apex of the arch formed by the rectum and turned-down sigmoid colon and the completely mobilized descending colon above. 4B, A long side-to-side rectosigmoidostomy is achieved with a GIA 80 or 90 instrument by placing one arm of the instrument transanally into the rectum and placing the other arm through the anus and previous fistula (now end-to-side rectosigmoidostomy) into the sigmoid colon. (From Steichen, F.M.: Bricker-Johnston sigmoid colon graft for repair of postradiation rectovaginal fistula and stricture performed with mechanical sutures. Dis. Colon Rectum, *35:* 599, 1992, with permission.)

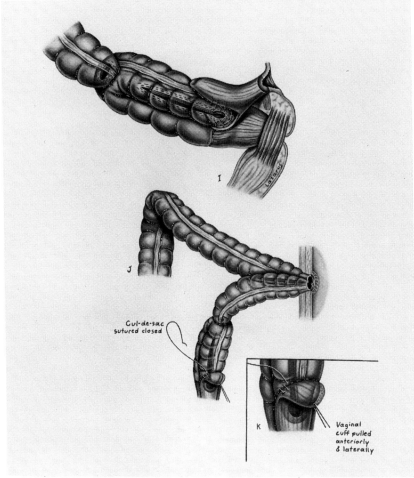

FIGURE 32-21. 5A and 5C, The posterior vaginal opening is sutured to the anterior sigmoid wall. 5B, The proximal descending colon is provided with a vented colocolostomy. (From Steichen, F.M.: Bricker-Johnston sigmoid colon graft for repair of postradiation rectovaginal fistula and stricture performed with mechanical sutures. Dis. Colon Rectum, *35:*599, 1992, with permission.)

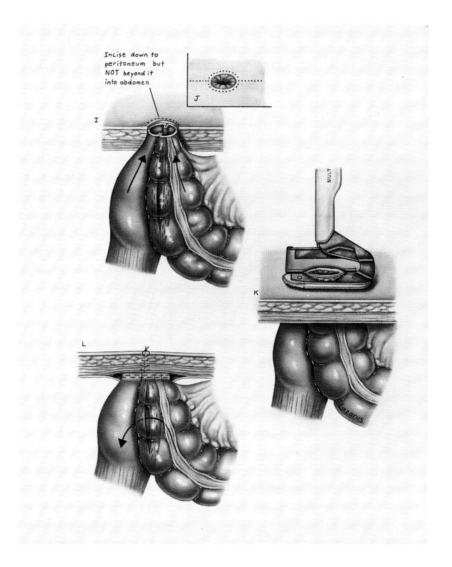

FIGURE 32-22. The third stage is accomplished under local anesthesia and on an ambulatory basis. The stoma or the colocolostomy is dissected, freed down to the peritoneum, and then closed extraperitoneally with a linear stapler, and the skin is approximated over this staple line. (From Steichen, F.M.: Bricker-Johnston sigmoid colon graft for repair of postradiation rectovaginal fistula and stricture performed with mechanical sutures. Dis. Colon Rectum, *35*:599, 1992, with permission.)

cence, 9.5%; and poor functional result, 5.3%. The mortality rate is up to 4.8%.[6] Nonetheless, in a subsequent, small-group study, Bricker reported satisfactory to excellent results in 19 of 26 patients.[7]

REFERENCES

1. Aartsen, E.J., and Sindram, I.: Repair of the radiation induced rectovaginal fistulas without or with interposition of the bulbocavernous muscle (Martinus procedure). Eur. J. Surg. Oncol., *14*: 171, 1988.
2. Allen-Mersh, T.G., Wilson, F.J., Hope-Stone, H.F., et al.: The management of late radiation induced rectal injury after treatment of carcinoma of the uterus. Surg. Gynecol. Obstet., *164*:521, 1987.
3. Anesline, P.F., Lavery, I.C., Fazio, V.W., et al.: Radiation injury of the rectum: Evaluation of surgical treatment. Ann. Surg., *194*: 716, 1981.
4. Bourne, R.G., Kearsley, J.H., Grove, W.D., et al.: The relationship between early and late gastrointestinal complications of radiation therapy for carcinoma of the cervix. Int. J. Radiat. Oncol. Biol. Phys., *9*:1445, 1983.
5. Bricker, E.M., and Johnston, W.D.: Repair of postirradiation rectovaginal fistula and stricture. Surg. Gynecol. Obstet., *148*:499, 1979.
6. Bricker, E.M., Johnston, W.D., and Patwardhan, R.V.: Repair of postirradiation damage to colorectum: A progress report. Ann. Surg., *193*:555, 1981.
7. Bricker, E.M., Kraybill, W.G., and Lopez, M.J.: Functional results after postirradiation rectal reconstruction. World J. Surg., *10*: 249, 1986.
8. Browning, G.G.P., Varma, J.S., Smith, A.N., et al.: Late results of mucosal proctectomy and coloanal sleeve anastomosis for chronic irradiation rectal injury. Br. J. Surg., *74*:31, 1987.
9. Buchler, D.A., Kline, J.C., Peckham, B.M., et al.: Radiation reactions in cervical cancer therapy. Am. J. Obstet. Gynecol., *111*: 745, 1971.
10. Cooke, S.A.R., and Wellsted, M.D.: The radiation damaged rectum: Resection with coloanal anastomosis using the endoanal technique. World J. Surg., *10*:220, 1986.
11. Cunningham, I.G.E.: The management of radiation proctitis. Aust. N. Z. J. Surg., *50*:172, 1980.
12. DeCosse, J.J., Rhodes, R.S., Wentz, W.B., et al.: The natural history and management of radiation induced injury of the gastrointestinal tract. Ann. Surg., *170*:369, 1969.
13. Deveney, C.W., Lewis F.R., and Schrock, T.R.: Surgical management of radiation injury of the small and large intestine. Dis. Colon Rectum, *19*:25, 1976.
14. Drake, D.B., Pemberton, J.H., Beart, R.W., et al.: Coloanal anastomosis in the management of benign and malignant rectal disease. Ann. Surg., *206*:600, 1987.
15. Galland, R.B., and Spencer, J.: Surgical management of radiation enteritis. Surgery, *99*:133, 1986.
16. Gazet, J.C.: Parks' coloanal pull-through anastomosis for severe, complicated radiation proctitis. Dis. Colon Rectum, *28*:110, 1985.
17. Gordon, P.: Ulcerative colitis in principles and practice of surgery

for the colon, rectum, and anus. St. Louis, Quality Medical Publishing, 1992, p. 686.

18. Harling, H., and Balsev, I.: Surgical treatment of radiation injury to the rectosigmoid. Acta Chir. Scand., 152:691, 1986.
19. Hatcher, P.A., Thomson, H.J., Ludgate, S.N., et al.: Surgical aspects of intestinal injury due to pelvic radiotherapy. Ann. Surg., 201:470, 1985.
20. Kagan, A.R., DiSaia, P.J., Wollin, M., et al.: The narrow vagina, the antecedent for irradiation injury. Gynecol. Oncol., 4:291, 1976.
21. Kaplan, A.L., Hudgins, P.T., and Wall, J.A.: Postradiation pelvic fibrosis simulating recurrent cacinoma. Am. J. Obstet. Gynecol., 92:117, 1965.
22. Kimose, H.-H., Fischer, L.F., Spjeldnaes, N., et al.: Late radiation injury of the colon and rectum. Dis. Colon Rectum, 32:684, 1989.
23. Kinsella, T.J., and Bloomer, W.D.: Tolerance of the intestine to radiation therapy. Surg. Gynecol. Obstet., 151:273, 1980.
24. Knight, C., and Griffen, F.: An improved technique for low anterior resection of the rectum using the EEA stapler. Surgery, 88:710, 1980.
25. Knight, C., and Griffen, F.: Techniques of low rectal reconstruction. Curr. Probl. Surg., 20:391, 1984.
26. Kottmeier, H.L., and Gray, M.J.: Rectal and bladder injuries in relation to radiation dosage in carcinoma of the cervix: A five year followup. Am. J. Obstet. Gynecol., 82:74, 1961.
27. Lee, K.H., Kagan, A.R., Nussbaum, H., et al.: Analysis of dose, dose rate and treatment time in the production of injuries by radium-treatment for cancer of the uterine cervix. Br. J. Radiol., 49:430, 1976.
28. LoIudice, T., Baxter, D.O.D., and Balint, J.: Effects of abdominal surgery on the development of radiation enteropathy. Gastroenterology, 73:1093, 1977.
29. Lucarotti, M.E., Mountford, R.A., and Bartoloi, D.C.C.: Surgical management of intestinal radiation injury. Dis. Colon Rectum, 34:865, 1991.
30. Marks, G., and Mohiudden, M.: The surgical management of the radiation injured intestine. Surg. Clin. North Am., 63:81, 1983.
31. Novak, J.M., Collins, J.T., Donowitz, M., et al.: Effects of radiation on the human gastrointestinal tract. J. Clin. Gastroenterol., 1:9, 1979.
32. Nowacki, M.P., Szawlowski, A.W., and Borkowski, A.: Parks' coloanal sleeve anastomosis for treatment of postirradiation rectovaginal fistula. Dis. Colon Rectum, 29:817, 1986.
33. O'Connor, J.J.: Argon laser treatment of radiation proctitis. Arch. Surg., 124:749, 1989.
34. Palmer, J.A., and Bush, R.S.: Radiation injuries to the bowel associated with the treatment of carcinoma of the cervix. Surgery, 80:458, 1976.
35. Perez, C.A., Breaux, S., Bedwinek, J.M., et al.: Radiation therapy alone in the treatment of carcinoma of the uterine cervix: Analysis of complications. Cancer, 54:235, 1984.
36. Pourquier, H., Dubois, J.H., and Delard, R.: Cancer of the uterine cervix: Dosimetric guidelines for prevention of late rectal and rectosigmoid complications as a result of radiotherapeutic treatment. Int. J. Radiat. Oncol. Biol. Phys., 8:1887, 1982.
37. Reichelderfer, M., and Morrissey, J.F.: Colonoscopy in radiation colitis. Gastrointest. Endosc., 26:41, 1980.
38. Rubinstein, E., Ibsen, T., Reimer, E., et al.: Formalin treatment of radiation induced hemorrhagic proctitis. Am. J. Gastroenterol., 81:44, 1986.
39. Russell, J.C., and Welch, J.P.: Operative management of radiation injuries of the intestinal tract. Am. J. Surg., 137:433, 1979.
40. Seon-Choen, F., Goh, H.S., Eu, K.-W., et al.: A simple and effective treatment for hemorrhagic radiation proctitis using formalin. Dis. Colon Rectum, 36:135, 1993.
41. Sher, M., and Bauer, J.: Radiation induced enteropathy. Am. J. Gastroenterol., 85:121, 1990.
42. Steichen, F.M., Barber, H.K.R., Loubeau, J.M., et al.: Bricker-Johnston sigmoid colon graft for repair of postradiation rectovaginal fistula and stricture performed with mechanical sutures. Dis. Colon Rectum, 35:599, 1992.
43. Unal, A., Hamberger, A.D., Seski, J.C., et al.: An analysis of the severe complications of irradiation carcinoma of the uterine cervix: Treatment with intracavitary radium and parametrial irradiation. Int. J. Radiat. Oncol. Biol. Phys., 7:999, 1981.
44. van Nagell, J.R., Parker, J.C., Maruyama, Y., et al.: Bladder or rectal injury following radiation therapy for cervical cancer. Am. J. Obstet. Gynecol., 119:727, 1974.
45. Varma, J.S., Smith, A.N., and Busuttil, A.: Function of the anal sphincters after chronic radiation injury. Gut, 27:528, 1986.
46. White, A.J., Buchsbaum, H.J., Blythe, J.G., et al.: Use of the bulbocavernosus muscle (Martius procedure) for repair of radiation induced rectovaginal fistulas. Obstet. Gynecol., 60:114, 1982.
47. Yeoh, E.K., and Horowitz, M.: Radiation enteritis. Surg. Gynecol. Obstet., 165:373, 1986.
48. Zoetmulder, F.A., Gortzak, E., den Hurtog Jager, F.C., et al.: Surgical repair of radiation damage of the rectum: A systematic approach to a difficult problem. Eur. J. Surg. Oncol., 14:479, 1988.

Chapter 33

WOUNDS, FOREIGN BODIES, AND FECAL IMPACTION

WILLIAM F. FALLON, JR.

WOUNDS OF THE ANORECTUM

Physical force from within the rectum or applied to the rectum from an external source can cause injury to the rectum and anus, as well as to the muscular sphincter apparatus surrounding the distal rectum and anus. Many of the types of injury to the anorectum are of sufficient force that the rectal injury is part of a pattern that is multisystemic in nature, often associated with shock at the time of presentation, and with a significant risk for infectious sequelae if the injury is not identified early or treated aggressively.

In general, trauma to the rectum occurs relatively infrequently.[7,16,17,30,38] Penetrating trauma is the usual mechanism and can occur from gunshot wounds to the lower torso, buttock, or perineal area. Penetrating injury can also occur from stab wounds to the buttock or perineum, impalement, or the insertion of objects into the rectum under a variety of circumstances. Blunt trauma occurs less frequently, usually as a result of motor vehicle crash or pedestrian vehicular accidents, and is most commonly seen with associated pelvic fractures.[27,37,40,49,58,59]

As the terminating point of the gastrointestinal tract, the anorectum and the associated muscular sphincter apparatus play an important role in the control of waste elimination. Injury, either blunt or penetrating, often disrupts this normal function, with incontinence as a potential outcome. As with other types of rectal pathology, anatomic considerations are important in planning a diagnostic and therapeutic approach to the patient with a rectal injury. Familiarity with the anatomy of the anorectum is essential.

The relationship of the anorectum to the visceral layer of the peritoneum is depicted in Figure 33–1. The overall length of the rectum is 12 to 15 cm. The upper portion of the rectum is within the peritoneal cavity, completely covered by peritoneum. The middle portion is only covered by peritoneum over its anterior surface and thus has a retroperitoneal portion. The distal portion of the rectum is completely below the peritoneum. Because of the lateral bends in the rectum, the distance from the external anal orifice to the peritoneal reflection over the anterior aspect of the midportion of the rectum is relatively short, only 3 to 5 inches. All of the sphincter muscles, the puborectalis muscle, and the levator ani are below the peritoneal reflection.

In addition to the lateral turns in the rectum, the distal rectum has an acute angulation from anterior to posterior through the puborectalis as it becomes the anal canal. The action of the puborectalis and the normal resting sphincter tone keep the anal canal closed and the walls of the distal rectum in apposition. This, coupled with intra-abdominal pressure pushing down on the rectosigmoid angle acts as a valve to maintain competent closure of the rectum.[6] Distention of the rectum over time that overcomes resting sphincter tone; direct sphincter injury that interrupts competent closure; and traumatic disruption of normal functional relationships, blood supply or innervation may lead to incontinence.

The majority of wounds to the anorectum involve the intraperitoneal or retroperitoneal portions of the rectum.[24] Penetrating trauma can have a trajectory through all layers of the rectum (Fig. 33–2), involve the sphincter muscles, penetrate the peritoneum causing contamination, and be associated with multiple intra-abdominal or pelvic organ injury in addition to the rectal injury.[7,13,18,29,30,41,66] These injuries occur as a consequence of gunshot wounds to the lower abdomen, pelvis, buttocks or gluteal region, perineum, and upper thighs. Penetrating trauma due to stab wounds or impalement usually is associated with entrance wounds through the anus, perineum, or buttocks and can cause a pattern of injury similar to that seen with gunshot wounds, depending upon the length of the weapon or the impaling object. Due to the close proximity of the

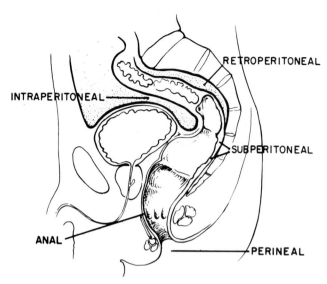

FIGURE 33-1. Anatomic classification of types of injuries of the bowel below the promontory. (From Haas, P.A., and Fox, T.A., Jr.: Civilian injuries of the rectum and anus. Dis. Colon Rectum, *22*:17, 1979, with permission.)

anterior peritoneal reflection to the external anal orifice and to the acute angulation in the distal rectum, intraperitoneal injury is possible even with short objects.

The rectum and anus can be caught in the trajectory of a wounding projectile or be the primary object of attack. Injury can occur during violent sexual assault, sodomy, rape, or homosexual or autoerotic activity with or without ancillary devices, the nature of which is limited only by the imagination of the participants.[2,15,24,36,50,68] These injuries may present in a delayed fashion, are more subtle in their presentation, and may have a higher risk for sphincter injury as well as injury to the rectum below the peritoneal reflection. There may be a higher risk of infectious complications.

Blunt injury to the pelvis and lower abdomen as seen with pelvic fractures and pelvic crush can cause anorectal laceration and injury to the sphincter mechanism. These injuries can occur as a result of motor vehicle crash, rollover injury, and falls, particularly the straddle type injury. Injury occurs due to penetration of bony fragments through the wall of the rectum, disruption of the blood supply, or as a result of shear injury from the strong muscular attachments to the surrounding bony pelvis.[14,37,46,64] Rectal injury from pelvic fracture is almost always below the peritoneal reflection.

Iatrogenic injury is typically penetrating in nature. Rectal injury has been reported with peritoneal contamination following contrast enema examination, therapeutic enema insertion, and the use of rectal thermometers.[11,15,21,25,28,39,50,53,56,60] Endoscopic polypectomy can increase the risk of rectal perforation due to contrast enema examination if performed within a short period after the polypectomy.[9,44,45,48,57] Due to the close proximity of the rectum to the vagina and the prostatic urethra, rectal injury has been reported following or during urologic, obstetric, and gynecologic procedures.[5,22,43]

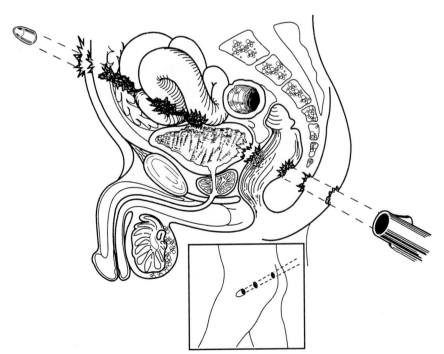

FIGURE 33-2. Rectal injury from gunshot wound to the buttock. (From Maull, K.I., Snoddy, J.W., and Haynes, B.W., Jr.: Penetrating wounds of the buttock. Surg. Gynecol. Obstet., *149*:856, 1979, with permission.)

These types of injuries generally are below the peritoneal reflection. Although polypectomy-related barium contrast perforations can occur throughout the colon, the circumstances of increased risk with biopsy obtained via the rigid proctoscope make this injury more likely to be above the peritoneal reflection in the rectosigmoid region.

Management of rectal injury evolved from the military experience with rectal trauma.[16,17,33,50,51,67] Military wounds to the rectum were most often high-velocity gunshot or fragmentation wounds with extensive tissue destruction and contamination. Septic complications were a frequent source of morbidity and mortality.[17] Gradual improvement in outcome occurred during successive military campaigns culminating in the results of treatment employed during the Vietnam conflict.[33] Rectal injury management consisted of laparotomy with diverting colostomy, washout of the distal defunctionalized limb of the colon and the rectum, repair of the rectal injury, including sphincter repair if possible, and dependent presacral drainage. Wounds were handled by the technique of delayed closure. The improvement in outcome associated with this policy of management was substantial, resulting in its virtual uniform adoption in combat casualty care.[33,67]

The spectrum of anorectal injury encountered in civilian practice includes a variety of injuries not typically seen in the military setting.[3,8,16,24,30,38,50] Injury can occur to the mucosal surface of the rectum without full-thickness involvement. In some types of injury occurring as a complication of elective surgery, the bowel may have been cleansed preoperatively. Repair of the rectal injury may not require proximal diversion in this situation.[2,5,43,50] In civilian penetrating rectal trauma, gunshot wounds are often of a lower velocity, with less extensive tissue loss or fecal contamination than combat injury. Treatment with colostomy is still an essential component; however, the remaining tenets are less than uniformly practiced.[7,8,55,62,65]

The most significant factors in the development of infectious complications in the management of civilian rectal injury are delay in the detection of the rectal injury or a delay in the performance of the diverting colostomy. Controversy surrounds the role of distal washout or presacral drainage. Clinical judgment and experience with the management of rectal injury become important in the decision to use such steps as distal rectal washout, presacral drainage, or in deciding which type of diverting colostomy to employ.

TYPES OF ANORECTAL INJURIES

The majority of injuries occurring to the rectum and anus from outside the lumen are due to gunshot wounds. Stab wounds, shotgun wounds, and impalements are seen less frequently.[24,38,58,62,65] Gunshot wounds encountered in civilian practice are usually low velocity, most often single missiles that have entrance sites in the lower abdomen, buttock, gluteal area, or perineum.[3,41,66] The trajectory of these wounds can traverse the rectum at any level but usually involves the intraperitoneal or middle portion of the rectum and so can be both intraperitoneal as well as extraperitoneal in its course. Multisystem injury is frequent due to the large number of organ systems in close proximity within the pelvis.[18,24,29,30] Vascular injury may be present and should be suspected in those who present in shock.[13,19] The extent of fecal contamination may be variable. Shotgun injuries are associated with much more local tissue destruction at the site of entry.

Stab wounds to the rectum usually originate in the buttocks, perineum, or gluteal region, and may involve the intraperitoneal portion of the rectum if the wounding agent was of sufficient length. A similar spectrum of injury to that seen with gunshot wounds can result.

Penetrating rectal injury also may be seen as a result of surgery within the pelvis, abdomen, or perineum. Any process resulting in the adherence of the rectum to adjacent structures, such as endometriosis, pelvic inflammatory disease, neoplastic disorders, or radiation therapy, increases the risk of such operative injury. Preoperative preparation of the bowel in patients thought to be at risk for rectal injury from these procedures makes sense and can help reduce the risk of pelvic sepsis following accidental injury to the rectum. Rectal injury occurring in this setting, if detected immediately, can almost always be treated with primary repair without diversion.

Rectal injury occurs in a small number of patients undergoing urologic surgical procedures. The complication is most frequently reported during open prostatic surgery.[5,43] These injuries are almost always detected at the time of the operative procedure. Two-layer, primary repair of the rectal injury has been successfully employed, with fecal diversion reserved for those in whom there is a delay in diagnosis.

Injury to the anorectum or to the muscular sphincter apparatus, and rectovaginal fistula, are recognized complications of obstetric or gynecologic procedures.[6,22,23,62] Factors associated with an increased risk of rectal injury during vaginal delivery include midline episiotomy, nulliparity, complicated delivery, and large fetal size.[22] The use of forceps in the delivery process may increase the risk as well. The majority of obstetric injuries are third degree (i.e., injury only to the muscular sphincter apparatus). Full-thickness, fourth-degree injury involving the rectal mucosa is seen less frequently. These lesions correspond to the grade-three and -four rectal injury scale of the Organ Injury Scaling Committee of the American Association for the Surgery of Trauma.[22,42] Tears of the anal sphincter and those through the anal mucosa should be repaired immediately following delivery. The rectal mucosal laceration is repaired with interrupted absorbable sutures placed in the submucosal layer. The muscular sphincter apparatus is repaired by placing interrupted sutures through the sheaths of the sphincter muscles and repairing the remainder of the injury in layers. Fecal diversion is seldom needed.

Rectovaginal fistulas have multiple causes.[23,62] Primary transanal repair in those patients with this condition as a complication of gynecologic surgery is possible. Fistulas occurring due to or as a consequence of malignancy or irradiation will require fecal diversion with colostomy as well.

Intraluminal rectal full-thickness injury is a known occurrence following endoscopic procedures using both rigid proctoscopic and flexible endoscopic instruments.[9,25,44,45,48,57] Procedures associated with injury when using the rigid proctoscope are more often emergent; are associated with some degree of bowel obstruction, vovlulus, or both; and tend to be performed in elderly patients and with poor colonic preparation. The usual point of perforation is in the intraperitoneal portion of the rectum at or around the rectosigmoid junction. Flexible endoscopic instruments may have a somewhat lower incidence of perforation, but this may be due to their infrequent use in these settings.

Biopsy procedures performed through rigid proctoscopic instruments have a greater propensity to be deeper tissue samples with an associated greater risk for perforation. Heat injury causing a full-thickness injury can occur as a result of electrocautery snare or biopsies done via flexible endoscopic instruments as well as via rigid proctoscopes. Contamination associated with these injuries is usually minimal as a result of preprocedure bowel cleansing. When recognized immediately, surgical repair and diversion of the fecal stream is associated with good overall results.

Diagnostic contrast evaluation of the colon and rectum (barium, gastrograffin, or triple-contrast computed tomography [CT] enema) can cause rectal injury and perforation. Risk factors for the occurrence of rectal perforation during barium contrast studies include using inflatable balloon-tipped catheters and performing a study immediately following proctosigmoidoscopy, especially when a biopsy was obtained.[11,21,25,60] In those instances when the tip of the enema device has been responsible for the injury, perforation occurs most frequently in the anterior portion of the rectum at the point where it angles sharply posteriorly, just above the puborectalis muscle. Perforation can also occur at sites of previous, recently performed biopsies or where the rectum is involved in inflammatory disease processes. Most of these perforations involve the extraperitoneal rectum, and have been documented by both plain radiographs and CT as well as diagnostic endoscopy.[21] Injury can also involve the middle portion of the rectum, with extension directly into the peritoneal cavity. The effect of barium sulfate contrast extravasation into the peritoneal cavity is well documented both in the laboratory and in clinical practice.[11] A marked inflammatory response with diffuse peritonitis rapidly ensues following peritoneal contamination with barium contrast. A synergistic effect is noted when fecal contamination is also present. Mortality associated with this event is significant, warranting prompt diagnosis, aggressive resuscitation, and early surgical intervention. At the time of surgery, repair of the rectal injury if possible and diverting colostomy with distal washout should be performed. A vigorous attempt to remove as much of the barium precipitate as possible should be carried out as well. Interestingly, extraperitoneal barium extravasation from rectal injury does not appear to elicit the same degree of systemic inflammatory response and has been reported

to have been successfully managed nonoperatively.[21] Clinical judgment must be used regarding the role of this alternative management method of care, however.

Prevention of this occurrence is the best policy. The radiologist should be told of any previous biopsy or proctoscopic procedure, whether rectal inflammatory disease is present or suspected, and if previous pelvic surgery or irradiation has occurred. Barium contrast studies following biopsy procedures should be delayed 7 to 10 days to decrease the likelihood of perforation during the procedure. Careful evaluation of the precontrast scout film for the presence of extraperitoneal or extraluminal air is recommended as well.[25]

Therapeutic enema administration may cause intraluminal rectal injury in several ways. In a manner similar to that seen with injury following contrast enema performance, insertion of a firm enema nozzle tip into the rectum anteriorly can result in a rectal wall injury that can range from partial-thickness mucosal injury to a full-thickness perforation. Perforations can be confined to the extraperitoneal space or extend into the peritoneum. The chemical content of substances delivered to the rectum for therapeutic or other purposes may cause chemical burn injury to the mucosal layer if intact or into deeper layers if there is an associated perforation.[25,53,56] Detection may be difficult, as many patients who receive enemas are old and debilitated. Others may be reluctant to admit that the event occurred in the first place and only seek care when forced to by progressive symptoms. Delay in diagnosis is frequent and must be considered when planning therapy. Some patients will require fecal stream diversion as part of the treatment. Most mishaps with therapeutic enema administration can be avoided with adherence to the proper technique of administration. Rectal thermometers may also cause rectal injury if inserted improperly.

Intraluminal impalement injury may range from minor lacerations of the mucosa that are not full thickness to severe, full-thickness injury that is extraperitoneal or that has an intraperitoneal component.[15,24,39,50] Impalement injuries mostly involve falls onto objects such as fence spikes, broom handles, or fixed posts. Soldiers have been reported having been impaled on their rifles as they dismount from vehicles.[31] Criminal assault may also involve impalement, with knives or other weapons penetrating the rectum as a target, with extensive injury.[15] Sexual activity involving the rectum from auto-erotic stimulation using a variety of instruments to more dangerous practices of fist fornication or hand balling can result in major injury as well.[15,36,50,68] Treatment will most often involve diverting colostomy, although some injuries that are not full thickness may be observed.

Insufflation injury of the rectum involves the delivery of air or water, usually under high pressure, into the rectum. The force of this injection is responsible for the injury, which may include rectal rupture, retroperitoneal hematoma and contamination, as well as intra-abdominal perforation and injury.[34] Treatment almost always involves fecal stream diversion.

Blunt trauma is an infrequent cause of rectal injury. However, the amount of energy associated with this mechanism of injury is so great that the rectal injury is often only one component of multisystem injury, associated soft tissue injury, and hemorrhagic shock.[7,27,59] The cause of this type of injury is usually a motor vehicle, motor cycle, or pedestrian-vehicular crash.[59] Any patient with a pelvic fracture, particularly an open pelvic fracture, has the potential for a rectal injury. Severe, comminuted fractures of the pelvis may cause extraluminal rectal injury through penetration of the wall of the rectum by fragments of bone. Hemorrhage is a frequent associated finding as is the presence of urologic injury.[49,52] Rectal tears can also occur with less severe injury to the bony pelvis either as a result of a fall or after a straddle injury to the perineum.

Rectal injury occurs due to the disruption of the attachments to the pelvis of the muscular sphincter apparatus or from shear forces. These rectal injuries are usually below the peritoneal reflection and may be either partial thickness or full thickness. Often, the exact location of the injury may be uncertain, and only the presence of extraperitoneal, retroperitoneal air on plain radiography, subcutaneous emphysema on physical examination, or the presence of pelvic hematoma or abscess on CT of the pelvis indicates the presence of an injury.[14,37,46,63]

A rare type of rectal injury following pelvic fracture is devascularization injury in which full-thickness rectal necrosis follows disruption of the blood supply to the rectum.[64] The rich, collateral blood flow through the pelvis and the dual mesenteric and systemic blood supply to the rectum make this an unusual event. Embolization of the internal iliac vessels to control hemorrhage, or operative exposure of the pelvic skeleton for internal fixation, may compromise blood supply that is already limited due to the nature of the pelvic injury or pre-existing vascular disease.

Rectal injury encountered in these circumstances is treated with proximal diversion and washout. Even without a documented rectal injury, these complex pelvic or perineal injuries may require diversion of the fecal stream to control septic sequelae.[4,17,32,40]

SYMPTOMS AND DIAGNOSIS

Because of the several mechanisms that can cause rectal injury and because of variation in the time of presentation to the hospital, the pattern of symptoms and physical findings associated with rectal injury can be variable. Penetrating injury from gunshot wounds, stab wounds, and certain types of impalement may suggest rectal injury due to the location of the entrance wounds, exit wounds, or the suspected trajectory of the wounding object through tissues. Penetrating injury to the lower abdomen, lower back, buttock, gluteal region, perineum, or upper thighs should suggest the possibility of a rectal injury. These patterns of wounding frequently injure the intraperitoneal rectum, have a high incidence of associated injury, and may be accompanied by shock.[7,13,19,29,41] Signs of peritoneal irritation are typically seen. Most authorities recommend proceeding directly to the operating room to complete the diagnostic work-up

and to continue resuscitation in those patients with signs of hemodynamic instability.

In patients with penetrating trauma who are stable and who have an injury pattern suggestive of rectal injury, it is appropriate to proceed with a careful history and physical examination. These patients may complain of abdominal, pelvic, or rectal pain and, often, tenesmus. Many of the events leading to rectal injury are embarrassing or are events of abuse. The buttocks, gluteal region, and perineum should be carefully inspected for evidence of open wounds or rectal bleeding. A digital rectal examination is performed to evaluate resting sphincter tone. Severe pain on examination, a palpable defect or mass within the rectum, and evidence of either gross blood or occult blood within the stool,[8,13,18,20,24,29,35] or the presence of intraluminal blood is highly suggestive of rectal injury regardless of the vector of wounding. Its absence, however, does not reliably exclude the presence of rectal injury.[35,41] In patients with suspicious trajectory or entrance wounds, proctosigmoidoscopy is essential. While not perfect, the combination of digital rectal examination and proctosigmoidoscopy has an acceptable overall diagnostic accuracy and should be performed in combination in every patient with a suspected rectal injury from penetrating trauma. If a rectal injury is diagnosed by physical examination and proctosigmoidoscopy, the patient is prepared for the operating room with the further evaluation of associated at-risk systems deferred or performed in that setting.

Blunt injury from a motor vehicle, motorcycle, or pedestrian-vehicular accident with associated pelvic, perineal, lower abdominal, or hip injury may be associated with extraluminal injury to the rectum. These injuries may be open or closed, with rectal injury due to laceration by bony fragments, shear injury from pelvic structural deformation, or extension of the perineal lacerations through the wall of the rectum itself. In this group of patients, the presence of shock is an extremely important consideration, as the overwhelming cause of death seen early in this injury pattern is from exsanguination.[32,40,49,52] The management of the shock takes precedence and may include pelvic fixation, angiography, and laparotomy to achieve hemorrhage control. Symptoms of rectal injury may be minimal in an unresponsive, hypotensive patient and signs of injury may not initially be detected because of the urgency associated with the need for hemorrhage control. Rectal examination is performed when feasible in this sequence of events. Careful inspection of the anus and perineum is important to identify any lacerations with extension into the anus or rectum. Wounds are not probed or vigorously explored, as this may cause severe bleeding. Next, digital examination of the rectum is performed to identify the adequacy of sphincter tone and contraction, the presence of gross blood, palpable rectal wall defects, or bony fragments projecting into or pressing against the rectal wall. Fecal stream diversion with colostomy is an important component in the management of many types of injury within this setting. Documented rectal injury is only one such indication. Most surgeons have a low threshold for performing diversion, and further diagnostic evaluation of the full extent of the rectal injury is often deferred until later in the patient's hospital course.

When there is a delay in presentation to the hospital, the pattern of signs and symptoms associated with rectal injury is somewhat different. Penetrating injury that may fall into this category includes minor impalement injury, and autoerotic or homosexual activity with injury. Blunt injury of this type includes minor falls or straddle injury. Sexual assault, anal rape, and child abuse may also be associated with a delayed presentation due to the individual's reluctance or fear about admitting the occurrence of the event. These injuries are predominantly intraluminal in nature. Falls and straddle injury to the pelvis may injure the rectum by the action of shear forces at the level of the puborectalis. These injuries are almost always below the peritoneal reflection. Symptoms include abdominal pain, tenesmus, and rectal bleeding.[10,15,36,37,50,68] There is usually evidence of sepsis with either systemic signs or leukocytosis. Examination of the peritoneum is important. In children who are suspected victims of abuse, clothing, diapers, and so forth should be inspected for blood as well. The anus is inspected for fissures, swelling, bruising, and prolapse. Digital examination is performed to evaluate the sphincter and assess for the presence of blood, a rectal wall mass, or a rectal mural defect. Plain radiographs of the pelvis may reveal extraluminal gas or extraperitoneal dissection of air into the chest or abdomen. Free intraperitoneal air may also be seen and is indicative of free perforation into the abdomen, regardless of the symptoms of the patient.[45] Minor falls have been reported to cause a similar clinical picture on presentation, and there may not be any evidence of rectal injury on clinical examination. Signs and symptoms of pelvic or extraperitoneal infection or abscess may be the only indication that an injury has occurred.[46,63]

In this delayed-presentation group of patients, CT of the abdomen and the pelvis may be extremely useful in identifying the presence of extraluminal septic sequelae, such as pelvic or ischiorectal abscess.[10,14,21,37,45,46] The anus, rectum, and perineum are always evaluated first. The intraluminal evaluation of the rectum is first done by digital exam to evaluate the sphincter and to check for blood. The rectal mucosa is then inspected visually by endoscopic measures in an attempt to identify the presence of injury. This examination in children or in those who cannot cooperate may have to be done under anesthesia in order to be complete. Intrarectal contrast studies must be used cautiously in patients who are suspected of having a rectal injury. The dangers of intraabdominal contamination with barium extravasation through a rectal tear have been previously described. Foreign body contamination of the extraperitoneal tissues with contrast may worsen septic complications. Abdominal sonography and CT scanning of the abdomen and pelvis can be helpful in defining the full extent of pelvic sepsis, reduce the risk of contrast contamination of extraluminal tissues, and provide a therapeutic option in the form of percutaneous drainage if accessible by location.

Iatrogenic rectal injury may be recognized at the time it occurs or after a variable delay. Patients with rectal injury that occurs in the course of an operative procedure will not show any symptoms because they are anesthetized. In this group, careful inspection of the area of the rectum close to the operative site is essential. In those patients who are not anesthetized, injury that is recognized at the time of occurrence usually is associated with signs and symptoms of peritoneal irritation, pelvic pain or tenderness, and signs of systemic toxicity. The longer the delay in the detection of the injury, the more likelihood that signs and symptoms of toxicity will predominate.

Every patient being evaluated for the possibility of rectal injury must have an adequate evaluation of the bladder and urethra.[13,18,29,40,41] Contrast urethrography is done in male patients suspected of having a urethral disruption. The bladder is evaluated by cystography in both male and female patients. All female patients must have a thorough vaginal examination. Diagnostic peritoneal lavage is useful to evaluate these patients for the presence of associated intra-abdominal injury. In the case of major impalement injury, the portion of the object extending into the tissues must be left in place and removed only under controlled circumstances, usually in the operating room, to prevent death from sudden, unexpected exsanguination.

TREATMENT OF ANORECTAL INJURY

The operative evaluation and treatment of rectal injury should proceed after adequate preoperative preparation has been accomplished. Due to the nature of these injuries, the risks for peritonitis and sepsis, and the possibility of fluid sequestration from peritonitis, the preparation must be expeditious and aggressive. If not already present, intravenous lines are established and volume resuscitation is begun with warm crystalloid solutions. Blood is drawn for laboratory studies and for crossmatching. Supplemental oxygen is delivered via mask. Bladder catheterization is accomplished to ensure adequate urine output in response to volume resuscitation. A nasogastric tube is placed to decompress the stomach. Once volume resuscitation is under way, empiric antibiotic therapy is started that provides broadspectrum coverage for the organisms likely to be encountered, including *Bacteroides* species as well as other enteric organisms.[3,46,50] A variety of acceptable antibiotic regimens are available to choose from. Because contamination is already present or has already potentially occurred, these antibiotics should be delivered rapidly in full doses.

Preparation for operation includes notification of the operating room (OR) of the urgent nature of the case and the details of the procedure so that the room can be properly prepared. The patient will be placed in the modified lithotomy position if at all possible. Patients with rectal injury and exsanguination may not tolerate this position and the supine position can be used initially with the patient positioned during the procedure once control of hemorrhage is achieved. If not already performed, the OR personnel will need to obtain and prepare a rigid proctoscope for use during the procedure.[7,20,24,29,35,41]

The abdominal approach is through a long midline incision for those with rectal injury due to trauma. For patients with other types of rectal injury, the incision can begin as a lower midline incision with extension above the umbilicus as necessary for exposure or treatment. The nature and location of the rectal injury, the extent of intra-abdominal contamination, the presence of associated injuries, and the stability of the patient once under anesthesia will determine how the injury is approached intraoperatively. Each aspect of the treatment of rectal injury—colostomy for fecal diversion, distal segment washout, drainage of the presacral or pararectal spaces, and sphincter repair—must be carefully considered during the procedure. In those patients with blunt injury and open, complex perineal or soft tissue injury with or without associated rectal injury, daily débridement and dressing changes are an essential additional adjunct to their treatment.[4,32,40,49,52]

In some circumstances, the choice may be made not to operate. This is a decision in which patient selection is critical. The types of patients potentially suitable for nonoperative management are those who have sustained extraperitoneal iatrogenic injury from diagnostic procedures, minor impalement that is not full thickness on proctoscopic examination, and selected patients who have free intraperitoneal air but no abdominal symptoms following endoscopic procedures.[9,44,45,48,50,57] Often, the reason nonoperative treatment is elected is because the patient is stable and asymptomatic when evaluated by the surgeon. These patients must be followed closely with serial examinations and careful attention to changes in the vital signs. Broad-spectrum antibiotic therapy should be employed similar to that used when an operation is planned. Gastrointestinal tract rest is established and intravenous fluid replacement is begun. Delay in abdominal exploration when symptoms develop can be fatal.

WOUNDS OF THE INTRAPERITONEAL OR RETROPERITONEAL RECTUM

After exploration of the abdomen, and when treatment of higher priority conditions has been completed, wounds of the intraperitoneal or retroperitoneal portions of rectum should be addressed. The nature of the injury will determine how it is treated. Simple perforations can be débrided and closed in layers. More extensive injury or destruction may require resection. Simple iatrogenic injury above the peritoneal reflection without fecal contamination, treated immediately or soon after the incident, is managed by primary closure.[5,24,43,50] Similarly, discrete injury due to a low-velocity penetrating missile, associated with little or no peritoneal soilage, has been successfully managed with primary repair alone.[24,30,38,39] More extensive injury to the rectum, significant intra-abdominal contamination by feces in combination with blood or barium, and delay in operation due to late presentation or detection all warrant conservative treatment with colostomy formation. The rec-

tal injury is repaired or resected. A diverting sigmoid colostomy is fashioned in the left lower quadrant. When repair has been performed, this colostomy can be a diverting loop colostomy fashioned over a bridging device.[8,40,55] In cases of resection of the rectal injury, the colostomy is fashioned as an end sigmoid colostomy.[8] The distal, defunctionalized segment may be of variable length depending on the location of the injury requiring resection.

Once the colostomy has been placed, a decision must be made to proceed with the other components of rectal injury treatment: presacral drainage, distal segment washout, and wound care. Those who have primary repair without colostomy receive no further treatment of their rectal injury. Those with injury treated by colostomy and resection, whose injury was above the peritoneal reflection, also require no further treatment. Those who may need further treatment are patients with injury involving the midportion of the rectum who had mobilization of the retroperitoneal portion of the rectum as part of their treatment. Depending on the extent of the retroperitoneal, presacral, and pararectal dissection done to treat the rectal injury, drainage of the retrorectal space may be indicated.[3,7,8,13,16,30,33,38,39,62,65,67] Drainage may be via the perineum or transabdominally using Silastic closed suction drainage devices.[24] Typically, two drains are used. The drainage route originally described was via the perineum using Penrose drains brought out through stab incisions near the anococcygeal raphe.[33] Many still employ this route, although using the Silastic, closed suction drainage devices now available.

The value of distal rectal washout in penetrating trauma is more problematic.[55,65] The potential for increasing fecal contamination of the extrarectal soft tissues has prompted some to caution against its use.[65] Others have noted a decreased incidence of infectious sequelae following its use in penetrating trauma.[55] Distal rectal washout plays an important role in decreasing the incidence of infectious sequelae in those with rectal injury from blunt trauma, open pelvic fracture, and major perineal soft tissue injury.[4,17,32,40,49,52,55,59] When distal washout is used, it is performed at the termination of the abdominal portion of the procedure. In patients in whom a diverting loop colostomy has been performed, the fascia is closed and the abdominal incision packed. For those with an end colostomy, the washout must be performed with the abdomen open to provide access to the distal defunctionalized limb. In this situation, the abdominal cavity is protected with laparotomy pads to prevent soilage during the washout. A pursestring suture is placed in the wall of the distal colon and tied around a large mushroom-type catheter through which the irrigation is performed. Simultaneously, with the patient in the modified lithotomy position, anal sphincter dilatation is performed by another member of the operating team and gentle manual removal of stool in the rectal vault is accomplished. Following this, several liters of warm crystalloid solution is introduced through the mushroom catheter to irrigate the distal colon and rectum. The effluent is directed into large holding containers away from the patient's wounds. Several liters may be needed to accomplish satisfactory cleansing, and the operative team must persist until clear effluent exits the anus. At the conclusion of the rectal washout, if not already accomplished, the abdominal fascia is closed and the colostomy appropriately matured. The skin and subcutaneous layers of the abdominal incision are then packed and protected for delayed primary closure at a later date. If necessary, perineal soft tissue wounds can be irrigated, débrided, and packed at this time.

WOUNDS OF THE SUBPERITONEAL RECTUM

Subperitoneal rectal injury may range in severity from incomplete rectal wall injury, minor full-thickness iatrogenic injury, to more severe full-thickness injury with tissue destruction and fecal contamination.[2,24,36,50,68] Treatment is tailored to the type and extent of injury encountered. A good visual inspection of the rectal injury via the proctoscope is essential. Incomplete rectal wall injury can be managed by observation in the hospital, gastrointestinal tract rest, and appropriate antibiotic therapy. Some types of iatrogenic injury, such as enema tips or thermometers with complete rectal penetration, can be managed this way as well. More extensive injury should be treated as are those injuries in the intraperitoneal portion of the rectum with diverting colostomy and selection of those other facets of rectal injury treatment deemed appropriate.

The subperitoneal category of rectal injury presumes no associated intra-abdominal injury, although intraperitoneal contamination can still result because of the close proximity of the peritoneal reflection to the anal verge. Patients operated upon for apparent subperitoneal rectal injury who require diverting colostomy must have a thorough abdominal exploration to exclude intraperitoneal contamination. A diverting sigmoid loop colostomy is most frequently used in these patients because there is often no need for resection of the injury. Similarly, when the injury is below an intact peritoneal reflection, it may not be necessary to accomplish presacral drainage.[62] Distal rectal washout is frequently used in this group of patients in order to minimize the risk of ongoing fecal contamination of the extraperitoneal tissues.

Rectal injury repair is difficult with subperitoneal rectal trauma because exposure is so limited. Most surgeons would defer repair until the risks of fecal contamination and infection are minimal. Rarely is further dissection for exposure of the injury indicated in the acute setting.

Patients with severe rectal destruction because of blunt or penetrating injury to the perineum and pelvis represent a small but critical subset of patients with subperitoneal rectal injury. These patients have such extensive injury that there is significant tissue loss to the surrounding pararectal structures or to the rectum itself. In this group of patients, more extensive local débridement is needed. Every effort should be made to conserve structures that may be important functionally once the patient recovers but also to remove potential sources of infection. Occasionally, abdominoperitoneal resection is required.[8,33,59] More likely is the need for a Hartmann's procedure to isolate the distal rectal stump.[8] An end sigmoid colostomy is fashioned and distal washout is accomplished by local irrigation via the perineum.

INJURY TO THE PERINEUM AND MUSCULAR SPHINCTER APPARATUS

Damage from blunt or penetrating trauma to the perineum or pararectal soft tissues may also involve the sphincter apparatus, either directly or indirectly via disruption of nerve or vascular supply. The risks associated are infections early and incontinence later in the patient's course.[6,24,27,32,40,49,52,64] Injury to the muscular sphincter apparatus can also occur following complicated childbirth, some types of child abuse, and anal assault or rape. These also have early infectious sequelae and later risks for incontinence.[6,12,15,50]

Careful inspection of the perineum in these patients will identify lacerations, bruising, rectal prolapse, or eversion. Digital rectal examination in the awake and cooperative patient can determine the status of resting sphincter tone and the strength of voluntary sphincter contraction. Most open wounds of the perineum and all open pelvic fractures with lacerations close to the rectum will require a proximal diverting loop colostomy and distal washout of the defunctionalized segment. The diverting loop colostomy is particularly attractive in this regard because it can be performed expeditiously with a minimal abdominal incision when there is no risk of an associated intra-abdominal injury. Wounds are always left open, and repeated débridement may be required.

Iatrogenic rectal injury recognized at the time of occurrence should be repaired immediately.[12] Such injury most often occurs during childbirth or with gynecological and urologic procedures. Repair should be performed in layers with absorbable suture. A diverting colostomy usually is not necessary. When the rectal injury is not identified immediately, infection occurs and incontinence may result.[6] Repairs attempted in this setting are less than satisfactory in terms of overall success, and may require a diverting colostomy as well.

FOREIGN BODIES OF THE RECTUM

Rectal foreign bodies usually are introduced from below. A small percentage of objects are ingested and are subsequently passed per rectum without incident, usually in children or accidentally, or in those with behavior disorders. The smuggling of drugs packed into body cavities, particularly the rectum, has been described as well. Almost all rectal foreign bodies seen in large series have been introduced as part of autoerotic or homosexual activity in men.[2,15,24,39,50,68] A variety of devices have been found retained in the rectum at the time of evaluation in the hospital. There is often a delay in presentation to the hospital because of reluctance on the part of the patient to admit to such behavior.

Patients with retained foreign bodies usually complain of abdominal pain at the time of presentation. The exact cause may not be initially volunteered by the patient. Oftentimes, plain abdominal radiographs may be the first indication that the foreign object is within the rectum. Patients may also complain of other symptoms related to rectal injury, such as rectal or perineal pain and tenesmus.

Evaluation of the patient with a rectal foreign body can initially be started in the emergency department. Most foreign bodies can be removed and many minor rectal injuries treated on an outpatient basis.[2,50] Evaluation of the rectum commences with determination of the patient's vital signs. Delayed presentation of patients with perforation following foreign body insertion is usually associated with signs of toxicity or shock. In stable patients, the rectum and perineum are carefully examined for external signs of trauma or abnormal sphincter protrusion. Those who practice rectal sex usually have a relaxed sphincter and consequently less likelihood of sphincter trauma. In contrast, the forcible insertion of objects into unwilling participants, as part of anorectal assault or child abuse, is associated with a more significant risk of sphincter damage. A digital rectal examination is then performed to evaluate the sphincter, identify the location of the foreign body, and determine the presence of intraluminal blood. No attempt is made to remove the foreign body at this time unless it can be grasped easily at the level of the anal canal and can be removed without injury to the wall of the anorectum. Plain radiographic studies with both anteroposterior and lateral views of the abdomen and pelvis are also obtained in order to help localize the foreign body. These films should also be evaluated for the presence of free intra-abdominal or retroperitoneal air that may suggest perforation.

The patient usually will undergo proctoscopic examination without enema preparation in the emergency department or clinic area. Gentle technique and a certain amount of ingenuity are basic requirements for the atraumatic removal of foreign bodies from the rectum. Blind use of grasping forceps should be avoided and every effort made to remove the object without injuring the mucosa of the rectum. Following removal of all foreign objects, a thorough inspection of the anal canal and rectum with the proctoscope is essential to be sure that no other objects are retained and that there is no evidence of significant injury to the rectal wall. Following successful removal of the foreign body, most patients can be treated on an outpatient basis.[2]

Admission to the hospital and extraction in the operating room with general anesthesia are necessary for those who have foreign objects that are large, have sharp edges, or that have become lodged high in the rectum or rectosigmoid junction. Often, with adequate anesthesia and relaxation, foreign objects deemed difficult to remove in the outpatient setting become relatively easy to extract. Others have reported spontaneous passage of large objects just with admission and bedrest.[2] The operation is performed in the modified lithotomy position under general anesthesia. The patient is prepared for an abdominal laparotomy should this become necessary. Proctoscopic examination proceeds and attempts are made to extract the object facilitated by closed abdominal manipulation or pressure applied over the lower abdomen. In the unusual instance when the foreign body cannot be removed, a laparotomy is performed. Then the object can be manipulated into range of the proctoscope for grasping and removal. Rarely, this will be unsuccessful and the colon will have to be opened and the object extracted via the colotomy. This colotomy can then be closed; a diverting loop colostomy with distal rectal washout may be needed. Once the foreign body has been removed, thorough proctoscopic examination is completed to exclude rectal wall injury. Perforations encountered in the course of the removal of rectal foreign bodies either by the surgical team or the patients themselves should be treated by repair, washout of the distal rectum and diverting colostomy.

Even without gross perforation of the rectum, the severe mechanical trauma associated with the insertion of large foreign objects into the rectum can result in signs of sepsis localized to the pelvis or more generalized in nature. The syndrome seems to result from severe mechanical trauma and transmural inflammation. Affected patients should be admitted to the hospital and treated with broad-spectrum antibiotics, gastrointestinal tract rest, and intravenous fluid resuscitation. They need to be followed closely to monitor development of a pelvic abscess or other septic sequelae.

FECAL IMPACTION

Fecal impaction involves a mechanical obstruction caused by a large, compacted mass of feces in the rectal ampulla. Occasionally, the impaction may extend proximally in the colon. A variety of conditions can be associated with fecal impaction.[1,26,28,47,53,54] Impaction seems to occur most commonly in the elderly, those bedridden by medical, orthopedic, or neurologic conditions, the chronic use of medications such as antacids or narcotics, and as a complication of cystic fibrosis with inadequate enzyme replacement. Patients who have surgical procedures or pathology involving the anorectum, such as acute fissures, surgical procedures for hemorrhoids, and so forth, may have constipation from pain leading to impaction.

Fecal impaction is the clinical manifestation of prolonged fecal loading.[28] The most severe complication is bowel obstruction with perforation. Symptoms of fecal impaction include cessation of regular bowel function and defecation with lower abdominal distress, distention, and pain. Paradoxically, many patients then exhibit feculent diarrhea resulting from loss of rectal sphincter tone caused by chronic distention of the rectal ampulla. Digital examination will identify the hard fecal mass. Abdominal examination may also detect palpable stool within the colon indicative of fecal loading. Plain abdominal radiographs may help to rule out mechanical bowel obstruction or perforation and may serve to identify a dangerous degree of bowel distention.

The treatment of most impactions should involve digital removal of the fecal bolus. This is usually accomplished at the bedside, but may require anesthesia and, occasionally, laparotomy to manipulate the stool out through the rectum. Patients may also require nasogastric decompression, intravenous rehydration, and agents to loosen and break up stool.[1] Enemas to aid in disimpaction must be used carefully to avoid complications.[28] Pulsed irrigation devices have been used successfully as a means of rehydrating stool to promote removal.[47] For most patients, such as the elderly, bedridden, and those with spinal cord injury or congenital diseases such as cystic fibrosis, prevention is extremely important. Intake of sufficient dietary fiber and fluid is essential. Agents designed to promote evacuation may need to be used regularly. Medications that are constipating should be avoided. Periodic abdominal and rectal examinations should be considered for those under medical care who are at risk.

A rare complication of fecal impaction is stercoral perforation.[54] Pressure necrosis and erosion of a large, hardened mass of stool can occur anywhere in the colon. Mucosal ulceration precedes the perforation and may be manifest by signs and symptoms of acute or chronic blood loss. Ulcerations may be multiple. Patients who present with a long history of fecal impaction and complain of abdominal distention with signs of peritonitis require documentation of perforation, aggressive resuscitation, and urgent laparotomy. Fecal contamination is controlled by identification and isolation of the injured segment. The abdomen is cleansed with copious amounts of warm fluid. Resection of the segment of injured bowel should be performed along with the removal of as much of the fecal load in the colon as is possible. An end colostomy should be fashioned. The distal rectal segment should also be irrigated clear of any fecal load. These patients may be difficult to manage postoperatively because of general colonic dysfunction from chronic fecal loading. More extensive resection may be necessary to definitively treat the underlying problem.[26]

REFERENCES

1. Apelgren, K.N., and Yuen, J.C.: Distal colonic impaction requiring laparotomy in an adult with cystic fibrosis. J. Clin. Gastroenterol., 11(6):687, 1989.
2. Barone, J.E., Yee, J., and Nealon, T.F., Jr.: Management of foreign bodies and trauma of the rectum. Surg. Gynecol. Obstet., 156: 453, 1983.
3. Bartizal, J.F., Boyd, D.R., Folk, F.A., et al.: A critical review of management of 392 colonic and rectal injuries. Dis. Colon Rectum, 17:313, 1974.
4. Birolini, D., Steinman, E., Utiyama, E., et al.: Open pelviperineal trauma. J. Trauma, 30:492, 1990.
5. Borland, R.N., and Walsh, P.C.: The management of rectal injury during radical retropubic prostatectomy. J. Urol., 147:905, 1992.
6. Browning, G.G.P., Motson, R.W., and Henry, M.M.: Combined sphincter repair and postanal repair for the treatment of complicated injuries to the anal sphincters. Ann. R. Coll. Surg. Engl., 70:324, 1988.
7. Brunner, R.G., and Shatney, C.H.: Diagnostic and therapeutic aspects of rectal trauma: Blunt versus penetrating. Am. Surg., 53: 215, 1986.
8. Burch, J.M., Feliciano, D.V., and Mattox, K.L.: Colostomy and drainage for civilian rectal injuries: Is that all? Ann. Surg., 209: 600, 1989.
9. Carpio, G., Albu, E., Gumbs, M.A., and Gerst, P.H.: Management of colonic perforation after colonoscopy. Report of three cases. Dis. Colon Rectum, 32:624, 1989.
10. Chen, Y.M., Davis, M., and Ott, D.J.: Traumatic rectal hematoma following anal rape. Ann. Emerg. Med., 15:850, 1986.
11. Cordone, R.P., Brandeis, S.Z., and Richman, H.: Rectal perforation during barium enema: Report of a case. Dis. Colon Rectum, 31: 563, 1987.
12. Critclow, J.F., Houlihan, M.J., Landolt, C.C., et al.: Primary sphincter repair in anorectal trauma. Dis. Colon Rectum, 28:945, 1985.
13. Duncan, A.O., Phillips, T.F., Scalea, T.M., et al.: Management of transpelvic gunshot wounds. J. Trauma, 29:1335, 1989.
14. Ebraheim, N.A., Savolaine, E.R., Rusin, J.R., et al.: Occult rectal perforation in a major pelvic fracture. J. Orthop. Trauma, 2:340, 1989.
15. Eckert, W.G., and Katchis, S.: Anorectal trauma. Am. J. Forensic Med. Pathol., 10:3, 1989.
16. Falcone, R.E., and Carey, L.C.: Colorectal trauma. Surg. Clin. North Am., 68:1307, 1988.
17. Fallon, W.F., Jr.: The present role of colostomy in the management of trauma. Dis. Colon Rectum, 35:1094, 1992.
18. Fallon, W.F., Jr., Reyna, T.M., Brunner, R.G., et al.: Penetrating trauma to the buttock. South. Med. J. 81:1236, 1988.
19. Feliciano, D.V., Burch, J.M., Spjut-Patrinely, V., et al.: Abdominal gunshot wounds. Ann. Surg., 208:362, 1988.
20. Ferraro, F.J., Livingston, D.H., Bdum, T., et al.: The role of sigmoidoscopy in the management of gunshot wounds to the buttocks. Am. Surg., 59:350, 1993.
21. Gardner, D.J., and Hanson, R.E.: Computed tomography of retroperitoneal perforation after barium enema. Clin. Imaging, 14: 208, 1990.
22. Green, J.R., and Soohoo, S.L.: Factors associated with rectal injury in spontaneous deliveries. Obstet. Gynecol., 73:732, 1989.
23. Greenwald, J.C., and Hoexter, B.: Repair of rectovaginal fistulas. Surg. Gynecol. Obstet., 146:443, 1978.
24. Haas, P.A., and Fox, T.A., Jr.: Civilian injuries of the rectum and anus. Dis. Colon Rectum, 22:17, 1979.
25. Harned, R.K., Williams, S.M., Maglinte, D.D., et al.: Clinical application of in vitro studies for barium enema examination following colorectal biopsy. Radiology, 154:319, 1985.
26. Heine, J.A., Wong, W.D., and Goldberg, S.M.: Surgical treatment for constipation. Surg. Gynecol. Obstet., 176:403, 1993.
27. Howell, H.S., Bartizal, J.F., and Freeark, R.J.: Blunt trauma involving the colon and rectum. J. Trauma, 16:624, 1976.
28. Huang, A.R., and Bergman, H.: Complications of the "Mayo" enema. J. Am. Geriatr. Soc., 38:470, 1990.
29. Ivatury, R.R., Rao, D.M., Nallathambi, M., et al.: Penetrating gluteal injuries. J. Trauma, 22:706, 1982.
30. Ivatury, R.R., Licata, J., Gunduz, Y., et al.: Management options in penetrating rectal injuries. Am. Surg., 57:50, 1991.
31. Jackson, D.S., Maj.: Accidental impalement injuries of the intraperitoneal rectum caused by the barrel of the self loading rifle. J. R. Army Med. Corps, 131:164, 1985.
32. Kudsk, K.A., McQueen, M.A., Voeller, G.R., et al.: Management of complex perineal soft-tissue injuries. J. Trauma, 30:1155, 1990.
33. Lavenson, G.S., and Cohen, A.: Management of rectal injuries. Am. J. Surg., 122:226, 1971.
34. Lee, R.Y., Miller, S., and Thorpe, C.: Intrarectal tear from water skiing. Am. J. Gastroenterol., 87:662, 1992.
35. Levine, H., Simon, R.J., Smith, T.R., et al.: Guaiac testing in the diagnosis of rectal trauma: What is its value? J. Trauma, 32:210, 1992.
36. Lischick, W.P., Knoll, S.M., and Isaacson, N.H.: Rectosigmoid perforations in homosexual patients. Am. Surg., 51:602, 1985.
37. Magen, A.B., Moser, R.P., Woomert, C.A., et al.: Septic arthritis of the hip: A complication of a rectal tear associated with pelvic fractures. AJR, 157:817, 1991.
38. Mangiante, E.C., Graham, A.D., and Fabian, T.C.: Rectal gunshot wounds. Am. Surg., 52:37, 1986.
39. Marti, M.C., Morel, P., and Rohner, R.: Traumatic lesions of the rectum. Int. J. Colorect. Dis., 1:152, 1986.
40. Maull, K.I., Sachatello, C.R., and Ernst, C.B.: The deep perineal laceration—an injury frequently associated with open pelvic fractures: A need for aggressive surgical management. J. Trauma, 17:685, 1977.
41. Maull, K.I., Snoddy, J.W., and Haynes, B.W., Jr.: Penetrating wounds of the buttock. Surg. Gynecol. Obstet., 149:855, 1979.
42. Moller, B.K., and Laurberg, S.: Intervention during labor: Risk factors associated with complete tear of the anal sphincter. Acta Obstet. Gynecol. Scand., 71:520, 1992.
43. Moore, E.E., Cogbill, T.H., Malangoni, M.A., et al.: Organ injury

scaling, II: Pancreas, duodenum, small bowel, colon, and rectum. J. Trauma, *30*:1427, 1990.

44. Morse, R.M., Spirnak, J.P., and Resnick, M.I.: Iatrogenic colon and rectal injuries associated with urological intervention: Report of 14 patients. J. Urol., *140*:101, 1988.

45. Nivatvongs, S.: Complications in colonoscopic polypectomy: Lessons to learn from an experience with 1576 polyps. Am. Surg., *54*:61, 1988.

46. Nguyen, B.D., and Beckman, I.: Silent rectal perforation after endoscopic polypectomy: CT features. Gastrointest. Radiol., *17*:271, 1992.

47. Nolan, J.F.: Delayed Presentation of Rectal Perforation. J. R. Soc. Med., *83*:744, 1990.

48. Puet, T.A., Phen, L., and Hurst, D.L.: Pulsed irrigation enhanced evacuation: New method for treating fecal impaction. Arch. Phys. Med. Rehabil., *72*:935, 1991.

49. Reiertsen, O., Skjoto, J., Jacobsen, C.D., and Rosseland, A.R.: Complications of fiberoptic gastrointestinal endoscopy—five years' experience in a central hospital. Endoscopy, *19*:1, 1987.

50. Richardson, J.D., Harty, J., Amin, M., et al.: Open pelvic fracture. J. Trauma, *22*:533, 1982.

51. Robertson, H.D., Rax, J.E., Ferrari, B.T., et al.: Management of rectal trauma. Surg. Gynecol. Obstet., *154*:161, 1982.

52. Roettig, L.C., Glasser, B.F., and Barney, C.O.: Definitive surgery of the large intestine following war wounds. Ann. Surg., *124*:755, 1946.

53. Rothenberger, D., Velasco, R., Strate, R., et al.: Open pelvic fracture: A lethal injury. J. Trauma, *18*:184, 1987.

54. Salzstein, R.J., Quebbeman, E., and Melvin, J.L.: Anorectal injuries incident to enema administration. Am. J. Phys. Med. Rehabil., *67*:186, 1988.

55. Serpell, J.W., and Nicholls, R.J.: Stercoral perforation of the colon. Br. J. Surg., *77*:1325, 1990.

56. Shannon, F.L., Moore, E.E., Moore, F.A., et al.: Value of distal colon washout in civilian rectal trauma—reducing gut bacterial translocation. J. Trauma, *28*:989, 1988.

57. Smith, I., Carr, N., Corrado, O.J., and Young, A.: Rectal necrosis after a phosphate enema. Age Aging, *16*:328, 1987.

58. Soon, J.C.C., Shang, N.S., Goh, P.M.Y., and Rauff, A.: Perforation of the large bowel during colonoscopy in singapore. Am. Surg., *56*:285, 1990.

59. Steele, M., and Blaisdell, F.W.: Treatment of colon injuries. J. Trauma, *17*:557, 1977.

60. Strate, R.G., and Grieco, J.G.: Blunt injury to the colon and rectum. J. Trauma, *23*:384, 1983.

61. Tadros, S., and Watters, J.M.: Retroperitoneal perforation of the rectum during barium enema examination. Can. J. Surg., *31*:49, 1988.

62. Tancer, M.L., Lasser, D., and Rosenblum, N.: Rectovaginal fistula or perineal and anal sphincter disruption, or both, after vaginal delivery. Surg. Gynecol. Obstet., *171*:43, 1990.

63. Thomas, D.D., Levison, M.A., Dykstra, B.J., et al.: Management of rectal injuries. Am. Surg., *56*:507, 1990.

64. Thomas, P.R.S.: Ano-rectal injury causing extraperitoneal and subcutaneous emphysema. Injury, *18*:426, 1987.

65. Tomkins, R.G., McCabe, C.J., Burke, J.F., et al.: Rectal necrosis after pelvic crush injury. J. Trauma, *28*:697, 1988.

66. Tuggle, D., and Huber, P.J.: Management of rectal trauma. Am. J. Surg., *148*:806, 1984.

67. Vo, N.M., Russell, J.C., and Becker, D.R.: Gunshot wounds to the buttocks. Am. Surg., *49*:579, 1983.

68. Whelan, T.J., Jr.: Surgical lessons learned in the care of the wounded. Med. Bull. U.S. Army, Europe, *38*:4, 1981.

69. Witz, M., Shpitz, B., Zager, M., et al.: Anal erotic instrumentation. Dis. Colon Rectum, *27*:331, 1984.

Chapter 34

PILONIDAL DISEASE, PRESACRAL CYSTS AND TUMORS, AND PELVIC AND PERIANAL PAIN

STEVEN D. WEXNER / SANDER R. BINDEROW

PILONIDAL DISEASE

Pilonidal cysts or sinuses represent an acute or chronic infection of the natal cleft. The disease generally occurs in young adults and teenagers, with a 3:1 male:female predominance. The condition was originally reported by Anderson in 1847 and subsequently by Hodges in 1880.[8,35] The original use of the term pilonidal sinus referred to a "nest of hair." The derivation of this term comes from the fact that the epithelial-lined sinus almost always contains hair. If the sinus becomes infected, it can drain from one or several openings in the area of the natal cleft. During World War II, more than 77,000 soldiers were admitted to Army hospitals for pilonidal sinus problems, and they remained hospitalized an average of 44 days.[2] In the early part of the Viet Nam conflict, the United States Navy reported that during a 1-year period, 2,075 men spent almost 91,000 sick days out of work directly attributable to pilonidal disease.[78] The problem of pilonidal disease is a large-scale problem that consumes many health care dollars and results in a large loss of productive time.

Etiology

Originally, pilonidal disease was thought to be congenital in origin. In 1946, however, Patey and Scarff first advanced the view, now more commonly accepted, that pilonidal disease arises from a chronic foreign body reaction resulting from penetration of the subcutaneous tissues by hair shafts that come from the surrounding skin.[63] This theory has led to the appellation of jeep drivers disease, as it is often associated with young hir-

sute men who have occupations that require prolonged periods of sitting in moving vehicles.

The other theory is that the pilonidal sinus represents a fused remnant of the caudal end of the medullary canal. A reasonable view is probably that most pilonidal cysts and sinuses are acquired by a combination of poor hygiene, local trauma, and the presence of a deep natal cleft. There may be, however, a few pilonidal sinuses that develop from a pre-existing congenital sinus or subcutaneous space.

Pathologic Features

The most constant finding related to pilonidal disease is the presence of one or more midline pits lined by skin in the sacrococcygeal area. There is often loose hair beneath these midline depressions, but hair follicles are rarely seen. The sinus wall may be lined with either granulation tissue or squamous epithelium. The inflammation usually proceeds in a cephalad and lateral direction, often forming secondary pits and openings. Carcinoma has occurred in long-standing pilonidal sinuses, although this finding is rare. Squamous cell carcinoma predominates in these rare cases and is probably analogous to the skin tumors associated with burns, skin grafting, and chronic scar formation.

Symptoms and Diagnosis

Pilonidal disease can be categorized into three distinct stages.[73] The first and most common during initial presentation is the acute pilonidal abscess. Chronic pilonidal disease, the next stage, is the residual anatomic defect that results from abscess drainage. Chronic disease can also be present in the patient without the acute abscess, but with a chronically draining fistula. The last stage, and the most difficult to treat, is the chronic recurrent pilonidal sinus. Treatment for the latter involves advanced plastic surgery flap techniques as discussed later in the chapter.

Most patients present in the acute stage with pain, swelling, and purulent discharge. Fever and leukocytosis may be physical findings. A careful history often reveals that the presentation was precipitated by mechanical trauma. Some feel that such trauma may convert the lesion from an asymptomatic chronic inflammation to an acute fulminating process. In the active phase, mixed infections are found with such pathogenic organisms as *Staphylococcus aureus* and *Streptococcus*. Anaerobes and gram-negative rods also may play a role, as *Bacteroides* species can often be detected on culture.[36] The chronic variety of pilonidal disease causes a persistent painful sensation at or overlying the coccyx. Patients occasionally experience painless intermittent drainage. Some patients may have already had multiple recurrent abscesses in the sacrococcygeal area either spontaneously or surgically drained. These areas heal for only a short time and subsequently break down again. These patients are in the complex category.

Physical examination may reveal some surrounding cellulitis or tenderness around the natal cleft or sacrococcygeal area. Almost always, one or several dimples or sinuses will be found either along or immediately adjacent to the midline natal cleft. Frequently, a tuft of hair will be seen extruding from the external orifice. If present, this sign is virtually diagnostic. If no hair is present, a probe can be gently placed into the opening and its course determined. If the patient has already undergone incision and drainage of abscesses in this area, the characteristic dimples may not be present. Differential diagnosis includes anorectal fistula, simple abscess, inflammatory bowel disease with a complex fistula, hidradenitis suppurativa, actinomycosis, and tuberculosis.

Methods of Treatment

The treatment of a pilonidal cyst or sinus is usually surgical, but the choice of treatment varies with the extent of the lesion and whether it is complicated by acute or chronic infection. From the perspective that it is an acquired disease, the assessment of underlying factors such as poor hygiene, excessive hairiness, and mechanical trauma is worthwhile. With the view that the lesion is essentially a chronic foreign body reaction, the least complicated surgical approach is best.

Asymptomatic Lesions

An asymptomatic pilonidal dimple found in a child or young adult requires no treatment. In cysts and sinuses that are infected but not purulent when first seen, the infection should be controlled by treatment with hot compresses and appropriate antibiotics before excision is undertaken. If abscess formation or inadequate drainage of the infection is present, immediate incision and drainage of the lesion should be employed and the inflammation should be allowed to subside before pro-

ceeding with a planned excision of the cyst or sinus tract.

Acute Pilonidal Abscess

There is general agreement that acute abscess formation should be treated by immediate incision and drainage, usually as an outpatient procedure and with the use of local anesthesia. In cases in which the degree of cellulitis is minimal or moderate and the abscess cavity is not unusually extensive, a simple yet definitive operation can be undertaken. Such an operation should involve excision of the midline sinus with narrow margins and curettage of the wall of the abscess cavity. A specimen of the abscess contents can be taken for culture, but the use of antibiotics in most cases is not necessary. Postoperative wound care should be meticulously carried out and should employ wet dressings and hot sitz baths in the early phases. In addition to standard sitz baths, a jet stream of water is a very effective means of maintaining a clean wound. Either a shower attachment or a portable Water-Pik, as used for dental care, is an excellent adjunct. If these implements are unavailble, scrubbing the edges and the base of the wound with a toothbrush is also helpful. Hair around the edges of the wound should be shaved weekly until the wound is completely healed, and granulation tissue should be cauterized or curetted away and the wounds loosely packed open to encourage rapid epithelization. Although healing usually occurs within 2 to 4 weeks, only one third of patients will be free of recurrence. Success is related to prolonged meticulous wound care and healing from the base of the wound to the top.

Chronic Pilonidal Disease

Persistence of the underlying pilonidal sinus is likely in cases involving a large abscess for which only simple incision and drainage has been carried out. Definitive treatment for moderately symptomatic chronic pilonidal sinus should, in most cases, be conservative, involving small-scale procedures and deliberately avoiding hospitalization and loss of time from work. The patient should be instructed about the nature of the lesion, and the importance of meticulous local measures should be stressed. Follow-up should be done on a regular outpatient basis.

Patients with chronic pilonidal disease may be treated conservatively, but are usually treated with surgery. The surgical procedure involves excision of the diseased tissue; a variety of options are available for wound management. The wound may be (1) left open to close by secondary intention, (2) marsupialized, (3) closed primarily, (4) closed using skin grafts, or (5) closed using flaps.

Obviously, a wound left open will drain and thus an abscess will not form provided that healing occurs in the appropriate geometric fashion. However, the length of time to complete healing can be quite prolonged. Conversely, primary closure obviates continued drainage and the need for frequent dressing changes and wound surveillance. However, the risks of abscess formation and wound breakdown with recurrence are greater after primary closure than after excision without closure.

Barcia retrospectively analyzed data on 330 consecutive military personnel treated by one surgical group over a 2-year period.[9] Of these, 229 patients were treated by 240 formal extirpative procedures; all operations were performed in the operating room, and after 4,760 bed days there was a significant prevalence of unhealed wounds. The other 101 patients were treated by weekly shaving of the natal cleft and incision and drainage of any acute suppuration. None of these procedures was done in the operating room and all wounds healed in these patients. This study highlights the importance of meticulous depilatory technique in preventing disease progression.

Perhaps the simplest definitive procedure for chronic pilonidal disease is pilonidal cystotomy, which can be done in most instances in an outpatient setting using local infiltration anesthesia. In this procedure, the primary and secondary tracks are probed and laid open. The contained hairs and granulation tissue are removed along with the midline dimples to the underlying cavity. The walls of the sinus or cyst, however, are not removed; the skin edges adjacent to the incision are trimmed and beveled quite conservatively. Control of oozing from the edges is best accomplished with cautery and the application of a dressing. Shaving of the wound edges in the follow-up period is very important. The majority of these wounds heal within 2 months, but in some cases a longer period will be required. A prolonged healing period may be the chief disadvantage of this approach compared with the combination of excision and skin grafting. Reported recurrence rates are not significantly greater for cystotomy than for more elaborate surgical procedures.

The indications for the use of the various other methods of definitive treatment involving surgical excision include, most obviously, failure of pilonidal cystotomy and other conservative measures to control the inflammation. The degree of lateral extension and the formation of secondary skin openings will also favor the use of more radical operations to some extent.

The wounds created by completed excision of pilonidal disease of average extent tend to be difficult to close because of their anatomic location. A variety of techniques, most of them employing flaps, have been suggested to overcome this difficulty.[24,53,70] Without flaps or grafts, these wounds are notably slow to heal by secondary intention, and they tend to gape widely around the exposed sacrum and coccyx. On average, they take between 2 and 3 months to close, so that various surgical compromises, including partial closure, skin grafting, and marsupialization may need to be employed to accelerate achievement of wound closure. Closing the skin primarily, while reducing healing time, results in a higher incidence of wound infection and breakdown. However, some authors have recently reported better results by primary closure of small pilonidal disease wounds after excision.[74,91] We feel the best compromise between leaving the wound open and primary closure is marsupialization.

General Surgical Tips

ANESTHESIA FOR SURGICAL TREATMENT. These operations are performed electively with general or regional block anesthesia. The presence of cellulitis or active infection is a contraindication to regional anesthesia. Local infiltration anesthesia is generally unsatisfactory.

POSITION AND INCISIONS. The ideal placement of the patient is the prone–jackknife position with the table slightly flexed at the level of the hips and the buttocks taped apart. The hips must be elevated on a Kraske-type roll (Fig. 34–1). The skin is carefully shaved and cleansed with an antiseptic. The use of a fiberoptic operating headlight facilitates the search for granulation tissue; this method is often the best way to follow and unroof side tracks. A set of fistula probes, such as Lockhart-Mummery probes, and a grooved director are helpful in the search for side tracks. In addition, a set of bone curettes must be on the operating room tray, as these are useful to débride the cysts and tracks. Electrocautery is the optimal method of hemostasis.

The exact shape and location of the incision depends on the type of operation to be employed and the extent of tissue and contour of the area to be excised. Usually

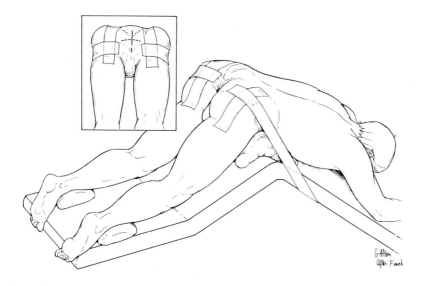

FIGURE 34-1. The prone–jackknife position for pilonidal cystotomy or cystectomy.

a narrow elliptic incision, extending entirely around the pilonidal lesion and with the long axis of the ellipse vertical and parallel to the spine, is employed (Fig. 34–2).

Marsupialization

Marsupialization consists of incising the pilonidal cyst, emptying its contents, excising its walls, and suturing the edges of its floor to the edges of the skin incision so that the wound can heal by secondary intention.

If the epithelial lining of the floor of the pilonidal cyst has not been destroyed by infection, it resembles true skin histologically and functions as such. If the epidermoid lining has been destroyed, the resulting granulation epithelializes to form a substantial scar.

Buie and Curtiss believe that the treatment of pilonidal disease by marsupialization has the following advantages[14]:

1. The residual epithelial lining stabilizes the wound edges just as in the technique of anal fistulotomy and thus reduces the overall size of the wound.

2. Unnecessary amounts of normal tissue are not sacrificed.

3. Recurrences are rare.

4. The time required for complete healing following operation is satisfactory.

5. Preoperative preparation is minimal.

6. Postoperative bed confinement is reduced.

7. Special postoperative management including bed rest, special diet, and intentional constipation is avoided.

8. Postoperative discomfort is minimal.

9. The operation is technically easy to perform, and deep wounds that involve the sacral fascia or periosteum are avoided.

10. Adherent, immovable, painful scars do not develop.

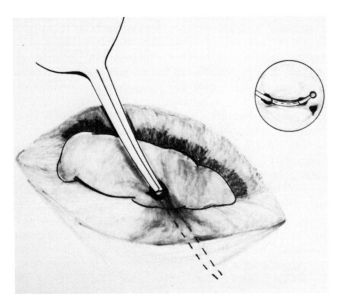

FIGURE 34–2. The use of a curved probe or a grooved director to unroof side tracks.

11. The operation can be employed in almost all patients with pilonidal disease.

TECHNIQUE. When an undrained pilonidal abscess is present, an attempt is made to remove the entire dome of the abscess instead of merely performing incision and drainage. Such a procedure may exteriorize the abscess cavity sufficiently to produce a cure, or the wall of the abscess may be so close to the skin edge that uniting the two with a few sutures may be all that is necessary to exteriorize the abscess cavity completely.

In the usual subject, in whom there is no undrained abscess, marsupialization is accomplished by inserting a probe or a grooved director into each side track and incising over it. If more than one sinus is present, the others are treated in a similar manner until all the subsidiary tracks and the entire cavity have been opened widely. Methylene blue is unnecessary because the appearance of the tissue involved by pilonidal disease can be easily distinguished from normal tissue, and subsidiary tracks can be discovered by curetting the residual wall of the cyst after the cavity has been opened widely. The opening of a subsidiary track is often revealed by the persistence of granulation and detritus at that point despite vigorous scrubbing. A probe is inserted into all primary subsidiary tracks that are discovered, and they are opened widely and similarly examined for any secondary subsidiary tracks. Following the granulation tissue is usually the easiest way to find these side tracks.

The overhanging edges of the incised skin, along with the external and lateral walls of the cysts and sinuses, are cut away, leaving the floor of the cyst or abscess and its branching tracks intact. After hemostasis has been achieved with electrocautery, the skin edges are then sutured to the cut margins of the remaining floor of the cyst and its branching sinuses with a continuous lock stitch of 3-0 chromic or 3-0 polyglycolic acid suture. In some cases the skin cannot be approximated to the lining membrane along its entire margin: when this occurs, the skin margin in that area must be sutured to the thickened fibrous integument usually found adjacent to inflamed pilonidal lesions, or even to the subjacent fat. These alternatives are not preferred, but it is said that they do not interfere with a favorable result.[14]

We do not pack these wounds, as packing prevents drainage and can be uncomfortable. We recommend laying a single folded gauze pad loosely across the base of the wound and taping it in place. The dressing is removed the evening of surgery, and sitz baths are begun. Patients should take three sitz baths daily and can cover the wound loosely with a gauze pad to prevent soilage of clothing. The wound should be examined at weekly intervals in the office. Water-Pik and toothbrush débridements by the patient and curettage by the physician at each office visit will help expedite the healing process. Most wounds should heal within 4 to 6 weeks, and the recurrence rate should be less than 7% at 8 years.[2]

Chronic Recurrent Pilonidal Disease

A wide array of techniques exists for operative eradication of pilonidal disease. Larger wounds can be cov-

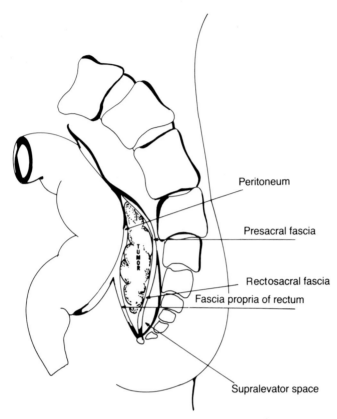

FIGURE 34-3. The anatomy of the presacral space and its relationship to surrounding structures.

ered with a split-thickness skin graft at the initial operation to speed the healing process. A variety of flap techniques are useful in complex, recurrent pilonidal disease. All of the flap procedures first involve deep excision of the pilonidal disease down to the prevertebral fascia. A flap consisting of skin, subcutaneous tissue, and sometimes muscle or fascia is then created and rotated to fill the defect. Gluteus maximus myocutaneous flap, Z-plasty, and rhomboid fasciocutaneous flap have been used with success rates of 90%.[4,53,64,69,84] Flaps can also be used as a means to close a large pilonidal wound primarily.[39,51]

All of these techniques have limited usefulness, since most cysts are cured by simpler, more conservative procedures. However, one very useful technique for the treatment of recurrent pilonidal cysts that are refractory to other forms of surgical extirpation is the cleft closure. This technique essentially consists of obliteration of the midline by rotating a cross-natal cleft flap. The procedure is performed in the same-day surgery unit. Bascom reported 30 consecutive patients in whom a total of 68 "curative" pilonidal procedures had failed (one to six procedures per patient).[11] All 30 wounds healed after cleft closure. The median number of office visits was two visits, and the mean number of lost days of school or work was 4 days. There were five early postoperative complications: one wound infection, one delayed healing, and three small areas of flap necrosis. Only one case recurred, 2 years later. We have used this procedure with good success.

Summary

Acute abscesses should be drained without any excision. Chronic sinuses should be conservatively excised, either as a cystotomy or as narrow excision with marsupialization. Postoperative wound care is the key to successful healing. However, despite meticulous attention to hygiene, nonhealing lesions may be encountered. These sinuses should again be treated by conservative excision and marsupialization. Further failure to heal or recurrence dictates an alternate approach. Any of the complex rotation flaps can be used. Alternatively, we prefer the Bascom cleft closure procedure.

PRESACRAL CYSTS AND TUMORS

Anatomy

The retrorectal or presacral space is the area between the upper two thirds of the rectum anteriorly and the sacral vertebrae posteriorly (Fig. 34-3). The other anatomic boundaries are the ureters and internal iliac vessels laterally, the pelvic peritoneal reflection superiorly, and the rectosacral fascia inferiorly. The rectosacral fascia originates at the periosteum of the fourth sacral vertebra and runs inferoanteriorly to meet the rectum, 3 to 5 cm cephalad to the anorectal ring.[18,27] The presacral space is really a potential space that normally contains mesenchymal tissue, the middle sacral artery, the superior hemorrhoidal vessels, and branches of the sympathetic and parasympathetic nerves. Caudal to the rectosacral fascia is the supralevator space, a U-shaped space bordered by Denonvilliers' fascia anteriorly and the levator ani muscles inferiorly. Many lower presacral cysts and tumors are actually in this space (Fig. 34-4).

Incidence and Classification

Because these lesions are seldom seen by most practitioners, very large populations must be studied to estimate their true incidence. Spencer and Jackman reported three presacral cysts found during 20,851 routine adult proctosigmoidoscopic examinations.[75] Also from the Mayo Clinic, Whittaker and Pemberton reported one presacral tumor in 40,000 hospitalizations.[90] Thus, these two retrospective studies estimate the incidence to be from 0.0025 to 0.014%. The incidence of presacral teratomas is 1 in 40,000 births.[29,62] Table 34-1 lists the various lesions that have been reported in the presacral space.[22,43,48,68,85] In considering the differential diagnosis of a presacral lesion, the basic tenet to recall is that any tissue line that inhabits the boundaries of the space may be the parent cell line for both benign and malignant growths. Therefore, the simplest means of constructing a comprehensive table of tumor types is to systematically list the cell lines found in the space (Table 34-1). Despite an extensive variety of possible lesions, the majority are either congenital lesions, of which developmental cysts are the most common, or neurogenic tumors.[38,85]

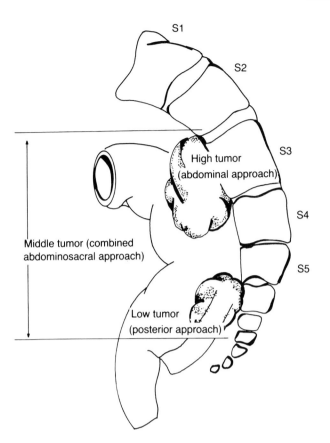

S1

S2

S3

High tumor
(abdominal approach)

S4

Middle tumor (combined
abdominosacral approach)

S5

Low tumor
(posterior approach)

FIGURE 34–4. The location of high and low presacral cysts and tumors. Note that many low-lying lesions are actually in the supralevator space.

Pathologic Features

Finne has established certain criteria that are helpful in determining both the type of tumor likely to be present in a given patient and the likelihood of malignancy.[23] He found that presacral lesions diagnosed in the neonatal period carry a 4% risk of malignancy, whereas those diagnosed in the postnatal and pediatric period are associated with a 95% rate of malignancy. In adults, only 10% of cystic lesions are malignant, whereas solid lesions carry a 60% rate of malignancy. Finne also noted that when all malignant lesions are considered, the female:male ratio is 1:1.

History

The first report of a presacral lesion was by a seventeenth century French obstetrician named Peu.[33] The term sacral teratoma was coined in 1869 by Virchow.[87] The first documentation of the surgical extirpation of a presacral lesion was published by Middeldorpf in 1885.[52] Because of this, many authors in the earlier part of the twentieth century referred to presacral teratoma as Middeldorpf's tumors.[90]

Congenital Lesions

More than half of all presacral tumors are congenital and two thirds of them are developmental cysts.[23] Jao

and co-workers retrospectively reviewed 129 patients with primary presacral tumors.[38] Of these tumors, 79 (61%) were congenital, and 49 of the congenital lesions were cystic (62%). There is a female predominance that ranges from 4:1 to 15:1.[23,38,75] These cysts usually contain columnar or cuboidal mucus-secreting epithelium and have elements of squamous and transitional epithelia.

TABLE 34–1. CLASSIFICATION OF PRESACRAL CYSTS AND TUMORS*

I. Congenital
  A. Developmental cysts
    1. Epidermoid
    2. Dermoid
    3. Mucus-secreting
    4. Teratomas
  B. Teratocarcinoma
  C. Chordoma
  D. Anterior sacral meningocele
II. Nerve
  A. Ganglioneuroma
  B. Ependymoma
  C. Neurilemmoma
  D. Neurofibroma
  E. Neurofibrosarcoma
III. Cartilage, Bone, and Muscle
  A. Benign
    1. Osteoma
    2. Osseous cyst
      a. Simple
      b. Aneurysmal
    3. Chondroma
    4. Leiomyoma
  B. Malignant
    1. Osteogenic sarcoma
    2. Ewing's tumor
    3. Chondrosarcoma
    4. Giant-cell tumor
    5. Leiomyosarcoma
IV. Adipose, Fibrous, and Endothelial
  A. Lipoma and liposarcoma
  B. Fibroma and fibrosarcoma
  C. Endothelioma and hemangioendothelial sarcoma
  D. Myelolipoma
V. Hematologic and Lymphatic
  A. Lymphangioma and lymphangiosarcoma
  B. Plasmacytoma
  C. Hemangioma and hemangiosarcoma
  D. Pericytoma
  E. Lymphoma
VI. Traumatic and Inflammatory
  A. Hematoma
  B. Abscess
    1. Perineal
    2. Pelvic
    3. Perirectal
    4. Enteric with fistula
  C. Granuloma
VII. Miscellaneous
  A. Desmoid
  B. Endometrioma
  C. Mesenchymoma
  D. Metastatic carcinoma
  E. Recurrent pelvic carcinoma
    1. Rectal
    2. Prostatic
    3. Cervical
    4. Other

*Modified from Uhlig, B.E., and Johnson, R.L.: Presacral tumors and cysts in adults. Dis. Colon Rectum, *18*:581, 1975, with permission.

Although both endodermal and ectodermal layers are present, the histologic picture is different from that of a teratoma. A variety of terminologies are commonly used to classify these mucus-secreting cysts. These terms include dermoid, cystic teratoma, cystic hamartoma, enterogenic cyst, and simple cyst.[92]

Uhlig and Johnson classified these presacral developmental cysts based on histopathologic characteristics.[85] They noted that mucus-secreting cysts are usually lined with columnar mucus-secreting epithelium; however, squamous or transitional epithelium may be present. The cysts are often multiloculated and thin walled and contain a clear to light green mucoid material. Epidermoid cysts have squamous epithelium but lack skin appendages. Dermoid cysts have sweat glands, hair follicles, and sebaceous glands in addition to a stratified squamous lining. Teratomas have two or more germ-cell layers and may contain hair, brain, cartilage, kidney, teeth, or other tissue types. Indeterminate cysts are those that become so inflamed that histopathologic categorization is not possible. The great majority of these cysts are benign, although malignant degeneration is possible.[23,75]

Although most congenital lesions are asymptomatic and are found on digital rectal examination, they also can become infected, and present as an abscess. Several authors have cited criteria for suspecting the diagnosis of a presacral developmental cyst.[75,85] These criteria include the presence of a presacral mass, the presence of a postanal dimple or sinus, history of recurrent perianal suppuration, history of multiple failed fistulotomies, hair or sebum exuding from a perianal sinus, and an inability to find an anorectal cryptoglandular source for the preceding symptoms. Moreover, if the patient is female, the index of suspicion should be even higher.

Presacral Teratoma

Although rare, the presacral teratoma is the most common teratoma of infancy and the most common extragenital teratoma in all ages. Its incidence has been reported as 1 in 40,000 births.[31,38] The lesion is much more common in females than in males at all ages, with 60 to 90% of the cases occurring in females.[23,90]

Presacral teratomas contain tissue from two or more germ cell layers; the degree of differentiation of the elements varies. Benign lesions tend to contain well-differentiated, mature elements such as hair, bone, and teeth. In addition, benign tumors are usually cystic, whereas their malignant counterparts are frequently solid.[23]

The largest series of presacral teratomas is that of Altman and colleagues.[5] They surveyed the members of the surgical section of the American Academy of Pediatrics for the frequency with which they encountered all such lesions between 1962 and 1972; 405 cases were reported. Seventy-four per cent of the patients were females and more than 90% were full-term, vaginally delivered infants. More than half of the patients were diagnosed on the first day of life, although 18% were not diagnosed within the first 6 months of life. Of the total cases reported, 18% had associated anomalies, musculoskeletal and renal being the most common.

The tumors were grouped according to their location. Type I tumors (186 patients) were predominantly external with only minimal presacral components. Type II tumors (138 patients) had a nearly equal external and presacral distribution. Type III tumors (35 patients) were externally visible tumors and predominant masses located in the pelvis with intra-abdominal extension. Type IV tumors (39 patients) were presacral masses only with no external presentation. This classification is shown diagrammatically in Figure 34–5.

Eighty-two per cent of the tumors were histologically benign and 18% were malignant. Distant metastases were present at initial diagnosis in none of the type I lesions, in 6% of the type II lesions, in 20% of the type III lesions, and in 8% of the type 4 lesions. The size of the tumor had no bearing on the incidence of malignancy. However, the most consistently significant correlate with malignancy was age. Only 7% of girls and 10% of boys diagnosed prior to 2 months of age had malignant lesions, whereas 48% of girls and 67% of boys older than 2 months had malignancy at diagnosis. The occurrence of radiographically visible calcification (33 to 50%) has no relation to malignancy.[29]

The findings of Grosfeld and Billmire were similar, with 67 to 76% of patients with presacral teratomas 1 to 4 weeks old at the time of diagnosis.[29] Most of the remaining patients will have presented by the age of 4 years. Most of the newborns are asymptomatic with a prominent external mass. Associated anomalies are seen in 12 to 18% of patients with presacral teratomas. Although these anomalies have involved all organ systems, the most striking association has been with anorectal malformations, including rectal stenosis and imperforate anus.[20,41,56]

In the adult population, the tumors may be associated with necrosis, infection, and the clinical signs of anorectal suppurative disease. If the teratoma is cystic, it can rupture intrarectally, evert, and grow into a pedunculated intraluminal tumor.[25] Most reported cases in adults have been in young females, in whom the tumor presents as either hair growing out of the anus or prolapse of the everted pedunculated growth.[90]

Chordoma

The chordoma is a malignant tumor that arises from the remnants of the fetal notochord. In the adult, the nucleus pulposus of the intervertebral disk is the only normal notochordal remnant. However, chordomas appear to arise from the vertebral bodies rather than from the disks. Although they can arise anywhere along the vertebral column, the presacral area is most common.[40]

Chordomas have a male/female ratio of 5:1 and a peak incidence in the fifth and sixth decades of life.[38,40] In the Uhlig and Johnson series, chordomas were the second most common type of primary presacral lesion after developmental cysts.[85] Overall, they are the most common primary presacral malignancies, representing 10 to 25% of presacral lesions in most series.[37,38]

Chordomas are of low-grade malignancy, growing

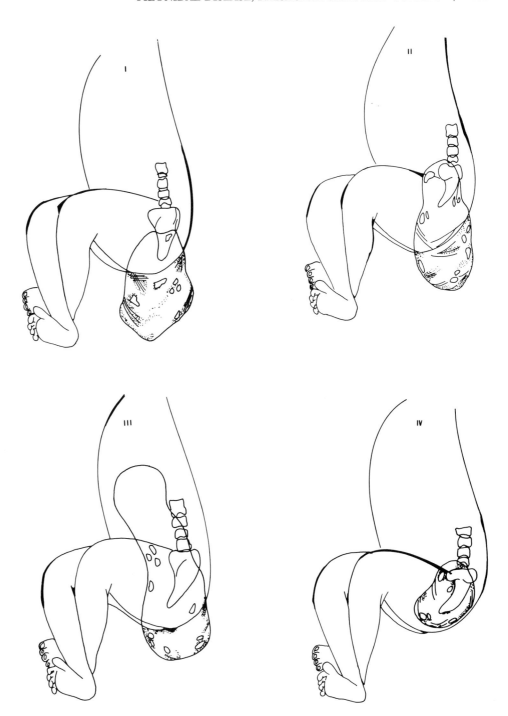

FIGURE 34-5. The Altman classification of teratomas. Type I tumors are predominantly external (sacrococcygeal), with only a minimal presacral component. Type II tumors present externally and also have a significant intrapelvic extension. Type III tumors are apparent externally, but the predominant mass is pelvic and also extends into the abdominal cavity. Type IV tumors are presacral with no external component. (From Altman, R.P., Randolf, J.G., and Lilly, J.R.: Sacrococcygeal teratoma: American Academy of Pediatrics Surgical Section Survey—1973. J. Pediatr. Surg., *9*:389, 1974, with permission.)

slowly and destroying neighboring tissue. Grossly, the lesion is hard, rubbery, nontender, and is almost always palpable transrectally.[38] Grossly, the chordoma is a lobulated, well-defined mass composed of soft gelatinous tissue, often with areas of hemorrhage and necrosis. Microscopically, the cells are clustered in irregular groups separated by gelatinous stroma that closely resembles the stages of notochord development.

Symptoms are caused by the persistent growth of these lesions that invade and replace bone, nerve, and soft tissue as they expand. Because of this method of growth, the presenting symptoms are usually pain or neurologic manifestations such as lower extremity weakness, fecal or urinary incontinence, or sexual dysfunc-

tion. Ten to 40% of chordomas are associated with distant metastases.[49] Metastases can be to lymph nodes, lungs, liver, skin, and skeletal muscle.

In the series by Jao and co-workers, two thirds of patients with chordomas had radiographic findings.[38] The four criteria for roentgenographic diagnosis of chordoma are rarification or destruction, trabeculation, calcification, and expansion of bone.

Anterior Sacral Meningocele

Anterior sacral meningoceles are anterior herniations of the meningeal sac, usually through a sacral defect, which communicate with the subarachnoid space. These rare, benign lesions are congenital, occur in women, and are associated with sacral anomalies, most commonly a scimitar sacrum (Fig. 34–6). Since these lesions rarely contain neural elements, they are not associated with a neurologic defect.

Oren and colleagues reviewed 120 cases of anterior sacral meningocele reported since 1837.[61] They reported a female:male ratio of 3:1, with the peak incidence occurring during the childbearing years. Most clinical manifestations were caused by pressure from the mass on adjacent structures such as the rectum, bladder, uterus, and sacral nerve roots. In addition to constipation, urinary symptoms, dyspareunia, dysmenorrhea, and dystocia, a pelvic mass is occasionally present.[40] Some patients present with headaches caused by compression of the sac itself.[61] Approximately 10 to 20% of patients with anterior sacral meningoceles have associated teratomas and cysts that cloud the diagnosis. As noted previously, the Currarino triad is an anorectal malformation—usually an imperforate anus, a sacral bony defect, and a presacral mass.[20] The mass can be an anterior sacral meningocele, a teratoma, or a developmental cyst.

Other Presacral Lesions

The most common "other" tumors found in the presacral space are neurogenic. They account for approximately 15% of presacral lesions.[37] These tumors encompass a broad spectrum of peripheral nerve tumors. A solid lesion in children or young adults is highly suggestive of a ganglioneuroma; presacral neurogenic tumors are not usually associated with von Recklinghausen's disease. Although the majority of neurogenic lesions are benign, they can cause significant local nerve damage because of the proximity of the cauda equina. They are indolent and often reach a large size prior to diagnosis. In a recent review of presacral lesions, 15% of malignant tumors were neurogenic.[17] Although the prognosis for survival is good, the morbidity can be significant.

Primary osseous neoplasms in the presacral area are less common than are metastatic ones. The lesions are often discovered because of persistent skeletal pain or peripheral neuropathy secondary to pressure on the sacral nerve roots. Malignant sarcomas derived from cartilage or bone, such as Ewing's sarcoma, have a poor prognosis. Most of these lesions are widespread and inoperable.

Benign tumors can be resected en bloc, if possible. However, locally advanced neoplasms may be difficult to resect because of the involvement of high sacral and lumbar nerve roots. Retrorectal and supralevator abscesses are a rare cause of a presacral mass. "Spontaneous" presacral hematomas are also occasionally seen.[22] They can result from external trauma or childbirth. In this miscellaneous category of presacral lesions, one must consider metastases from distant tumors and recurrences of pelvic malignancies.

Leiomyoma of the rectum is aggressive and associated with at least a 30% rate of recurrence.[23] The majority of recurrences occur between 4 and 8 years after primary

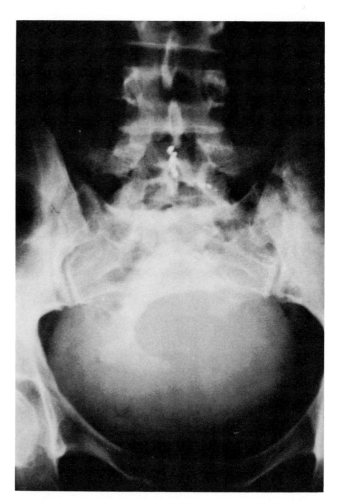

FIGURE 34–6. A radiograph of the typical "scimitar sacrum" seen with an anterior sacral meningocele. (Courtesy of Charles O. Finne III, M.D.)

resection. Large leiomyomas must be followed aggressively, as those larger than 5 cm have a significantly higher incidence of local recurrence.[23]

Symptoms

The symptoms depend on the size and location of the tumor. Generally, malignant tumors cause more symptoms than do their benign counterparts. Although Spencer and Jackman found that only 45% of presacral cysts caused symptoms, Cody and associates found that 95% of presacral malignancies were symptomatic.[17,75]

Pain is the most common symptom, being associated with 40% of benign and 90% of malignant tumors.[38] Although the pain may radiate to the pelvis or legs, it is usually localized in the lower back. Abdominal, perineal, and rectal pain are all less common.[40,85] Patients can present with symptoms similar to sciatica; these symptoms are secondary to either compression or direct invasion of the nerve. Some patients relate the onset of the pain to direct trauma.

Constipation and tenesmus are present in 23 to 33% of patients[17,38]; they result from direct tumor compression of the rectum. Less frequently, incontinence is seen because of malignant invasion of sacral nerve roots. Other less frequently seen symptoms include urinary retention and incontinence. These manifestations are due to the effect of the mass on the bladder neck and to sacral nerve invasion, respectively. Dystocia can be caused by pelvic outlet obstruction. This finding has been reported in 4% of all female patients and in 20% of female patients with anterior sacral meningoceles.[23,85]

Infected developmental cysts may present with perineal pain, fever, or purulent discharge. Although these manifestations have been discussed in the section on developmental cysts, all patients in whom multiple procedures for perianal suppuration have failed should be evaluated for a presacral cyst. This axiom is even more important in females, given their predilection for these tumors.

Since anterior sacral meningoceles communicate with the subarachnoid space, activities that increase intra-abdominal pressure can cause headaches. These actions include the Valsalva maneuver and other straining. Thus, patients may present with headaches during bowel evacuations. Rarely, patients present with meningitis caused by enteric pathogens that have infected the dural sac.[61]

Diagnosis

Perhaps more than with any other gastrointestinal disease, a thorough physical examination in these cases is almost always more rewarding than are all exhaustive sophisticated tests. The perianal area should be inspected to identify any postanal dimple. In addition, although it is infrequently seen, anesthesia of the perineum indicates nerve involvement. A rectal examination is the cornerstone of diagnosis. Of the 120 presacral lesions seen at the Mayo Clinic, 97% were palpable on rectal examination.[38] Uhlig and Johnson noted that many presacral lesions were soft and compressible.[85] Therefore, it is necessary to rotate the examining finger a full 360 degrees around the anus to obtain an accurate assessment of the presacral space. The examiner should note the consistency, size, and exact location of the lesion, as this will help plan subsequent operative extirpation. Lesions are almost never transabdominally palpable.

Although sigmoidoscopy may show extrinsic compression when a large lesion is present, small tumors have no such effect. The mucosa is usually normal. Cody and co-workers performed 12 open biopsies (14 transacral and 8 transabdominal) and 15 needle biopsies (15 transacral and 3 transrectal) in 39 patients with no complications.[17] However, Jao and associate found that patients who had preoperative biopsy of chordomas had a markedly higher local recurrence rate than did those whose lesions were not biopsied.[38] Finne also points out that there is a risk of infection, fistula formation, and tumor cell spread secondary to biopsy.[23] Verazin and colleagues reported a case of a death after transrectal needle biopsy of a presacral tumor.[86] The cause of death was septic shock secondary to *Escherichia coli* and *Clostridium perfringens* bacteremia. Because of this and similar cases, several authorities condemn preoperative biopsy of a pre-

sacral lesion.[21,23,40] They feel that the best biopsy is total surgical excision. Only if the lesion is inoperable is biopsy useful to plan adjuvant therapy and to avoid unnecessary surgery. In these selected instances, the two possible paths of biopsy are transrectal and extrarectal. The latter approach is simple, effective, and associated with fewer complications.[23] The tip of the needle can be safely guided by a finger in the rectum.

Radiologic Studies

Plain pelvic radiographs should be obtained routinely. Jao and co-workers at the Mayo Clinic found that all of their 120 patients had the presacral tumor identified with only a digital rectal examination and an abdominopelvic roentgenogram.[38] As previously mentioned, the scimitar sacrum, as shown in Figure 34–6, is an almost pathognomonic finding. Other bony abnormalities, both destructive and congenital, may be present. The more common causes of bony destruction are malignant presacral tumors and metastatic lesions. Teeth or other osseous tissue associated with teratomas may be present.

If the cyst is small and low-lying, further evaluation is unnecessary. As discussed, an excisional biopsy is the next step. If, however, the lesion is large or high or if osseous changes are evident, some of the tests to be discussed will be of benefit.

Barium enema is useful to exclude mucosal disease and to document extrinsic rectal wall involvement. The lateral view shows the width of the retrorectal space. However, the combination of digital examination, proctosigmoidoscopy, intrarectal ultrasound, and computed tomography (CT) scan is probably superior. Many authors consider CT scan with intrarectal contrast to be mandatory in the preoperative evaluation of these patients.[23,38,42,46,47] The CT scan clearly shows the size of the lesion and its spatial relationship to the sacrum, bladder, ureters, and iliac vessels. The CT scan also can differentiate solid from cystic lesions. As Finne has pointed out, 60% of solid lesions in adults are malignant.[23] In addition to intrasacral contrast, intravenous contrast should be used to assess the position of the kidneys and ureters, as a pelvic kidney is a rare cause of a presacral mass. Moreover, hydronephrosis and bladder involvement can be excluded. If suspicion exists about a pelvic kidney, an intravenous pyelogram (IVP) can be obtained. The IVP is not necessary in patients with small low-lying lesions, but is helpful with large high-lying tumors. The CT scan has essentially replaced the IVP.

Magnetic resonance imaging (MRI) is currently used in conjunction with CT scan to help further define the extent of the lesion. Saggital and coronal plane images of the tumor and surrounding structures allow the surgeon an appreciation of the extent of the tumor that is not possible with CT scan alone. Moreover, excellent quality images show the tumor in relation to the pelvic bones, spinal column structures, and central nervous system.[16] MRI is now a routine radiologic modality in the work-up of many patients with a presacral tumor.

A myelogram should be performed in all patients in whom an anterior sacral meningocele is suspected. In addition, patients with a presacral lesion and central nervous system symptoms should have myelography. The myelogram should show the relationships among the sacral nerve roots, tumor, and central nervous system.

Conventional transabdominal ultrasound is not helpful because of the deep posterior location and numerous overlying structures. Transrectal ultrasound, however, is useful in determining the depth of rectal tumors and is useful for extrarectal lesions as well.[66] Transgluteal ultrasound across the ischial foramen is another promising technique, although the interpretation is more difficult.[32] Transrectal ultrasound (US) can image any mass within 15 cm of the anus. The technique, performed with a 7.0-mHz intrarectal probe, can easily, quickly, and in a relatively noninvasive manner distinguish cystic from solid lesions. Moreover, no complications have been reported to date. Transrectal US is also useful to establish the degree of infiltration into the rectal wall and perirectal fat. It thus helps to identify the degree of invasion and determine whether or not rectal resection is a necessary adjunct to surgical excision.[16,66] Since the technique is simple and requires only a dispos-

able phosphate enema for preparation, it can often be performed at the time of initial diagnosis, immediately following digital examination and proctosigmoidoscopy.

A fistulogram may be helpful in a case of draining sinus, an angiogram will be useful if proximal sacral resection is necessary, and a bone scan might be indicated if destructive lesions of the sacrum are noted on plain films. Figure 34–7 presents a simple algorithm for the diagnosis and treatment of presacral tumors.

Surgical Treatment

There are essentially three approaches to these lesions: posterior, anterior or abdominal, and combined. The approach chosen is best determined by a consideration of size, location, and the type of lesion. Although the posterior approach is ideal for distal lesions and infected cysts, high-lying lesions without sacral involvement are best treated transabdominally. The combined technique is best for malignant lesions that involve the sacrum. Regardless of the surgical approach, full mechanical and antibiotic bowel preparation is nec-

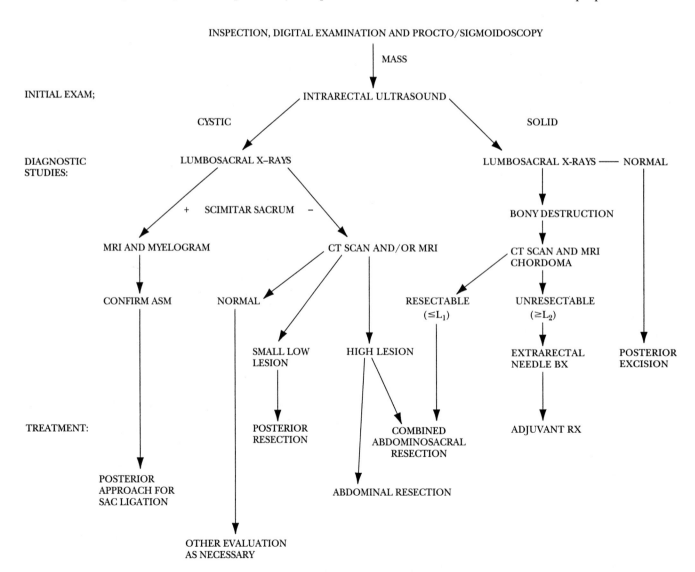

FIGURE 34–7. An algorithm for the diagnosis and treatment of presacral cysts and tumors.

essary. This precaution allows safe rectal repair or resection if necessary. Additional technical details are found in Chapter 21.

Posterior Approach

The posterior approach is excellent for the majority of presacral cysts and teratomas. Most developmental cysts have no osseous involvement, and their excision is easily accomplished in this manner. A coccygectomy is required because it adds little morbidity to the procedure and improves exposure and because without it the recurrence rates are significantly higher.[19,45]

The technique for excision is to place the patient in the modified prone–jackknife position on a Kraske roll with the buttocks taped apart (see Fig. 34–1). The incision is made over the lesion, generally at the level of the coccyx. A variety of incisions are available, including paracoccygeal, transcoccygeal, T-shaped, and curvilinear (Fig. 34–8). We generally use a paracoccygeal incision on the ipsilateral side of the lesions. The incision is deepened to the coccyx and through the anococcygeal ligament. The levator ani muscles are then reflected laterally to enter the supralevator space, and dissection commences inferolaterally (Fig. 34–9). At all times, care must be taken to avoid injury to the rectal wall while separating it from the cyst. A finger in the rectum during this part of the dissection is a helpful adjunct. The coccyx is disarticulated from the sacrum, its superior attachments are divided with electrocautery, and the specimen is removed (Fig. 34–10). Hemostasis must be meticulous, as a large dead space remains after this procedure. The middle sacral artery occasionally bleeds briskly if not adequately coagulated. The consistent location of the artery on the anterior surface at the midpoint of the sacrococcygeal junction helps in the effort for hemostasis. A suction catheter should be placed through a separate stab wound, and the subcutaneous tissue and skin should be closed.

The fourth and fifth sacral segments and their associated nerve roots can be resected via the perineal approach to permit access to the presacral space and resection of low presacral tumors that do not involve the sacrum. Preservation of the second and third sacral roots and vertebrae ensures adequate neurologic function.[31,76] If necessary, the resection can encompass both nerve roots at S2, and one at S3. However, a neurogenic rectum and bladder, as well as other adverse neurologic sequelae, will result. The S1 vertebra must remain fixed for skeletal stability.

If an infected cyst has ruptured into the rectum, transrectal drainage is the procedure of choice. This includes curettage of the cavity and enlargement of the drainage point. The lesion is excised as a second stage after the acute inflammation has resolved.

Anterior Approach

This approach is best for high presacral tumors that do not involve the sacrum. The advantages of transabdominal exposure are direct visualization and protection of the pelvic structures and early ligation of the

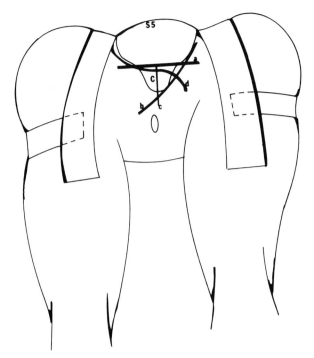

FIGURE 34-8. Various incisions for resection of presacral cysts and tumors with an en bloc coccygectomy. *a*, Transverse at the level of the sacrococcygeal joint. *b*, Curvilinear paracoccygeal (unilateral). *c*, Midline. *d*, Bilateral "lazy-S."

sigmoid vascular pedicle. After entering the abdomen and confirming the diagnosis, the rectosigmoid is visualized and reflected to the right. The presacral space is exposed, and the relationship of the tumor to the ureters and iliac vessels is determined. The sigmoid artery and vein and the middle sacral vessels are ligated. Posteriorly, the presacral fascia must not be violated, as massive bleeding will result from the presacral vessels. This type of bleeding is difficult to control, as the severed vessel retracts into the sacrum (Fig. 34–11). Nivatvongs has designed a titanium thumbtack that is both easy to use and effective in controlling sacral hemorrhage.[59] Others have commercialized the availability of the tack and confirmed its applicability.[77]

Combined Abdominoposterior Approach

The combined abdominoposterior approach offers excellent visualization of the ureters and iliac vessels. If it is synchronously performed by two surgical teams, the patient must be in the lateral decubitus position. Alternatively, a staged procedure with supine positioning for the abdominal approach followed by the prone–jackknife position for the pelvic approach can be used. The proper position for the synchronous approach is shown in Figure 34–12. The abdominal incision can be either midline or oblique, and the posterior incision should be either transverse or curvilinear.

The gluteus maximus and erector spinae muscles are detached from the sacrum and reflected laterally. After division of the anococcygeal ligament inferiorly, the posterior rectal wall is seen; the coccyx can be excised for additional exposure. At this point, the abdominal and posterior dissections meet.

Sacral mobilization is begun by inferior division of the sacrospinous and sacrotuberous ligaments bilaterally. The sciatic nerve and inferior gluteal vessels run anterior to the piriformis muscle. If division of the piriformis is necessary, these structures must be protected. The last step prior to sacral resection is superior division of the bilateral paired sacroiliac ligaments. The abdominal viscera and ureters must be protected and the common iliac arteries temporarily occluded while a transverse sacral osteotomy is made. After division of the tethering anterior longitudinal ligament, the specimen is removed. A large suction-type drain should be left in place.

Sacral Resection

In the case of chordoma, en bloc resection of the tumor and affixed sacral segments is necessary to resect the tumor with an adequate margin. The limitations to the proximal level of sacral resection are sacroiliac and spinal instability and the neurologic sequelae associated with the division of sacral nerve roots. MacCarty and co-workers recommend preservation of the upper two sacral vertebral bodies and the upper three sacral nerve roots.[50] Gunterberg and associates found that skeletal stability was adequate with preservation of the proximal half of the first sacral vertebra only.[31] However, they also

noted that although bilateral sacrifice of the second through fifth sacral roots caused severe impairment of anorectal function, unilateral loss of all five sacral roots produced no measurable abnormalities or symptoms. Cody and colleagues had four instances of permanent neurologic damage, all in patients who had sacrectomies at or proximal to S2.[17] These data support aggressive surgical management when a cure can be reasonably expected. Although this goal is ideal in chordoma patients, only 4% of such patients actually undergo total extirpation.[7,65] Radiation therapy, therefore, remains an important alternative.

Radiation Therapy

Multiple trials with radiation therapy in patients with chordoma have recently been reported. Lybeert and Meerwaldt reported 18 patients with chordoma.[49] Fourteen patients underwent surgical excision, but only two of the procedures were curative. Ten patients received between 40 and 70 Gy radiation; six patients had early recurrences, and only one survived longer than 4 years without evidence of recurrence. Reddy and co-workers reviewed ten patients with chordomas.[65] Three patients had biopsy and radiation, six patients had subtotal tumor resection and radiation, and four patients had radiation alone. The radiation dose ranged from 65 to 70 Gy; the mean time to recurrence was lengthened from 2.5 years in the nonirradiated group to 4 years in the

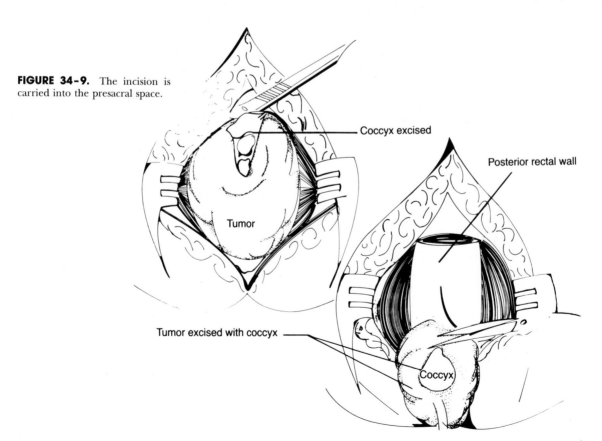

FIGURE 34-9. The incision is carried into the presacral space.

Coccyx excised

Tumor

Tumor excised with coccyx

Posterior rectal wall

Coccyx

FIGURE 34-10. The coccyx is disarticulated, and the specimen is removed.

irradiated group. Only three patients (33%) were alive and free of disease at 5 years.

Amendola and associates studied 21 patients treated with between 50 and 60 Gy and concluded that the combination of high-dose radiation therapy and complete or subtotal surgical resection offered the best chance for cure.[7] However, survival rates at 5 and 10 years were only 50 and 20%, respectively. Cummings and colleagues reported similar survival rates in their 24 patients treated with biopsy or incomplete resection and 40 to 55 Gy of radiation.[19] Specifically, the uncorrected 5- and 10-year survival rates were 62 and 28%, respectively, and most patients had clinically detectable chordomas at the time of reporting.

Anterior Sacral Meningocele

After appropriate myelographic diagnosis, a multidisciplinary surgical team should prepare for resection in anterior sacral meningocele. Both a neurosurgeon and a colorectal surgeon should be involved. The basic treatment technique is ligation and resection of the neck of the cyst through a posterior approach.

Prognosis

The prognosis after complete resection of benign lesions is excellent, especially if coccygectomy has been performed. The Mayo Clinic reported a 15% recurrence rate for benign lesions; 60% of these cases were developmental cysts and 40% were giant cell tumors.[38] The recurrence rate after excision of infected cysts is higher.[23]

The prognosis for malignant presacral tumors, including teratocarcinoma, osteosarcoma, malignant giant cell tumor, and Ewing's sarcoma, is poor. Cody and associates reported survival rates at 5, 10, 15, and 20 years of 69, 50, 37, and 20%, respectively.[17] Local recurrence occurred in 48% of their patients. Recurrences are poorly

managed by any technique. Chordomas grow slowly and can recur at any time.

POSTERIOR PELVIC AND PERIANAL PAIN

There is a great deal of overlap within the spectrum of posterior pelvic and perianal pain syndromes. The most important aspect in the diagnosis of posterior pelvic and perianal pain is the exclusion of treatable causes for such pain. Inspection and digital, anoscopic, and sigmoidoscopic examinations must be done. Fissures, fistulas, perirectal and perianal abscesses, and thrombosed hemorrhoids must be excluded.

There is, unfortunately, no uniform symptom or symptom complex that is diagnostic of posterior pelvic or perianal pain. The pain can be throbbing or burning, constant or intermittent, and radiating or nonradiating. The pain can occur during activity or can awaken patients from sleep. Some patients gain relief from a positional change or activity, whereas in others the pain is exacerbated by such maneuvers. Simpson originally described coccygodynia as a vague ache or tenderness in the sacrococcygeal area associated with simultaneous rectal or perianal pain.[71] The pain can radiate to the buttocks or posterior thighs and can be worse when the patient has been sitting for a long time.[82] The pain may be exacerbated, ameliorated, or unchanged by bowel evacuation. This chronic spasm theory led to the use of the term levator syndrome.[28] Levator spasm should be accompanied by a tender levator muscle noted during digital evaluation. Moreover, continued massage during the exam may offer some symptomatic relief.[77]

Causes of posterior pelvic and perianal pain include proctalgia fugax.[1,81] Proctalgia fugax produces spontaneous, nonradiating, severe, crampy pain, which is either constant or intermittent. Although some episodes resolve spontaneously after a few minutes, positional changes can also help. Although levator spasm has been reported to have a large female predominance, proctal-

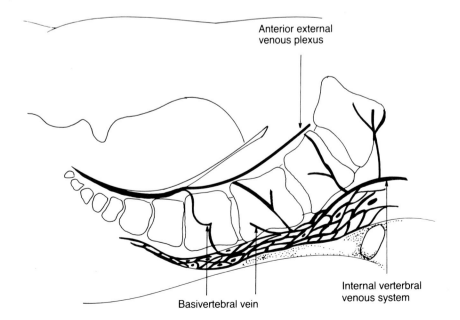

FIGURE 34-11. The relationship of the presacral veins to the sacrum. When torn, these veins retract into the bone, and hemostasis is difficult to achieve.

Anterior external
venous plexus

Internal verterbral
venous system

Basivertebral vein

gia fugax has been reported more commonly in men.[1,81] These same authors found a slightly younger age group of patients afflicted with the latter syndrome. Thompson reported a high incidence of the irritable bowel syndrome in patients with proctalgia fugax.[83]

Other causes of pain exist and may include intussusception, descending perineum syndrome, and paradoxical puborectalis contraction. These latter three causes, however, are usually associated with pain only on defecation. Moreover, the pain may be due to adhesions from previous surgery. Neill and Swash found that 20 of their 35 patients with chronic perianal pain (57%) had surgery of the pelvic viscera, lumbar spine, or anal canal prior to the onset of pain.[57] In addition, 13 patients (37%) had a history of sciatica. All of these idiopathic pain syndromes can be referred to as chronic idiopathic rectal pain (CIRP).[26]

Diagnosis

The first step is to obtain a careful history in which the characteristics and qualities of the pain are sought. This assessment must include location, radiation, type of pain, relationship of onset to position and activity, relief by positional changes, effect and relationship of defecation to pain, and a thorough standard colorectal history. Examination must include inspection and digital examination to exclude pruritus ani, fissures, fistulas, abscesses, thrombosed hemorrhoids, and levator spasm. Sigmoidoscopy should be done to look for intussusception, solitary rectal ulcer, and arteriovenous malformation, in addition to other intraluminal pathologic conditions. A gynecologic examination must exclude pelvic malignancy. Oliver and associates reported several patients with "levator spasm" who actually had recurrence of pelvic cancer, prostatic cancer, or vaginal abscess.[60] Success will be achieved by adhering to a protocol for evaluation and treatment as presented in Figure 34–13.

If no cause for the pain is found after the preliminary examination, anorectal physiologic tests may be pursued. Cinedefecography electromyography (EMG) can exclude intussusception and nonrelaxing or paradoxically contracting puborectalis syndrome.[10] Electromyography, including pudendal nerve terminal motor latency evaluation, helps to give an assessment of the function of the pelvic floor musculature and its nerve supply. Electromyography will reveal either increased activity, or failure to relax in the external sphincter, if nonrelaxing puborectalis or paradoxical puborectalis contraction are present. Anal manometry seldom reveals any cause for CIRP.[26,89] Intrarectal ultrasound, used commonly for staging of rectal tumors, has been utilized more frequently in the diagnosis of benign anorectal conditions.[55] Its applicability extends to patients with CIRP. The examination will occasionally reveal a perirectal abscess that was not apparent even on examination under anesthesia.[15] These abscesses can then be drained to provide patients with relief of their previously undiagnosed pain.[34]

In a recent review by Wexner and associates, colorectal physiologic testing (CPT) was itself evaluated as a means of diagnosing various anorectal conditions.[89] Unlike the success reported for patients with incontinence and constipation, the ability of CPT to demonstrate a diagnosis for patients with CIRP was disappointing. Only 18% of patients with CIRP had a diagnosis established on the basis of CPT. Of the 82% of patients in whom a diagnosis was not able to be elucidated, 23% had levator spasm diagnosed on physical exam that was not appreciated with CPT. While these tests can be performed with essentially no morbidity, they will be able to assist only a small group of patients.

At this point, neurologic evaluation is necessary to exclude spinal cord tumors, sciatica, and sacral root irritation. The ultimate assessment is performed by a psychiatrist and should include the Minnesota Multiphasic

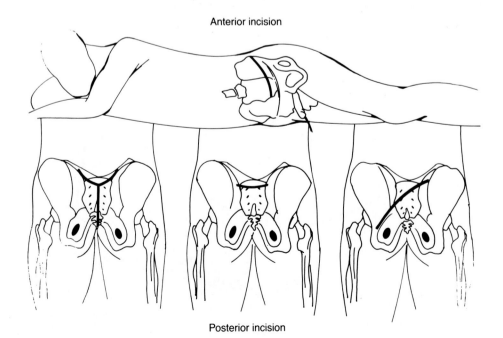

Anterior incision

Posterior incision

FIGURE 34-12. Lateral decubitus position for the combined abdominoposterior approach. Also shown are a variety of useful incisions.

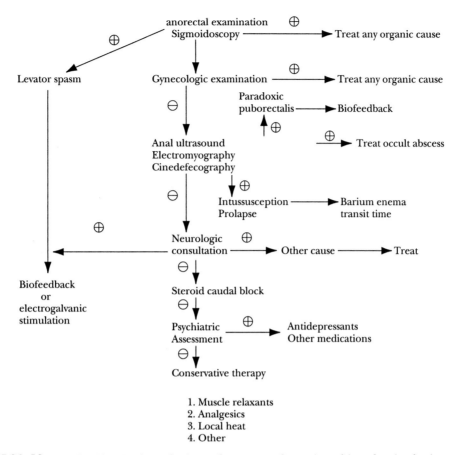

FIGURE 34–13. An algorithm for the evaluation and treatment of posterior pelvic and perianal pain.

Personality Inventory (MMPI) or a similar psychosocial evaluation. The psychiatrist plays an important role in the treatment of idiopathic pain syndromes and in prescribing phenothiazines, benzodiazepines, and antidepressants when indicated. This counseling and support are very valuable.[28] A study evaluated the personality differences of patients with levator spasm using the MMPI.[34] Hypochondriasis, depression, and hysteria scores, the so-called neurotic triad, were significantly elevated for the levator spasm patients. Thus, these subjects may be manifesting their psychologic distress as the physical symptom of levator spasm.

Treatment

Various treatments exist, and they should be tailored to the cause of the pain. Obviously, surgically correctable causes of posterior pelvic and perianal pain should be definitively addressed. Patients in whom no cause for pain is readily identified and those who exhibit pelvic floor dynamic abnormalities must be referred to a specialty center equipped to perform comprehensive anorectal physiologic evaluation.[10]

Conservative treatment includes the administration of acetaminophen, muscle relaxants, codeine, local anesthetics, local heat, sitz baths, systemic muscle relaxants, analgesics, and other similar measures.[80] Swash has been disappointed with the use of pudendal nerve blocks and pelvic floor massage.[80] If levator spasm can be diagnosed

by electromyography, cinedefecography, or balloon proctography, electrogalvanic stimulation (EGS) or biofeedback should be used. Oliver and co-workers reported a 77% rate of improvement of levator spasm with EGS.[60] These data were similar to those previously reported.[58,72] Bleijenberg and Kujpers reported a 70% rate of success when biofeedback was used to treat the nonrelaxing puborectalis syndrome.[13] Although the nonrelaxing puborectalis syndrome is not a cause of posterior pelvic and perianal pain per se, biofeedback may be useful in the treatment of levator spasm. Initial enthusiasm for EGS has been tempered somewhat after the report by Billingham and colleagues that reviewed the long-term results of this therapeutic modality.[12] While 60% of patients reported "excellent" or "good" results immediately after the treatment, only 25% remained in these categories on long-term telephone follow-up.

In a recent study of 60 patients with CIRP, biofeedback and EGS were assessed. The treatment of CIRP indeed proved a frustrating endeavor. Successful pain relief was reported by 38% of patients who underwent EGS, and 43% of patients who had biofeedback. Over 50% of patients continued to have pain.

For pain due to levator spasm that persists after failed biofeedback or EGS, caudal epidural block may offer still another alternative.[6] We recently studied eight patients who underwent steroid caudal block for intractable pain.[93] All of the patients had been previously treated with analgesics, antidepressants, EGS, and biofeedback without success. The procedure was performed under local anesthesia and intravenous sedation by an anesthesiologist specializing in pain management. The caudal epidural space was entered with a 22-gauge needle passed through the sacral hiatus. Short- and long-acting local anesthetics and a long-acting steroid were then injected. The procedure was performed on an outpatient basis and was repeated one time if necessary.

Pain relief was described by the patient as "excellent" or "good" in 75% of cases. While further studies of long-term benefit are needed, initial results show steroid caudal block as a promising new technique in the treatment of chronic intractable rectal pain.

Regardless of treatment suggested, some patients will never be relieved of their pain. These patients must be counseled about the lack of any identifiable organic, anatomic, or physiologic cause. Absence of neoplasia must be stressed. Encouragement that surgery is not needed or of any value should be emphasized. Patients like these are best managed not by a surgeon, but by a psychiatrist.

REFERENCES

1. Abrahams, A.: Proctalgia fugax. Lancet, 2:444, 1935.
2. Abramson, D.J.: Outpatient management of pilonidal sinuses: Excision and primary closure. Mil. Med., 143:753, 1978.
3. Abramson, S.J.: Excision and delayed closure of pilondal sinuses. Surg. Gynecol. Obstet., 144:205, 1977.
4. Allen-Mersh, T.G.: Pilonidal sinus: Finding the right track for treatment. Br. J. Surg., 77:123, 1990.
5. Altman, R.P., Randolf, J.G., and Lilly, J.R.: Sacrococcygeal teratoma: American Academy of Pediatrics Surgical Section Survey—1973. J. Pediatr. Surg., 9:389, 1974.
6. Amarnath, L.A., and Wexner, S.D.: Caudal epidural block in the management of proctalgia fugax. Am. J. Pain Management, 4: 153, 1994.
7. Amendola, B.D., Amendola, M.A., Oliver, E., and McClatchey, K.D.: Chordoma: Role of radiation therapy. Radiology, 158:839, 1986.
8. Anderson, A.W.: Hair extracted from an ulcer. Boston Med. Surg. J., 36:74, 1847.
9. Barcia, P.J.: Pilonidal disease: A conservative approach. In Goldberg, S.M. (ed.): Principles of Colon and Rectal Surgery. Minneapolis, University of Minnesota Press, 1985, p. 208.
10. Bartolo, D.C.C., Bartralam, C.I., Ekberg, O., et al.: Proctography, symposium. Int. J. Colorectal Dis., 3:67, 1988.
11. Bascom, J.U.: Repeat pilonidal operations. Am. J. Surg., 154:118, 1987.
12. Billingham, R.P., Isler, J.T., Friend, W.G., and Hostetler, J.: Treatment of levator syndrome using high-voltage electrogalvonic stimulation. Dis. Colon Rectum, 30:584, 1987.
13. Bleijenberg, G., and Kujpers, H.C.: Treatment of the spastic pelvic floor syndrome with biofeedback. Dis. Colon Rectum, 30:108, 1987.
14. Buie, L.A., and Curtiss, R.K.: Pilonidal disease. Surg. Clin. North Am., 32:124, 1952.
15. Cataldo, P.A., Senagore, A., Luchtefeld, M.S., et al.: Intrarectal ultrasound in the evalution of perirectal abscesses. Dis. Colon Rectum, 36:554, 1993.
16. Christensen, M.A., and Blatchford, G.J.: Presacral tumors in adults. In Beck, D.E., and Wexner, S.D. (eds.): Fundamentals of Anorectal Surgery. New York, McGraw-Hill, 1992, p. 386.
17. Cody, H.S., III, Marcove, R.C., and Quan, S.H.: Malignant retrorectal tumors: 28 years' experience at Memorial Sloan-Kettering Cancer Center. Dis. Colon Rectum, 24:501, 1981.
18. Crapp, A.R., and Cuthbertson, A.M.: William Waldeyer and the retrorectal fascia. J. Surg. Gynecol. Obstet., 138:252, 1974.
19. Cummings, B.J., Hodson, I., and Bush, R.S.: Chordoma: The results of megavoltage radiation therapy. Int. J. Radiat. Oncol., 25: 41, 1986.
20. Currarino, G., Coln, D., and Votteler, T.: Triad of anorectal, sacral, and presacral anomalies. AJR, 137:395, 1981.
21. Dozois, R.R.: Presacral cysts and tumors. In Goldberg, S.M. (ed.): Principles of Colon and Rectal Surgery. Minneapolis, University of Minnesota Press, 1987, p. 321.
22. Farkas, A.M., Quevedo-Bonilla, G., Gingold, B., et al.: Presacral hematomas, diagnosis and treatment. Dis. Colon Rectum, 30: 130, 1987.
23. Finne, C.O., III: Presacral tumors and cysts. In Cameron, J.L. (ed.): Current Surgical Therapy—2, Toronto, B.C. Decker, 1986, p. 482.
24. Fishbein, R.H., and Handelsman, J.C.: A method for primary reconstruction following radical excision of sacrococcygeal pilonidal disease. Ann. Surg., 190:231, 1979.
25. Fried, H., and Stone, H.B.: Four rare rectal tumors. Surg. Gynecol. Obstet., 50:762, 1930.
26. Ger, G.C., Wexner, S.D., Jorge, M.N., et al.: Evaluation and treatment of chronic intractable rectal pain—a frustrating endeavor. Dis. Colon Rectum, 36:139, 1993.
27. Goligher, J.: Surgery of the Anus, Rectum, and Colon, 5th ed. London, Balliere Tindall, 1984, p. 5.
28. Grant, S.R., Salvati, E.P., and Rubin, R.J.: Levator syndrome and analysis of 316 cases. Dis. Colon Rectum, 18:161, 1975.
29. Grosfeld, J.L., and Billmire, D.F.: Teratomas in infancy and childhood. Curr. Probl. Cancer, 9:1, 1985.
30. Gross, R.E., Clatworthy, H.W., Jr., and Meeker, I.A.: Sacrococcygeal teratomas in infants and children. A report of 40 cases. Surg. Gynecol. Obstet., 92:341, 1951.
31. Gunterberg, B., Kewenter, J., Petersen, I., and Stener, B.: Anorectal function after major resections of the sacrum with bilateral or unilateral sacrifice of sacral nerves. Br. J. Surg., 63:546, 1976.
32. Heckemann, R., Wernecke, K., Hezel, J., and Magnus, L.: Transgluteal ultrasonography. Radiology, 147:587, 1983.
33. Hennig, L.: Quoted by Jao, S.W., Beart, R.W., Spencer, R.J., et al.: Retrorectal tumors, Mayo Clinic Experience, 1960–1979. Dis. Colon Rectum, 28:644, 1985.
34. Heyman, S., Wexner, S.D., and Gulledge, A.D.: MMPI assessment of patients with functional bowel disorders. Dis. Colon Rectum, 36:593, 1993.
35. Hodges, R.M.: Pilonidal sinus. Boston Med. Surg. J., 103:485, 1980.
36. Hodgeson, W.J.B.: Pilonidal sinus and cyst. In Cameron, J.C. (ed.): Current Surgical Therapy—2. Philadephia, B.C. Decker, 1986, p. 150.
37. Jackman, R.J., and Clark, P.L.: Retrorectal tumors. JAMA, 145:956, 1951.
38. Jao, S.W., Beart, R.W., Spencer, R.J., et al.: Retrorectal tumors, Mayo Clinic Experience, 1960–1979. Dis. Colon Rectum, 28: 644, 1985.
39. Jiminez-Romero, C., Alcalde, M., Martin, F., et al.: Treatment of pilonidal sinus by excision and rhomboid flap. Int. J. Colorect. Dis., 5:200, 1990.
40. Johnson, W.R.: Retrorectal tumors. In Goldberg, S.M., Gordon, P.H., and Nivatvongs, S. (eds.): Essentials of Anorectal Surgery. Philadelphia, J.B. Lippincott, 1981, p. 215.
41. Kirks, D.R., Merten, D.F., Filston, H.C., and Oakes, W.J.: The Currarino triad: Complex of anorectal malformation, sacral bony abnormality, and presacral mass. Pediatr. Radiol., 14:220, 1984.
42. Krestin, G.P., Beyer, D., and Steinbrich, W.: Computed tomography in the differential diagnosis of the enlarged retrorectal space. Gastrointest. Radiol., 11:364, 1986.
43. Labow, S.B., Hoexter, B., and Susin, M.: Presacral myelolipoma: Report of a case and review of the literature. Dis. Colon Rectum, 20:606, 1977.
44. Lahr, C.L., Rothenberger, D.A., Jensen, L.L., and Goldberg, S.M.: Balloon proctography. A simple method of evaluating anal function and diseases. Dis. Colon Rectum, 29:1, 1986.
45. Law, A.A.: Pelvic tumors with sacral attachments. Surg. Gynecol. Obstet., 35:593, 1922.
46. Levine, E., and Batnitzky, S.: Computed tomography of sacral and presacral lesions. Crit. Rev. Diagn. Imaging, 21:307, 1984.
47. Localio, S.A., Eng, K., and Coppa, G.F.: Anorectal, Presacral and Sacral Tumors. Philadephia, W.B. Saunders, 1987, p. 153.
48. Lovelady, S.B., and Dockerty, M.B.: Extra-genital pelvic tumors in women. Am. J. Obstet., 58:215, 1949.

49. Lybeert, M.L.M., and Meerwaldt, J.H.: Chordoma: Report on treatment results in eighteen cases. Acta Radiol. Oncol., 25:41, 1986.

50. MacCarty, C.S., Waugh, J.M., Mayo, C.W., and Coventry, M.B.: The surgical treatment of presacral tumors; a combined problem. Mayo Clin. Proc., 27:73, 1952.

51. Manterola, C., Barroso, M., Araya, J.C., and Fronseca, L.: Pilonidal disease: 25 cases treated by the Dufourmental technique. Dis. Colon Rectum, 34:649, 1991.

52. Middeldorpf, K.: Quoted by Jao, S.W., Beart, R.W., Spencer, R.J., et al.: Retrorectal tumors, Mayo Clinic Experience, 1960–1979. Dis. Colon Rectum, 28:644, 1985.

53. Middleton, M.D.: Treatment of pilonidal sinus by Z-plasty. Br. J. Surg., 55:516, 1968.

54. Mills, S.E., Walker, A.N., Stallings, R.G., and Allen, M.S.: Retrorectal cystic hemartoma. Arch. Pathol. Lab. Med., 108:737, 1984.

55. Milsom, J., and Gaffner, H.: Intrarectal ultrasonography in rectal cancer staging and in the evaluation of pelvic disease. Am. Surg., 212:602, 1988.

56. Moazam, F., and Talbert, J.L.: Congenital anorectal malformations, harbingers of sacrococcygeal teratomas. Arch. Surg., 120:856, 1985.

57. Neill, M.W., and Swash, M.: Chronic perianal pain: An unsolved problem. J. R. Soc. Med., 75:96, 1982.

58. Nicosia, J.F., and Abcarian, H.: Levator syndrome; a treatment that works. Dis. Colon Rectum, 28:406, 1985.

59. Nivatvongs, S., and Fang, D.T.: The use of thumbtacks to stop massive presacral hemorrhage. Dis. Colon Rectum, 29:589, 1986.

60. Oliver, G.C., Rubin, R.J., Salvati, E.P., and Eisenstat, T.E.: Electrogalvanic stimulation in the treatment of levator syndrome. Dis. Colon Rectum, 28:662, 1985.

61. Oren, J., Lorber, B., Lee, S.H., et al.: Anterior sacral meningocele: Report of five cases and review of the literature. Dis. Colon Rectum, 20:492, 1977.

62. Pantoj, A.E., and Rodrigues-Ibanez, I.: William Waldeyer and the retrorectal fascia. Surg. Gynecol. Obstet., 138:252, 1974.

63. Patey, D.H., and Scarff, R.W.: Pathology of postanal pilonidal sinus: Its bearing on treatment. Lancet, 2:484, 1946.

64. Perez-Gurri, J.A., Temple, W.J., and Ketcham, A.S.: Gluteus maximus myocutaneous flap for the treatment of recalcitrant pilonidal disease. Dis. Colon Rectum, 27:262, 1984.

65. Reddy, E.K., Mansfield, C.N., and Hartman, G.V.: Chordoma. Int. J. Radiat. Oncol. Biol. Phys., 7:1709, 1981.

66. Rifkin, M.S., and Marks, G.J.: Transrectal ultrasound as an adjunct in the diagnosis of rectal and extra-rectal tumors. Radiology, 157:499, 1985.

67. Sanchez, J., Nigro, M.F., and Colvin, D.: Congenital pelvis arteriovenous malformation: An unusual cause of rectal pain. Dis. Colon Rectum, 33:327, 1990.

68. Schittek, A., Clausen, K.P., and Minton, J.P.: Mesenchymoma of the rectrorectal space: A case report and review of the literature. J. Surg. Oncol., 25:85, 1984.

69. Sherief, A., Kamal, M.S., El Bassyoni, F.: The rationale of using the rhomboid fasciocutaneous transposition flap for the radical cure of pilonidal disease. Dermatol. Surg. Oncol., 12:1295, 1986.

70. Shute, F.C., Jr., Smith, T.E., Levine, M., et al.: Pilonidal cysts and sinuses. Ann. Surg., 118:706, 1943.

71. Simpson, J.Y.: Coccygodynia and diseases and deformities of the coccys. Med. Times Gazette, 40:1009, 1859.

72. Sohn, N., Weinstein, M.A., and Robbins, R.D.: The levator syndrome and its treatment with high voltage electrogalvanic stimulation. Am. J. Surg., 144:580, 1982.

73. Solla, J.A., and Rothenberger, D.A.: Chronic pilonidal disease. Dis. Colon Rectum, 33:758, 1990.

74. Sondenaa, K., Andersen, E., and Soreide, J.A.: Morbidity and short term results in a randomized trial of open compared with closed treatment of chronic pilonidal sinus. Eur. J. Surg., 158:351, 1992.

75. Spencer, R.J., and Jackman, R.J.: Surgical management of precoccygeal cysts. Surg. Gynecol. Obstet., 115:449, 1962.

76. Stener, B., and Gunterberg, B.: High amputation of the sacrum for extirpation of tumors. Principles and technique. Spine, 3: 351, 1978.

77. Stolfi, V.M., Milsom, J.W., Lavery, I.C., et al.: A newly designed occluder pin for presacral hemorrhage. Dis. Colon Rectum, 35: 166, 1992.

78. Stephens, F.O., and Sloane, D.R.: Conservative management of pilonidal sinus. Surg. Gynecol. Obstet., 129:786, 1969.

79. Swash, M., and Snooks, S.G.: Electomyography in pelvic floor disorders. In Henry, M.J., and Swash, M. (eds.): Coloproctology and the pelvic floor; pathophysiology and management. Cambridge, England, University Press, 1985, p. 88.

80. Swash, M.: Chronic perianal pain. In Henry, M.M., and Swash, M. (eds.): Coloproctology in the Pelvic Floor; Pathophysiology and Management. Cambridge, England, University Press, 1985, p. 388.

81. Thaysen, T.E.H.: Proctalgia fugax. A little known form of pain in the rectum. Lancet, 2:243, 1935.

82. Thiele, G.H.: Coccygodynia cause and treatment. Dis. Colon Rectum, 6:422, 1963.

83. Thompson, W.G.: Proctalgia fugax. J. R. Coll. Phys., 14:247, 1980.

84. Toubanakis, G.: Treatment of pilonidal sinus disease with the Z-plasty procedure (modified). Am. Surg., 52:611, 1986.

85. Uhlig, B.E., and Johnson, R.L.: Presacral tumors and cysts in adults. Dis. Colon Rectum, 18:581, 1975.

86. Verazin, G., Rosen, L., Khubchandani, I.T., et al.: Retrorectal tumor: Is biopsy risky? South. Med. J., 79:1437, 1986.

87. Virchow, R., Quoted in Jao, S.W., Beart, R.W., Spencer, R.J., et al.: Retrorectal tumors, Mayo Clinic Experience, 1960–1979. Dis. Colon Rectum, 28:644, 1985.

88. Wexner, S.D., Marchetti, F., Salanga, V.D., et al.: Neurophysiologic assessment of the anal sphincters. Dis. Colon Rectum, 34:606, 1991.

89. Wexner, S.D., Jorge, J.M., Nogueras, J.J., et al.: Colorectal physiologic testing: Use or abuse of technology. Eur. J. Surg., 160:167, 1994.

90. Whittaker, L.D., and Pemberton, J.D.: Tumors ventral to the sacrum. Ann. Surg., 107:96, 1938.

91. Williams, R.S.: A simple technique for successful primary closure after excision of pilonidal sinus disease. Ann. R. Coll. Surg., Engl., 72:313, 1990.

92. Woolley, M.M.: Malignant teratomas in infancy and childhood. World J. Surg., 4:39, 1980.

93. Yoon, K.S., Choi, S.K., Amaranth, L.A., et al.: Caudal epidural block with methylprednisolone acetate in the management of chronic idiopathic rectal pain. Coloproctology, 16:161, 1994.

Chapter 35

ANORECTAL ANOMALIES

JAY L. GROSFELD

Malformations of the anorectum are relatively common congenital anomalies. The vast majority of experience in the management of these lesions has been obtained at specialized children's hospitals dealing with disorders of the newborn. The reported incidence of anorectal anomalies ranges from 1 in 3,500 to 1 in 5,000 live births. Malformations occur more commonly in boys than in girls; however, this may vary according to the level of the defect. Imperforate anus may be associated with other congenital anomalies, including duodenal atresia, esophageal atresia with tracheoesophageal fistula, rare instances of coexisting aganglionic megacolon, urinary tract abnormalities, exstrophy of the bladder or cloaca, sacral defects, presacral lesions (teratomas, anterior meningocele), congenital heart defects, and chromosomal syndromes including trisomy 13-15, trisomy 16-18, Down's syndrome (trisomy 21), the cat-eye syndrome (otic atresia and colobomas), and the VATER association (vertebral defects, imperforate anus, tracheoesophageal fistula, esophageal atresia, radial limb anomalies, and renal dysplasia).[32]

EMBRYOLOGY

Although the embryology of the anorectal area has been alluded to earlier in this volume, we will address some aspects of development that have generated some controversy. There is general agreement that the cloaca is noted in the 12- to 15-day embryo. The cloacal membrane is defined as that area between the primitive streak and the body stalk where endoderm and ectoderm fuse without intervening mesoderm. The allantois is an extension of gut endoderm that becomes part of the bladder and extends up to the amnion. The allantois marks the ventrocephalic limits of the cloaca. Cloacal folds (or genital folds) are mesoblastic proliferations that surround the cloacal membrane.

The mesonephric ducts join the superior lateral wall of the cloaca just inside the cloacal membrane at 28 days of gestation. The cloaca is now a large chamber into which the hindgut enters superiorly and the tailgut exits inferiorly. Just in front of the hindgut, the allantois projects ventrally and superiorly. The ventral body wall develops and displaces the upper end of the cloaca. Anal tubercles (mesoblastic structures) form on both sides of the cloaca at its junction with the tailgut and impinge on the lumen at this junction. The anal tubercles fuse centrally, displacing the cloacal orifice of the involuting tailgut dorsally away from the cloacal membrane.[6]

The urorectal septum descends to demarcate the cloaca into a ventral urogenital sinus and a dorsal hindgut. By the middle of the seventh week of gestation, the anus and rectum are completely divided from the urogenital tract. The anal membrane then breaks down. The mesodermal perineal body extends to about the same level of the anal folds (hillocks). The cloaca is completely divided and no external cloaca exists. The anal tubercles unite behind the cloaca and form a U-shaped fold dorsally and laterally between the tail and the anus. The dorsal cloacal wall evaginates just above the margin where the anal tubercle impinges on the lumen at the future site of the crypts and columns of Morgagni. The anorectal musculature becomes defined and arises from the third sacral to the first coccygeal myotonic hypomeres, starting at the eighth week of gestation.[2] The anal portion of the rectum is initially long and of endodermal origin (hindgut origin). Beginning in the ninth week of gestation, the external sphincter, levator ani (particularly the puborectalis muscle), and even the ganglia and plexuses of the rectum are well defined.

In a 55-mm fetus, the anal portion of the rectum is reduced in length by a gradual shortening and broadening. According to studies of human embryos in the Carnegie collection by deVries,[7] no proctodeum is seen. This observation contradicts the time-honored role of the anal pit (or proctodeum of ectodermal origin) in the development of the anal canal as demonstrated in other mammalian species (e.g., chick embryo). Further, it questions the rationale that anorectal malformations are the result of a failure of the anal pit (proctodeum) to become continuous with the hindgut cavity. Addi-

450

TABLE 35-1. INTERNATIONAL CLASSIFICATION OF ANORECTAL ANOMALIES (1970)*

Level	Male	Female
High Deformities (Supralevator)		
Anorectal agenesis	Without fistula	Without fistula
	With fistula	With fistula
	rectovesical	rectovesical
	rectourethral	rectovaginal (high)
		rectocloacal
Rectal atresia male and female		
Intermediate Deformities (supra- and translevator)		
Anal agenesis	Without fistula	Without fistula
	With fistula	With fistula
	rectobulbar	rectovaginal (low)
		rectovestibular
Anorectal stenosis, male and female		
Low Deformities (infralevator)		
At normal anal site male and female		
covered anus—complete		
anal stenosis		
At perineal site	Anterior perineal anus	Anterior perineal anus
	Anocutaneous fistula	Anocutaneous fistula
	(covered anus—	(covered anus—incomplete)
	incomplete)	
At vulvar site	Nil	Vulvar anus
		Anovulvar fistula
		Anovestibular fistula
Miscellaneous Deformities		

*After Stephens, F.D., and Smith, E.D.: Anorectal malformations in children. Chicago, Year Book Medical Publishers, 1971, with permission.

tional studies in human embryos are required to further elucidate the exact cause of the myriad anorectal anomalies.

CLASSIFICATION

Anorectal malformations are classified according to their anatomic level of presentation and occurrence by sex. An important classification was developed by Stephens, Smith, and others at an international workshop on anorectal malformations in 1970 (Table 35–1).[28,29] Although this classification was used extensively (particularly in Australia and New Zealand), it was considered too complex and detailed by many surgeons.

In 1984, the Wingspread classification was developed by Stephens, Smith, and others to address only the commonly observed anorectal anomalies (Table 35–2).[27] The newer classification used similar terms and was based on anatomic levels but excluded important anomalies such as rectocloacal defects and anterior ectopic anus. Cloacal malformations are listed separately under the new classification system.

The major differentiation among lesions is whether they occur as high-, intermediate-, or low-lying anomalies with or without an associated fistula. High lesions indicate that the end of the rectal atresia is located in a supralevator location, intermediate lesions indicate that the end is in a translevator position, and low-lying (infralevator) lesions indicate that the end of the atresia has passed beyond the levator (through the puborectalis) to lie below the lowest portion of the ischium.

TABLE 35-2. WINGSPREAD CLASSIFICATION OF ANORECTAL ANOMALIES (1984)*

Level	Female	Male
High	Anorectal agenesis	Anorectal agenesis
	with rectovaginal fistula	with rectoprostatic urethral fistula
	without fistula	without fistula
	Rectal atresia	Rectal atresia
Intermediate	Rectovestibular fistula	Rectobulbar urethral fistula
	Rectovaginal fistula	
	Anal agenesis without fistula	Anal agenesis without fistula
Low	Anovestibular fistula	Anocutaneous fistula
	Anocutaneous fistula	Anal stenosis†
	Anal stenosis†	
Cloacal malformations		
Rare malformations		Rare malformations

*Developed by Stephens, F.D. et al., at the Symposium on Anorectal Anomalies. Wingspread Report, Racine, WI, 1984.
†Previously called covered anus.

High lesions lie above the pubococcygeal line, intermediate lesions lie between the pubococcygeal line and the lower ischium, and low lesions (infralevator) lie below the lowest ischium ossification (Fig. 35–1). Recently, Peña has suggested that the appearance of the sacrum should be included in the classification, as more than two missing sacral vertebrae alters the prognosis and may play a role in the decision-making process.[19]

More than 80% of patients have a fistulous connection with the genitourinary tract or the perineum (Fig. 35–2). Boys with high rectal atresia have a fistula to the urethra at the level of the verumontanum in 80% of cases and to the bladder in 6% of cases.[32] In boys with a low-lying lesion, 70% have an anocutaneous fistula that presents anterior to the external sphincter along the midline raphe of the perineal body as it extends up to the scrotum (Fig. 35–3). In 20 to 30% of cases, an anal membrane (complete), anal stenosis, or an anteriorly displaced anal orifice is noted. Direct injection of contrast material into the fistula site is often useful in delineating the exact nature of the anomaly. Contrast will also allow detection of the unusual rectal atresia with a long fistulous tract to the perineum.

In girls, the easiest way to clinically assess the anatomy is by direct visualization during physical examination of the perineum in the lithotomy position. Little girls present with variants of the normal three perineal orifices: (1) urethra, vagina, and a third opening representing an imperforate anus with associated perineal or recto-fourchette fistula (Fig. 35–4); (2) two openings, the urethra and vagina in a baby with an imperforate anus and a rectovaginal fistula; and (3) one perineal opening, an imperforate anus with a cloaca and vesicocloacal and rectocloacal fistulas. Of girls with high anomalies, 80% have an associated fistula (usually to the lower third of the vagina), whereas more than 93% with low rectal atresia have a fistula.

Of interest is the fact that babies with Down's syndrome often do not have a fistula and present with low- or intermediate-level rectal atresia. In patients with a "flat"-appearing bottom, with little or no buttock crease and no anal skin features, one can presume there is an associated sacral defect (dysgenesis or agenesis), and a high lesion can usually be predicted. Sacral nerve branches S1, S2, and S3 are necessary for anal continence. Such patients have a poor prognosis in regard to continence developing. At times, the perineal fistula is not always apparent immediately after birth. Since this is a very low-lying cause of neonatal intestinal obstruction, the physician usually can wait 18 to 24 hours to observe development of a bulging anal membrane darkened by meconium, or a fistula passing meconium, prior to subjecting the neonate to a preliminary colostomy.

Colostomy should be performed to relieve intestinal obstruction in the newborn period for cases of high and intermediate rectal atresia. Perineal fistulas in boys and girls almost always indicate a low lesion. Passage of meconium via the vagina or penis (Fig. 35–5) or air passed at urination in boys usually signifies rectovaginal or rectourethral or bladder fistulas, respectively, and indicates the presence of a high or intermediate lesion requiring a colostomy.

Diagnostic studies may be helpful in delineating the anatomy. Electrical anorectal sphincter muscle mapping can accurately determine the site and activity of the external sphincter muscle and locate the central complex to house the anoplasty. This can be done in the newborn period as a prognostic indicator of potential sphincter function and is extremely helpful in the operating room at the time of definitive surgery. Lumbosacral radiographs should be obtained to evaluate the sacral anatomy. Many babies have spinal dysraphic syndromes.[9] In the neonate, ultrasound examination of the lumbosacral spine is useful in identifying spinal cord lesions. In older infants, magnetic resonance imaging (MRI) studies are superior in detecting abnormalities, including tethered cord, lipomeningocele, and the like. Thirty-eight per cent of infants with high imperforate anus and 5% of those with low-lying atresias may have spinal cord abnormalities.[33] Occult spinal lesions can be suspected by the presence of a subcutaneous sacral mass, dimple, sinus tract, hemangioma, nevus, or area of hypertrichosis over the sacral region.[9] Infants with cloacal exstrophy have a very high risk of spinal defects.

Urinalysis may detect the presence of meconium consistent with a rectourinary fistula. Renal ultrasound is useful to detect associated urinary tract anomalies in

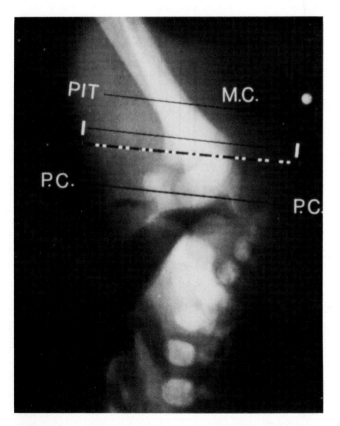

FIGURE 35–1. Lateral invertogram in a patient with anorectal agenesis and a rectourethral fistula. Air shadow is above the pubococcygeal line (*P.C.*). Air is noted anteriorly in bladder. *I* is the line of the ischial ossification site (the level of translevator lesion), whereas *M.C.* is the mucocutaneous line, the level of low (infralevator) lesions. (From deVries, P.A.: The surgery of anorectal anomalies: Its evolution with evaluations of procedures. Curr. Probl. Surg., *21*(5):1, 1984, with permission.)

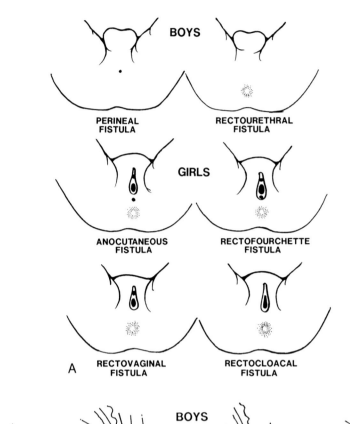

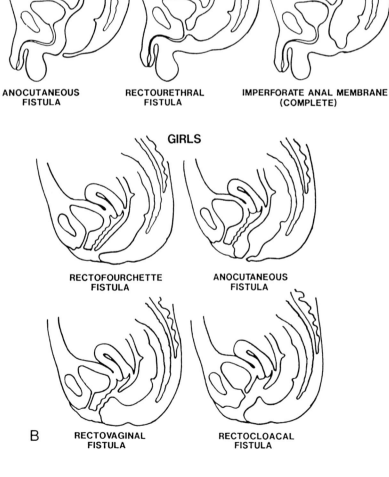

FIGURE 35-2. *A*, Perineal appearance of anorectal anomalies in boys and girls. *B*, The lateral view of the same defects.

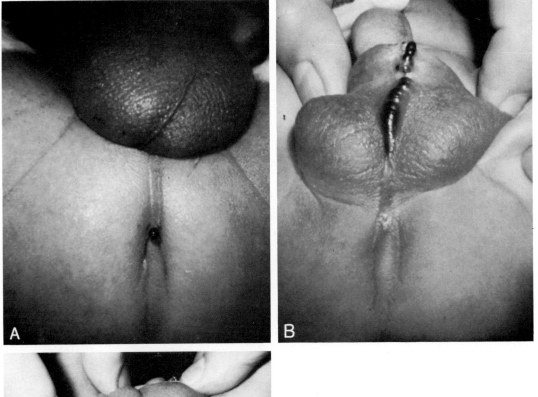

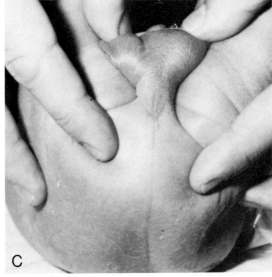

FIGURE 35-3. *A*, Appearance of little boy with an infralevator (low) lesion and anocutaneous fistula with small amount of meconium. *B*, Fistulous tract filled with meconium that extends anteriorly along the scrotal raphe. *C*, Perineum of a baby boy with imperforate anus and a rectourethral fistula. No cutaneous fistula site is observed.

the newborn, which may occur in up to 40% of cases. Recent experience with perineal ultrasonography has been useful in detecting low rectal atresia lesions, whereas computed tomography (CT) scan[8,31] and MRI[21] of the pelvic musculature are helpful in determining the status of the pelvic muscular diaphragm and its relationship to the end of the rectal atresia and the position of the pubococcygeal line. These tests are more correctly interpreted when performed 18 to 24 hours after birth.[19] A retrograde cystourethrogram is an accurate method of delineating an associated rectourethral fistula in boys.

Diagnostic endoscopic evaluation in girls with a cloacal defect is essential prior to any definitive repair. It will demonstrate instances of vaginal septation, vaginal atresia, and duplex uterus (double cavity). The upside-down invertogram x-ray study so often used to determine the level of the rectal atresia in the past is relied on less completely today. More contemporary modalities of diagnostic testing that are complementary to that study are now available and, when used in combination, are more precise in determining the exact anatomy.

PELVIC MUSCULAR ANATOMY AND PHYSIOLOGY OF CONTINENCE

We will briefly review the normal anatomy of the rectum and pelvic musculature and mechanisms of continence (as they relate to congenital disorders of this region) in order to attempt to understand the current methods of reconstruction of complex anorectal anomalies. The normal rectum is divided at its angulation by the contraction of the puborectalis muscle into an am-

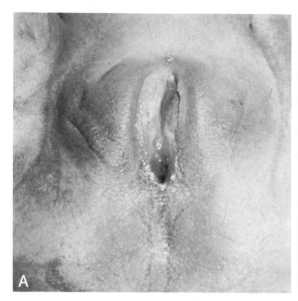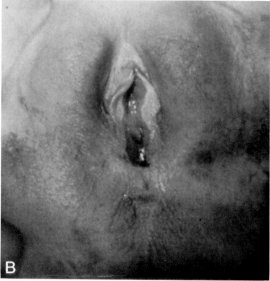

FIGURE 35-4. *A* and *B*, Perineal examinations in two different girls show the presence of imperforate anus and a rectofourchette fistula.

pulla above and an anal canal below. The posterior rectal wall is acutely indented by the anterior pull of the puborectalis muscle and overhangs the rest of the levator diaphragm. The anal canal is surrounded by sphincter muscles and is tethered to a concentrically arranged internal (involuntary) sphincter and an external (voluntary) sphincter. The skin-lined anal canal has intrinsic sensory receptors with conventional nerve endings that detect pain, touch, temperature, tension, and friction. There are no sensory receptors per se in the ampulla that are sensitive to distention (stretch). The puborectalis muscle is the key sensor at the entry of the anal canal from the ampulla.[27] This governs both unconscious and conscious opening and closing of the canal and gives warnings of impending defecation.

Continence is maintained normally by a combination of resting tone in all the sphincters and both reflex and voluntary contraction of the puborectalis muscle and deep external sphincter. The resting tone in the internal sphincter occludes the lumen of the perineal part of the anal canal but relaxes just ahead of the peristaltic contraction in the adjoining ampulla and pelvic portion of the anal canal. As an increase in the intraluminal pressure in the rectum rises to the level of the resting pressure of the canal, the spinal reflex operates to maintain closure by contraction of the puborectalis sling and maintains continence during the relaxation phase.[13] Higher propulsion pressure waves in the rectum force the entrance of stool into the anal canal. This activates stretch receptors of the puborectalis and initiates an afferent impulse to the spinal and cortical centers and an awareness of rectal distention. The voluntary sphincters and regulation of anorectal continence are then under conscious control.

The relaxation of the internal sphincter in response to rectal distention in normal patients is referred to as the rectoanal reflex and is lacking in patients with Hirschsprung's disease. The internal sphincter is under control of the parasympathetic nervous system through the spinal arc at S2, S3, and S4, which contains nerve centers that coordinate rectal peristaltic activity and involuntary (unconscious) sphincter control. The pudendal nerve supplies the sympathetic stimulus that causes constant contraction of the internal sphincter and produces the "continent slit" shape of the anus. This cortical arc is called into play when increased intraluminal pressure exceeds the resting pressure. The afferent pathway is via the pudendal nerve to the spinal center and cerebral endings in the cortex that activate the efferent pathway controlling the voluntary muscle sphincters.

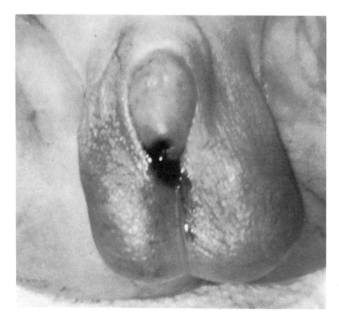

FIGURE 35-5. Meconium is seen coming from the penile urethral orifice. This is consistent with a rectourethral fistula.

The entire length of the anal canal is surrounded by voluntary muscles. The funnel-shaped musculature compresses the upper anal canal on three sides by the anterior pull of the puborectalis sling, whereas the lower skin-lined aspect of the anal canal is squeezed by the barrel-shaped external sphincter. The levator ani muscle complex is composed of four muscles (the pubococcygeus, ileococcygeus, puborectalis, and coccygeus). These structures form the complete muscle floor of the pelvis and in addition provide a portal of exit from the anal canal and prevent herniation of the pelvic contents alongside the canal by blending with the smooth muscle coats of the rectum.

The pubococcygeus muscle forms a cone, the apex of which grips the anal canal and suspends it as it passes from the pelvis to the perineum. The puborectalis forms a collar behind the pelvic portion of the anal canal and around the cone of the pubococcygeus muscle, causing an acute angulation of the back wall of the canal at its junction with the rectal ampulla. The ileococcygeus muscles unite in the midline behind the rectum and counter the impact of downward abdominal pressure.

The external sphincter is a barrel-shaped muscle that lies outside the internal sphincter in continuity with the puborectalis sling and surrounds the anal canal from the pectinate line to the anal orifice. Shafik[26] described the anal sphincter as a triple-loop system. The superior or upper loop is composed of the deep external sphincter, which joins or fuses with the inferior edge of the puborectalis. The middle portion is that segment of the external sphincter that is attached to the coccyx, and the lower loop is the subcutaneous or superficial striated muscle that encircles the anal canal and is fixed anteriorly to the perineal skin by fibrous septa. The longitudinal septum is a continuation of the longitudinal smooth muscle of the rectum that extends downward and passes between the internal and external sphincters; its tendrils (as well as the ileococcygeus fibers) penetrate the internal and external sphincters, the ischiorectal muscle, and perianal fat.[12] The internal sphincter is the thickened segment of circular smooth muscle ending at the anal orifice. The circular muscle is penetrated by the tendinous aspect of the longitudinal layer and the pubococcygeus, which fan out and penetrate the superficial external sphincter and attach to the skin, resulting in the puckering effect. These coattails bind the internal and external sphincters and anchor them to one another, yielding a firm muscular contraction to allow defecation.

Although Stephens[29] stressed the importance of the puborectalis muscle in regard to the development of continence in patients with imperforate anus, he also considered the internal and external sphincter muscles to be of little value. Stephens theorized that the puborectalis provided the main sphincter mechanism available for continence in these cases. DeVries and Peña,[4] however, demonstrated that the external sphincter played an important role in the development of fecal continence. In their careful dissections during the performance of posterior sagittal anoplasty for imperforate anus, they failed to detect an isolated puborectalis muscle but referred to a striated muscle complex that represents a fusion of the puborectalis portion of the levator ani and the external sphincter muscle (particularly the deep portion). They further state that dorsal to the muscle complex are the superficial and subcutaneous external sphincter muscles that extend upward to the coccyx as a separate layer of longitudinal muscle fibers. The point at which the external sphincter muscle fuses with the levators marks the beginning of the striated muscle complex.

Many patients with imperforate anus have problems with continence. There is great variability in the presence of striated muscle from patient to patient. Some patients have weak musculature, whereas some have nearly normal muscle. The presence or lack of underlying sacral and neurologic abnormalities also plays a role in the success or failure in any specific case. Additionally, a major problem in many cases (particularly in infants with high imperforate anus) is the lack of an internal sphincter muscle. An internal sphincter can be identified in some instances of low imperforate anus with an anterior ectopic opening or perineal fistula. When the location of the imperforate anus is higher, however, the important "message center" for the rectoanal reflex is lacking, leading to the frequent complaint among some of these patients that they are unaware of the presence of feces in the anus, which results in soiling. Sections taken through the site of a rectourethral fistula indicate that the remnant of the internal sphincter muscle may be within the fistula itself.[35] Since most surgical procedures for imperforate anus leave this area in place to reduce the chance of injury to the urethra, the internal sphincter in these cases is often not of use to the patient. The goal for patients with high imperforate anus is to perform a procedure as carefully as possible to preserve whatever sphincter and levator muscles are available and to place the rectum within the muscle complex to allow the best opportunity for development of *socially acceptable continence.*

OPERATIVE TECHNIQUE

As a general rule, infants with low anomalies can be treated definitively in the neonatal period. Babies with a complete anal atretic membrane can be managed by incising the skin (bulging with meconium behind it) to relieve the obstruction. Dilations (using Hegar dilators, Nos. 9 to 12, on a daily basis) for 3 to 4 months will maintain an adequate anal orifice. Passage of more formed stools in later infancy maintains the opening.

Infants with an anocutaneous fistula are managed by a cutback perineal anoplasty (Fig. 35–6). A Y-V technique that creates a U-shaped superficial external sphincter and widened skin orifice is employed. The puborectalis and deep external sphincter muscles are carefully identified by electrostimulation and are preserved. A portion of the posterior fistula wall is incised and sutured to the skin edges with interrupted 4-0 absorbable suture (Vicryl or Maxon). The new anoplasty site should be sized to a No. 10 Hegar dilator. Postoperatively, bowel contents are gently dabbed from the perianal skin with moist cotton balls. Vigorous wiping techniques should

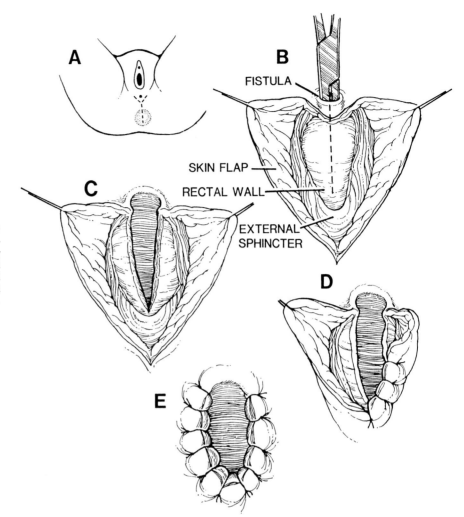

FIGURE 35–6. Y-V cutback anoplasty for anal atresia with anocutaneous fistula. Following Y incision (*A*), skin flaps are carefully raised, and the sphincter is identified and preserved (*B*). The rectal pouch is incised (*C*), and the edges of the rectum are sutured (full-thickness) to the skin edges (*D* and *E*).

be avoided in the first week. Gentle tepid water skin irrigations can be employed after 48 to 72 hours to clean the skin. Daily dilations with a No. 10 Hegar dilator are initiated 10 days after the procedure and are continued for a 6-month period. The dilator size is gradually increased to a No. 13 or No. 14 dilator.

Although Smith[27] suggests a cutback anoplasty for girls with an anovestibular fistula to the extravaginal fourchette, we believe these patients require a transplant anoplasty to preserve the perineal body and adequately separate the vaginal and anal orifices. The little girl can be decompressed through the rectofourchette fistula by daily dilation, and definitive surgery can be delayed until the perineal and vaginal tissues become more sturdy (age 3 to 6 months). Accurate diagnosis of the level of the atresia is important, as an intermediate-level (translevator) rectovestibular fistula in a girl is similar to a rectourethral fistula at the level of the verumontanum in a boy and would require a preliminary colostomy.

Transplant anoplasty is begun by placing a series of 4-0 silk traction sutures at the 12-, 3-, 6-, and 9-o'clock positions of the fistula opening (Fig. 35–7). Using a fine curved tenotomy scissor, the fistula is carefully dissected free close to its wall (in four quadrants). The anterior dissection in the common wall between the fistula and posterior vaginal wall is tedious. Appropriate fine aspirators,

a fine-tip electrocoagulator, and wide-angle magnifying loupes (2.5 to 3.5×) are useful adjuncts. Once above the fistula site, the anterior and lateral dissection is more easily accomplished. Posteriorly, careful perineal dissection also is required to prevent injury to the striated muscle complex. The superior extent of the posterior dissection is taken well up within the puborectalis–deep external sphincter muscular sling. The site of the new anal orifice is identified by electrical muscle mapping to demonstrate the "pucker site." A skin incision is made at this point, and careful dissection through the center of the subcutaneous and superficial external sphincter muscle, to join the posterior dissection of the fistula tract within the muscular sling, is performed. The opening is gently dilated with Nos. 7, 8, and 9 Hegar dilators. The fistula is then transplanted to the new anal orifice site using the previously placed traction sutures. The fistula site is narrow enough to enter this area without tapering. The posterior smooth muscle rectal wall 2 cm above the orifice is sutured to the muscle complex with interrupted 4-0 silk sutures to prevent prolapse. The anoplasty is completed by suturing the anal orifice (full thickness) to the edges of the anal skin with interrupted 4-0 Vicryl or Maxon sutures. Hemostasis (in the fourchette incision) is ensured, and the previous fistula site at the fourchette is closed with interrupted 4-0 Vicryl or Maxon sutures. A Foley catheter is left

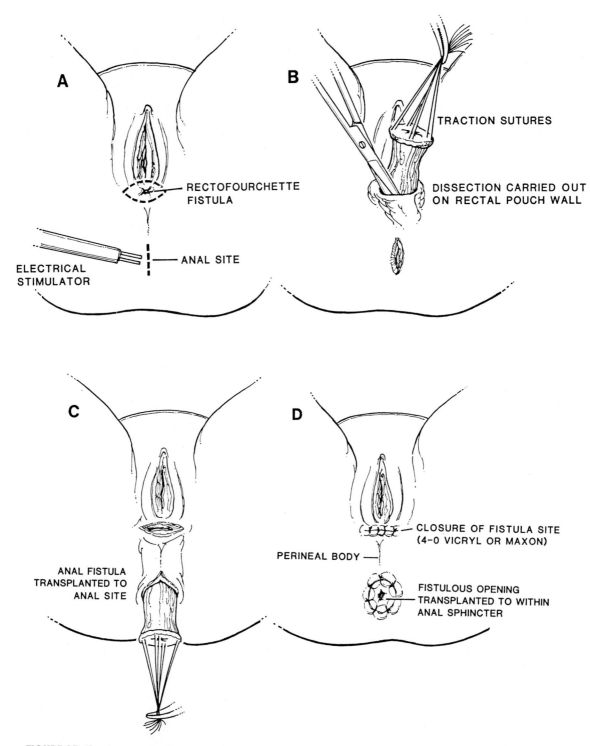

FIGURE 35-7. Correction of imperforate anus with rectofourchette fistula. The anal site is selected with the aid of an electrical stimulator (*A*). Traction sutures are placed. The fistula is carefully dissected free with tenotomy scissors (*B*). The traction sutures are used to guide the opening to a transplanted anal location within the sphincter complex. Interrupted 4-0 Maxon sutures are used (*C*). The fistulous site is closed with interrupted 4-0 suture. Note the preservation of the perineal body (*D*).

in place for 72 hours to prevent urine from bathing the new suture lines. Perianal skin care is similar to that noted previously for the cutback anoplasty.

Alternative techniques to repair rectofourchette and anovestibular fistula have been described by Peña[19] and Okada and associates.[17] Peña prefers to place a prelim-

inary sigmoid colostomy at birth and perform a posterior sagittal anorectoplasty at 4 to 8 weeks of age.[19] Okada and associates recommend using an anterior sagittal anorectoplasty, dividing the anterior sphincter in the midline through a perineal incision and placing the transplanted rectal fistula site within the sphincter muscle. The anterior margin of the sphincter is resutured around the rectum.[17] No colostomy is employed.

Infants with intermediate or high anorectal agenesis or rectal atresia, with or without a fistula to the genitourinary tract, and all patients with cloacal anomalies will require a temporary colostomy. We usually prefer a high sigmoid colostomy, whereas others routinely employ a right transverse colostomy. Either is acceptable. However, the sigmoid colostomy results in a more formed stool and fewer peristomal skin complications than does diversion at a more proximal site. Infants grow quite normally with a colostomy, and since they are incontinent of feces in the first year or two of life, a colostomy bag may actually be more simple to change and easier to manage than a diaper (albeit more expensive). The colostomy should be divided to ensure complete diversion of feces and avoidance of contamination of the urinary tract or vagina through spillover of fecal material into the efferent limb and the rectal fistula. It is important to leave the distal limb long enough to perform a sacroperineal pull-through procedure without a laparotomy if possible.[18]

Even if the sigmoid stoma is maintained as a loop colostomy, the relatively shorter distal segment allows for irrigation of the distal colon and avoids the occurrence of hyperchloremic acidosis. This electrolyte abnormality is occasionally seen in patients with a transverse colostomy caused by absorption of potentially infected urine from the mucosa of a long segment of unused distal colon.[32] In every case, infants with a fistula to the urinary tract benefit from urinary tract prophylaxis using trimethoprim-sulfamethoxazole, 2 mg/kg/day given orally in two divided doses, or other similar medications.

A distal "loop-o-gram" (loop colostomy) or distal colostogram (divided colostomy) can also be performed with contrast material through the sigmoid stoma to more clearly define the site of rectourethral, rectovesical, rectovaginal, or rectocloacal fistula.

The colostomy is left in place for 2 to 12 months prior to a definitive repair according to the practice of the specific surgeon, the type of anomaly, and the general condition of the patient. Although some authors have recommended repair in the neonatal period, this is associated with a higher complication rate and we usually perform this procedure between 6 and 9 months of age.

In the past two decades, a multiplicity of techniques have been advocated for the "modern" operative correction of high and intermediate anorectal anomalies. They include the abdominoperineal pull-through procedures[30]; a sacroperineal or sacroabdominoperineal pull-through procedure as advocated by Stephens[29] and his Australian colleagues, which delineates the puborectalis muscle and divides the rectourethral fistula from within the rectal atresia; and modifications of the Stephens procedure by Kiesewetter[11] and by Rehbein,[22,23] in which a submucosal resection is performed to allow for an abdominoperineal pull-through procedure within a muscular sleeve of the original rectal atresia. An anterior transperineal rectoplasty was advocated by Mollard[13,14] and associates to identify the puborectalis and the fistula, and then the Kiesewetter abdominoperineal technique was used. In 1982, deVries and Peña[4] described the posterior sagittal anorectoplasty (sacroperineal approach), which divides each of the striated muscles in the midline sagittal plane, divides the fistula from within the rectal atresia lumen, and significantly tapers the distal bowel to fit snugly within the muscle complex, which is then reconstituted around the rectum and anoplasty site. More recent innovations from Japan by Yokoyama[35] and, especially, modifications from Australia by Smith[27] combine the excellent exposure afforded by the Peña[18] sagittal anoplasty (which avoids laparotomy and gains excellent exposure to divide the fistula) with the modifications of keeping the combined puborectalis, pubococcygeus, and deep external sphincter intact and minimally tapering the bowel. The Peña procedure is the most popular operation currently employed for intermediate and high lesions. We will present the technique of the Peña[18] operation and Smith's[27] modifications in detail.

In preparation for a definitive procedure, the distal bowel segment is prepared with 0.25% neomycin solution. Preoperative antibiotics are started 2 hours prior to the procedure. The baby is placed in a jackknife position with careful padding of the groin. A urinary catheter is inserted, the operative field is prepared with iodophor, and appropriate drapes and linens are applied. The proposed anal site is determined by electrical muscle stimulation.

A sagittal midline incision is placed on the lower sacrum just above the coccyx and is carried to the anticipated anal site; all of the levator ani and sphincter muscles are divided posteriorly, including the puborectalis and deep external sphincter (Fig. 35–8). Smith[27] modifies this procedure by dividing the superficial and subcutaneous parts of the external sphincter and the diaphragmatic portion of the levator (iliococcygeus, ischiococcygeus) muscles sagittally but not dividing the puborectalis, pubococcygeus, and deep external sphincter muscles, which are kept intact.

The rectal pouch is identified and carefully mobilized circumferentially above the fistula site by blunt dissection close to the bowel wall to avoid injury to neural structures and the prostatic plexus. The distal rectal pouch is entered and the fistula is identified from within the lumen. A submucosal plane is developed around the fistula to avoid injury to the seminal vesicles and prostate. The fistula is closed with interrupted 4-0 Vicryl or Maxon sutures. The rectal pouch is then carefully mobilized, keeping the dissection in the plane of the bowel wall and using a fine-tip electrocoagulator to cauterize multiple vessels (from the middle hemorrhoidal artery) just beyond the rectal wall. In the vast majority of cases associated with a rectourethral fistula, rectal mobilization is more than adequate through the sacroperineal approach, and a laparotomy is unnecessary. However, laparotomy may be required in cases of imperforate anus with high rectal atresia and a rectovesical fistula. In these latter cases, the rectum may not be identified through the usual posterior sagittal incision.

The distal bowel is tapered, if necessary, to comfortably fit within the reconstituted muscle complex without causing injury to the essential muscles. Tapering is accomplished by excising a V-shaped wedge of the poste-

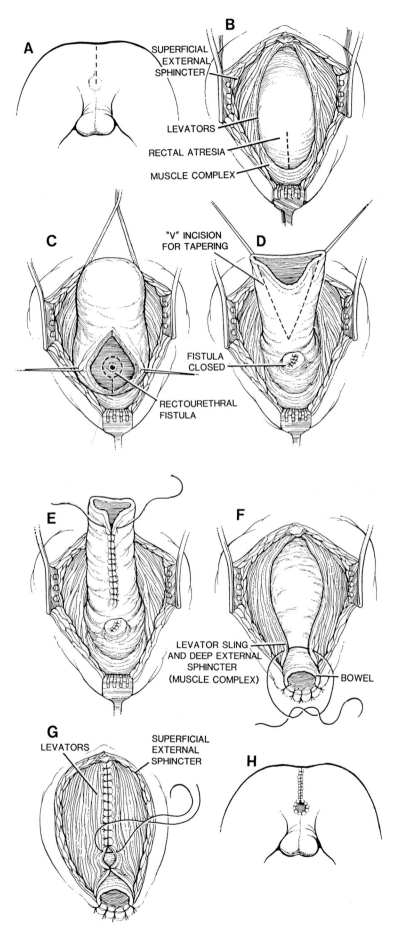

A

B

SUPERFICIAL
EXTERNAL
SPHINCTER

LEVATORS

RECTAL ATRESIA

MUSCLE COMPLEX

C

D

"V" INCISION
FOR TAPERING

FISTULA
CLOSED

RECTOURETHRAL
FISTULA

E

F

LEVATOR SLING
AND DEEP EXTERNAL
SPHINCTER
(MUSCLE COMPLEX)

BOWEL

G

LEVATORS

SUPERFICIAL
EXTERNAL
SPHINCTER

H

FIGURE 35-8. Posterior sagittal anorectoplasty. In the prone position, an incision is made in the midline from the lower sacrum to the selected anal site (*A*). The levator and sphincter muscles are divided posteriorly in the midline. The rectal pouch is identified (*B*). The pouch is opened and the rectourethral fistula is identified within the rectal lumen (*C*). Submucosal resection frees the bowel from the fistula, which is closed with interrupted sutures (*D*). The bowel is tapered to a No. 12 Hegar size (*E*). The muscle complex is reconstituted starting at the deepest portion of the puborectalis muscle and the deep external sphincter (*F*). Levators and superficial external sphincters are then reapproximated with interrupted sutures (*G*). The tapered anoplasty is sutured to the skin with interrupted 4-0 Vicryl or Maxon (*H*).

rior wall of the rectal atretic segment and using a two-layered inverting closure with a 4-0 Vicryl or Maxon inner layer and an outer layer of nonabsorbable 4-0 silk or Prolene. It is important to avoid excessive tapering, which may result in a severe stricture. We usually perform the tapering over a No. 12 Hegar dilator.

The tapered rectum is then placed within the divided muscular complex, which is reconstituted around the rectum with fine interrupted silk or Prolene sutures. The deepest suture begins at a point at which the distal portion of the levator ani joins the external sphincter layers, bringing the rectum close to the urethra or vagina. Electrical muscle stimulation is employed to carefully identify the structures. The wall of the rectum is tacked to the muscle complex in a few places in an attempt to reincorporate the longitudinal smooth muscle of the rectum with the striated muscle complex, causing a tethering effect. The proximal margins of the levators are closed with interrupted 4-0 silk or Prolene. The course of the tapered anoplasty then passes more posteriorly to the site of the new anal opening. The anoplasty is completed by securing the end of the tapered bowel (full thickness) to the skin exit with interrupted 4-0 sutures, incorporating the subcutaneous sphincter in the bites.

In Smith's modification[27] of the Peña procedure (in which the puborectalis is kept intact), a Penrose drain is passed through the sling below the fistula site, and the tapered bowel is then passed through the sling anterior to the drains with the aid of traction sutures. The distal bowel is placed within the divided levator muscles and superficial and subcutaneous external sphincter muscles, which are accurately reconstituted around the bowel with interrupted 4-0 silk sutures. Saeki and colleagues recently described the use of an intraoperative ultrasound probe to guide the bowel through the center of the muscle complex during Smith's procedure.[25] The anoplasty Smith advocates is a skin-lined tract originally credited to Nixon,[3,16] which avoids anocutaneous stenosis. Skin closure in both techniques is with subcuticular suture and Steri-strips.

The colostomy is left in place for 3 to 6 months to allow complete healing and adequate dilation of the new anoplasty. Dilations are initiated at 10 days to 2 weeks following the procedure (the first dilation is usually under anesthesia) using Nos. 8, 9, and 10 Hegar dilators initially and then advancing to larger sized dilators (e.g., Nos. 11 and 12, then 13 and 14) with time. The parents of the child must be carefully instructed regarding the importance of the dilations, which must be performed twice a day at home to avoid stenosis. Relatively frequent follow-up visits to the surgeon's office in the first few weeks to months following the procedure to monitor progress are important. Dilations may be necessary for 6 to 12 months following closure of the colostomy; however, the frequency of dilatation can gradually be diminished.

Repair of cloacal anomalies are more complex and should be left to experts in the field with considerable experience in the management of such cases. Cloacal anomalies vary widely in their presentation and all require a preliminary colostomy. In approximately 40% of cases, hydrocolpos may coexist resulting in bladder trigone compression and urinary tract obstruction.[19] Although the goals of treatment include obtaining urinary continence, fecal control, and normal sexual function, these are not easily achieved. Performing the procedure using a posterior approach (''sky-diver's position'') has been useful in obtaining a satisfactory anatomic repair. However, the functional outcome is often less than desirable, especially in cases with coexisting sacral abnormalities.[19]

POSTOPERATIVE COMPLICATIONS

Postoperative complications related to the anoplasty include anoplasty dehiscence, mucosal prolapse, and stricture. These problems are often related to infection, excess rectal mobilization and redundant mucosa, failure to create a skin-lined anus, and inadequate postoperative dilatation. Techniques for revision anoplasty described by Nixon and Yazbeck and associates result in a satisfactory outcome in most cases.[16,34] Many infants develop perianal skin excoriation that usually resolves with local care (sitz baths, protective ointment application [laser's paste, ilex cream]).

Although deVries and Peña[4] reported only minor postoperative complications, others have described a number of serious complications following posterior sagittal anoplasty. Nakayama and associates[15] reported major complications in 6 of 23 patients (26%), including sacral wound dehiscence, femoral nerve palsy, leakage of the tapered rectoplasty, recurrent urethral fistula, multiple rectocutaneous fistulas, and a supralevator fistula. Most of these complications were related to technical errors and are probably avoidable. Genitourinary complications, including neurogenic bladder, urethral stricture, and urethral diverticulum, also are observed and are often related to technical errors at the time of the pull-through procedure.

FUNCTIONAL RESULTS

Because of variability in anatomy and sacral deformity, the wide spectrum of anorectal disorders managed by different surgical techniques, and dissimilar criteria for success, the results occasionally have been difficult to compare and interpret. As a general rule, fecal continence following correction of low anomalies is quite good. The rectal tissues have already passed through the muscular complex in an orderly fashion, and a simple cutback or transplant anoplasty for a low fistula will often result in a good outcome. The higher the rectal atresia, the worse the functional outcome. In some reports, girls have better fecal continence results than boys, possibly because of the increased incidence of low- and intermediate-level anomalies in girls.

A number of methods to assess continence have been developed and include subjective (e.g., good, fair, poor); numerical (e.g., the Kelly score based on fecal leakage, sensation, and contrast enema findings)[10]; and a variety of physiologic evaluations, including balloon anorectal manometrics, electrical sphincter muscle mapping, anorectal angulation, and the like.[27] The bottom line, however, is whether the patient is clean or soiled and malodorous.

Long-term results for patients with high imperforate anus indicate that a good result will be obtained in approximately 50% of patients, whereas the remaining half will have a fair or poor (incontinent) outcome.[11,32] The best results have been achieved by Mollard,[13] with 80% of patients being continent. However, this study involved a relatively small number of patients (15 cases). Recent studies suggest that the short-term functional results following the Peña procedure and its modifications have achieved good results in 60% of cases with a normal sacrum.[19]

Children with imperforate anus may have significant deficiencies in sensation, the capacity to hold (inadequate sphincter), and ability to evacuate (poor motility) stool. Most children with imperforate anus are born without normal anal canal sensation.

Patients can often manage to stay clean with a formed solid stool but cannot manage to control liquid stools and/or gas. Due to poor motility, many patients do not completely empty the rectum in a single bowel movement and are prone to soil. Patients with a normal sacrum, a well-located anal orifice, some sensation, and an adequate sphincteric mechanism will usually respond to a training program and achieve socially acceptable continence. After posterior sagittal anorectoplasty, some patients develop severe constipation due to hypomotility characterized by poor propulsion and poor peristalsis that results in megarectum and megasigmoid.[1,20] This is more common in patients with low malformations. Cheu and Grosfeld, and Peña and El Behery have reported significant improvement after low anterior resection and/or sigmoid resection, leaving the sphincters and previously performed anoplasty in place.[1,20] Although one might anticipate that tapering the rectum during analorectoplasty would improve motility, Rintala showed no improvement in sphincter activity or rectal motility following posterior sagittal anoplasty procedures.[24]

Patients who remain incontinent should be carefully re-evaluated. Careful study of the pelvic musculature and sacral spinal anatomy (using CT, MRI, contrast defecography, and so on), the urinary tract, and electrical sphincter mapping should be performed. Reoperative procedures are most useful for instances of "missed-muscle complex" or a misplaced anal orifice. The Peña posterior sagittal anoplasty and the Mollard anterior perineal procedure have been used successfully (in 33% of patients) as secondary operations.[28] It is wise to protect a secondary procedure with a proximal diverting colostomy to ensure healing without fecal contamination.[18] A careful bowel preparation is also essential in these cases.

In instances of incontinence that occur despite a proper pull-through procedure, a bowel management program to completely empty the rectum and colon may be useful. This requires daily colon (washout) irrigations, and a constipating diet often supplemented by Imodium or Lomotil. Both the parent and child must be motivated to ensure the best chance for success of this type of program.

Gracilis muscle sling operations have been employed in an attempt to improve voluntary muscle tone, but the long-term success rate is less than 50%. In addition, enemas are often required for complete evacuation. In some instances in which incontinence is inevitable (e.g., sacral agenesis, failure of previous surgical procedures, and reoperations), an end colostomy may be the most appropriate long-term procedure to achieve a socially acceptable status.

Management of patients with variants of imperforate anus is difficult and carries with it a significant degree of physician responsibility, often requiring long-term follow-up into adulthood. A concise understanding of the anatomy and the surgical techniques are essential. These are procedures that should not be attempted by the "occasional surgeon" who rarely deals with neonatal anomalies. The first operation done well by an experienced surgeon most often allows the child the best chance for successful bowel control.

REFERENCES

1. Cheu, H.W., and Grosfeld, J.L.: The atonic baggy rectum: A cause of intractable obstipation after imperforate anus repair. J. Pediatr. Surg., 27:1071, 1992.
2. Crelin, E.S.: Development of the musculoskeletal system. CIBA Clin. Symp., 33:31, 1981.
3. Davies, M.R., and Cywes, S.: The use of a lateral skin flap perineoplasty in congenital anorectal malformations. J. Pediatr. Surg., 19:577, 1984.
4. deVries, P.A., and Peña, A.: Posterior sagittal anorectoplasty. J. Pediatr. Surg., 17:638, 1982.
5. deVries, P.A., and Cox, K.L.: Surgery of ano-rectal anomalies. Surg. Clin. North Am., 65:1139, 1985.
6. deVries, P.A., and Friedland, G.W.: The staged sequential development of the anus and rectum in human embryos and fetuses. J. Pediatr. Surg., 9:755, 1974.
7. deVries, P.A.: The surgery of anorectal anomalies: Its evolution with evaluations of procedures. Curr. Probl. Surg., 31:1, 1984.
8. Ikawa, H., Yokoyama, J., Sanbonmatsu, T., et al.: The use of computerized tomography to evaluate anorectal anomalies. J. Pediatr. Surg., 20:640, 1985.
9. Karrer, F.M., Flannery, A.M., Nelson, M.D., et al.: Anorectal malformations: Evaluation of associated spinal dysraphic syndrome. J. Pediatr. Surg., 23:45, 1988.
10. Kelly, J.H.: The clinical and radiological assessment of anal continence in childhood. Aust. N. Z. J. Surg., 42:62, 1972.
11. Kiesewetter, W.B.: Imperforate anus II. The rationale and technic of the sacra-abdomino-perineal operation. J. Pediatr. Surg., 2: 106, 1967.
12. Localio, S.A., Eng., K., and Coppa, G.F.: Anatomy, physiology of the anus and rectum. Anorectal, Presacral and Sacral Tumors. Philadelphia, W.B. Saunders, 1987, p. 16.
13. Mollard, P., Marechal, J.M., and Jaubert de Beaujen, M.: Surgical treatment of high imperforate anus with definition of the puborectalis sling by an anterior perineal approach. J. Pediatr. Surg., 13:499, 1978.
14. Mollard, P., Marechal, J.M., and Jaubert de Beaujen, M.: Le reperage de la sangle du releveur au cours du traitement des imperforations ano-rectales hautes. Ann. Chir., 16:461, 1975.
15. Nakayama, D.K., Templeton, J.M., Ziegler, M.M., et al.: Complications of posterior sagittal anoplasty. J. Pediatr. Surg., 21:488, 1988.
16. Nixon, H.H.: A modification of the proctoplasty for rectal agenesis. Pamietnik I-Go Zjazdu, 10:5, 1967.
17. Okada, A., Kamada, S., Imura, K., et al.: Anterior sagittal anorectoplasty for rectovestibular and anovestibular fistula. J. Pediatr. Surg., 27:85, 1992.

18. Peña, A., and deVries, P.A.: Posterior sagittal anorectoplasty: Important technical considerations and new applications. J. Pediatr. Surg., 17:796, 1982.

19. Peña, A.: Current management of anorectal malformation. Surg. Clin. North Am., 72:1393, 1992.

20. Peña, A., and ElBehery, M.: Megasigmoid: A source of pseudoincontinence in children with repaired anorectal malformation. J. Pediatr. Surg., 28:199, 1993.

21. Pringle, K.C., Sato, Y., and Soper, R.T.: Magnetic resonance imaging as an adjunct for planning and anorectal pullthrough. J. Pediatr. Surg., 22:571, 1987.

22. Rehbein, F.: Zur operation der hohen Rectumatresie mit Recto-urethral-fistel. Abdomino-sacro-perinealer Durchzur. Z. Kinderchir., 2:503, 1965.

23. Rehbein, F.: Imperforate anus: Experiences with the abdominoperineal and abdomino-sacral-perineal pull-through procedures. J. Pediatr. Surg., 2:99, 1967.

24. Rintala, R.: Postoperative internal sphincter function in anorectal malformation—a manometric study. Pediatr. Surg. Int., 5:127, 1990.

25. Saeki, M., Kazvhiko, H., Nakano, M., et al.: Sacroperineal anorectoplasy using intraoperative ultrasonography: A preliminary report. J. Pediatr. Surg., 28:779, 1993.

26. Shafik, A.: A new concept of the anatomy of the anal sphincter mechanism and the physiology of defecation. The external anal sphincter: A triple-loop system. Invest. Urol., 12:412, 1975.

27. Smith, E.D.: The bath water needs changing, but don't throw out the baby: An overview of anorectal anomalies. J. Pediatr. Surg., 22:335, 1988.

28. Smith, E.D.: The identification and management of ano-rectal anomalies. In Smith, E.D. (ed.): Progress in Pediatric Surgery, Vol. 9, Munich, Urban-Schwarzenberg, 1976, p. 7.

29. Stephens, F.D., and Smith, E.D.: Anorectal Malformations in Children. Chicago, Year Book Medical Publishers, 1971.

30. Swenson, O., and Donnellan, W.L.: Preservation of puborectalis sling in imperforate anus repair. Surg. Clin. North Am., 47:173, 1967.

31. Tam, P.K.H., Chan, F.L., and Saing, H.: Direct sagittal CT-scan: A new diagnostic approach for surgical neonates. J. Pediatr. Surg., 22:397, 1987.

32. Templeton, J.M., and O'Neill, J.A., Jr.: Anorectal malformations. In Ravitch, M.M., Welch, K., Randolph, J.G., et al. (eds.): Pediatric Surgery. Chicago, Year Book Medical Publishers, 1985, p. 1022.

33. Tunnel, W.D., Austin, J.C., Barnes, P.A., and Reynolds, A.: Neuroradiologic evaluation of sacral abnormalities in imperforate anus complex. J. Pediatr. Surg., 22:58, 1987.

34. Yazbeck, S., Luks, F.I., and St. Vil, D.: Anterior perineal approach and three flap anoplasty for imperforate anus: Optimal reconstruction with minimal destruction. J. Pediatr. Surg., 27:190, 1992.

35. Yokoyama, J., Hyashi, A., Ikawa, H., et al.: Abdominoextended sacroperineal approach in high-type anorectal malformations and a new operative method. Z. Kinderchir., 40:151, 1985.

Index

Note: Page numbers in *italics* refer to illustrations; page numbers followed by t refer to tables.

465

ISBN 0-7216-4986-6